CLASSIFICATION OF NURSING DIAGNOSES
Proceedings of the Fifth National Conference

CLASSIFICATION OF NURSING DIAGNOSES

Proceedings of the Fifth National Conference

Edited by

MI JA KIM, R.N., Ph.D., F.A.A.N.

Associate Professor, College of Nursing,
University of Illinois at Chicago,
Health Sciences Center,
Chicago, Illinois

GERTRUDE K. McFARLAND, R.N., D.N.Sc.

Nurse Consultant, Division of Nursing,
USPHS, Health Resources and Services Administration,
U.S. Department of Health and Human Services,
Rockville, Maryland

AUDREY M. McLANE, R.N., Ph.D.

Professor, College of Nursing
Marquette University,
Milwaukee, Wisconsin

with 31 illustrations

The C. V. Mosby Company
ST. LOUIS   TORONTO   1984

MOSBY

A TRADITION OF PUBLISHING EXCELLENCE

Editor: Barbara Ellen Norwitz
Assistant editors: Sally Gaines, Terry Young
Manuscript editor: Margaret Ann Weeter
Design: Jeanne E. Bush
Production: Carol O'Leary, Judith A. England, Kathleen L. Teal

Printed in the United States of America

The C.V. Mosby Company
11830 Westline Industrial Drive, St. Louis, Missouri 63146

Library of Congress Cataloging in Publication Data
Main entry under title:

Classification of nursing diagnoses.

    Proceedings of the 5th National Conference on
the Classification of Nursing Diagnoses, held in St. Louis,
Mo., April 14-17, 1982.
    Bibliography: p.
    Includes index.
    1. Diagnosis—Congresses. 2. Nursing—Congresses.
I. Kim, Mi Ja. II. McFarland, Gertrude K.
III. McLane, Audrey M. IV. National Conference on the
Classification of Nursing Diagnoses (5th : 1982 :
St. Louis, Mo.) [DNLM: 1. Nursing process—Congresses.
W3 NA435D 5th 1982c / WY 100 C614 1982]
RT48.C553   1984   610.73   83-24950
ISBN 0-8016-2668-4

C/VH/VH 9 8 7 6 5 4 3 2   03/A/327

CONTRIBUTORS

RUBY AMOROSO-SERITELLA, R.N., M.S.N., F.A.A.N.
Hines Veterans Administration Hospital, Hines, Illinois; University of Illinois at Chicago, Health Sciences Center, Chicago, Illinois

CAROL A. BAER, R.N., M.S.N.
New England Deaconess Hospital, Boston, Massachusetts

CAROLINE S. BAGLEY, R.N., M.S.N.
The Catholic University of America, Washington, D.C.

TONY M. BALISTRIERI, R.N., M.S.N.
Mount Sinai Medical Center, Milwaukee, Wisconsin

KATHRYN BARNARD, R.N., Ph.D., F.A.A.N.
University of Washington, Seattle, Washington

PATRICIA D. BARRY, R.N., M.S.N.
St. Francis Hospital and Medical Center, Hartford, Connecticut

ANN MARIE BECKER, R.N., M.S.N.
St. Louis University, St. Louis, Missouri

BARBARA BERKOWICH, R.N.
Shock Trauma Center, Maryland Institute for Emergency Medical Services Systems, University of Maryland, Baltimore, Maryland

BARBARA BURKE, R.N., M.S.N.
Harper Grace Hospital, Detroit, Michigan

LYNDA J. CARPENITO, R.N., M.S.N.
Wilmington Medical Center, Wilmington, Delaware

JANET R. CARSTENS, R.N., M.S.N.
Southwest Missouri State, Cape Giradeau, Missouri

ANNE MARIE CHENEY, R.N., M.S.N.
Consultant, Wauwatosa, Wisconsin

KENNETH L. CIANFRANI, R.N., Ph.D.
University of Illinois, Rock Island, Illinois

PATRICIA CLUNN, R.N., Ed.D.
University of Miami, Coral Gables, Florida

MARGA SIMON COLER, R.N., Ed.D.
College of Our Lady of the Elms, Chicopee, Massachusetts

DENISE COST, R.N., CCRN
Shock Trauma Center, Maryland Institute for Emergency Medical Services Systems, University of Maryland, Baltimore, Maryland

NAOMI DAVENPORT, R.N., M.N.
Dammasch State Hospital, Wilsonville, Oregon

SANDRA DELI, R.N.
Shock Trauma Center, Maryland Institute for Emergency Medical Services Systems, University of Maryland, Baltimore, Maryland

MARCIA DELOREY, R.N., M.S.N.
Children's Hospital Medical Center, Boston, Massachusetts

RICHARD J. FEHRING, D.N.Sc., R.N.
Marquette University, Milwaukee, Wisconsin

JOAN B. FITZMAURICE, R.N., M.S.
Boston College, Chestnut Hill, Massachusetts

GARYFALLIA L. FORSYTH, R.N., Ph.D.
Rush University, Chicago, Illinois

JACQUELINE D. FORTIN, R.N., M.S.
University of Rhode Island, Kingston, Rhode Island

CLAUDIA GAMEL-BENTZEL, R.N., B.S.N., CCRN
Neurological Referral Center, Boston, Massachusetts

GRAMATICE GAROFALLOU, R.N., M.S.
The Hospital of the Albert Einstein College of Medicine, Bronx, New York

KRISTINE M. GEBBIE, R.N., M.N.
Human Resources, Oregon State Health Division, Portland, Oregon

MARJORY GORDON, R.N., Ph.D., F.A.A.N.
Boston College, Boston, Massachusetts

MEG GULANICK, R.N., M.S.N.
Michael Reese Hospital, Chicago, Illinois; University of Illinois at Chicago, Health Sciences Center, Chicago, Illinois

SUZANNE KRYSTON GUZELAYDIN, R.N., M.S.
The University of Michigan, Ann Arbor, Michigan

BARBARA HAAS, R.N., M.S.N.
TRICE, Yarmouth, Maine

TERESE M. HALFMAN, R.N., M.S.N.
University of Wisconsin—Milwaukee, Milwaukee, Wisconsin

LEONA CARLSON HAYES, R.N., M.S.N.
Olivet Nazarene College, Kankakee, Illinois

LOIS M. HOSKINS, R.N., Ph.D.
The Catholic University of America, Washington, D.C.

KATHY HUBALIK, R.N., M.S.N.
Westside Veterans Administration Medical Center, Chicago, Illinois; University of Illinois at Chicago, Health Sciences Center, Chicago, Illinois

CAROL A. HUNT, R.N., M.S.N.
University of Wisconsin—Milwaukee, Milwaukee, Wisconsin

DOROTHEA F. JAKOB, R.N., M.A.
Department of Public Health, Toronto, Canada

MARY K. JIRICKA, R.N., M.S.N.
Mount Sinai Medical Center, Milwaukee, Wisconsin

PHYLLIS E. JONES, R.N., M.S.
University of Toronto, Toronto, Canada

MARY A. KELLY, R.N., Ed.D
Clemson University, Clemson, South Carolina

BARBARA KEYES, R.N., B.S.
Shock Trauma Center, Maryland Institute for Emergency Medical Services Systems, University of Maryland, Baltimore, Maryland

MI JA KIM, R.N., Ph.D., F.A.A.N.
University of Illinois at Chicago, Health Sciences Center, Chicago Illinois

PHYLLIS B. KRITEK, R.N., Ph.D., F.A.A.N.
Center for Nursing Research and Evaluation, University of Wisconsin—Milwaukee, Milwaukee, Wisconsin

SHEILA LaFORTUNE-FREDETTE, R.N., M.S.
Fitchburg State College, Fitchburg, Massachusetts

FRANCES M. LANGE, R.N., D.S.N.
The University of Alabama in Birmingham, Birmingham, Alabama

MARGARET C. LANNON, R.N., M.S.
Boston University Medical Center, Boston, Massachusetts

MARILYN LEWIS LANZA, R.N., M.S.
Edith Nourse Rogers Memorial Veterans Hospital, Bedford, Massachusetts; Boston University, Boston, Massachusetts

PRISCILLA A. LOGUE, R.N., M.A.
Chinle IHS Clinic, Chinle, Arizona

VIRGINIA LUETJE, R.N., M.S.N.
St. Louis University, St. Louis,
Missouri

MARGARET LUNNEY, R.N., M.S.N.
Hunter College—Bellevue School of
Nursing, New York, New York

MARGARET D. McCOMB, R.N., B.S.
Dammasch State Hospital, Wilsonville,
Oregon

GERTRUDE K. McFARLAND, R.N.,
D.N.Sc.
Division of Nursing, USPHS Health
Resources and Services Administration,
U.S. Department of Health and Human
Services, Rockville, Maryland

ELIZABETH A. McFARLANE, R.N.,
D.N.Sc.
The Catholic University of America,
Washington, D.C.

AUDREY M. McLANE, R.N., Ph.D.
Marquette University, Milwaukee,
Wisconsin

RUTH E. McSHANE, R.N., M.S.N.
University of Wisconsin—Milwaukee,
Milwaukee, Wisconsin

MARYELLEN McSWEENEY, R.N.,
Ph.D.
St. Louis University, St. Louis,
Missouri

PATRICIA A. MARTIN, R.N., M.S.
Miami Valley Hospital, Dayton, Ohio

CATHY D. MEADE, R.N., M.S.
Milwaukee County Medical Complex,
Milwaukee, Wisconsin; University of
Illinois at Chicago, Health Sciences
Center, Chicago, Illinois

CHRISTINE MIASKOWSKI, R.N.,
M.S.N.
The Hospital of the Albert Einstein
College of Medicine, Bronx, New York

JUDITH FITZGERALD MILLER, R.N.,
M.S.N.
Marquette University, Milwaukee,
Wisconsin

WINNIFRED C. MILLS, B.Sc.N., M.Ed.
University of British Columbia,
Vancouver, Canada

KAREN MOYER, R.N., M.S.N.
Michael Reese Hospital, Chicago,
Illinois

CAROLYN A. NOWAK, R.N., M.S.N.
University of Wisconsin—Milwaukee,
Milwaukee, Wisconsin

ELINOR PARSONS, R.N., M.S.N.
Hines Veterans Administration
Hospital, Hines, Illinois

KAREN K. PERET, R.N., M.S.,
C.N.A.A.
Monson Developmental Center,
Palmer, Massachusetts

SUSAN KEIL PFOUTZ, R.N., M.S.
The University of Michigan, Ann
Arbor, Michigan

JANICE S. PIGG, R.N., B.S.N.
Columbia Hospital, Milwaukee,
Wisconsin

SUE POPKESS-VAWTER, R.N., Ph.D.
University of Kansas Medical Center,
Kansas City, Kansas

SISTER CALLISTA ROY, R.N., Ph.D.,
F.A.A.N.
Mount St. Mary's College, Los Angeles,
California

M. GAIE RUBENFELD, R.N., M.S.
The Catholic University of America,
Washington, D.C.

WANDA B. RUTHVEN, R.N., c.,
P.H.N., M.S.
Case Manager, Fremont, California

LAURA RYAN, R.N., M.S.N.
National Institutes of Health, Bethesda,
Maryland

JANET SCHERBEL, R.N., M.S.N.
University of Illinois at Chicago,
Health Sciences Center, Chicago,
Illinois

ANN M. SCHREIER, R.N., Ph.D.
The Catholic University of America,
Washington, D.C.

JOYCE K. SHOEMAKER, R.N., Ed.D.
Temple University, Philadelphia,
Pennsylvania

SALLY McDONALD SILVER, R.N.,
M.S.N.
University of Wisconsin—Milwaukee,
Milwaukee, Wisconsin

SUSAN SIMMONS, R.N., M.S.N.
National Institutes of Health, Bethesda,
Maryland

MAXINE SLIEFERT, R.N., M.S.
University of Wisconsin—Milwaukee,
Milwaukee, Wisconsin; University of
Illinois, Health Sciences Center,
Chicago, Illinois

SANDRA SPANGENBERG, R.N., M.A.
CBS, Inc., New York, New York

BARBARA STACHOWIAK, R.N., B.S.
Monson Developmental Center,
Palmer, Massachusetts

MARGARET J. STAFFORD, R.N.,
M.S.N., F.A.A.N.
Hines Veterans Administration
Hospital, Hines, Illinois; University of
Illinois at Chicago, Health Sciences
Center, Chicago, Illinois

ROSEMARIE SUHAYDA, R.N., M.S.N.
University of Illinois at Chicago,
Health Sciences Center, Chicago,
Illinois

LYNN TOTH, R.N., B.S.N.
Shock Trauma Center, Maryland
Institute for Emergency Medical
Services Systems, University of
Maryland, Baltimore, Maryland

ROSALINDA M. TOTH, R.N., M.A.
Newark Beth Israel Medical Center,
Newark, New Jersey

SALLY TRIPP, R.N., M.S.
University of Massachusetts, Amherst,
Massachusetts

MADELINE WAKE, R.N., M.S.N.
Marquette University, Milwaukee,
Wisconsin

MARY B. WALSH, R.N., M.S.N.
The Catholic University of America,
Washington, D.C.

JUDITH WARREN, R.N., M.S.
University of Hawaii at Manoa,
Honolulu, Hawaii

GLENN A. WEBSTER, Ph.D.
University of Colorado, Denver,
Colorado

SUSAN L. WESSEL, R.N., M.S.
The Jewish Hospital of Cincinnati,
Cincinnati, Ohio; University of Illinois
at Chicago, Health Sciences Center,
Chicago, Illinois

CAROLYN J. YOCOM, R.N., M.S.N.
University of Illinois at Chicago,
Health Sciences Center, Chicago,
Illinois

KAREN A. YORK, R.N., M.S.N.
Miami Valley Hospital, Dayton, Ohio

SHIRLEY MELAT ZIEGLER, R.N.,
Ph.D.
Texas Women's University, Dallas,
Texas

PREFACE

Between the Fourth and Fifth National Conferences the accelerated growth of nursing diagnosis in literature and use was unprecedented both in academia and in the clinical settings. Scholarly articles appeared in both clinical and research journals, attesting to the maturity of the subject matter, and five books and one manual on nursing diagnosis providing a wide theoretical base have been published. Such activity lent strength to the Fifth National Conference. The Conference was held in St. Louis, its birthplace, from April 14 to 17, 1982, with leadership provided by Karen Murphy, Administrator Coordinator; A. Becker and M. Gordon, the co-conference directors; G. McFarland, A. McLane, and M. Kim, members of the steering committee; along with input from Task Force members. A total of 199 nurses, from 28 states and Canada, attended the Conference.

This Conference distinguished itself from others by accepting bylaws for the first time in the history of the organization. The Conference group also chose a new name, North American Nursing Diagnoses Association (NANDA). As the name signifies, the organization duly recognizes the significant contribution made by Canadian nurses.

To fulfill the major function of the organization—to develop nursing diagnosis classification systems—the Conference continued to provide two tracks for participants. Small groups in the first track examined new nursing diagnoses (supported by clinical and/or research data) that were submitted before the Conference. They generated issues and research questions for each nursing diagnosis approved at the Fourth National Conference. Although no conscientious effort was given to refining previously accepted nursing diagnoses, some revision of defining characteristics ensued while the diagnoses and issues were examined. This process differed from small group work at previous conferences. It was intended to improve the output of the Conference and signaled the commitment of the Conference group to research on nursing diagnoses. K. Gebbie, with the assistance of Sr. C. Roy, played a major role in orchestrating multiple small groups involved in this task. The report is included in Chapter 6.

The second track consisted of one small group whose members examined the nursing diagnosis taxonomical system itself in light of the proposed theorists' framework. This important piece of work was led by P. Kritek with the assistance of Sr. C. Roy. It is included in Chapter 2. Such avenues of participation allowed a meaningful dialogue between clinicians, theorists, and educators, producing a significant piece of work that will serve us well.

In particular, the taxonomy developed by P. Kritek's group pointed out the incompleteness and inadequacies in our current system. The logic of the system and the levels of abstraction of the diagnostic labels should be the focus of our concern and debate in the future as the organization continues its struggle to develop rational taxonomical systems.

If there were one single force that gave a major boost to the Fifth National Conference Group on Classification of Nursing Diagnoses, it was the publication of the American Nurses' Association Social Policy Statement in which the definition of nursing explicitly included "diagnosing" as an expected function of a nurse (1980). Wide circulation of this document and acceptance of its content by nurses employed in various roles and work settings may indicate that the profession is at a point where the formulation of its language is of prime concern. The formation of the American Nurses' Association Steering Committee for the Development of a Classification System, which presumably will address this issue, supports this observation.

This Conference was fortunate to have K. Barnard as the keynote speaker. She was one of seven task force members who developed the ANA Social Policy Statement. Her paper, "The American Nurses' Association's Social Policy Statement, Nursing: Implications for the Conference Group's Work on Classification of Nursing Diagnosis," presented in Chapter 1, sets the stage for both professional organizations, ANA and NANDA, to work effectively for the benefits of the nursing profession. As she indicates in her paper, the decision of the ANA Congress for Nursing Practice (September 1981) to delete the statement, "Nurses diagnose and treat these (human) responses, not the health problem themselves" warrants attention and further study. As the Congress reasoned, "it is clear that nurses do diagnose and treat selected health problems." The questions K. Barnard poses are thought-provoking for all who are concerned with the progress of the nursing diagnosis taxonomy.

Chapter 2 begins with a paper by G. Webster. His topic, "Nomenclature and Classification System Development," is not only timely, but is enriched by his prior experience as a member of the Task Force that developed the ANA Social Policy Statement. He provides the reasons and the need for standardization of nomenclature and offers suggestions for conceptualizing the framework for empirical sciences such as nursing. His recommendations to keep nursing diagnoses in an alphabetical order for the present time and to make the nursing diagnosis list more inclusive are just two of many that are certain to be helpful in our continuing work on classification of diagnostic labels.

Sr. C. Roy in her paper, "Framework for Classification Systems Development Progress and Issues," in Chapter 2, addresses commonly held concerns about the unitary man/human framework. She places emphasis on the assumptions underlying the theorists' conceptualization of unitary man as an open system, rather than on the word itself. Sr. Roy reported that one of the reasons that the concepts of the framework are not workable is that they lack empirical anchorage. Several nurse-theorist task force members point out that the nine patterns do not reflect the rules for categorization. This raises a serious question as to the usefulness of the patterns for ordering the phenomena of nursing. It appears that the framework needs additional theoretical development and clinical testing. Suggestions offered by Sr. Roy in her paper amply demonstrate a critical evaluation of the theorists' work.

Members of the small group who worked on the taxonomy generated a significant piece of information that will serve as the cornerstone for future taxonomy development. Their attempt to classify nursing diagnoses according to four levels of abstraction, and to parallel these to nine patterns proposed by nurse theorists, is an ambitious one and deserves further scrutiny by expert taxonomists.

Chapter 3 begins with a paper by M.J. Kim that presents a point of view on the need for and role of physiologic nursing diagnoses in a nursing taxonomy. As a nurse-physiologist with several years of critical care nursing experience, Kim argues for the National Conference Group to be open minded and include those nursing diagnoses that have interdependent nursing interventions. She painstakingly points out that a nursing taxonomy cannot at present be limited to only those diagnoses that nurses treat independently. Such an approach would eliminate a vast number of diagnoses from even the current list. Besides, the definition and practice of independence vary depending on geographic regions, institutions, and individual nurses.

Next, G. Forsyth's paper entitled "Etiology: In What Sense and of What Value?" points out that "conceptualization of etiology for nursing science cannot be approached directly. Too many a priori concerns lie in the way." A diagram depicting various ways of delineating cause and effect relationships reflects the complexity of the issue facing the current structural definition of nursing diagnosis. A model using multiple correlation for relating risk or predictive factors has been proposed as a useful approach.

A scholarly treatise by P. Kritek on issues pertinent to current nomenclature and classification systems demonstrates that problems of nursing diagnoses are inseparably linked to the problems of nursing science and the profession. Comparison of a taxonomy of nursing diagnoses with that of chemistry and physics may appear almost unfair, yet the logic behind their classification scheme may be all the more pertinent to our way of thinking. Her thorough examination of different conceptualizations of the phenomena of nursing as depicted in various classification schemas provides a broad base for intellectual debate and exploration by all nurses. Her quotation of Albert

Einstein's letter to Solovine (1949), ". . . there is not a single concept of which I am convinced that it will stand firm, and I feel uncertain whether I am in general on the right track" leaves us food for thought.

A powerful presentation by R. Toth on the use of nursing diagnoses for prospective reimbursement for nursing services in conjunction with Diagnoses Related Groups (DRGs) increases our sensitivity to the importance of active involvement in fiscal management. It is reassuring to hear from a current nursing administrator that incorporating nursing diagnosis into the DRG system is not only feasible but also necessary if nursing wants to provide "planned professional therapy rather than routine hospital tasks based on traditional time frames and services." She correctly forewarns of the resistance that will confront nurses when they try to use a reimbursement system for nursing services. Her successful use of the DRG system for nursing service is, indeed, a model to follow.

Chapter 4 is composed of 21 research papers that were presented in the formal session ($n = 7$), small group sessions ($n = 3$), and poster session ($n = 11$). Diverse inquiries into the identification, validation, and use of nursing diagnoses were reported by researchers using multiple methods. The findings have implications for practice, education, and taxonomy development.

Although each paper carries its own merit, doctoral dissertations by J. Shoemaker and K. Cianfrani deserve special attention. Shoemaker uses Soltis' framework for analysis of concepts and the Delphi format to produce group consensus in identifying the essential and variant features of nursing diagnoses. The attributes of the definition of nursing diagnosis she found in the study should be useful in clarifying the concept of nursing diagnosis. K. Cianfrani, on the other hand, carried out a study examining the diagnostic process and found that increased amounts of data and low relevant data were associated with more errors in making correct health problem diagnosis. Through these research projects, numerous new nursing diagnoses and defining characteristics for existing diagnoses were created, and these should be examined by an appropriate body of the NANDA in order to be included in the approved list.

Twenty-four papers related to practice and education are included in Chapter 5. Although some papers have a research component, the editors judged them to fit best under the rubric of practice and education with the firm belief that research is (should be) an inherent component in these areas as well. Six papers were presented in the formal sessions, nine in the small group sessions and nine in the poster session. Again, doctoral dissertations by M. Lanza and P. Clunn are noted. Their contributions are singled out to illustrate further need for research at doctoral or postdoctoral levels. Certainly the field will become even more fertile when the scholarly outputs such as these increase.

Several issues, dilemmas, and ideas surface in this chapter. Invariably, the nature of nursing diagnosis is addressed from several vantage points. Several authors, linking nursing diagnosis with the autonomy of the profession, express the notion that independent nursing treatment/therapies must be possible for a nursing diagnosis to be within the domain of nursing. M. Lunney believes that if nursing diagnoses refer to only parts of a system, they do not reflect nursing's unique focus on the whole person. To bring the issue into focus, one must raise the question of how to strike a balance between the need for specificity and sensitivity in the diagnostic categories and the importance of maintaining the unique focus of nursing. The need for and role of health and strength-oriented nursing diagnoses are addressed, directing our attention to the health arena in the health-illness continuum with which nurses deal. As described in W. Ruthven's paper, priority setting by risk category, such as at risk, high risk, low risk and no risk, may help address some of these concerns.

Another dilemma facing some of us is that nursing is trying to identify its own domain and map out its own scope of practice at a time when the multidisciplinary approach to health problem solving is in vogue. M.L. Lanza, who presents nursing staff as victims of violence, presents a different perspective on nursing diagnosis. Data presented may contribute to the development of the nursing diagnosis *violence (or victim reaction)* assuming the experiences of nurses are viewed as those of patients/clients. Possible implications of such an approach to the definition of nursing diagnoses need to be examined.

Chapter 6 begins with the list of nursing diagnoses labels that have been approved by the National Conferences to date. Etiologies and defining characteristics of all nursing diagnoses are found in the *Pocket Guide*, which is being published with this book. The *Pocket Guide* also includes selected prototype nursing care plans using nursing diagnoses. The need for a pocket-sized manual for everyday practice was expressed by many practicing nurses, and the editors believe that such a guide will promote wider use of nursing diagnoses. It is followed by K. Gebbie's summary of the work of small groups that examined the diagnostic labels. Three new mechanisms used in this conference need to be noted. First, the small groups generated ideas and made recommendations to the task force group that made final decisions about proposed changes and approval of new nursing diagnoses. Second, selected research papers were presented in the small groups before the group examined any new nursing diagnoses or suggestions to refine existing defining characteristics. Third, the group made a conscientious effort to relate existing diagnoses to the nine patterns of unitary man whenever possible. The defining characteristics that were related to one of the nine unitary man patterns are listed separately under each nursing diagnosis for those who may want to pursue a study in this area.

Issues, research questions, and reference lists for each diagnosis are also included in the chapter.

Chapter 7 contains the state of the art of nursing diagnoses as gleaned from the literature. A. McLane and R. Fehring provide a critical review of the nursing diagnoses literature. Reviews of six books on nursing diagnoses are presented by A. Becker, G. McFarland, A. McLane, F. Lange, and M.J. Kim. This chapter is supplementary to the National Conference and is intended to broaden the readers' knowledge and interject critical evaluations of books that were written about nursing diagnosis. The views expressed in this section are those of the individual authors and do not necessarily reflect the opinions of NANDA.

Chapter 8 covers events that occurred before and during the Fifth National Conference. M. Gordon presents a report of task force group activities between national conferences and discusses the rationale and planning of the Fifth Conference. This is followed by a report by L. Carpenito on the Continuing Education workshop that was held one day before the Conference. A. Becker, who participated in the workshop, presents a summary of her paper, "Nursing Diagnosis and History."

Evaluation of the National Conference and the work on nursing diagnosis was obtained from 25 participants who were selected by the editors to represent different regions and varied backgrounds. G. McFarland and M.J. Kim analyzed the responses to a two-page questionnaire and their summary is presented in Chapter 9. As the regional representation of participants was examined, the absence of USPHS Region VIII (Colorado, Montana, South Dakota, North Dakota, Utah, and Wyoming) became apparent and may reflect the need for wider and more even distribution of nursing diagnosis work. Recommendations stemming from this survey will serve as valuable bases for the planning of future conferences.

The editors wish to express their appreciation for the support of the Clearinghouse that facilitated the editing process of the *Proceedings*. We are especially thankful for the hard work of the Task Force members who approved the nursing diagnoses, for the faithful reports of group leaders who made the *Proceedings* so valuable, for the scholarly presentations of all authors who made the Conference so stimulating, and for the staunch support of all conference attendees without whose active participation this Conference would not have existed. Last, but not least, the editors owe immeasurable thanks to Janet Larson and Chi Weh Loh, doctoral students of M.J. Kim at University of Illinois at Chicago, College of Nursing, for their faithful and efficient assistance. The editors are likewise deeply appreciative of the support given by the College of Nursing, University of Illinois at Chicago, during the editing process of this *Proceedings*.

The editors extend their best wishes to the newly formed organization, NANDA, and to those officers who were elected. May their contribution be a cornerstone for the nursing profession.

MI JA KIM, R.N., PH.D., F.A.A.N.
GERTRUDE MCFARLAND, R.N., D.N.SC.*
AUDREY MCLANE, R.N., PH.D.

---

*The contents of this book reflect the author's ideas and are not necessarily those of the U.S. Department of Health and Human Services, USPHS, Health Resources and Services Administration.

CONTENTS

Appendixes

CHAPTER 1

Keynote address: social policy statement—implications for nursing

Since the American Nurses' Association (ANA) resolution supporting the use of nursing diagnoses in the Nurse Practice Act in 1976, the ANA Social Policy Statement (1980) has made another historical contribution to nursing, particularly to the North American Nursing Diagnosis Association. The ANA Social Policy Statement has become an integral aspect of nursing by stating that the diagnosis of patients' health problems is a part of nursing. Dr. K. Barnard, a member of the Task Force that developed the statement, was the keynote speaker for this conference. The discussion that followed her presentation further illuminates the articulation of the two organizations and the diversity of nursing's concern, perception, and interpretation of the work of nurse theorists and that of the National Conference Group.

The ANA's social policy statement on nursing—implications for the conference group's work on classification of nursing diagnoses

KATHRYN BARNARD, R.N., Ph.D., F.A.A.N.

It is a pleasure to bring greetings from the ANA, particularly from the Congress for Nursing Practice, which formulated *Nursing: A Social Policy Statement*. I would like to recognize the effective leadership of Dr. Norma Lang who served as both the chairperson of the Congress for Nursing Practice and the chairperson of the Task Force on the Nature and Scope of Nursing Practice and Characteristics of Specialization in Nursing during the time the Social Policy Statement was formalized.

Membership in this Task Force was an interesting experience. The task of developing a statement that represented the nature and scope of nursing practice was a challenge, because of the diversity within the professional society.

For the past 6 years, I have served on the executive committee of the Division of Maternal-Child Health of the ANA. During this time I have developed a clearer perspective of the practice issues in relation to contemporary nursing. I have also taught a course in our parent-child master's program on the nursing process in parent-child nursing. I am actively doing research on nursing care with high-risk infants and families, and I teach core courses in our doctoral program about family adaptation to health problems and about environments, supporting and nonsupporting. From these multiple perspectives I see that nursing, both as a profession and as a discipline, is moving rapidly, is dynamic, and is an increasingly forceful element of society. Through recent experiences with the Task Force, I realize the richness and complexity of the issues facing nursing and have, therefore, developed patience with our course of development and our emerging knowledge base for practice.

It is my responsibility to share with you the scope of the Social Policy Statement and, as much as possible, to share with you some of the developing views of the statement. I will comment on what future course of action might be pursued by the ANA and the Conference Group on Classification of Nursing Diagnosis. The ANA has already put into place a steering committee for the development of classification systems dealing with nursing phenomena. Norma Lang is the chairperson of this committee. Members are Marjory Gordon, representing your nursing diagnosis group; Roberta Thiry, the liaison with your group and the ANA Congress for Nursing Practice; Ada Sue Hinshaw; Marleen Ventura; Jean Steel; and myself. I can assure you that there is a basis for a future relationship between the ANA and your organization. One strong implication of the Social Policy Statement is support for your activities.

Let me tell you a little about the process the Task Force went through in developing the statement. In addition to the chairperson Norma Lang, the members of the Task Force were Nina Argondizzo, Hildegard Peplau, Maria Phaneuf, Jean Steel, Glenn Webster and myself. Research for the statement meant reaching back in history to examine the documentation of nursing and analyzing the relationship of the profession to society and to health care, with sensitivity to the ethical, legal, and political issues. The ANA has made several attempts to publish a definition of nursing. The complexity of the issues and the level of conceptual clarification about nursing practice had precluded any agreement on this issue. However, many successful definitions had been offered by individual nurse philosophers. From these writings, starting with Nightingale's *Notes on Nursing* (1859), the Task Force attempted to make a cohesive statement about what nursing has been and is, rather than what it may be in the future.

After reviewing the proceedings of your first four conferences, I am impressed by how you have dealt with the definitions of nursing. I see a great deal of similarity in the way you, as a group of colleagues, scholars, clinicians, and researchers, have dealt with the central theme of what nursing is— caring for individuals in relation to their health; promoting, maintaining, or restoring their behavior. On this focus, there is not much disagreement. Disagreement comes only when specific definitions emerge, dealing with boundary questions within or at the edge of nursing practice.

The Social Policy Statement defining nursing practice is made in recognition of society's right to know how nursing's social responsibility is exercised in practice. "Nursing, like other professions, is an essential part of society, out of which it grew, and out of which it has been evolving. Nursing can be said to be owned by society in the sense that all of nursing's professional interests must be and must be perceived as serving the interests of the larger whole of which it is a part" (ANA, 1980, p. 3). As far as we are aware, nursing is the only health profession that has formally issued a public statement about its practice as an affirmation of social accountability.

Nursing must view and must be viewed in the context of the entire health care arena, a major focus of public attention in the United States at this time. A national transition is occurring in which our society is moving from a disease-oriented system of care to health-oriented system of care. Issues such as organization, delivery, and financing of care, development of health resources, provision of public health through prevention and environmental measures, increased responsibility by individuals for self-care, development of new knowledge and technology through research, and health care planning as a matter of national policy are all relevant to the definition of contemporary nursing. Nursing serves society's interests in the area of health. The professional has taken the initiative and continues to make a major contribution to the evolving health-oriented system of care. The contract of nursing to society is honored by the ANA through work derived from the collective expertise of its members: establishing a code of ethics, establishing standards of practice, fostering development of nursing theory, establishing educational requirements for entering professional practice, developing certification processes for the profession, and, now, defining the nature and scope of nursing practice.

The 1981 definition of nursing honors the historic orientation at the same time that it reflects the influence of nursing theory that is part of nursing's evolution. According to this definition, nursing is the diagnosis and treatment of human responses to actual or potential health problems. The definition differentiates the scope of nursing practice from that of medical practice, which is to diagnose and treat disease and trauma in human beings, and demonstrates the development of the independent role of nursing when compared with a 1955 statement issued by the ANA Board of Directors. The 1955 definition of nursing had been submitted by the ANA committee on legislation. In essence, it said that the practice of professional nursing meant the performance of acts involved in the observation, care, and counsel of the ill, injured, or infirm. It ended with the statement that "the definition shall not be deemed to include acts of diagnosis or prescriptions of therapeutic or corrective measures." Nursing has come a long way in less than 30 years to the present definition and statement, which is reflected in the laws in many states and which gives nurses the independent function of diagnosing and treating patient conditions when they are trained to do so.

It is useful to clarify several terms in the 1981 definition, beginning with health. The statement uses health as a qualifier of the type of problems with which nurses deal. *Health* in the Social Policy Statement is defined as a "dynamic state of being in which the developmental and behavioral potential of an individual is realized to the fullest possible extent" (ANA, 1980, p. 5). The definition also states that "each individual possesses various strengths and limitations and that the relative dominance of either the strengths or the limitations determines the individual's place on the health continuum. A person's health is his biological and behavioral integrity, his wholeness", (ANA, 1980, p. 5). Therefore when we evaluate nursing's definition of health and resulting health problems, it is obvious that the perspective is inclusive rather than exclusive. Health is a dynamic state of being, involving the developmental and behavioral potential of the individual and biologic and behavioral integrity. With this broad definition of health, how do we come to a manageable clinical perspective? In my own specialty area of parent-child nursing, I have identified some of the frequent and more important health problems with which nurses deal: pregnancy and complications of pregnancy, parenting and alterations in parenting, attachment disorders, prematurity, developmental disabilities, chronic illness in children, high life change, strains in transitions of the developmental phases, abuse and neglect and accidents. All these situations are significant as health problems having an actual or potential influence on the developmental and behavioral state of individuals and on their biologic and behavioral integrity.

Another way of looking at health problems less tied in to the standard terminology might be to look at major constructs, such as role change or role assumption, that might be required. Examples are the transition involved in becoming a parent, the transition of becoming ill or becoming well, and the transition involved in changing family membership. Thus the definition of health, as relayed in the actual wording and in several examples, is broad and demands that individual nurses must, by reason of their own preparation or interests, define the type of health problem with which they are dealing.

The next term to consider in the definition is *human responses.* The responses, the phenomena of concern to nurses, are responses to actual health problems. The phenomena, as defined in the Social Policy Statement, are "any observable manifestation, need, concern, event, dilemma, difficulty, occurrence, or fact, that can be described or scientifically explained as a phenomenon that lies within the nursing practice target area" (ANA, 1980, p. 4). Nursing is concerned with a wide range of health-related responses observed in sick and in well persons. The responses can be reactions to an actual problem such as a disease, or they can anticipate potential health problems. Nurses diagnose and treat the responses. Phaneuf (1982) states, "The patient has the health problem; the responses are the nursing problem." Human responses that are the focus of nursing include (1) self-care limitations; (2) impaired functioning in areas such as rest, sleep, ventilation, circulation, activity, nutrition, elimination, skin, and sexuality; (3) pain and discomfort; (4) emotional problems related to illness and treatment, life-threatening events or daily experiences such as anxiety, loss, loneliness, or grief; (5) distortion of symbolic functions, reflected in interpersonal and intellectual processes such as hallucinations; (6) deficiencies in decision making and ability to make personal choices; (7) self-image changes required by health status; (8) dysfunctional perceptional orientations to health; (9) strains related to life processes such as birth, growth and development, and death; and (10) problematic affiliative relationships.

Studying the work of your Conference Group, I decided that what the Social Policy Statement calls human responses you call the defining characteristics of the nursing diagnosis; they are the behaviors or cues. The nurse theorist group refers to human responses as the empirical indicators of a pattern.

As for the term *diagnosis,* we have drawn from the work of the Nursing

Diagnosis Conference Group, literature, and standard meanings of diagnosis. In the Social Policy Statement, we said, "Diagnosis is an effort to objectify a perceived difficulty or need by naming it as a basis for understanding and taking action to resolve the concern" (ANA, 1980, p. 11).

We define the *theoretic base* in nursing as partially self-generated and partially drawn from other fields, recognizing that nursing is primarily an applied science, that it uses the results of nursing research, and that it selects theories from many other sciences on the basis of their explanatory value in relation to the phenomena that nurses diagnose and treat. Nurses use intrapersonal, interpersonal, and systems theories. Intrapersonal theories explain phenomena within persons, interpersonal theories aid in understanding interactions between two or more people, and systems theories provide explanations of complex networks or organizations and the dynamics of their parts in the processes in interaction. This range of theories is necessary because the various conditions within the scope of nursing cannot be understood in terms of cause-and-effect relationships only but also require knowledge of system dynamics, patterns, and process interactions.

The Social Policy Statement discusses *treatment* in relation to the actions of nursing.

> The aims of nursing actions are to ameliorate, improve, or correct conditions to which those practices are directed to prevent illness and to promote health. Ideally, actions are taken on the basis of understood fact in carrying out nursing care. Highly developed technical and interpersonal skills are equally important as are the sensitive observations and intellectual competencies required for the nurse in the nursing situation to arrive at a diagnosis and to determine a beneficial nursing action. Treatment of a diagnosed condition involves nursing actions that can be described and explained theoretically as to their relation to phenomena and expected outcome (ANA, 1980, p. 12).

Also related to and implicit in the definition is that nursing actions are intended to produce beneficial effects in relation to identified responses. It is the result of the evaluation of outcomes of nursing actions that suggests whether or not those actions have been effective in improving or resolving the conditions to which they were directed.

The Social Policy Statement in its initial form was reviewed at the 1981 biennial convention of the ANA and has been reviewed by numerous groups since it was published in 1980. Approximately 1500 copies a month are distributed through the Publications Department of the ANA. The reaction has been generally positive. The one issue consistently regarded as a problem is the emphasis on the nurse's diagnosis and treatment of human responses to health problems, rather than the health problem. In fact, the statement as originally proposed did indicate in the text accompanying the definition

(ANA, 1980, p. 10) that the nurse diagnosed and treated the responses, not the health problems. This distinction raised a number of questions in the nursing community, particularly by nurses trained in nurse practitioner skills. Many nurses in primary health care do in fact treat health problems in addition to the responses. In considering the balance of emphasis, nurses deal more often with the human responses. However, this is still an open question. Clarification will come from questioning and debate. You should note that in September 1981 the ANA Congress on Nursing Practice voted to delete the statement, "nurses diagnose and treat these responses, not the health problems themselves," because it is clear that nurses do diagnose and treat selected health problems.

Dealing with the question of the scope of nursing practice is an ongoing challenge. I have noticed that in your literature you have also dealt with the question of appropriate diagnoses that nurses make. If we look at health care provided to society through the services of many professions, each has its own defining characteristics and independent functions. Characteristics of the various professionals can be described by looking at the scope of practice in terms of the boundary, the intersections with other health professionals, the core that distinguishes it from other professions, and the various dimensions within itself.

As one of the professions in the health care system, nursing can be described by its boundaries, intersections, core, and dimensions. The nursing segment of the health care system has an external boundary that expands outward in response to changing needs, demands, and capacities of society and is a result of the advances in nursing research.

The scope of nursing practice intersects with that of other health care professions. The interprofessional intersections are the meeting points at which nursing extends its practice into the domain of other professions. The intersections are not hard and fast lines, separating nursing from other professions; they should allow for expansion and flexibility. All health care professionals interact in practice, share the same overall mission, have access to the same published scientific knowledge, and to some degree overlap their activities.

The diagnosed human responses to actual or potential health problems are the core of nursing practice. The core distinguishes nursing professionals from other health care professionals. Diagnosis of the phenomena within the scope of nursing practice leads to the application of theory to explain the response and to determine actions to be taken to improve it. Through the ongoing process of identifying and classifying human responses to health problems, the range of diagnostic categories within the scope of nursing practice is constantly expanding. Thus through nursing research and professional practice, the core of nursing is being refined.

The following example will help characterize human responses. Typical human responses to pregnancy include fatigue, anxiety, maintenance of normal body functioning, possible lack of knowledge, possible role changes, and capacity for self-care. An even more specific level of human response, possible role changes, might include information-seeking behavior, role rehearsal, denial of role change, support-seeking, and anticipation of such role changes. I am reminded as I list these specific human responses to pregnancy that the phenomena on which nurses focus are often multiple, episodic, continuous, fluid, and varying. Therefore we need to develop diagnostic criteria that take into account these characteristics of the human responses. The diversity of approaches that is possible within your own conference group, the nurse clinician group, the nurse theorist group, and the ANA all have value.

I draw on Kritek's statement (1982, p. 22-23) that the

uniqueness of nursing is tied intimately to the dilemma created by a holistic view of persons and that the inferential process arising out of our holistic data . . . is both the heart of the nature of nursing and one of our biggest challenges because it is this inferential process that we know the least about.

The nurse theorist group seems to be talking about a conceptualization of the synthesis of patterns of behavior coming from empirical indicators. In fact, in 1980 they defined nursing diagnosis as a term that synthesized a cluster of empirical indicators describing characteristics of unitary man, or what some prefer to call the biologic and behavioral integrity or wholeness of the human being (Roy, 1982). The entire conference group's definition of nursing diagnosis involves the judgment or conclusion that occurs as a result of the nursing assessment. The components of diagnosis include a statement of the problem, its etiologies, and its signs and symptoms, which constitute defining characteristics. The defining characteristics, to use your terminology— human responses, as stated in the ANA Social Policy Statement—provide a basis for a mutually beneficial and collaborative effort to take place between the Nursing Conference Group and the ANA.

Enmeshed in our dialogue is the question of boundaries. Research studies such as those reported by Nicholetti, Reitz, and Gordon (1982) demonstrate that as we study nursing practice such as they did in obstetric nursing, we will begin to see the clustering of cues, observations, or indicators that nurses use. In their study they found that a majority of the cues were related to the roles and relationships of the pregnant or newly delivered mother.

The ANA Steering Committee asked all practice divisions within the ANA to provide by November 1982 a list of the phenomena of human responses to actual and potential health problems with which their practice division deals, based on their scope and standards of practice statements and the classifications of nursing diagnosis. The committee has also asked for a listing of the actual or potential health problems in their domain of practice. We hope to use this in further work in which we will be determining strategies to further our collective efforts to clarify nursing diagnosis. These activities should lead to state of the art papers and conferences about the phenomena with which nursing deals. We anticipate establishing liaisons with some of the published literature and hope to facilitate conferences about human responses and health problems with respect to both their diagnosis and treatment.

A diversity of approaches will provide a strong base for us to continue to clarify the nature of nursing practice. I agree with Gordon's statements (1982) encouraging the standarization of an assessment structure of certain health-related behavioral patterns. She proposes that by so standardizing we could clarify the domain of accountability, which could then be the focus of clinical studies and the focus of development of expertise in assessment and diagnosis. Gordon proposes the domains of interest for her and other clinicians with whom she has worked to be health perception–health management patterns, nutritional-metabolic patterns, elimination patterns, activity-exercise patterns, cognitive-perceptual patterns, sleep-rest patterns, self-perception–self-concept patterns, role-relationship patterns, sexuality-reproductive patterns, coping-stress-tolerance patterns, and value-belief patterns. In my opinion this serves as a good orientation. I have recommended to the Standards Revision Committee of the ANA, Division of Maternal-Child Health, that they incorporate use of this typology and appropriate diagnostic terms from your group in revising the standards in relation to the new scope of practice statements.

We have structures in our respective organizations to aid us in defining the practice of nursing. The ANA has the scope of practice statements for generic nursing and also for specialty areas that must begin to incorporate the inferential process involved in making assessments and determining a diagnosis that provides a framework for nursing action and evaluation of that action. This is the next frontier in nursing. We therefore can build on what the nurse theorist group has discussed concerning the synthesis of patterns from empirical indicators. I encourage a consideration of their definition of synthesis of clusters of empirical indicators, describing characteristics in unitary man, or of biologic and developmental wholeness. Our next challenge is to develop the criterion for the clustering of phenomena or indicators that will lead to accurate and reliable diagnoses, setting the framework for an expansive phase in nursing when we begin to look carefully at our therapeutic acts. By defining, synthesizing, and refining our work, we will be able to test the theory that nurses diagnose and treat human responses to health problems.

In summary, when viewed from the perspective of the ANA Social Policy Statement and definition of nursing, the work of the National Conference

Group on the Classification of Nursing Diagnosis is impressive and highly relevant to the larger whole. Your work serves to enrich our professional ability to identify standards of nursing practice with respect to diagnosis. The identification and classification you have done serve to focus nursing research and theory construction. Nursing diagnosis will be an increasingly important vehicle for fostering the independent contribution of nursing and providing a basis for clarifying issues of financing health care services.

We have challenges ahead, for example:

1. How much of professional nursing is diagnosis? Is diagnosis the basis of all our actions?
2. Is there a knowledge base for health restoration distinct from health promotion?
3. How do we develop criteria for diagnostic categories that enable reliable diagnosis in view of human responses that are multiple, episodic, continuous, fluid, varying, less discrete?
4. How do we clarify boundaries without setting them?
5. How do we communicate the work of nursing to our various publics— our clients, our colleagues, and our neighbors?

Speaking for the ANA, we look forward to future collaborative efforts. We each have mechanisms to use. You have an effective continuing education network. You have established a national resource to foster the development of nursing diagnosis. The ANA has the statements of practice, the standards, and the quality assurance programs. We now have a Steering Committee. I envision conference groups dealing with one diagnosis: specifying, clarifying, researching, and establishing criteria for the diagnosis, treatment, and evaluation. We will be testing whether nursing is the diagnosis and treatment of human responses to health problems.

REFERENCES

American Nurses' Association: Nursing: a social policy statement, Kansas City, Mo., 1980, The Association.

Gordon, M.: Nursing diagnosis process and application, New York, 1982, McGraw-Hill Book Co.

Kritek, P.B.: The generation and classification of nursing diagnosis: toward a theory of nursing. In Kim, M.J., and Moritz, D.A., eds.: Classification of nursing diagnosis, proceedings of the third and fourth national conferences, New York, 1982, McGraw-Hill Book Co.

Nicoletti, A.M., Reitz, S.E., and Gordon, M.: A descriptive study of parenting diagnosis. In Kim, M.J., and Moritz, D.A., eds.: Classification of nursing diagnosis, proceedings of the third and fourth national conferences, New York, 1982, McGraw-Hill Book Co.

Nightingale, F.: Notes on nursing: What it is and what it is not, London, 1859, Harrison & Sons.

Phaneuf, J.: Personal communication, Spring 1982.

Roy, Sister C.: Historical perspective of the theoretical framework for the classification of nursing diagnosis, in Kim, M.J., and Moritz, D.A., eds.: Classification of nursing diagnosis, proceedings of the third and fourth national conferences, New York, 1982, McGraw-Hill Book Co.

Discussion

Gertrude Torres: I got from your talk a sense of camaraderie and commitment to a common core understanding between ANA, this group, and the theorists. I would like to say I don't see it that way. I think the theorist group is more, and I use the words carefully, "holistic, pattern oriented and nonproblem oriented." The ANA is still going with its specialty councils and the problem-oriented approach to a social policy statement, which I have difficulty with at present. And then I see this particular group going into empirical data without a clear-cut system by which they are linked to the nurse theorists. However, I think it is healthy and reasonable that at this point in our development, we are off on little different paths and that we will collide at some point, I hope in a positive way. But I do not take the position that we need to think now that we are all together in one happy family, because I do not perceive we are. I don't think we could be. Thank you.

Kathryn Barnard: The message I was trying to convey was that there is diversity and that, in fact, I see diversity as the strength. As long as we can maintain important touchpoints so that we can make relationships among the points of view expressed in the work that various groups are doing, we can be open and receptive to input and use that for changing course. I do not see any value in working toward unity at this point. I think there is much more strength to be gathered from diversity. In the marketplace the clarity and point of view that is most important in practice will emerge. There will always be groups breaking off to deal with particular perspectives and points of view; we have to expect this and try to accommodate them within the larger group.

Jane Lancour: Could you clarify for me what you said about the Social Policy Statement referring to human responses? I thought I understood you to say that you saw similarity between the defining characteristics as used by the National Conference Group and the empirical data as defined by the nurse theorist group. Would you explain that a little more?

Kathryn Barnard: As I studied the published diagnostic statement, I determined much of what is labeled as defining characteristics is in my perception classified as human responses in the Social Policy Statement.* I understand that the Theorist Group is classifying these phenomena as empirical indicators. The Theorist Group goes on to say some very important things about the synthesis of patterns of these phenomena. I think essentially the diagnosis involves this synthesis of patterns. For instance, criteria for making a diagnosis should include historic data, developmental data, observational data, interview data, and standardized testing so that it is only on the basis of multiple indicators that a nursing diagnosis would be possible. Therefore there may be a need to better define some of the defining characteristics. As it is now practiced, the chance level, the probability of coming up with different nursing diagnoses for the same client by different nurses, may be a real problem. Nursing deals with phenomena that are fluid and that change. We deal with people who are in a transitional stage. I first became aware of this lack of stability while doing research on children. Change is a psychometric nightmare, but it is part of human adaptation. We are dealing with unstable phenomena; this will be a challenge for us in developing diagnostic criteria.

---

*American Nurses' Association: Nursing: a social policy statement, Kansas City, Mo., 1980, The Association.

As I look at the current practice of nursing, one thing that is happening is "doing assessments." I think the next step is to encourage nurses who are collecting data to use the inferential process and develop a statement of a problem or a diagnosis. What we do is so much of an unconscious part of our behavior that nurses have a great deal of difficulty knowing or being able to tell you what they do. Nurses seldom wait until they complete an assessment. They are doing a physical assessment on a newborn or the mother, they are teaching, and they are clarifying. They are talking about diaper change. They are doing all sorts of things all the time while they are doing a physical assessment. And it is quite different from watching the same kind of physical assessment being done by a physician. At least that has been my experience in observing.

CHAPTER 2

Nursing diagnosis, nursing theory, and framework

The need for a standardized nomenclature has been both implicitly and explicitly expressed by the National Conference Group since its inception. Webster presents a comprehensive theoretic foundation for the needs and reasons for standarization of nomenclature and brings out some pragmatic points that must be considered in developing a nursing diagnosis taxonomy. Sister Callista Roy presents a discussion of the framework for classification systems development. She updates the activities of nurse theorists and brings a proper perspective of their relationship to the National Conference Group, now called the North American Nursing Diagnosis Association. She addresses some key issues related to the framework and provides some insights into the scope and magnitude of the task at hand. Kritek presents a report of a small group who worked on the taxonomies during the conference. Her synthesis of the group discussion illustrates the inadequacies and incompleteness of the current taxonomy system.

Nomenclature and classification system development

GLENN A. WEBSTER, Ph.D.

REASONS FOR STANDARDIZATION

The major reasons for standarization of nomenclature and classification of nursing diagnoses are (1) facilitation of communication, (2) computer stores and access of information, (3) political and legal needs, (4) advancement of nursing theory and science, and (5) education. All these reasons encourage the establishment of a usable classification system for nursing diagnoses as soon as possible. Some qualification is needed in the case of the fourth reason. A premature and misunderstood classification system would hinder more than it would help the development of nursing theory and science.

These reasons are not neatly separable; communication, education, computer access, and the advancement of the political and legal interests of nursing are related activities. What is not so obvious at first is the connection between theory, science, and communication. Nomenclature and classification are essential for the intellectual discernment of the individual practitioner and scientist, not just for communication with others. Common nouns and other general terms allow us to attend to interesting and significant aspects of our phenomena of concern. Conscious awareness is the result of the successful use of symbols, for example, our labels for nursing diagnoses. The better the classifications and nomenclature, the better will we be able to see "what needs fixing" and what we need to carefully "allow nature to fix."*

DIFFICULTIES THAT MUST BE OVERCOME

Following are the principal difficulties to be overcome in the development of a standard nomenclature and classification system for nursing diagnoses.

1. The first difficulty is the unrivaled complexity of nursing's phenomena of concern: human responses to health conditions (ANA, 1980) run the gamut from what appears to be the purely physical, through the psychobiologic and psychosocial, to what appears to be the purely spiritual.
2. As an empirical science, nursing shares the limitation to nominal rather than real essences, which is characteristic of all empirical science.

---

*Florence Nightingale used the concept of *nature* in this Renaissance-Enlightenment sense. She was aware that the health practitioner was in most instances just a facilitator, that nature was the causal agent responsible for the successful recovery of the patient.

3. Complete success in naming coordinate species and mutually exclusive and jointly exhaustive classes is possible only in the formal and not in the empirical sciences.
4. Nursing is a young empirical science presently in a phase of very rapid change and development. The classifications suggested by future theories are likely to be quite different from those suggested by its current theories.
5. Nursing as a practice or profession is closer to history than to most other natural and social sciences. Nursing and history are concerned with the individual and nonrepeatable, rather than just with the general and repeatable (Collingwood, 1943). The patient looks to the nurse for recognition as a person and not just as an example of a kind of disease or problem.

PRELIMINARY RECOMMENDATIONS

When the reasons for developing a classification system of nursing diagnoses are compared with the difficulties that must be overcome in the development of such a system, an open, tentative, provisional, alphabetic system, which includes diagnoses suggested by differing theoretic perspectives and diagnoses based on recent and contemporary practice, seems best for the present time and for the future (Kim and Moritz, 1982). Such a dictionary of diagnoses should be reviewed periodically to ensure that the labels for diagnoses are definable in terms that allow successful use by the practicing nurse. At the same time, insistence on definitions in terms of real essences is out of place in all empirical science, including nursing. The possible definitions are nominal rather than real or essential; that is, they will provide suggestions for the use of the label rather than the full essence of the label. When the meaning for a diagnostic label is derived from theory, it should be noted as part of the definition. Deriving meanings from theory is acceptable as long as a nurse, using the theoretic perspective behind the label, can successfully use the label. Success is defined as discerning objective features of the phenomena of concern by means of the label or diagnostic category.

NOMINALISM AND ESSENTIALISM

The belief that communication presupposes the ability to name general types, which in turn presupposes the ability to recognize these types, leads easily though not necessarily to essentialism. *Essentialism* is the belief that there are natural types or essences that we must learn to recognize and discriminate from one another, that failure to recognize these natural types will result in inelegance if not nonsense. In contrast, *nominalism* maintains that we are free to group phenomena together in an unending variety of ways, that the concept of a natural kind is a delusion that leads us to attempt impossible tasks. For the realist or essentialist, science and knowledge progress by discerning an order that is really in the phenomena of concern and that is fundamental to the phenomena independent of experience and concepts. For the nominalist, who is one kind of idealist, the order discerned is relative to his concepts, theories, and language. There is no way of knowing whether the order is actually in the phenomena; but if it is, it is likely to be of little importance rather than fundamental.

The distinction between essentialism and nominalism is illustrated by a change in attitudes concerning the nature of physics during the past 20 years. Earlier we were essentialistic; we believed that physics would provide a common language for communication with extraterrestial technical civilizations. We believed that no matter how different the persons of another civilization were from humans, they at least would have discovered the same fundamental regularities in nature that we discerned through our best physical theory. During the 1970s we came to a radically different position concerning physics. We now believe that 10,000 different technical civilizations will probably have 10,000 different systems of physics and that the fundamental regularities and facts discerned by these systems will also be different, though relatable given enough time and intelligence. We believe that the world is the *same* world, though viewable from radically different theoretic and conceptual perspectives. A change of perspective changes what is discerned and what is considered fundamental. Only now in the 1980s is our imagination beginning to be wild enough to give us an idea of how very different the same world can look from different perspectives (Laudan, 1981; Newton-Smith, 1981).

The medieval debate between classical realism (forms or universals are most real) and nominalism (only words are universals, actual entities are all irreducibly particular) ended in the realization that the only solution was a modification of both theories. Similiarly in the debate concerning the relationship between a common noun and its referent within the world, nominalism and essentialism, the solution will be a position somewhere between the two extremes. Order obviously exists within the phenomena of concern that is independent of a scientist's ability to perceive it. Just as obviously, the order that is perceived by a scientist is only a small part of the order that is actually within the phenomena. The history of science provides strong inductive evidence for the belief that the order the scientist perceives as fundamental is probably not fundamental for the phenomena themselves. This statement needs qualification. "Fundamental for the purpose of organizing theory about the phenomena of concern" must be distinguished from "fundamental within the phenomena of concern as things in themselves are independent of the fact that they are discerned." These two kinds of fundamentals will merge when we achieve omniscience concerning the phenomena.

Until that time, the distinction allows us to see the truth in the nominalists' position. Our terms allow us to focus on a kind of order within the phenomena that is sufficient for our purposes in planning interventions and communication, including computer access and the like, but that is most likely not the most fundamental and certainly not the only kind of order within the phenomena. Locke's distinction (1959) between nominal and real essences is in agreement with these distinctions. Locke believed that we know nominal rather than real essences, that the nominal essence is related to the real essence as part to whole, and that nominal essences are sufficient to allow us to use abstract or general terms.

The preceding distinctions are directly relevant to the problem of nomenclature and the development of a classification system for nursing diagnoses. Nursing science and nursing theory are only beginning their most fruitful and progressive periods. The nominal essences that nursing currently recognizes through theory and nomenclature are more unclear and more distant from the heart of real essences than will be the case in a few more decades, let alone several more centuries. Nevertheless, the gap between nominal and real essences will never be closed, not in any empirical science developed by finite persons.

However, the fact that empirical science necessarily deals with nominal rather than real essences must be distinguished from the fact that nursing can expect rapid progress toward the grasp of much more useful and cognitively insightful nominal essences in the near future. Nursing must, by its nature, avoid strict categories. Nurse theorists and practitioners need the freedom to view their phenomena of concern from new perspectives. Whatever classification system for nursing diagnoses is adopted should preserve as much of that freedom as possible.

FORMAL AND EMPIRICAL CONCEPTS

The distinction between formal and empirical concepts is related to the preceding discussion of essentialism and nominalism and real and nominal essences. In mathematics and symbolic logic, the concepts are formal and the essences are real. These are the sciences in which are found paradigmatic classification systems, with their clear distinctions between genera and species, coordinate classes, and kinds that are mutually exclusive and jointly exhaustive. In the formal sciences, definitions can state real essences, rather than merely provide suggestions for the successful use of the common nouns in question.

Outside the formal sciences, ideal classification systems are seldom found. Everyone is familiar with the difficulties that biology has faced in distinguishing animate from inanimate, organic from inorganic, plants from animals. But its species, genera, and families work well enough for the sake of the advancement of the science. We are beyond the kinds of mistakes that were made by many biologists in medieval times. We know that the classifications we establish are only partially reflected by nature itself, that nature is not so interested in neat and tidy distinctions as are we who are trying to make sense of it. The territory is much more unclear and more complicated than the maps that we have constructed for the purpose of finding our way about the territory. We know that the map is not the territory, though we hope that the features we discern by successful use of the map are actually features of the territory. That is not the issue. The issue is whether our maps are the final maps and the best maps. We know that they are not. So long as this knowledge is not forgotten, we can proceed with the wise development of classification systems, which are one kind of map.

If we forget the limits of our knowledge in the empirical sciences, we may believe that our nomenclature and classifications are final and authoritative, when in fact they are only tentative and provisional. This is not a peculiarity of nursing alone; it is a peculiarity of all empirical science. Our nomenclature allows us to discern by focusing our attention, which is more negative than positive. (We see by ignoring the infinite complexity of our phenomena of concern and by concentrating on a finite and partial aspect of those phenomena that is simple enough to be grasped by our finite intellects.) If we forget what we are doing in intellectually discerning by means of terms, concepts, and theories, the result is what Whitehead (1967) labeled the *fallacy of misplaced concreteness*, the fallacy of mistaking the abstract for the concrete. Reality is always much richer than we are able to discern by means of the empirical concepts we possess at some stage of our development. Our concepts are like searchlights picking out those aspects of things on which they happen to focus, while leaving most aspects of things in darkness. The human responses to health conditions that are the phenomena of concern of nursing are much more complex than the sorts of phenomena of interest to most of the older empirical sciences. For nursing practice and nursing science to advance, any classification system adopted at this stage of nursing's history must be deliberately designed to be open, provisional, and tentative.

THE MATHEMATICAL MODEL OF CLASSIFICATION

The simplest and most easily understood classification is the type that has been achieved in number theory and other branches of mathematics and logic. This is a classification system, hierarchically arranged, in which the classes at each level pack into the preceding level and are mutually exclusive and jointly exhaustive. The nature of this type of system is best understood by the following illustration:

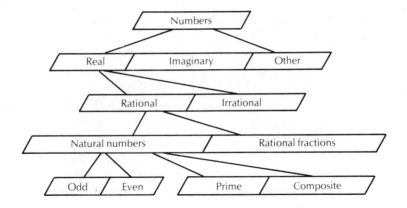

This is among the simplest of all classification systems because it deals with the abstract and ideal rather than the concrete and actual and because the entities to be classified are eternal and universal rather than temporal and individual. When the subject matter is of this type, science can be exact. Of course, there are problems that have not been solved in mathematics. The task of discovering all possible branches of mathematics will never be completed because there is no such thing as *all* possible branches of mathematics. Consider, for example, the class labeled other in the initial division of numbers into the subclasses real and imaginary. Even in an exact science one often cannot close a classification system.

Another interesting feature about the classification of numbers is that there is often more than one possible subdivision of a generic class, for example, real numbers can be divided into negative and positive real numbers, into rational or irrational real numbers, or into fractions and whole numbers (with the fractions including the irrationals). Another division is that of natural numbers into primes and composites, rather than into odd and even numbers. The division that one chooses depends on one's interest and purpose.

In mathematics, *monothetic* definitions of classes are usually possible; for example, a rational number is a real number that can be expressed as the ratio between two whole numbers. Also in mathematics one expects to be able to achieve a precision in classification that produces classes that are *mutually exclusive* (no member of the generic kind belongs to more than one subclass) and *jointly exhaustive* (each member of the generic class belongs to at least one of the subordinate classes).

Mathematics represents one extreme as far as classification is concerned. Precise definitions of its classes are usually possible. Simple criteria for determining class membership, criteria that are algorithmic, again are possible.

Hierarchies in mathematics are obvious. Inability to achieve mutually exclusive and jointly exhaustive classifications is unusual. It is no wonder that mathematics is used as a model for classification.

CLASSIFICATION IN THE EMPIRICAL SCIENCES

As we move away from mathematics into the empirical sciences, we lose the neatness and ease of the classifications of mathematics. We enter a world in which the phenomena of concern are concrete and infinitely complex and in which our knowledge and understanding are limited. Here we start with empirical concepts that are the products of history and common sense and refine them by developing theory. These empirical concepts give us slices of the phenomena of concern that overlap or that leave large gaps. Our first reaction is to attempt to achieve the precise mutually exclusive, and jointly exhaustive classifications that are possible in mathematics.

But we soon discover that our empirical concepts are allowing us to manipulate that which remains for the most part unknown to us. We develop theories to extend our knowledge and alleviate our ignorance. At first it seems that the theories will allow us to achieve what the original empirical concepts failed to provide—classifications like those of mathematics.

But as theories advance and compete, we discover that the phenomena of concern were much more complex than we at first imagined. It also becomes apparent that our classification schemes are functioning for the purposes of communication and the advancement of knowledge in spite of the fact that they fall short of the ideals provided by mathematics. Alternate theories lead to alternate classification schemes. Sometimes the alternatives are reduced to a single one that is clearly superior. This does not often occur; rather we have different perspectives on the same phenomena—perspectives that complement each other and that together provide us with a more complete understanding of the phenomena. The wave versus the particle analyses of matter in physics is among the most famous instances of competing but complementary perspectives.

In sciences in which generalization is the goal, classification is more serious because of its connection with the development of theory. Insofar as nursing is concerned with appropriate responses to particular human situations, its classification of those situations is important. The practicing nurse would be helped by algorithms for the proper classification of phenomena. But algorithms are possible in only some of the branches of the exact sciences, such as mathematics and logic. Strictly speaking there are no algorithms, decision procedures, in the empirical sciences. Instead, there are procedures that work in most cases. Nursing should seek such tests or procedures; they are essential for effective treatment. But the wise nurse knows that the individual case is much more complex than the theories and tests that are available. If nursing were merely a science and not also a profession, the element of irreducible individuality would not be so distressing. The problem is that the nurse must act—often nothing more than look and give reassurance, which is a definite form of action.

CRITICAL REALISM OR MODIFIED ESSENTIALISM

The essentialist believes that the phenomena of concern possess a natural structure independent of the scientific investigator that is to be discovered by that investigator and properly reflected in the classification scheme of the science. A question often posed by a biologist is, "Are the individual living organisms members of one species or two species?" The Aristotelian biologist believed in the eternalness of the species and in its givenness as something to be discovered. In more recent times biologists have been forced to recognize that there is an element of fuzziness about the idea of one species—that borderline individuals, mutant or otherwise, will often defy classification. Nature is too rich and inventive for any one neat classification system, yet such systems are important for the progress of science.

Consider the following example from astronomy. The distinction between *planet* and *star* seems clear and unambiguous. A star is defined as a self-luminous body with a mass larger than that of a planet. If we include nucleosynthesis as the source of energy among our defining criteria for a star, we run into immediate difficulty. White dwarfs are stars that have exhausted their thermonuclear fuels and are shining by gravitational energy alone. The heat and light they radiate is produced by their contraction in size. But if we admit that white dwarfs are stars, what do we do about bodies like the planet Jupiter? Careful measurement of the energy radiated by Jupiter reveals that it is emitting twice the energy that it receives from the Sun. It is therefore self-luminous. Is Jupiter a planet or a star? Wisdom dictates that we acknowledge the existence of borderline cases, ones that do not clearly fit either category.

These examples point away from simple essentialism toward some sort of modified essentialism or critical realism. The extreme nominalist maintains that our classifications reflect only our own conventions and not the nature of the phenomena of concern. Wisdom seems to dictate some sort of intermediate position. Insofar as our classification schemes are useful and especially insofar as they can be justified by a coherent body of theory, they probably do give us a perspective on order within the phenomena that is independent of our theories and classifications. But the perspective we have achieved is only one of many possible perspectives, and the order we have discovered, though it be real, may turn out to be relatively trivial and inconsequential compared with the order that might be discovered with an alternate set of theories and classifications.

Nursing's phenomena of concern are far more complex than those of physics and astronomy; hence, the inability to resolve the present incoherence among existing nursing theories. Better theory is needed to achieve hierarchical ordering of classes of phenomena. But no matter how good the theory, classes will overlap and gaps will exist. Also, it will be a very long time before the various theoretical perspectives are reconciled and coordinated in an integrated perspective.

Fear and anxiety are examples of nursing diagnoses that illustrate many of the above concerns (Kim and Moritz, 1982). Fear is a more commonsense empirical concept; anxiety is a more theory-laden empirical concept. Anxiety has its theoretic base in Freudian psychoanalytic theory (Freud, 1926). There is no reason why both terms should not be included among recognized nursing diagnoses, contrary to the decision of the 1980 conference to delete anxiety from the list. Nursing should not exclude diagnostic labels simply because those labels are grounded in theories developed outside nursing. The relevant factor should be the usefulness of the label for discerning features of interest to the nurse. Fear has identifiable objects. Anxiety is like fear, but without identifiable objects. This fact is interesting and sometimes quite important for proper treatment. Currently, neither category seems reducible to the other, though there is overlap and a certain lack of coordination. More work must be conducted on theory. Meanwhile, nurses should be allowed to use those diagnostic terms they find helpful, and some type of instruction should be provided for successful use of the term.

FINAL RECOMMENDATIONS

Nursing must compromise between the needs of practice and science. The needs of nursing practice require classification. The needs of nursing science would be better met by postponing any authoritative classification indefinitely. The compromise that suggests itself is to simply alphabetize existing classes of diagnoses, with room in such a classification for many different sorts of phenomena and for classes that we know overlap. The list should be inclusive rather than exclusive. For the more theory-laden categories, universal acceptance of the related theory should not be demanded for inclusion of the diagnostic category. Rather, the definitions of such diagnostic categories should specify the related theory. The compilers of such a list can make it clear that they are not endorsing the equal worthiness of all diagnostic terms and categories in the list.

Such a system should contain classes that are definitely not coordinated. When a better theory is developed, some classes will become genera in relation to others. From the point of view of science, this will be less than satisfactory; but the nurse scientist should find the list of diagnoses interesting. From the point of view of practice, the list must be developed at the same time that the science is developing. A multiplicity of perspectives enriches practice. Beware of false and troubling dichotomies; they are the result of attempting to use indistinct classes as though they were clear and precise or open classifications as though they were mutually exclusive and jointly exhaustive. In this situation, nursing's classes are in fact nominal and only very partially essential.

Classification systems are ancillary to nursing practice. Nursing practice uses knowledge of the universal to gain insight into the individual. For this reason, it is not essential that the classification systems be anything like those of mathematics. Nursing cannot achieve the precision of mathematics because no empirical science can and because empirical sciences that are more concerned with the individual are less like mathematics than those that are concerned primarily with the general or repeatable aspects of phenomena. Physics is closer to mathematics than is history. Nursing is halfway between sciences like physics and history. History is unique among the sciences because its phenomenon of concern is the individual. Historians may use lawlike statements, but they are not concerned with their truth or falsehood. Historians do not study wars as such but some particular war such as World War II.

Nursing is more interested in the general than is history. Without knowledge of the general, nursing practice would be completely intuitive. Without knowledge of the general, no nurse would have any idea what sorts of interventions are appropriate for particular diagnoses. Nor would a diagnosis be possible, for it consists of the recognition of some complex universal in the particular.

But in the end the nurse is concerned with a particular patient (or a particular community) at some particular time. The essence of nursing is concern with persons as such rather than merely with abstract aspects of them. This makes nursing more like history than like the usual empirical sciences. It also makes nursing more complex than most empirical sciences because persons are the most complex phenomena in any science.

Insofar as nursing cannot ignore the universal or general, it must be able to classify. But insofar as nursing science is as yet embryonic as a result of the unsurpassed complexity of nursing's phenomena of concern, the classes or kinds with which the nurse presently works are more unclear and more temporary than in almost any other science. Classify, but only provisionally, and with openness to a variety of practical and theoretical perspectives.

REFERENCES

American Nurses' Association: Nursing: a social policy statement, Kansas City, Mo., 1980, The Association.

Collingwood, R.G.: The idea of history, Oxford, 1946, The Clarendon Press.

Freud, S.: Inhibitions, symptoms, and anxiety, London, 1926, The Hogarth Press, Ltd. (Translated by Alix Strachey.)

Kim, M.J., and Moritz, D.A., eds.: Classification of nursing diagnoses: proceedings of the third and fourth national conferences, New York, 1982, McGraw-Hill Book Co.

Laudan, L.: Progress and its problems: towards a theory of scientific growth, Berkeley, 1977, University of California Press.

Locke, J.: Essay concerning human understanding, New York, 1959, Dover Publications, Inc.

Newton-Smith, W.H.: The rationality of science, Boston, 1981, Routledge & Kegan Paul.

Sokal, R.R., Classification: purposes, principles, progress, prospects, Science **185**(4157):1116, 1974.

Whitehead, A.N.: Science and the modern world, New York, 1967, Free Press.

Discussion

Kenneth Cianfrani: Some of the difficulties that you have discussed I heard as arguments against nursing diagnosis. And one of those is that if we are developing general categories, we are going to start categorizing or putting clients or patients into boxes. We would categorize the client as an instance of appendicitis or an instance of decreased cardiac output. Could you comment on that?

Glenn Webster: Your comment strikes right at the heart of the matter. I think what we need are diagnostic categories for the purpose of being able to see, but that is not the issue. The issue is what you do with them once you have them. And alongside that, how many of those diagnostic categories you possess. If you attempted to achieve standardization in the sense of just one closed list, with each term defined from one particular point of view, that would be better. But if you have an open list, with the terms defined from whichever points of view that are relevant to the definition, one of the results would be lack of standardization, missiveness. But another result would be a lot more richness in diagnostic categories than would otherwise exist. The open list could become a tool, and when nurses review the list of diagnostic categories, reading the instructions, the definitions, and the comments on the theoretic perspectives that are relevant for understanding a particular diagnosis, their practice would be enriched. I think whichever list is forthcoming, it should be a partial open list to which additions could be made. I am personally in favor of an alphabetic list, with willingness to be completely chaotic as far as mutually exclusive categories are concerned. There needs to be someone who can explain what a term means. For example, I noticed that anxiety was dropped from your list of nursing diagnoses at the last national conference. I find this deletion interesting in a strange way. Anxiety is not fear from a Freudian point of view. I think that particular diagnosis ought to be put back in with the references to Freud.

Marjory Gordon I think that is an interesting point. Probably that is partly true—that a lot of people have trouble with diagnoses such as noncompliance. I would never use that term, but I guess from a particular perspective, you are saying that it might be interesting to consider on an alphabetic list of diagnoses.

Glenn Webster: There might be some other diagnostic categories on the list that come out of areas of nursing practice that light has not been shed on theoretically. There is a wisdom in practice that the theories have not captured as yet. There is a wisdom in some of the theories that have not been captured in practice. You need it all.

Jacqueline Wylie: A lot of nurses have practiced from a very authoritative knowledge base that does not allow for change and flexibility. How do you help these nurses use a more tentative, open classification system? Is there a way to put the two together or help people move?

Glenn Webster: There is. It is a matter of going back to what you really know rather than what you are simply teaching. We do not want to be in the trap of the famous/infamous Oxford dons who maintain that what I do not know is not knowledge. That is the other side of the coin. What I know is knowledge, but what I do not know is not knowledge. There are a few elitists who support that very dogmatic position. It is a deadly position for nursing right now, which is changing rapidly. The theories will be much better 10 years from now than they are today. They are changing very rapidly. If you try to come up with closed categories prematurely, which we never will be able to do, any attempt to try to do it is an attempt to try to do the impossible. You are wasting energy. It is silly to try to square the circle when you know it cannot be done.

Wealtha Alex: We do know that there are several classification systems that are used within nursing, and I would like you to comment on an eclectic approach in which practitioners use a variety of classification schemes verus simply sticking to the lists that this conference group has prepared. Is there any value? What are the advantages and disadvantages?

Glenn Webster: I would see the list that came out of a group like this one as helpful, very useful for legal and computerization purposes, and so forth. But when it comes to the advantages to nursing knowledge, of course, you should be free of the "icon busters" to go ahead and create new categories. And then the next time the group meets, the newly created categories will be added to this list. In that sense, I think your list should always be open.

Framework for classification systems development: progress and issues

SISTER CALLISTA ROY, R.N., Ph.D. F.A.A.N.

In 1977 a group of nurse theorists was convened to assist the National Conference Group in developing a theoretic framework for classification of nursing diagnoses. This paper summarizes the historic background of the group and describes the framework that has evolved from the efforts of group members and their interaction with conference participants. Theorists' activities leading up to the Fifth National Conference and their postconference work are also discussed. Finally, the chairperson of the group presents reflections on the progress and issues of this 5-year project.

CONFERENCE REPORT
Historic background

Nursing is rapidly developing a theory base for practice and theoretic questions are being raised in every area of inquiry within the scientific and humanistic discipline of nursing. The approach of searching for theoretical links was already alive when the First National Conference on the Classification of Nursing Diagnoses was convened in St. Louis in 1973. The work groups of that conference proceeded inductively with the initial task of developing nursing diagnoses specific to the health, illness, functional ability, or disability of the individual (Gebbie and Lavin, 1975).

Conference participants in those groups began to suggest frameworks for categorization of nursing diagnoses. Two groups suggested inductive approaches including set theory and Venn diagrams to explain and illustrate the intersection of four domains of nursing problems—physical, cognitive, affective, and social. Four groups suggested deductive approaches. These approaches included use of Maslow's hierarchy of needs (1954); adaptation of the work of Abdellah and co-workers (1960); a three-step approach to needs, their immediacy, and degree of patient participation; and a focus on diagnoses as expressions of one's integrated human functioning.

While acknowledging the significant impact of the work of the First National Conference, concerns were expressed about the theoretic basis of the work and the resulting problems in the order of generality of the diagnostic labels. Sister Callista Roy articulated these concerns in her address at the opening of the Second National Conference in 1975. She noted that a taxonomy is a set of classifications that are ordered and arranged on the basis of a single principle or a consistent set of principles. The organizing principle determines the rules for eligibility into the system and the place the label will hold in the system. From the organizing principle, one can derive rules for the sets of labels and the subsets. Roy (1976) offered alternative suggestions for procedures to determine an organizing principle for the diagnostic classification system. The suggestions included looking at the frameworks suggested at the First National Conference, considering the available conceptual frameworks for nursing practice, and examining the more recent nurse practice acts.

To pursue this concern further, Sister Callista Roy drafted a proposal for a Task Force on Nursing Diagnoses in 1976 to convene a group of nurse theorists to assist with developing a framework for the classification system. The proposal was approved and of the 22 persons invited, 14 joined the group. Kim and Moritz (1982) have reported on the extensive work of this group. The work of this period focused on two major goals:

- To develop and present a theoretic framework to provide an organizing principle for the work of the conference
- To make recommendations to the Conference on the order of generality of the diagnostic labels

As an outcome of the theorists' participation in the Third and Fourth National Conferences, another goal was added to the initial goals:

- To correlate the theorists' work with the ongoing work of the conference and to clarify the relevance of the framework for nursing practice.

Work between the Fourth and Fifth Conferences

To continue work on the first two goals and to concentrate more on the third goal, several meetings of the nurse theorists were held between the Fourth and Fifth National Conferences. The results of these meetings are presented in this paper.

In the ongoing effort to demonstrate a relationship between the developing conceptual framework and the accepted classification of diagnoses, members of the group began with a list of defining characteristics of the nursing diagnoses as proposed by the Third and Fourth National Conferences (Kim and Mortiz, 1982). A total of 1051 defining characteristics were listed for the 42 accepted diagnostic labels. The rationale for returning to these defining characteristics was to see them as clinically based empirical data, that is, as the occurrences nurses observe in daily practice that lead them to make a particular diagnostic judgment. The theorists were to list under each of the nine pattern characteristics—exchanging, communicating, relating, valuing, choosing, moving, perceiving, knowing, and feeling—the numbers of all the diagnostic characteristics that seem to fit that pattern. For example, under *choosing* some of the defining characteristics that could be listed are as follows:

1. Not taking responsibility for self-care (from diagnosis of disturbance in self-esteem)

2. Inability to identify choices (from diagnosis of ineffective family coping patterns)
3. Adherence to fad diets (from diagnosis of alteration in nutrition: changes related to body requirements)
4. Discontinued religious participation (from diagnosis of spiritual despair)

In another approach to looking at the various levels of abstraction of the framework concepts and of the diagnostic labels for homework, the theorists also classified each of the 42 accepted diagnoses as empirical data, a summary concept, or a dimension. The results of this classification are also presented in this paper.

Description of the framework

The participants at the Fifth National Conference received a handout of the outline shown in Box 1. The highest level of the framework is the phenomenon of nursing—the health of unitary man/human. This term is made up of two concepts: unitary man/human and health.

For several years, the Theorist Group has struggled to reach a consensus and to articulate the meaning of the term *unitary man/human*. The term *unitary man* was introduced by Rogers (1970) in her science of unitary man. The Theorist Group has agreed on two basic assumptions about unitary man/human. First, they accepted the belief that unitary man/human is an open system, that is, a system in mutual interaction with the environment (see sections II,B and III in Box 1).

BOX 1   **Nurse theorist group report**

I. Diagram of diagnostic framework

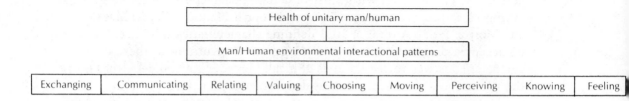

II. Diagnostic framework
   A. Phenomenon of nursing—health of unitary man/human
   B. Assumptions
      1. Unitary man/human
         a. Open system (negentropy)—mutual interaction with environment
         b. Four-dimensional energy field—pattern and organization

      2. Health
        a. Value
        b. Pattern of energy exchange that enhances field integrity
        c. Man/human–environment interactional patterns
   C. Conceptual framework
      1. Exchanging—mutual giving and receiving
      2. Communicating—sending messages
      3. Relating—establishing bonds
      4. Valuing—assigning relative worth
      5. Choosing—selection of alternatives
      6. Moving—activity
      7. Perceiving—reception of information
      8. Knowing—meaning associated with information
      9. Feeling—subjective awareness of information
III. Narrative about diagnostic framework

The first basic assumption about unitary man/human is the belief that unitary man/human is an open system, that is, a system in mutual interaction with the environment. Negentropy, a characteristic of open systems, is a process of continuous development toward increasing complexity and diversity. This process can be viewed from observations of individuals throughout the life process and observations from generation to generation.

The second basic assumption is that unitary man/human is a four-dimensional energy field characterized by pattern and organization. Each human field has a unique pattern. The uniqueness of the pattern and organization of each field is manifest in nine man/human–environment interactional patterns.

The basic assumptions about health are that (1) it is a value, (2) it is a pattern of energy exchange, (3) this pattern enhances field integrity of unitary man/human (field integrity is denoted by completeness, efficiency, clarity, accuracy, and authenticity), and (4) it is manifested through nine man/human–environment interactional patterns.

IV. Nursing diagnosis

Nursing is concerned with the health of unitary man/human. Nursing diagnosis is an integral component of the science and practice of nursing. It is a judgment about health based on data relevant to the conceptual framework of nine patterns. Diagnosis requires refinement of the patterns through identification of the characteristics.

    There is growing evidence of widespread acceptance of systems theory as an assumption within the discipline of nursing. In a survey of curriculum models in National League for Nursing accredited baccalaureate programs, DeBack (1981) reported that of 270 schools responding, 50% were categorized as systems models, 19% as developmental models, 6% as interaction models, and 24% as mixed models. Fitzpatrick and coworkers (1982) note that all the major nursing conceptual frameworks, that is, King, Orem, Rogers, and Roy, declare an underlying assumption encompassing systems theory. It is not surprising, then, that this group of nurse theorists agreed on the assumption that unitary man/human is an open system.

To further describe their concept of unitary man/human, the theorists note that negentropy is a characteristic of an open system. Negentropy is defined as the continuous development toward increasing complexity and diversity, such as occurred during the rapid growth of our schools of nursing and nursing service agencies. Structure, roles, functions, and services all became more complex and diverse. In an open system, this continuous development evolves along the space-time continuum. The Theorist Group report points out that this process can be viewed from observations of individuals throughout the life process and observation from generation to generation.

The second basic assumption according to the Theorist Group report is that unitary man/human is a four-dimensional energy field characterized by pattern and organization.* In exploring the idea of pattern, the theorists sought to differentiate between rhythm and pattern. The example of a kaleidoscope was used. As the kaleidoscope turns, the patterns change and the tempo of the change is its rhythm. Rhythm, then, is a characteristic of the pattern. Another example is crystals responding to sound waves. The theorists noted that the dimensions identified by the group are the "crystals" of unitary man. Each human field has a unique pattern of "crystals." This uniqueness is manifested in nine interactional patterns specific to the person.

The second major concept of the term *health of unitary man/human* is *health*. In an earlier work (Kim and Moritz, 1982), the Theorist Group had defined health as a rhythmic pattern of energy exchange that is mutually enhancing and expresses full life potential. In the deliberations preceding the Fifth National Conference, the Theorist Group agreed to accept three assumptions about health (see section II,B in Box 1): (1) value, (2) pattern of energy exchange that enhances field integrity, and (3) man/human–environment interactional patterns. The group, then, first recognized that values are involved in any discussion of health—the values of the nurse and the values of the person receiving nursing care. The referent for change, however, is the person's satisfaction with self or the person's own pattern as enhancing or self-destructive.

The second assumption notes that health signifies a pattern of energy exchange that enhances field integrity. Field integrity is denoted by completeness, efficiency, clarity, accuracy, and authenticity. This process of field integration moves one toward life's potential. Healthy exchanging then, for

---

*This assumption is not accepted as wholeheartedly as the first, either among the nurse theorists or the nursing community at large. Some believe that condensing an understanding of humans to an energy field is itself a reductionist approach.

example, is a pattern of energy exchanging that enhances the integrity of the field. Rate, duration, and amount (or quality and quantity) are evaluated.

This concept of health includes a third assumption that health involves the unitary man/human–environment interactional patterns, which has nine pattern characteristics (see Box 1). In seeking to further describe the nature of the unitary man/human–environment interactional patterns, the theorists had previously noted that human characteristics also include rational, sentient, goal-directed, purposeful, and functional in usual roles. These characteristics do not appear in the agreed on assumptions but seem basic in the thinking of some members of the Theorist Group.

The nine pattern characteristics are proposed as a conceptual framework for the diagnostic classification system. The concern, or phenomenon, of nursing has been identified as the health of unitary man/human as understood by the above assumptions. The Theorist Group recognizes nursing diagnoses as an integral component of the science and practice of nursing. Based on the framework presented, they view nursing diagnosis as a judgment about health that is based on data relevant to the nine pattern characteristics. In other words, the indices of the field pattern are the basis for diagnosis, and nursing diagnosis describes a health pattern at a point in time of an individual, family, or group.

In their discussion of nursing diagnoses from the viewpoint of unitary man/human, the theorists noted that diagnosis may begin with a given pattern such as moving. However, other patterns, such as choosing and knowing, are considered at the same time. Furthermore, physical motion does not wholly reflect the field notion. As the nurse collects data, information coalesces; that is, the pattern emerges. Diagnosis is the identification of the pattern of the person in interaction with an environmental pattern. Behavior is a manifestation of the field, and observations of behavior are indicators of the pattern of unitary man/human. The nurse constructs or recognizes the pattern.

The theorists are asserting that a unitary pattern emerges when one is working with a client. At the same time, they recognize that it is difficult to understand the information as it coalesces and to make references at broader, more general levels. Reducing the information the nurse obtains to rhythm and energy, a diagnosis such as the following might be made: *Conflict of person tempo in terms of actual movement and perceived tempo.* This nursing diagnosis would be based on the subjective report of how the person feels. During the nurse theorists' discussion, it was pointed out that the group must be consistent in definitions as they relate to unitary man and must emphasize that, in this approach, we look at individuals, not so-called norms. The group asserts that the nine pattern characteristics are always there and are always assessed.

The Theorist Group considered several basic questions related to the use of the nine pattern characteristics for nursing diagnosis in clinical practice. The question naturally arises as to whether or not the categories are mutually exclusive, and some members of the group believe that they are not. They are reflective of the whole, which is a unitary pattern. In dealing with the question of where do information, observations, and knowledge from physiology or medicine fit in the framework, the group suggested that they could be placed under the heading of additional relevant data. The group recognized that assessments for diagnoses are made on the basis of the empirical indications of the nine pattern characteristics. Although some exploratory reports on each pattern had been circulated among the group in 1980, the theorists believed that further discussion and research are needed to establish empirical indicators of the pattern characteristics. What may be needed is a way of identifying the trajectory of the person. These questions, as well as the entire framework described, are open for further study and clinical testing.

Levels of abstraction of accepted diagnoses

At the Fifth National Conference, the report of the Theorist Group in analyzing the levels of abstraction of the accepted nursing diagnoses was presented (Box 2). Seven of the accepted diagnoses were considered to be at the highest level of abstraction; that is, they were classified as constructs. Fifteen labels were at the concept level. The Theorist Group suggested that this is the same level as the nine pattern characteristics. Nineteen diagnostic labels were at the empirical level.

As noted in the report of the group work on taxonomies from the Fifth National Conference, practicing nurses have experienced problems in using the existing list. Many of these problems are a result of the lack of clarity in existing levels of abstraction. That group divided the labels into four levels of abstraction without naming each level. Their highest level, labeled Level I, was seen by the group as having a fairly high degree of parallelism with the nine pattern characteristics listed by theorists. This group also presented nine taxonomic trees, one for each pattern of unitary man/human.

In a general discussion of levels of abstraction for the framework, the theorists proposed the deductive approach shown in Fig. 1. Although this figure was simplified when the theoretic framework was presented, one can see that the Theorist Group has worked deductively to show levels of abstraction for the framework. They have also taken the inductively derived diagnostic labels and indicated orders of generality within them. The issue of levels of abstraction has not been settled, but the nurse theorists have presented their work at various stages of the project for consideration by the conference group and others.

BOX 2   **Levels of abstraction**

Constructs
  Comfort
  Communication
  Knowledge
  Noncompliance
  Thought process
  Spiritual distress
  Self-concept
Concepts
  Coping
    Ineffective, individual
    Ineffective, family, compromised
    Ineffective, family, disabling
    Family potential for growth
  Diversion activity
  Grieving, anticipatory
  Grieving, dysfunctional
  Mobility
  Parenting alterations—actual
  Parenting alterations—potential
  Rape trauma
  Self-care deficit
  Sensory perceptual alteration

  Sexual dysfunction
  Violence
Empirical data
  Airway clearance
  Bowel elimination
    Constipation
    Diarrhea
    Incontinence
  Breathing pattern
  Cardiac output
  Fluid volume deficit—actual
  Fluid volume deficit—potential
  Gas exchange
  Home maintenance
  Injury
  Nutritional—less
  Nutritional—more
  Nutritional—potential
  Tissue perfusion
  Urinary elimination—alteration
  Skin integrity
  Sleep patterning

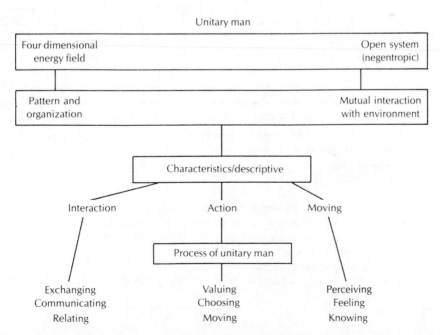

FIGURE 1   Proposed deductive approach regarding levels of abstractions agreed on by the group.

BOX 3   **Group activity**

Group number _____

Diagnostic label _____

Participant number _____

Task: Take all defining characteristics from the diagnostic label and identify by placing an X *under* the pattern each most appropriately represents. (Select only one pattern per characteristic.)
For those characteristics that do not seem to match a particular pattern, mark X under the category "Other."
Pattern definitions are noted on the diagnostic framework.

Patterns

Characteristics	Exchanging	Communicating	Relating	Valuing	Choosing	Moving	Perceiving	Knowing	Feeling	Other

Please complete the following on the other side of this sheet:
1. Which characteristics do not fit any particular pattern?
2. Which characteristics tend to fit multiple patterns?
3. Can you identify additional characteristics?
4. Do any new patterns emerge?
5. List any concerns/suggestions about using this diagnostic framework.

Group activity for conference participants

The work groups of the conference were asked to participate in further relating diagnostic framework to the work of the conference. The task was presented to conference participants as outlined in Box 3. Each of 12 work groups was assigned other tasks related to a limited number of accepted diagnoses with similar content areas (see Chapter 6). Within the time allotted for work group sessions, participants were asked to call on their expertise in the content areas of assigned diagnoses and complete the worksheets.

The group had already been assigned numbers, and each member of the group was then given a number as a participant in that group. A worksheet was to be filled out for each diagnostic label assigned to the group by each member. Thus, if a group of eight persons were examining four diagnostic labels, 32 worksheets would be completed by that group. In addition, the groups were asked to discuss their individual responses and turn in a sheet indicating a consensus of the group, if this was possible within the constraints of time and other commitments.

Specifically, the task involved taking all the defining characteristics for the diagnostic label and identifying, according to directions, the pattern each most appropriately represents. Participants were asked to select only one pattern per characteristic and to indicate those defining characteristics that did not seem to match a particular pattern.* The group activity assignment also included five questions that would help identify: (1) characteristics that did not fit any particular pattern, (2) charcteristics that tend to fit multiple patterns, (3) additional characteristics, (4) new patterns, and (5) any concerns or suggestions that emerged from using the diagnostic framework.

Summary of issues

The Theorist Group report to the conference summarized some major issues identified in the development of a framework for the classification system. The issues included the unanswered questions of defining characteristics for the nine patterns and of agreement on and consistent use of levels of generality within the framework and for the labels. Questions were also raised about mechanisms or structures for developing the clarification and validation of the framework by the National Conference Group and for continuing to develop the diagnostic nomenclature.

Discussion with the audience followed. Questions and comments centered on clarifying participants' understanding of the theorists' report and of the task assigned to the work groups. Information was provided to the audience on the process of concept development.

---

*It should be noted that to avoid the confusion that might have resulted from using the same word with both factors being related, defining characteristics were referred to as "characteristics" and pattern characteristics were called "patterns."

POSTCONFERENCE ACTIVITIES

Following the Fifth National Conference, activities of the Theorist Group centered on examining the result of the group activity that related the defining characteristics of the diagnosis to the nine patterns of unitary man/human. A volunteer task force of the theorists considered additional issues raised by the assignment, tasks still needed to accomplish the theorists' three stated goals, and structures that can be used to accomplish the tasks identified.

Conference work group review

An initial review of the conference work group responses to the task assigned by the theorists was conducted.* A total of 396 worksheets were in usable form. Summary sheets were prepared that noted the frequency with which a defining characteristic of a diagnosis was identified as matching a particular pattern. For example, on the summary sheet for Group 12, focusing on the diagnostic label of *self-concept, disturbance in self-esteem,* the defining characteristic of "lack of eye contact" was related to the pattern of exchanging by two participants; to communicating by four; to relating by two; and to choosing and moving by one each. Inspection of the summary sheets reveals a similar response of participant selections for many of the defining characteristics. In some cases the responses were more concentrated on one pattern. This was particularly true in the case of the physiologic characteristics. For example, for those participants considering *fluid volume deficit,* nine of the eleven participants identified "decreased urinary output" as most appropriately representing the exchanging pattern. However, even this tendency was not consistent. For example, in the diagnosis of *airway clearance, ineffective,* the defining characteristic of "dyspnea" had five selections of exchanging and five of feeling. Consistent with the premises of the framework, an indicator would reflect several "patterns" or reveal a whole pattern of the nine dimensions of the unitary person.

In considering the questions asked at the end of the worksheet, conference participants indicated that many defining characteristics fit into more than one pattern and many do not represent any of the defined patterns. Some participants believed that they were forcing fits into one category. Comments from group reports indicated that some participants believed that difficulty with the task resulted from a lack of understanding of the framework. Others believed that problems were a result of the inadequacies of the framework and its lack of utility for classifying nursing diagnoses. One particular inadequacy noted was the lack of clarity of the pattern definitions, which forced

---

*Sister Callista Roy acknowledges the assistance of Marguerite Eustace in organizing some of these data and preparing summary sheets sent to the Nurse Theorist Task Force.

respondents to use their own frames of reference. Concern was expressed for the reliability of the responses made by the same person over time or among respondents at a given time. In addition, the assignment prompted some participants to note that there is a difference between an organizing framework for diagnoses and theoretical frameworks for nursing practice. Individual participants also noted that the exercise pointed to inadequacies of the defining characteristics.

Nurse Theorist Task Force

A volunteer Task Force of the Nurse Theorist Group reviewed the Conference Work Group Summary Sheets, identified tasks remaining in accomplishing the goals of the Theorist Group, and suggested the best structure to accomplish the tasks identified. The Task Force members reviewed the summaries of data from the assignments completed by the work groups of the Fifth National Conference. They focused in a general way on what the data and the total 5-year project are saying about the framework and about the currently accepted list of diagnoses. Comments by the Task Force members at this time clearly revealed the incompleteness of the work on the framework and particularly the gap that remains between the framework and the nursing diagnoses that have been accepted by the National Conference.

Members acknowledged that the framework needs refinement. They identified specifically the need for defining key terms. The concept of pattern is basic to the framework and central to assessments for making nursing diagnoses. Yet, as one person noted, a definition of pattern that can be operationalized and is workable seems to be absent. Another need for better definitions is one for each identified pattern. For example, as defined, feeling implies cognition by the use of the term *information*, and emotions as nonrationalized feelings are not necessarily information processing. Once again, it was noted that the currently defined pattern categories are neither mutually exclusive nor jointly exhaustive.

The Theorist Group's efforts to articulate the holism of unitary man/human continue to raise questions. One member commented that she could not deal with the analyses that were done (one defining characteristic being related to one pattern) because of the original premise that the pattern characteristics, or dimensions, are relevant only in terms of the pattern of the whole person and not as entities that stand alone. We have stated that the patterns are dynamically interrelated and that it is this interrelatedness that differs for purposes of diagnoses. Does that mean that all patterns exist for typification on each characteristic or each diagnosis? Would each characteristic be assessed on all nine patterns? Do some characteristics have a greater alteration in some patterns relative to others? By the assumption of holism, we assert that all the patterns would be altered. From our current knowledge, there is no basis for predicting that one pattern would be altered more than any other; for example, in dealing with the area of *self-concept, disturbance caused by role performance,* valuing and choosing might be equally affected.

Several comments from Task Force members highlighted the discontinuity between the framework proposed by the theorists and the conference work on the nursing diagnoses. It seems clear that the concepts from the framework do not subsume all the constructs, concepts, and empirical data represented by the diagnostic labels. Conversely, all concepts from the framework do not have representation in the diagnoses. Thus, as one person succinctly noted, if the diagnoses do not "fit" in the conceptual framework, then probably we should not expect the characteristics to "fit."

Another member indicated that the difficulty with the concepts of the framework being unworkable is because they lack empirical anchorage. Observables, or phenomena, are not indicated nor do the assumptions convey the next steps to take in inquiring further about the key concepts and their empirical manifestations. This issue was further summarized by noting that the health of unitary man/human, our stated phenomenon of nursing, needs description, conceptualization, theorizing, and testing in the empirical research tradition.

In further considering the proposed framework as an organizing principle for a taxonomy of diagnoses, several Task Force members pointed out that the nine patterns do not reflect the rules for categorization. The lack of agreement in the multiple classifications we have attempted on the basis of the patterns is evidence that we do not have a typology or taxonomy. Perhaps we are not entirely clear about our principle for ordering. The patterns may not be the dimensions for ordering, but rather we may need to go back to some earlier work of the theorists where the patterns were being studied on variables such as time and rate. If the rules of categorization do not apply, it is possible that a phenomenon requires a new set of rules or a new paradigm.

Based on their critical reviews of theorists' work to date, the Theorist Task Force members made constructive suggestions about the remaining tasks to be done and approaches to accomplish these tasks. There was much agreement that the general tasks remaining are the tasks on which we have been working, that is, developing a framework, addressing orders of generality, and making this work useful for the conference and for nursing practice. The approaches suggested to move forward with these tasks included:

1. Refine and research the framework and the diagnoses in an organized way, for example, through our schools of nursing.
2. Rethink and refocus on what we are trying to build and what might be essential elements in the model we are developing; that is, address the issue of the difference between framework for practice and framework for diagnoses.
3. Clarify the framework's concept of nursing and relate this concept to

the criteria of social congruence, social utility, and social significance so that the conceptualization of nursing practice can give contextual meaning to the other concepts.

4. Decide on the level of diagnoses useful for practice and classify diagnoses above and below this level.

5. Identify diagnoses at the pattern-synthesis level to guide work on using the framework.

6. Try alternative ways of developing a typology such as:

   a. Develop matrixes for clinical data relevant to the patterns with dimensions of frequency, duration, quantity, quality, and rhythm against the descriptors for the pattern.

   b. Look at biopsychosocial levels separately for the nine patterns.

   c. Take the nine patterns as nine indicators of health status, that is, as single measures for the whole.

   d. Restrict exchanging to social interaction and have nine psychosocial patterns, then take the more physiologically oriented diagnoses and try by induction/retroduction to relate this level to the psychosocial patterns.

The Nurse Theorist Group faces the question of what structures are most appropriate to continue their tasks. The previous structure of the group convening independently for short, intensive work sessions seems no longer appropriate. Evidence for this fact comes from resignation letters from the members and from comments such as the following, "No structure can accomplish the task. It will take grey cells from the CNS in the human crania. Individuals or groups could work on it. But either way, in-depth scholarship is needed . . . something more than ad hoc brainstorming sessions will have to be occurring." There was support among the Task Force members that the time had come for the tasks of the Theorist Group to be carried out within the newly established structures of the North American Nursing Diagnoses Association. The Research and Taxonomy Committees seem most relevant. It is anticipated that the members of the Theorist Group will carry forward their agenda as their interests and resources dictate each one of them to do so within the new structure of the organization.

REFLECTIONS FROM THE CHAIRPERSON

Having served as chairperson of the Theorist Group for the past 6 years, I welcome the opportunity to offer my reflections on what the group has done. We set out with a gigantic task, and at present a gigantic task remains before us. Still, I believe that much has been accomplished between those two points. This group of highly talented nurses came to know one another better, to appreciate one another more, and to share some common understandings.

At the same time, our interactions have surfaced and placed in bold relief some of the key issues of our discipline today. How do we focus on the whole rather than the parts? How do we describe in observable terms what we believe the whole to be? How do we articulate our understandings and beliefs about holism? How does the vision of nursing focusing on unitary man/human relate to the world of nursing practice and to other health disciplines? Given the fact that nursing focuses on the complex phenomenon of the whole person, can diagnostic labels be developed and organized in a taxonomy to point out nursing judgments about the whole person or group? Can nursing demonstrate the social significance of its view of the health of unitary man/human? Can the dialectic tension between theory and practice provide creative energy for developing nursing knowledge? Is there some point of scientific revolution on the horizon that will resolve the struggles of our current phase of development?

We may not have the answers to those questions, but the mutual exchange between the Theorist Group and the past three National Conferences on the Classification of Nursing Diagnoses has served to clarify issues and to provide some direction for pursuing answers to these questions and other questions of mutual concern. Doctoral students and other scholars have begun to extend the study initiated by this project. I believe that the professional interests and commitments of all of us have been affected by this process. It is one contribution in a larger whole and cannot be judged only in the here-and-now. Rather, I choose to believe that the influence of the Theorist Group of the National Conference on the Classification of Nursing Diagnoses will be felt for a long time to come, in many ways. I am proud and grateful to have been a part of it.

REFERENCES

Abdellah, F. G., and others: Patient-centered approaches to nursing, New York, 1960, Macmillan Publishing Co., Inc.

DeBack, V.: The relationship between senior nursing students' ability to formulate nursing diagnoses and the curriculum model, Adv. Nurs. Sci. **3:**51, 1981.

Fitzpatrick, J. J., and others: Nursing models and their psychiatric mental health application, Bowie, Md., 1982, Brady Co.

Gebbie, K., and Lavin, M.A.: Classification of nursing diagnoses, St. Louis, 1975, The C.V. Mosby Co.

Kim, M.J. and Moritz, D.A., eds.: Classification of nursing diagnoses: proceedings of the third and fourth national conferences, New York, 1982, McGraw-Hill Book Co.

Maslow, A.: Motivation and personality, New York, 1954, Harper & Row, Publishers.

Rogers, M.E.: An introduction to the theoretical basis of nursing, Philadelphia, 1970, F.A. Davis Co.

Roy, Sister C.: Why are we here: opening address. In Gebbie, K.: Summary of the second national conference on classification of nursing diagnoses, St. Louis, 1976, The C.V. Mosby Co.

Discussion

Joanne McCloskey: I noticed in the exercise in the Kim and Moritz (1982)* book about which Sister Callista Roy spoke of earlier, when the diagnoses were put into the nine patterns, about 23 out of those 43 diagnoses were in the *exchanging* category. And I suspect that if we went through this exercise that you are suggesting, most of those 23 diagnoses that were in that *exchanging* category are physiologic. If we went through that exercise, I think we are going to get a lot of characteristics in the *exchanging* category. If that happens, do you think that this has implications for (1) including another pattern that is more physiologic in the unitary man framework and (2) redefining the goal of nursing since the focus now is on health? Do you see any implications for prevention of illness in there?

---

*Kim, M.J., and Moritz, D.A., eds.: Classification of nursing diagnoses: proceedings of the third and fourth national conferences, New York, 1982, McGraw-Hill Book Co.

Sister Callista Roy: I will try to answer that. There is a given in the question that we are breaking humans into biopsychosocial phenomena and that exchange is the physiologic phenomena. Because the patterns are not mutually exclusive, one would be tempted to put verbal or nonverbal communication under the *communication* pattern and put nutrition under *exchanging*. I think that it is not the quantity of defining characteristics under a pattern that is going to be significant, but it would clue us in if we had 1000 under *exchanging*, which has been part of our interest in the domain of the phenomena of nursing, and we had only a few under the other patterns. What we really recognize is that we have to keep treating people in a holistic manner. We may need to look at other patterns and merge other defining characteristics, and that would be a clue to us to move in that direction. What we are looking at is what we have been doing and what we theorists are saying that we need to be doing. The two may not be the same at this time. So let's deal with where we are, and when we analyze it, let us say to ourselves: Under *valuing*, we have a real vacuum of defining characteristics at which we have not really looked, to which we have not paid attention.

Margaret Hardy: I would just like to address the first question. I took the 1050 characteristics that you have developed and tried to categorize them into those patterns that you had in terms of everything going into *exchanging*, particularly if it was physiologic. At a point, I decided that it was not going to do justice to the pattern and I made a note that something has to be worked out that will include all those terms that really do not belong there. There were also some that crossed over, and I made a note that some defining characterisics fit both in the *perception* and the *communication* patterns, and this is something that we will have to deal with later. Just noting the problem you have is very helpful.

Cathie Guzzetta: I have been concerned for the last couple of years about how the work of the theorists can in fact be combined with what the National Conference Group has been doing since 1973. I am seeking clarification for the task that we are to complete this afternoon and what will happen as the end product of this task. I guess I am asking what is going to happen to those 42 diagnostic categories once we take 1400 defining characteristics and place them into patterns. Would you envision that those 42 categories would be eliminated after that point, and how would they fit in hereafter? How would we use the two?

Sister Callista Roy: I think I understand your question. First of all, this is only one task that the small groups are going to do. The small groups are continuing to work on those diagnostic labels from the point of view of the overall goals of the total conference. At some point, products of these exercises are going to merge, and it is hoped that those 42 diagnostic labels will be refined by moving up the scale of abstraction or moving down the scale, depending on where they already are. I think what we meant to say was: Please take what we did and consider it when you move forward with your task, which is to refine those labels. The 42 labels may become slightly changed. But that is the ongoing work of the conference, and we do not mean to be interfering with that. We mean to be enhancing that project by shedding some light on it. Because we operate under the premise that the refinement of each diagnosis is in process, we are not going to get upset that they are at different orders of abstraction. When you are doing the task with the defining characteristics as content experts, your products may be different from ours. One of the issues I want to raise at the end of this session is the mechanism whereby our joint goals will move forward. The implication of that is that we will have the summary of the small group work that will be published in the proceedings of this conference that will enchance the process. It is hoped that the newly formed organization will have a committee that will coordinate the activities of the two groups.

Cathie Guzzetta: Would you give me a little more reassurance? I think my concern is that once we complete this task, we will then reflect on the 42 diagnoses and see that they really are not useful for our purposes.

Sister Callista Roy: Okay. This is what I am saying. This total conference is not going to reflect on the 42 diagnoses. In your group, you will have four nursing diagnoses assigned to you or however many you do have. You need to take a hard look at those in the light of all the information we gave you today. At the 4:15 session this afternoon, you are going to be told what the rest of the tasks of those groups are. So the entire conference is not going to look at the 42 diagnoses. Each group is going to look at a small group of them, and yes, we hope there will be a change from the Fifth National Conference to the Sixth National Conference. Yes, we hope something different will come out of this. I really have tremendous hope that it will move us further along in the evolutionary stages. Just think where that is in relation to those of us who met in 1974. So, yes, we hope that what we are doing will have an impact on what comes out of the groups. Now you can understand why those groups are so important. So I will add a footnote again that your group leaders will be well-prepared to have you look at the whole process, but we meant this to be a working conference and not just hearing papers. I know you are absorbing a lot of content today. Given that information and given your expertise in the areas that you are assigned, we will continue to refine them.

Cathie Guzzetta: I am not trying to be a devil's advocate, but I just think that the group needs to be aware that some significant changes might occur as a result of this task and that the 42 nursing diagnoses could, in fact, change.

Sister Callista Roy: I agree that there could be changes based on a continuing look at the categories.

Marjory Gordon: Maybe you can address that later. There was an issue of making changes on the basis of clinical studies.

Sister Callista Roy: I think what we are getting into is the process of how the conference makes decisions about categories, and that would come later. What will come out of the small group work will be some recommendations. We are going to start out with some very specific tasks that will feed into our decision-making process about the labels.

Majory Gordon: The concern that Cathie raised is related to possible changes in the diagnostic categories. This concern needs to be addressed by the conference participants. Perhaps any change should be based on clinical studies rather than on opinions. People around the country have said, "Will you stop throwing those categories out and in and out?" Anxiety is a good example of this. I would like to stick to the criterion for change being clinical studies. One of the hopes is that the framework that has been developed by the theorists could potentially be a framework for research. Hence, the work of the National Conference Group and the theorists will be brought together by research.

Sister Callista Roy: Since I made the statement that the small group work could change the diagnostic labels, I need to emphasize that we are not going to come out of the Fifth National Conference with a new list. But we are going to come out with group work that has implications for the list.

Carol Hayes: It would seem to me that if you are going to put the characteristics within these nine patterns, your diagnoses then are going to be reflective of the pattern titles. You are going to have alterations in *exchange*, alterations in whatever these patterns are, and that is going to be quite different from the specificity we now have with current diagnostic labels. To me, the current labels are much more meaningful than the nine patterns.

Sister Callista Roy: We agree with you that the nine patterns are not specific enough, because they are at a more abstract level. This is the concept level, but concepts need to be explored, explicated, and developed. That is the next stage down the road. But we do not want to stay at that abstract level. We do not want the diagnosis to read, for example, *ineffective exchanging;* rather, once we have totally developed the concept of *exchanging*, there will be labels under the pattern.

Comment: I think you are counting your chickens before they hatch. From my framework in thinking this through, I do not get to alterations of things.

Comment: Well, that may be, but that is what the clinician has to deal with.

Comment: This may not be the theorists' idea but my own. I am very concerned that the Social Policy Statement is problem oriented and we are going "problem oriented" as if everything is a problem just like anything is a disease for medicine. When you look at things, there is the degree of something going on, more or less maladaptive, whatever it is. I don't think we are ready to label the thing in that way. The diagnosis would not be an *exchanging* problem. The diagnosis would be a statement of synthesis of information from all the patterns.

Sister Callista Roy: The labels are not going to be just one category, because human beings function as a whole. What we will do is merge a whole set of labels that cut across the nine patterns and create a holistic label at the concept level. It will have some specificity, because we do not want it just *exchanging*. We are in an evolutionary stage right now. We are not there yet. But, for sure, we are not going back to an ineffective pattern, because that is not how human beings operate.

Comment: I think you just raised an issue. I wonder since the questions now are coming on issues, if we should deal with our summary of issues.

Sister Callista Roy: Imogene also has made a suggestion that we deal with summarizing the issues that come out of this presentation of our progress. Our progress has to do with giving you a framework. We have offered a framework and a process for you to provide feedback to theorists for further development.

Imogene King: Some of the issues and problems have been recorded as homework, and some were recorded as I listened to this morning's discussion. The first issue is that the framework that has been developed by the Theorist Group deals with unitary man or holistic man, whichever term you prefer, whereas the diagnostic categories deal with interferences in that unitary man's health. That becomes an issue because if one group is dealing with interferences in health and another group is dealing with health, you really have a dichotomy. The second issue is that there are different levels of abstraction in terms of the 42 diagnostic categories that are currently published. When two or more people interact at different levels of abstraction, you have a problem in your group process. If you have two people at a level of concrete thinking, two at an intermediate level of abstraction, and three at a higher level of abstraction, you have no dialogue because nobody is listening to anybody. And I think we have to talk at this conference honestly about these kinds of issues. The third issue is that I do not see a common definition for all of us to use when we state defining characteristics. I have a definition I would like to share with you that could be used by this group if as a group you want it. I think if a common definition for defining characteristics is agreed on by this group, we would move forward much faster. The fourth issue is really a suggestion to use the current diagnostic labels and think of them as concepts. If you think of a diagnostic category as a concept, you will think differently about it, because if you develop the concept, you are developing the knowledge of it. When you develop the knowledge of it, you have the characteristics of the concept. From these characteristics, operational definitions can be formulated. This definition deals with a concept that is knowledge about the idea, whereas the diagnostic categories deal with a disturbance in something. If we do not understand what the process is for developing a concept, then it is very difficult to identify the characteristics of a concept. The fifth issue is a language issue. The unitary man framework uses the language of open systems, whereas the diagnostic format deals with other factors such as etiology, which is not systems language. Terms such as *disturbance* or *interference in health states* are systems terms. If we do not have clarity in the words we use, progress will be slow. The sixth issue is one of balance in the diagnostic categories. Some of us have attempted to fit the diagnoses into the nine patterns of human interactions and have found them to be primarily physiologically based. When you try to fit something that is physiologically oriented, you will probably place it under *exchanging* or *communicating*. I think these issues should be addressed as we continue with our efforts to identify a professional nursing language.

Sister Callista Roy: The group would like to have Imogene share the definition of defining characteristics.

Imogene King: This definition is not mine. It is a synthesis of many definitions from the philosophy of science. A defining characteristic is that which identifies the nature of something, whether it be an object, a person, or a thing. It is that which defines the nature of it. Now, in defining the nature of something, we also relate it to our own real world. We try to observe it and measure it. My test, when working with defining characteristics, is to ask questions. Can I observe it? Can I measure it? Can I do both? When I can observe it or measure it, then I can define it. We react holistically. When you try to define something, that definition is the holistic part of what we are trying to do. That sounds very confusing, but I cannot deal with human beings when I am trying to learn something about them. I have a conflict between what I know about learning and what I am thinking about holistic meaning. Maybe some of the rest of you have the same problem, analytic versus holistic. If I looked at pain, for example, which is a very complex concept, I would try to identify the nature of pain. There is a taxonomy of pain (Loeser and Black, 1975)[*] based on the published research studies on pain. Perhaps we need to look at the way the scientists developed a taxonomy of one concept—pain. They started by developing a measurement instrument and established some reliability and validity for the measurement instrument. Other scientists used the instrument, and more articles were published that demonstrated its reliability and validity. From the research (physiologic research, drug research, and research in human perceptions and suffering) they have now put together five levels of pain as a taxonomy. It is not a finished product. It really needs more extension, but it gives us some common language when we talk about pain. When we observe and measure it, we can do something about it.

Joan Fitzmaurice: This is a short question to Dr. King on the definition of defining characteristic. If I am correct now, you stated that the definition would define the nature of the thing. Are you suggesting that one characteristic equals one diagnosis?

Imogene King: No, there will be many characteristics.

Joan Fitzmaurice: Would it be a combination of characteristics?

Imogene King: Let me give you an example using one of the diagnostic categories,

---

[*]Loeser, J. and Black, R.A.: Taxonomy of pain, J. Pain **2**:81, 1975.

knowledge deficit. Those elements listed under *etiology* in my perception are defining characteristics. The defining characteristics that are listed under that concept are really the results of the elements listed under etiology. Concept development is identifying the knowledge of the term *knowledge*. So you identify characteristics that help you know what knowledge is. That is a bad example that I picked. But it seems to me, that we get the nature of the thing mixed up with the deviations from the nature of that thing. We are talking about knowledge deficit, but it seems to me that we have not yet talked about what knowledge is. If we know what knowledge is and we have the defining characteristics of knowledge, it is very easy to come up with a deficit.

Joan Fitzmaurice: I would probably find it more comfortable to talk about the characteristics that define the thing rather than the defining characteristics.

Imogene King: I agree with you and would delete the word defining.

Lynda Carpenito: This is a comment. We did a continuing education program yesterday. I am concerned that those people who were here yesterday who are leaving today might be getting an impression that unitary man (the unitary man framework) is in cement and that we are in the process of shortening or lengthening unitary man. No one ever said unitary man was in cement, and we do not know that it is our framework yet.

Margaret Lunney: I had some points of information that I wanted to clarify in reference to the levels of abstraction. Will you be sharing with us your criteria for deciding where the various terms fit in the levels of abstraction?

Imogene King: What the levels of abstraction deal with is theoretic work in terms of where some things fit relative to others, that is, where one set of terms fits relative to other sets.

Margaret Lunney: Do you foresee diagnostic labels at the construct level, concept level, or either one?

Imogene King: Yes. Concepts or constructs.

Margaret Lunney: With this so-called hierarchy, I think what could happen is that the ones that are fairly abstract might be broken into some smaller levels of diagnoses.

Comment: So in other words, you would foresee them to be more concepts than constructs. Constructs might be broken down to concepts.

Sister Callista Roy: Imogene said it is the development of the concept that will lead you. We are suggesting as theorists that the development of the concept across the patterns will lead you to the labels at a concept level. In addition, a new set of labels will emerge that will include all the current ones. The new set will be at an intermediate level of abstraction. I would like to add an issue to those you and Imogene raised. There is another basic issue and that is the mechanism or structure for moving forward, that is, the structure for clarifying and validating the framework and evolving diagnoses. We were given three tasks: first, to evolve a framework, which we did (whether it is accepted or not, it is there); second, to look at the labels and their levels of abstraction; and third, to try to relate the framework and diagnostic labels. We have done that. We as a conference group need to address the question of the mechanism or structure that will keep these three tasks moving.

Marjory Gordon: I think the theorists have put a great deal of work into their tasks, and we thank them for their contribution. As Sister Callista Roy very clearly said, the National Conference Group does not have a framework. There is a framework being developed by the Theorist Group that works with the National Conference Group. But right now, there is not a framework for the diagnostic categories. The proposed unitary man framework is an evolving theoretic perspective for looking at a human being.

Report of the group work on taxonomies

PHYLLIS B. KRITEK, R.N., Ph.D., F.A.A.N.

The task of the group on taxonomies was to generate an initial taxonomy for the labels that resulted from the work of the National Conference on the Classification of Nursing Diagnoses. A review of current nursing literature shows that numerous classification systems, with diverse organizing principles, are being developed. Some of these classification schema are attempts to develop a taxonomy of nursing diagnoses. Others used concepts from current diagnoses lists, but they were designed to organize collections of nursing interventions and assessments or were patient classification schema used in health care settings. In addition, the work of the nurse theorists within the total effort of the national conference, while greatly valued, had not yet been systematically explored for its taxonomic potential. The current list of nursing diagnoses is organized alphabetically. It was the task of the taxonomy group to address these developmental realities.

The group met three times, with a relatively stable set of participants and a high degree of group involvement. Decisions were made by consensus. Since this group, in contrast to other small groups, was engaged in a relatively unique task, ground rules were developed as work evolved. The group chairperson, in an effort to represent the nature of the group's task, outlined the following potential group activities:

1. Review the diverse, available taxonomies in current use and determine commonalities, levels of diagnostic categories, and levels of abstraction.
2. Examine available taxonomies to determine the feasibility of nursing diagnoses and/or unitary man concepts fitting into a current classification system.
3. Generate recommendations for making the taxonomy functional in the service setting.

The possibility of generating researchable ideas or questions was also discussed, since this was a task common to all conference groups.

☐Taxonomy group participants were Sally Aveni, Margaret Briody, Joan Crosley, Kathy Dickensheets, Julie Eddins (Recorder), Lucy Feild, Anne Marie Flaherty, Gary Forsyth, Margaret Hardy, Lois Hoskins, Florence L. Huey, Phyllis B. Kritek (Chairperson), Frances Lange, Nancy Lengel, Margaret Lunney, Joanne McCloskey, Karen Rieder, Barbara C. Rottkamp, Sister Callista Roy, and Carol Viamontes. The group acknowledges the contribution of Ms. Julie Eddins. Her careful notes made this detailed narrative report possible.

For a brief period, the group explored possible ways of approaching the task. Several members identified continuing problems experienced by practicing nurses using the existing National Conference list. Many of these problems focused on the lack of clarity in existing levels of abstraction and concreteness. Described another way, some existing labels seem to cover virtually hundreds of phenomena (for example, *alterations in self-concept*) while others seem quite discrete (for example, *potential for poisoning*). During this discussion, two members of the theorist group, Sister Callista Roy and Margaret Hardy, served as theory consultants to the group.

At this initial exploratory stage, the group decided to focus on the existing National Conference list of diagnoses, to use the theorists' patterns of unitary man as a potential classification schema, and to sort the existing list, first by levels of abstraction and second by patterns. It was observed that whereas levels of abstraction focus on vertical classification of phenomena, patterns of unitary man focus on a horizontal classification of phenomena. In addition, because several members expressed concern about the sexist language of patterns of unitary man, the phrase was revised to patterns of unitary persons.

Ground rules were quickly established. Group consensus would determine decision making, with majority rule deciding differences. When the group could not quickly agree on a concept, it was tabled and dealt with last. Only the labels themselves would be sorted, with little attention to related cues, interventions, research, and so forth. Qualifiers such as *actual, potential, deficit,* and *increased* would be deemphasized to facilitate focusing on the actual phenomena, for example, *grieving, pain, constipation.* The presence of such modifiers as possible organizing principles of classification was, however, noted. It was observed at this point that all phenomena did focus on some alteration and that this qualifier might best be addressed later in the process.

Given these ground rules, the labels were sorted into four levels of abstraction (Box 1). Level I was viewed as the most abstract and Level IV as the least abstract. The discussions that occured during this process brought to light several useful insights. Many members of the group noted that Level I phenomena appeared to be major categories of human response patterns related to the ANA Social Policy Statement's definition of nursing, "the diagnosis and treatment of human responses to actual or potential health problems" (ANA, 1980, p. 9). It was further noted that, having at least intuitively demonstrated that the existing National Conference list involved a minimum of four levels of abstraction, some diagnoses may be subsumed under some larger general category not yet named. Thus a Level III diagnosis may not actually be logically subsumed under any existing Level II or Level I labels but may provide direction on constructs that still need to be isolated, named and described. It was also noted that labels in Levels III and IV appeared more

BOX 1   **Classification by levels of abstraction**

Level I

Comfort	Fear	Nutrition	Spiritual
Communication	Knowledge	Self-concept	
Coping	Mobility	Thought processes	

Level II

Bowel elimination
Cardiac output, alterations
Pain
Verbal communication, impaired
Coping, ineffective family
Coping, ineffective individual
Impaired physical mobility
Parenting
Self-care deficit
Role performance
Sensory perceptual
Sleep pattern disturbance
Spiritual distress
Noncompliance
Airway clearance
Violence
Skin integrity, actual

Deficit diversional activity
Fluid volume deficit, actual
Fluid volume deficit, potential
Impaired gas exchange
Injury
Knowledge deficit
Alteration in nutrition
Body image
Self-esteem
Personal identity
Sexual dysfunction
Alterations in thought processes
Tissue perfusion
Urinary elimination
Grieving
Ineffective breathing
Skin integrity, potential

Level III

Constipation
Diarrhea
Incontinence
Cardiac output, decreased
Alteration in nutrition:
  More
  Less
  Potential for more than required
Sensory perceptual alteration
  Visual
  Auditory
  Kinesthetic
  Gustatory
  Tactile
  Olfactory
Tissue perfusion, alteration
  Cerebral
  Cardiopulmonary
  Renal
  Gastrointestinal
  Peripheral

Self-care deficit
  Feeding
  Bathing/hygiene
  Dressing/grooming
  Toileting
Potential for
  Injury
  Poisoning
  Suffocation
  Trauma
Alteration in parenting
  Actual
  Potential
Coping, family: potential for growth
Grieving
  Anticipatory
  Dysfunctional
Urinary elimination, alteration in patterns
Home maintenance management, impaired
Rape trauma syndrome

Level IV

Rape trauma syndrome
Rape trauma
Compound reaction
Silent reaction

useable because they became more concrete; that is, they named existing phenomena rather than a category of phenomena. It was noted that perhaps labels in Levels I and II are dysfunctional to practicing nurses because they name such category sets, rather than the actual phenomena. As several group members noted, Level I looked like assessment categories and Level III looked like the things we write a plan of care about. Finally, the group agreed that the sort into levels of abstraction had highlighted large gaps in the structure at all levels, that is, unnamed phenomena or categories of phenomena.

This last observation became even more apparent when the group began its vertical sort, categorization by patterns of unitary persons. Through a series of false starts, it became apparent that no single conceptual thread could be neatly traced through all four levels. Simply too many pieces were missing in the total puzzle. In every attempted tracing of a central theme, such as nutrition, pain, or learning, one or another portion was missing. Several group members noted that the Level I labels reflected a fairly high degree of parallelism with the patterns of unitary persons list. To resolve the impasse of the missing pieces, the group decided to first categorize all Level I labels as one of the nine possible patterns of unitary persons. That completed, the group decided to do the same with all four levels and generate nine sets of labels, each divided into four possible levels of abstraction. Once the nine sets of labels were generated, a process that evoked considerable conceptual struggling, the missing pieces became apparent. For example, although *grieving* appeared to fit into pattern nine, *feeling*, there was no Level I label appropriate to this phenomena. Yet in many cases the missing labels seemed apparent; that is, one could estimate an appropriate label.

By now, the group saw the clear potential for generating nine taxonomic trees, one for each pattern of unitary persons. The group agreed to do three

| TABLE 1 | Parallels of patterns and Level I content |

Patterns of unitary persons	Alterations in human responses (normless)
Exchanging	Nutrition, elimination, [oxygenation], [circulation], [physical integrity]
Communicating	[Communication]
Relating	[Role]
Valuing	Spiritual [state]
Choosing	Coping, [participating]
Moving	Activity, rest, [recreation] [activities of daily living], [self-care]
Perceiving	Self-concept, sensory/perceptual
Knowing	Knowledge, [learning], thought processes
Feeling	Comfort, [emotional integrity]

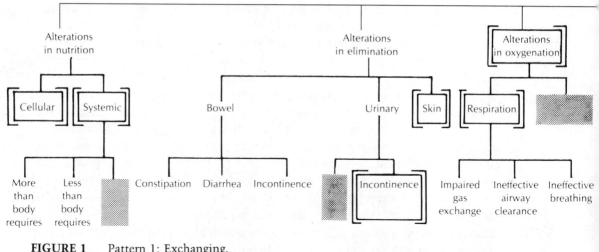

FIGURE 1   Pattern 1: Exchanging.

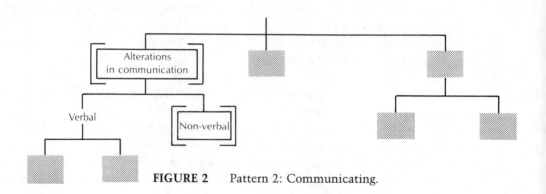

FIGURE 2   Pattern 2: Communicating.

things to make these trees maximally functional. First, when an approved diagnosis name needed slight modification for conceptual clarity, such modification would be made. Thus some concepts were used at two or more levels, with varying degrees of abstractness. Second, when a clear taxonomic omission created potential confusion, a proposed inclusion of a previously unnamed concept would when possible, be included. Third, some blank spaces would be built into the trees to accentuate the group's awareness of the marked incompleteness of the trees. It was the general aim to rough out a starting point for developing a taxonomy of the patterns of unitary persons as a classification schema. In finalizing the trees and subsequent taxonomy, the group began to view the nine trees as sets of phenomena, that is, those with common properties that related to the theorists' definitions of their nine patterns of unitary persons. While acknowledging some forcing of sets at this time and with recognition of continuous revision over time, the group be-

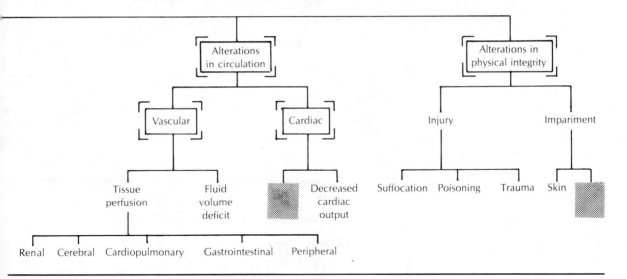

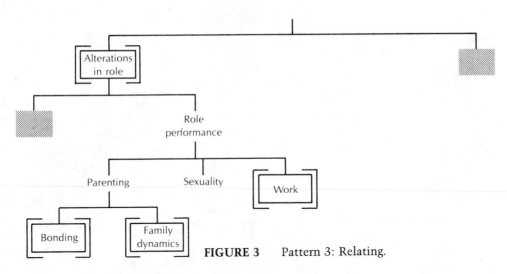

FIGURE 3   Pattern 3: Relating.

lieved the exercise of generating a beginning taxonomy was useful to the profession in directing discussion, exploration, investigation, and revision.

Table 1 presents the group's parallel of the nine patterns of unitary persons with nine categories of alterations in human responses. These alterations in human responses are presented as existing phenomena without norms of any kind implied. They are organizing labels for sets of nursing phenomena, that is, alterations in human responses. Thus, within the choosing pattern of a unitary person, an individual may experience an alteration in human response relative to a major category set called *coping.*

Figs. 1 through 9 present the nine taxonomy trees. Shaded areas indicate
Text continued on p. 57.

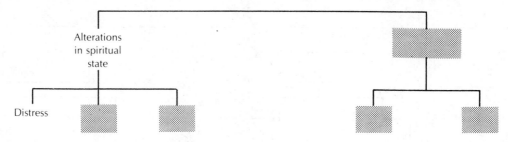

FIGURE 4   Pattern 4: Valuing.

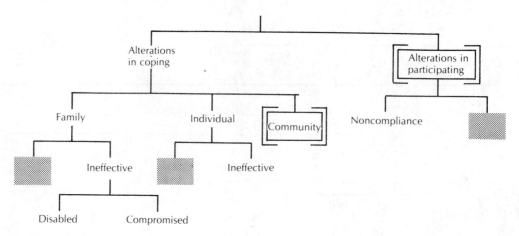

FIGURE 5   Pattern 5: Choosing.

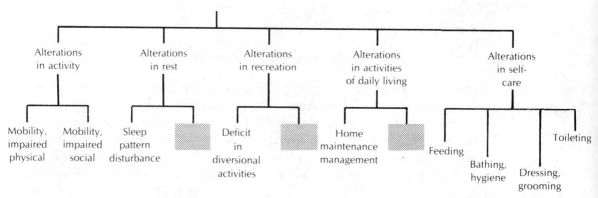

FIGURE 6   Pattern 6: Moving.

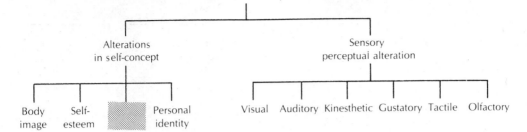

FIGURE 7   Pattern 7: Perceiving.

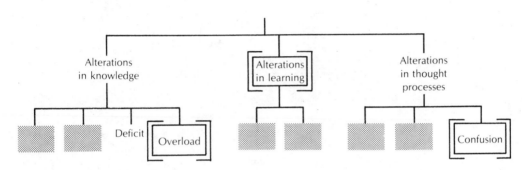

FIGURE 8   Pattern 8: Knowing.

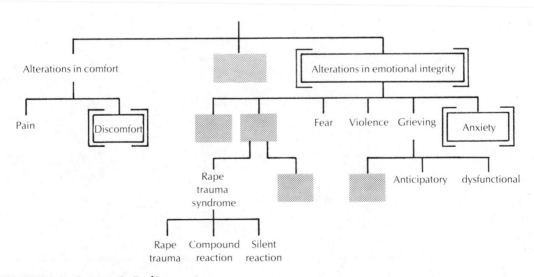

FIGURE 9   Pattern 9: Feeling.

```
1.  EXCHANGING
    1.1.  Alterations in Nutrition
          1.1. 1.  [Cellular]
          1.1. 2.  [Systemic]
                   1.1. 2.1.  More than body requires
                   1.1. 2.2.  Less than body requires
                   1.1. 2.3.  ▓▓▓▓▓▓▓▓
    1.2.  Alterations in Elimination
          1.2. 1.  Bowel
                   1.2. 1.1.  Constipation
                   1.2. 1.2.  Diarrhea
                   1.2. 1.3.  Incontinence
          1.2. 2.  Urinary
                   1.2. 2.1.  [Incontinence]
                   1.2. 2.2.  ▓▓▓▓▓▓▓▓
          1.2. 3.  [Skin]
    1.3   [Alterations in Oxygenation]

          1.3. 1.  [Respiration]
                   1.3. 1.1.  Impaired gas exchange
                   1.3. 1.2.  Ineffective airway clearance
                   1.3. 1.3.  Ineffective breathing
          1.3. 2  ▓▓▓▓▓▓▓▓
    1.4.  [Alterations in Circulation]
          1.4. 1.  [Vascular]
                   1.4. 1.1.  Tissue perfusion
                              1.4. 1.1. 1.  Renal
                              1.4. 1.1. 2.  Cerebral
                              1.4. 1.1. 3.  Cardiopulmonary
                              1.4. 1.1. 4.  Gastrointestinal
                              1.4. 1.1. 5.  Peripheral
                   1.4. 1.2.  Fluid volume deficit
          1.4. 2.  [Cardiac]
                   1.4. 2.1.  Decreased cardiac output
                   1.4. 2.2.  ▓▓▓▓▓▓▓▓
    1.5.  [Alterations in Physical Integrity]
          1.5. 1.  Injury
                   1.5. 1.1.  Suffocation
                   1.5. 1.2.  Poisoning
                   1.5. 1.3.  Trauma
          1.5. 2.  Impairment
                   1.5. 2.1.  Skin
                   1.5. 2.2.  ▓▓▓▓▓▓▓▓
```

FIGURE 10   Taxonomy structure.

2.   COMMUNICATING

    2.1. [Alterations in Communication]

        2.1. 1. Verbal

            2.1. 1.1. ▓▓▓▓▓

            2.1. 1.2. ▓▓▓▓▓

        2.1. 2. [Nonverbal]

    2.2. ▓▓▓▓▓

    2.3. ▓▓▓▓▓

        2.3. 1. ▓▓▓▓▓

        2.3. 2. ▓▓▓▓▓

3.   RELATING

    3.1. [Alterations in Role]

        3.1. 1. Role performance

            3.1. 1.1. Parenting

                3.1. 1.1. 1. [Bonding]

                3.1. 1.1. 2. [Family dynamics]

            3.1. 1.2. Sexuality

            3.1. 1.3. [Work]

        3.1. 2. ▓▓▓▓▓

    3.2. ▓▓▓▓▓

4.   VALUING

    4.1. [Alterations in Spiritual State]

        4.1. 1. Distress

        4.1. 2. ▓▓▓▓▓

        4.1. 3. ▓▓▓▓▓

    4.2. ▓▓▓▓▓

        4.2. 1. ▓▓▓▓▓

        4.2. 2. ▓▓▓▓▓

5.   CHOOSING

    5.1. Alterations in Coping

        5.1. 1. Family

            5.1. 1.1. Ineffective

                5.1. 1.1. 1. Disabled

                5.1. 1.1. 2. Compromised

            5.1. 1.2. ▓▓▓▓▓

        5.1. 2. Individual

            5.1. 2.1. Ineffective

            5.1. 2.2.

        5.1. 3. [Community]

    5.2. Alterations in Participating]

        5.2. 1. Noncompliance

        5.2. 2. ▓▓▓▓▓

FIGURE 10 cont'd   For legend see opposite page.
Continued.

```
6.  MOVING
    6.1.  [Alterations in Activity]
          6.1. 1.  Mobility, impaired physical
          6.1. 2.  Mobility, impaired social
    6.2.  [Alterations in Rest]
          6.2. 1.  Sleep pattern disturbance
          6.2. 2.  ▓▓▓▓▓▓▓
    6.3.  [Alterations in Recreation]
          6.3. 1.  Deficit in diversional activities
          6.3. 2.  ▓▓▓▓▓▓▓
    6.4.  [Alterations in Activities of Daily Living]
          6.4. 1.  Home maintenance management
          6.4. 2.  ▓▓▓▓▓▓▓
    6.5.  Alterations in Self-Care
          6.5. 1.  Feeding
          6.5. 2.  Bathing, Hygiene
          6.5. 3.  Dressing, Grooming
          6.5. 4.  Toileting
7.  PERCEIVING
    7.1.  Alterations in Self-Concept
          7.1. 1.  Body image
          7.1. 2.  Self-esteem
          7.1. 3.  Personal identity
          7.1. 4.  ▓▓▓▓▓▓▓
    7.2.  Sensory/Perceptual Alteration
          7.2. 1.  Visual
          7.2. 2.  Auditory
          7.2. 3.  Kinesthetic
          7 2. 4.  Gustatory
          7.2. 5.  Tactile
          7.2. 6.  Olfactory
8.  KNOWING
    8.1.  Alterations in Knowledge
          8.1. 1.  Deficit
          8.1. 2.  [Overload]
          8.1. 3.  ▓▓▓▓▓▓▓
          8.1. 4.  ▓▓▓▓▓▓▓
    8.2.  [Alterations in Learning]
          8.2. 1.  ▓▓▓▓▓▓▓
          8.2. 2.  ▓▓▓▓▓▓▓
    8.3.  Alterations in Thought Processes
          8.3. 1.  [Confusion]
          8.3. 2.  ▓▓▓▓▓▓▓
          8.3. 3.  ▓▓▓▓▓▓▓
```

FIGURE 10 cont'd   Taxonomy structure.

```
9.  FEELING
    9.1.  Alterations in Comfort
          9.1. 1.  Pain
          9.1. 2.  [Discomfort]
    9.2.  [Alterations in Emotional Integrity]
          9.2. 1.  [Anxiety]
          9.2. 2.  Grieving
                   9.2. 2.1.  Dysfunctional
                   9.2. 2.2.  Anticipatory
                   9.2. 2.3.  ▓▓▓▓▓▓
          9.2. 3.  Violence
          9.2. 4.  Fear
          9.2. 5.  ▓▓▓▓▓▓
                   9.2. 5.1.  Rape trauma syndrome
                              9.2. 5.1. 1.  Rape trauma
                              9.2. 5.1. 2.  Compound reaction
                              9.2. 5.1. 3.  Silent reaction
                   9.2. 5.2.  ▓▓▓▓▓▓
          9.2. 6.  ▓▓▓▓▓▓
    9.3.  ▓▓▓▓▓▓
```

FIGURE 10 cont'd   For legend see opposite page.

blank spaces, showing the tentative nature of these first trees. Bracketed terms have either been modified or inserted for the purposes of clarity. Fig. 10 shows these trees using a standard taxonomy structure. The shading and bracketing are repeated.

After completing the taxonomy, the group addressed several other issues. The taxonomy as devised has a limited number of levels. Several others may be necessary. The actual level of concreteness necessary for practice may not yet have been identified. This may explain the frustrations with the abstractness of some existing labels reported by many practicing nurses. The taxonomy does not possess conceptual purity. It requires work but is viewed as a starting point. Certainly the communication tree, by way of example, looks strikingly underdeveloped. The taxonomy is primitive and should be treated as such.

The group's taxonomy is an attempt to use the patterns of unitary persons as a principle of classification. Its first level of categorization involves alterations in human responses to health problems. The remaining portion of the ANA definition of nursing (actual or potential) may indeed be, by the group's observation, also present in this taxonomy. The question of having two identical taxonomies, one for actual phenomena and one for potential phenomena, was discussed. Each phenomena might also have a dichotomous categorization of actual or potential, since interventions would doubtless differ. Other classification principles that may need further exploration include levels of acuity, degree of risk, and intensity. These latter potential classification principles may clarify the qualifiers currently plaguing the National Conference list of diagnoses. Intensity may deal with terms such as greater, lesser, more, less, decreased, increased, deficit, and excess. Degree of risk may shed some light on qualifiers such as dysfunction, impaired, ineffective, disturbance in, compromised, distressed, and disabling. Distinctions between these terms are at best unclear, but some effort at refining classification principles may be helpful.

The content of this taxonomy reveals several patterns that require further investigation. The content does not clearly reflect any direct focus on health promotion or health maximization. The *exchanging* category is very complex already in comparison with most of the others. This complexity may indicate that phenomena that are less predominantly physiologic may be significantly more difficult to isolate, name, and describe. The categories of knowing and valuing also reflect this issue.

Finally, the *exchanging* category reflects an embedded classification principle of physiologic systems. Since the need to identify the involved physical system (renal, neurologic and so forth) is not always evident, the group questioned if this simply reflects nursing's persisting tendency to use medical conceptual schema and, hence, classification schema. The use of physical systems is further confounded when, for example, one scrutinizes tissue perfusion—when an alteration originates in cardiovascular dysfunction but expresses itself in genitourinary dysfunction. In all this, it is not entirely clear what is actually the nurse's phenomena of concern.

In conclusion, the taxonomy group offers a sketchy, initial, tentative taxonomy to be studied and tested in practice. Its use for research, computerization, and education requires assessment. This taxonomy should be measured against other existing classification schema in nursing and differences and commonalities identified and studied. The issues of missing levels and constructs, multiple classification principles, and unclear label modifiers must be discussed. The taxonomy is a beginning, not a conclusion. It is hoped that it is useful to nurses and nursing.

REFERENCE

American Nurses' Association: Nursing: a social policy statement, Kansas City, Mo., 1980, The Association.

CHAPTER 3

Issues related to nursing diagnoses

Four papers dealing with issues pertinent to nursing diagnosis taxonomy development are included in this chapter. The first paper focuses on the physiologic nursing diagnoses that have been questioned as to their relevance to nursing practice, hence to a nursing diagnosis taxonomy. The second paper explores the concept of etiology that has been challenged as to its need and usefulness for nursing diagnosis. The third paper discusses pertinent issues to current nomenclature and classification systems and raises the questions that should be considered for future development. The fourth paper discusses the advantages of using nursing diagnoses for prospective reimbursement for nursing service.

Physiologic nursing diagnosis: its role and place in nursing taxonomy

MI JA KIM, R.N., Ph.D., F.A.A.N.

The purpose of this paper is to examine the concept of nursing diagnoses, to explore controversies surrounding physiologic nursing diagnoses, and to provide insights regarding the role and place of such diagnoses in a nursing taxonomy. A physiologic nursing diagnosis is defined as an inferential statement made by a professional nurse that describes physiologic disturbances that impede optimum functioning and then direct the nurse to specific interventions, both independent and interdependent.

The major difference between this definition and others commonly offered is that it focuses on patients' physiologic problems that require interdependent nursing interventions in addition to independent decision making. An interdependent nursing intervention is that which the nurse makes on the basis of independent judgment and decision making to carry out medical orders (including standing orders) or to implement the medical regimen. Inherent in this definition is recognition of the reality that no health care discipline is truly independent of any other.

Furthermore, distinguishing physiologic nursing diagnoses from other types serves to illustrate the importance of and the critical need for having a taxonomy that incorporates the biophysical as well as the psychosociocultural and spiritual domains. It does not, by any means, indicate that physiologic diagnoses should constitute *the* major component of a nursing taxonomy. It needs to be affirmed that nursing diagnoses should encompass all pertinent domains of nursing care problems so that patient welfare can be addressed from a holistic perspective.

Since the inception of the National Conference on the Classification of Nursing Diagnoses, there have been implicit and explicit reservations about the role and place of physiologic diagnoses in a nursing taxonomy. Reactions have ranged from subtle discontent to frank rejection of certain diagnoses (Gordon, 1979). However, the studies of Wessel and Kim, Hubalik and Kim, and Suhayda and Kim* have demonstrated that physiologic diagnoses are considered clinically relevant by nurses and are well within the scope of nursing practice. In addition, the majority of nursing interventions based on

---

*See the following presentations in Chapter 4: Nursing Functions Related to the Nursing Diagnosis "Decreased Cardiac Output"; Nursing Diagnoses Associated with Heart Failure in Critical Care Nursing; and Documentation of Nursing Process in Critical Care.

physiologic nursing diagnoses are carried out independently by nurses without physician orders.

Three factors help explain the controversy surrounding physiologic nursing diagnoses. These factors relate to one's belief and understanding of the nature and scope of nursing practice. The first factor is the premise that nursing is concerned primarily with matters relevant to health rather than to illness, and physiologic diagnoses connote the latter. Few persons would argue against the concept of health-oriented nursing; indeed this has always been an integral component of nursing as evidenced by the teaching of preventive and rehabilitative measures in nursing courses and by the writings of Florence Nightingale (1969). Health-oriented nursing, however, cannot be the sole concentration of nursing since illnesses that require hospitalization of patients direct our attention to the care of the obviously ill as well at to that of the potentially ill. Not surprisingly, hospitals have long been the major stronghold of nursing practice and will probably continue to be the primary site of nursing practice for at least the foreseeable future. Thus care of ill persons who have altered physiologic functioning will demand the continued attention of the nursing profession.

The second factor is the belief that physiologic diagnoses are primarily within the realm of medicine based on the understanding that medicine is chiefly concerned with pathophysiologic phenomena. In fact, this frequently has been used as one of the major points to differentiate medical diagnoses from nursing diagnoses (Dodge, 1975; Durand and Prince, 1966; Mundinger and Jauron, 1975; Rothberg, 1967; Roy, 1975). Such a distinction, however, is presumptuous in that it too narrowly delimits the confines of medical practice. Certainly, this view is contrary to the belief of those physicians who ascribe to the concepts of holistic medicine.

Although some physiologic diagnostic terminology in nursing is similar to that in medicine, the conceptual (generic) approach to the patient's physiologic problem should not be regarded as a renaming of medical diagnostic effort. We need to remind ourselves that physiologic principles and terminology are for any profession to use; they certainly are not the exclusive right of medicine. Hence, equating physiologic nursing diagnoses with medical diagnoses is an ill-raised sophism at best. Such an intellectual artifact should not dictate the course and progress of the development of a taxonomy of nursing diagnoses.

The third factor related to this controversy is the puristic view of the independence of nursing practice. The concept of nursing diagnoses has been called a symbol of nursing autonomy; hence, in too many minds, independent nursing interventions are considered an intrinsic feature of nursing diagnoses. Such a purist approach would exclude from a nursing taxonomy any nursing judgments made in collaboration with medicine.

But the nature of nursing practice has been so intertwined with medicine that much of nursing judgment has been subsumed under medical care, thereby impeding attempts to delineate the scope of nursing practice. As previously noted, studies have shown that for any given physiologic nursing diagnosis, nursing interventions are often an admixture of independent and interdependent actions, with the independent action being the major component. Furthermore, as was shown in the ANA Social Policy Statement (ANA, 1980), the boundaries of nursing practice as compared with those of other health disciplines are not as distinct as one would like to think. Instead, large areas of overlap exist between disciplines. Moreover, I predict that the boundaries will get even less distinct as the interdisciplinary approach to health care becomes more of a reality. Any expansion of the scope of nursing practice invariably will result in increasingly blurred boundaries, which nursing taxonomy must be able to accommodate if it is to remain viable. Hence, any attempt at premature closure of a taxonomy of nursing diagnoses without incorporating physiologic diagnoses, in the name of independent nursing practice, may prove to have little resemblance to the current state of nursing practice.

In conclusion, a taxonomy of nursing diagnoses must reflect the interdependency of both basic and behavioral sciences to maintain a balanced science of nursing and to allow room for the inevitable expansion of nursing practice. Distortion in any direction will create an imbalance in the attempt to integrate scientific principles into nursing practice and will militate against the concept of holistic nursing. Hence, nursing diagnoses that describe patient problems, whether physiologic or behavioral, for which nurses carry out autonomous functions are too constrictive and therefore antithetical to the evolving nature of an applied science of nursing practice.

REFERENCES

American Nurses' Association: Nursing: a social policy statement, Kansas City, Mo., 1980, The Association.

Dodge, G.H.: What determines nursing vs. medical diagnosis? AORN J. **22**:23-24, 1975.

Durand, M., and Prince, R.: Nursing diagnosis: process and decision, Nurs. Forum **5**:50-64, 1966.

Gordon, M.: The concept of nursing diagnosis, Nurs. Clin. North Am. **14**(3):487-496, 1979.

Mundinger, M.O., and Jauron, G.D.: Developing a nursing diagnosis, Nurs. Outlook **23**:94-98, Feb. 1975.

Nightingale, F.: Notes on nursing, New York, 1969, Dover Publications, (Originally published in 1859.)

Rothberg, J.S.: Why nursing diagnosis? Am. J. Nurs. **67**:1040-1042, 1967.

Roy, C.: A diagnostic classification system for nursing, Nurs. Outlook **23**(2):90-94, Feb. 1975.

Etiology: in what sense and of what value?

GARYFALLIA L. FORSYTH, R.N., Ph.D

In the past decade, nurses have been involved in a national effort to identify, standardize, and classify health problems of particular concern in the practice of nursing. One of the troublesome issues has been the need for a comprehensive conceptualization of etiology. What is proposed is neither a truth statement nor a completed conceptualization; it may even be fiction. It represents one conceptualization, its genesis, and present status. It is offered as a beginning, to be critiqued, evaluated, refuted, or confirmed. A short segment from the historic and philosophic evolution of scientific theory that served as the antecedent framework for the paper is presented. A conceptualization of etiology with its value implications to nursing science follows.

ANTECEDENT FRAMEWORK

The concept of causality and the logic underlying causal analysis has been a productive area of discourse for early philosophers of science beginning with Newtonian physics through contemporary thought (Hanson, 1958; Gale, 1979; Shapere, 1977). Until recently, only the prevailing view of science was taught, and thus graduates from universities and professional programs more often than not accepted it as dogma. A cursory review of the advances in research and theory indicates that each advance initially was proposed as an alternative to the prevailing view and that each met with fierce resistance. For example, Lavoisier's proposal for oxygen theory stimulated a period of vigorous conceptual battle in chemistry; so did Copernicus' theory on astronomy, Pasteur's and Darwin's theories in biology, and others. Lessons were learned from examining the origin of these theories. As a result of examination of scientific advances, changes to prevailing views of science slowly and quietly emerged.

INSIGHTS FROM HANSON

The general perspective provided by Hanson's pattern of reasoning (1977) about the connection between conceptual organization and causality provides sufficient reason for pursuing causality. Hanson's statement (1958, p. 54), "The primary reason for referring to the cause of X is to explain X," holds

☐The author thanks Paula Meier, R.N., M.S.N., and Beverly Steele, R.N., M.S.N., D.N.Sc., students at the College of Nursing, Rush University, Chicago, for their assistance in ongoing critiques and suggestions in the preparation of this paper.

special meaning when considering the desired scope and purpose for the development of science for any discipline.

There are as many causes for X as there are explanations. For example, the cause of undernourishment may be identified by the nurse as alteration of nutrition—less than body requirement; by the parent as overactivity; and by the adolescent as ideal weight maintenance. Causes are certainly connected with effects because theories connect them. An explanation of X occurs when it falls into an interlocking pattern of concepts about other things, Y and Z. When X is related to other things, a completely novel explanation becomes a logical impossibility. *Cause* words are said to be charged since they carry a conceptual pattern. *Effect* words are less rich in theory and less able to serve as explanations of causes. As a result, causes explain effects, but not the reverse. Hanson (1958) asks, What is it to supply a theory? It is to offer an intelligible, systematic, conceptual pattern for the observed data. The value of this pattern is its capacity to unite phenomena that, without the theory, are either without form or wholly unnoticed. Hanson thus argues for a requirement of cause to achieve the development of knowledge to the level of explanation.

DOMAINS OF SHAPERE

Shapere (1977) proposed domain as a replacement for the observational-theoretic distinction as a body of information about which a problem has arisen. His analysis of domain recognizes the mutual interdependence of observation and theory rather than considering them as radically distinct types. To perform science using Shapere's philosophy requires ordering the domain, which in turn generates other problems of interest. Shapere (1977, p. 527) warns "that a body of information constitutes a domain is itself a hypothesis and may, ultimately, be rejected." Concepts would not necessitate reductionism and operationalism, required by the more logical positivist observational-theoretic distinction.

> The distinction between "observation" and "theory" has proved to be unclear, partly because what philosophers of science consider "observational" is found to be theory-laden in actual science usage, but also what they consider to be "theories" were treated in science the way "facts" or "observations" are treated and thus theories provided little or no insight into scientific reasoning, but even . . . obscured the character of that reasoning (Shapere, 1969, p. 115-163).

The demise of the observational-theoretic distinction as the base of truth about science and the acceptance of the mutual interdependence of observation and theory to provide meaning forecasts an ability to address and test questions of wholeness within a domain. Shapere's discussion also suggests new methodologic insights (Nickles, 1977). New methods will be found to match the newer epistemology.

THOUGHTS ON EPISTEMOLOGY

Gale (1979) addresses the two goals of science as (1) prediction and control and (2) explanation and understanding. The two goals are not absolutes for all sciences. Some sciences aim for only one of the two objectives. Behavioral psychologists usually seek only to discover correlations between behaviors that they use solely for prediction and control. Most behaviorists deny that their science will make any attempt to explain behavior in the sense that explain is usually meant—the sense that involves causal statements. Other sciences are mostly purely explanatory and do not allow for prediction and control. For example, the theory of biologic evolution can describe the course of biologic changes in the past but cannot be used to predict the future. A final general point concerns the logic of the two goals. Prediction and control can be distinguished from explanation and understanding by the use of correlation statements for the former and the use of causal connection statements for the latter. The "if . . . then" conditional statements are often read as if they were causal relations. This blurring becomes troublesome for science, as the controversy over smoking and lung cancer illustrates. The discovery of correlation is usually the first step in building a science, and the desire to find correlation arises from practical necessity. Both goals are seen as necessary elements of any whole science.

In his concluding remarks, Gale (1979) suggests that the preoccupation of science with practice, technology, prediction, and control has accounted for the pendulum swing too far toward the empirical pole of science. He confesses to a concentration on the conceptual system, the central element of the rationalist position, and believes that the weight of thought is now poised and ready for a rebound into a much more conceptualistic/rationalistic perspective of science. A story recounted by Gale (1979, p. 19) contrasts the difference between empiricist experimentation and rationalism. Albert Einstein's wife was invited by the director of one of the world's largest experimental laboratories to tour the site. She was escorted through acre after acre of huge, complicated, and expensive high-energy equipment. After the tour the director said to her, "This equipment, then, is what we are using to unlock the secrets of nature." Mrs. Einstein replied, "But that is what my husband does, too, he unlocks the secrets of nature. But he does it with a pencil on the back of an envelope."

CONCEPTUALIZATION OF ETIOLOGY FOR NURSING SCIENCE

Conceptualization of etiology for nursing science cannot be approached directly. Too many a priori conditions are in the way that are concerned with the broad area of philosophy of nursing science (Figure 1). What decisions have philosophers of nursing science made that are relevant to human beings—the focus of nursing? What are the patterns of interaction between human-to-human and human-to-environment? Will the assumptions held

FIGURE 1

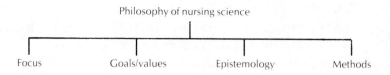

FIGURE 2

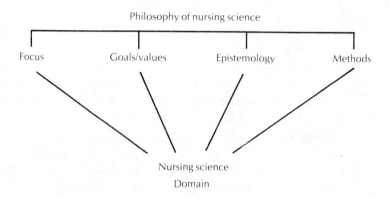

about human beings make a difference? Those of us who have worked in classification of nursing diagnoses with the Theorist Group would say, "Yes, it does make a difference." What about the purposes that nurses profess to espouse? Have we defined health? Will we strive for the goal of explanation and understanding as well as prediction and control? What perspective or perspectives of science will nursing scientists follow to identify nursing knowledge? Finally, what methods of science are acceptable to nurses as they pursue scientific knowledge? Are we building in freedom and flexibility consistent with the nature of nursing phenomena? The answers to these questions are important because they will provide the boundaries and direction for nursing science. Nurses need guidelines to make decisions about the questions they ask, such as, "Is this a nursing question? Does it overlap with another domain? Will the methods used provide answers with meaning to the problem studied?" Fortunately, there is evidence in the literature that some philosophic issues have been addressed (Meier, 1982; Silva, 1977; Watson, 1981; Webster, 1981).

The response of nurses to these questions will influence the nature, indeed the existence, of nursing science, as illustrated in Figure 2. Shapere (1977) indicated that the hypothesis that a domain has a deeper underlying unity may be proved false. The responses formulated, accepted, and reported within the nursing community answer domain problems that may or may not be expressed as theories. When the responses are expressed as theories, they are said to be the compositional theories of the domain. Whether or not

FIGURE 3

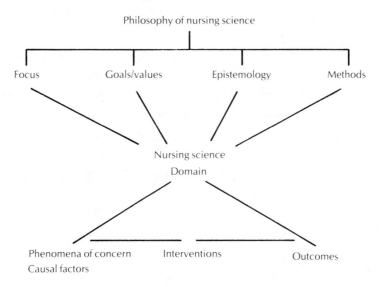

a domain actually exists depends on another level in the system of nursing science. It is at this lower level that theoretic problems that call for a deeper account of the domain will result in theories. The answers to these theoretic problems are evolutionary theories or nursing theories. I believe that nursing at this point meets all the characteristics of a domain. Nurses work at this level with the component parts (phenomena of nursing concern, nursing interventions, and client outcomes) to contribute to the body of nursing knowledge. These three components inform each other and in turn are informed by all four elements of the philosophic issues of focus, goals/values, epistemology, and methods (Figure 3).

The role of classification of nursing diagnoses in the identification of the phenomena of concern to nursing is particularly important (Gebbie, 1974; Roy, 1975). Decisions cannot be based on intuition or clinical experience but can be based on the analysis of observations of reality. Diagnosis occurs after assessment of specified criteria of a recognized clinical entity. The identification of each clinical entity, up to this time, depended on a clinician's subjective interpretation of visible, audible, or palpable clinical evidence. The goal of observer reliability requires that we accept specific validated criteria for diagnostic interpretation (Gordon, 1976). When the defining characteristics of a classified condition have been established, a more complex and confusing problem arises,—the many different properties and factors appear simultaneously in too many different combinations. Many persons who have worked on specific diagnoses have already experienced this fact. Difficulty arises in separating the different categories that seem to overlap; it is difficult to classify the overlap. This process is a complex one and is the first step in the structural definition of nursing diagnosis—naming or labeling the clinical entity with all its indicators. In addition to the first part of nursing diagnosis, which merely describes what is, a correlational model is needed for an explanation of how the indicators fit together. Etiology cannot be considered at this point, since the cause cannot be identified with certainty.

Cause and effect diagrammed says:

$$X \longrightarrow Y$$
$$\text{cause} \qquad \text{effect}$$

with a certainty that is uncharacteristic of association of variables where:

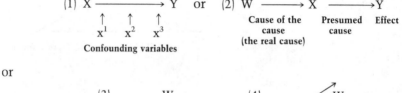

or

In the strictest sense, causality can be limited to X→Y. The other examples demonstrate the difficulties of attempting causal inference. The latter are more characteristic of clinical problems.

Prediction with a multivariate example does not approach causality:

$$Y = B_0 + B_1 X_1 + B_2 X_2 + B_3 X_3 \ldots B_n X_n$$

This formula simply states that Y is a function of the linear combination of the variables in that in combination they *predict* but do not necessarily *cause* Y to occur.

Blalock (1964) suggested processes for making causal inferences from correlation data and time sequencing (path analysis). Contemporary sociologic thought seems to question the applicability of these mathematical models and thus considers them irrelevant for discovering causes. They focus on the problem of interpretation (Duncan, 1966). The statisticians consider them invalid, and a philosophy of holism would find these mathematical models irrelevant. Blalock (1964, p. 5) himself states that "the best justification for attempting to deal with this difficult problem, perhaps somewhat prematurely, is that in actual research we find social scientists attempting to make causal inferences even when the underlying rationale is not at all clear."

There appears to be an inherent gap between the languages of research and theory that, according to Blalock (1964), can never be bridged in a completely satisfactory way.

If one admits that causal thinking belongs completely on the theoretic level and causal laws can never be demonstrated empirically, what is left to work with in carrying out the effort of building nursing science? First, I would argue for a multiple correlation model for relating and associating risk or predictive factors. Then for all entities for which there are enough data, a predictive model may be built and tested. Another major issue is whether or not nurses have been addressing a validity concern rather than causality. If a nursing diagnosis is thought of as the concept or construct, the variables called etiologic may be merely the indicators of the concept. The concept is then validly realized only through a combination of the referents or indicators. The relating/associating function becomes essential to understanding. Understanding is a very difficult process and may or may not result from the associations described. A further function of explanation is its ability to differentiate categories, which is particularly important to the clustering of categories.

Another methodology that has relevance for nursing, if we are serious about nursing's focus on unitary man, is the grounded theory method developed and refined by Glaser and Strauss (Glaser and Strauss, 1967; Glaser, 1978). Grounded theory may be used in relatively new areas as well as to gain a new perspective of a familiar situation. Some of our proposed nursing diagnoses would fit in either one or the other of these two situations. The elements of theory are generated by simultaneous collection of observational data and constant comparative analysis: (1) conceptual categories and their conceptual properties and (2) hypotheses or generalized relations among the categories and their properties (Glaser and Strauss, 1967). The procedures of this method are systematic and provide for empirical verification of the hypotheses and propositions developed during the research process. The final form emerging from the method is an integration of the conditions, contingencies, contexts, consequences, and strategies around one or more core variables rich in conceptual detail and adequate to develop testable hypotheses.

It should be obvious that we are suggesting that nurses make some decisions about methods consistent with the philosophy of nursing science and with the nature of the problems of concern. To continue to seek causes by using experimental methods is to compromise the principle of holism. To use causal inferences is to be aware that as of this point there are no wholly reliable, nonexperimental models to be used for the inferences. Nurses, as physicians do, will need to be aware of the limitations of making causal inferences. Although we may think in terms of a theoretic language containing words such as causal inferences, causes, and etiology, cause can never be demonstrated empirically. The processes of statistical inferences, of causal inference, and of judgment in decision-making overlap, but the principles that govern them are not the same. Observational data about how the problem acts, under what circumstances it exists, and by what measures it is controlled are required to support judgment in decision making. Susser (1977) makes a case for judgment and causal inference by citing three historic cases of smallpox vaccine, typhoid vaccine, and smoking in which issues were settled not by statistics but by rationalistic criteria for clinical decision making.

One of the cases concerned the exchange between Wright and Pearson in 1896 about the use of vaccine for typhoid fever. Pearson's statistical data did not agree with Wright's observational data. The issue was settled not by statistics but by political decision. Sir Richard Haldane, who was secretary of war and convinced that inoculation was useful and necessary, made Wright a knight to strengthen his (Wright's) reputation as a scientist, and the army proceeded using the vaccine. Subsequently, statistical data and Pearson's doubts were not ignored. Vaccine use was monitored for a long period with a variety of tests until the data had strengthened the case for the vaccine and inoculation was used regularly in the British and Irish armies.

Perhaps nurses can take pride in the effort to build science in that they are questioning their science claims. Nurses might draw support from Shapere who denies that all science at all times uses the same reasoning patterns or follows the same methodology. Nursing's focus on the wholeness of the human being requires a model of causality that will not minimize an individual's causal capacity, his actions, or his capacity to reflect on himself, on his situational environment, or on his attempts to transcend rather than to give in to the circumstances that shape and constrain him. It is becoming an increasingly dominant theme of Shapere (1977) that as sophisticated science proceeds, it develops improved patterns of reasoning not previously used in ways conditioned by the content of the science. Also, much of scientific progress in such development consists of increasingly subtle, improved patterns of reasoning for evaluating knowledge claims. Or, as Shapere (1977, p. 705) so aptly put it, "We learn how to learn as we learn."

CONCLUSIONS AND VALUE IMPLICATIONS

A summary of the foregoing thoughts serves little useful purpose, since the material represents excerpts from varied sources. Therefore a list of conclusions and value implications follows to highlight a personal assimilation and ordering of the information presented:

1. Causality for all theoretic and practical purposes of nursing is multifactorial. Etiology is a possibility when all possible information is gathered and analyzed, when the cause of an effect is isolated and can be stated with a certainty. It is a final stage in the conceptualization and reasoning process.

2. To be scientifically correct, nurses must speak of correlations, associations, or relationships that describe indicators, activities, and consequences of a particular conceptual system.

3. To the extent that reasoning allows for explanations of association (causal effect), the level of understanding about the entities being observed (nursing phenomena) is increased.

4. The reasoning process taken to the stage of identifying and testing correlational links will produce a tightly woven network of concepts, observations, and logical relations (descriptive and explanatory conceptual systems).

5. Nurses are concerned with concepts of pain, grieving, knowledge deficit, impaired mobility, and so forth. These conceptual systems are independent (unique) if they are derived from an agreed on philosophic framework addressing the focus, purpose, epistemology, and methods of nursing.

6. For every fully developed nursing phenomenon, including defining characteristics and causal factors, a conceptual system is being developed.

7. When clinical nursing management and evaluation strategies indicated by analysis of the evolving conceptual system are added to the model, a theory is developed that enables nurses to assume the validity of the construct, to explain, predict, and control the indicators, activities, and consequences of the health problem.

8. These theories developed out of the conceptual systems of nursing constitute the scientific domain of nursing.

9. Methods congruent with nursing's philosophy of science are available. The decision-making processes of nurses, enhanced by rigorous attention to conceptualistic/rationalistic development of the phenomena of concern, attract the respect of other scientific disciplines and, more to the point, the respect of those who constitute the focus of nursing's concern.

REFERENCES

Blalock, H.M.: Causal inferences in nonexperimental research, Chapel Hill, N.C., 1964, The University of North Carolina Press.

Duncan, O.D.: Path analysis: sociological examples, Am. J. Sociol. **72**(1):1, 1966.

Gale, G.: Theory of science, New York, 1979, McGraw-Hill Book Co.

Gebbie, C., and Lavin, M.A.: Classifying nursing diagnoses, Am. J. Nurs. **74**(2):250, 1974.

Glaser, B.G.: Theoretical sensitivity, Mill Valley, 1978, The Sociology Press.

Glaser, B.G., and Strauss, A.L.: The discovery of grounded theory: strategies for qualitative research, Chicago, 1967, Aldine Publishing Co.

Gordon, M.: Nursing diagnosis and the diagnostic process, Am. J. Nurs. **76**(8):1298, 1976.

Hanson, N.R.: Patterns of discovery, Cambridge, 1958, Cambridge University Press.

Hanson, N.R.: The waning of the Weltanschauungen views. In Suppe, F., ed.: The structure of scientific theories, Urbana, Ill., 1977, The University of Illinois Press.

Meier, P.: The observational-theoretical distinction of the received view: its influence upon nursing research, Unpublished paper, Chicago, 1982.

Nickles, T.: Heuristics and justification in scientific research: comments on Shapere. In Suppe, F., ed.: The structure of scientific theories, Urbana, Ill., 1977, The University of Illinois Press.

Roy, Sister C.: A diagnostic classification system for nursing, Nurs. Outlook 23(2):90, 1975.

Shapere, D.: Notes toward a post-positivistic interpretation of science. In Achinstein, P., and Barker, S., eds.: The legacy of logical positivism, Baltimore, 1969, The Johns Hopkins University Press.

Shapere, D.: Scientific theories and their domains. In Suppe, F., ed.: The structure of scientific theories, Urbana, Ill., 1977, The University of Illinois Press.

Silva, M.: Philosophy, science, theory: interrelationships and implications for nursing research, Image 9:59, 1977.

Susser, M.: Judgment and causal inference: criteria in epidemiologic studies, Am. J. Epidemiol. 105(1):1, 1977.

Watson, J.: Nursing's scientific quest, Nurs. Outlook 29:413, 1981.

Webster, G., Jacox, A., and Baldwin, B.: Nursing theory and the ghost of the received view. In Grace, H., and McCloskey, J., eds.: Contemporary issues in nursing, Boston, 1981, Blackwell Scientific Publications

Discussion

Gary Forsyth: I think that etiology of a particular diagnosis does have implications for the interventions that we design for the conceptualized problems. I do not necessarily believe that we are going to be able to say, without a doubt, it is this plus this that has caused this specific problem. But in the analysis of the defining characteristics of a particular problem, we will have some indication as to what intervention is needed. By testing and validating the outcome, we will become stronger and stronger in our reasoning power and in terms of gaining acceptance from our colleagues that particular interventions are appropriate for that series of defining characteristics of a particular problem.

Marjory Gordon: Would you, therefore, given that position, state that a medical diagnosis would not be an etiology? Because you are not, in a sense, treating a medical diagnosis.

Gary Forsyth: I would not consider any medical diagnosis as a nursing etiology. We would not have the knowledge in terms of what that is if it means adapting theories of medicine into nursing. I do consider that biopsychosocial human *responses* to pathology may contribute to problems that nurses define as nursing diagnoses. These various responses may become *the* etiology or the defining characteristic of a nursing problem.

Louette Lutjens: You spoke a great deal about causality. When I define etiology, I think about a cause and effect relationship; that is, what etiologic aspects can be identified as contributing factors. I do not know what your feelings are on that. But I think that is a little less strong than cause and effect, for sometimes we do not know the cause of the human response. I do think, however, that we can identify many contributing factors from our interviews.

Gary Forsyth: Yes, I indicated that we would be building a model for preventive, or risk factors, and those factors are considered the etiology of a conceptualized problem. You would be treating those factors after a period of further observation and investigation of clinical individuals. I indicated, as an example, the test cases of the link between lung cancer and smoking. They are still not saying that smoking is a cause, although they are approaching that. But it is a reason, and they have been able to supply us with a relationship or with a predictive model.

Current nomenclature and classification systems: pertinent issues

PHYLLIS B. KRITEK, R.N., Ph.D., F.A.A.N.

In 1973, when this collective effort took its first hesitant steps toward grappling with the hard question of taxonomy generation, the goal was more pragmatic than scientific. We have come a very long way in 9 short years and find ourselves confronted with new developmental tasks. Clearly these tasks are making demands on us, asking that we now be more scientific than pragmatic. This paper seeks to address this demand and to move us toward fresh directions of effort. It is my aim to point to the next set of questions, to ask rather than to prematurely foreclose on answers. I wish therefore to preface my comments with a personally valued insight from Albert Einstein, "One thing I have learned in a long life: that all our science, measured against reality, is primitive and childlike—and yet it is the most precious thing we have" (Hoffman, 1972).

It is in this spirit that I wish to share with you the assumptions that have guided my comments:

1. All knowledge is tentative.
2. Today's best answer to any question contains, in the answer, the seeds of its own demise; that is, it highlights, by its very articulation, its incomplete or tentative nature.
3. It is inherently more reassuring to force an answer to appear complete and final than it is to struggle to keep questions open: the tentativeness of knowledge can be painful.
4. This resistance to critical inquiry (perhaps antiintellectualism in a uniquely virulent form) functions as a covert value in professional nursing.
5. Various subgroups in nursing are eager to challenge and critique this covert value.
6. The formal efforts to label and categorize nursing's phenomena of concern have participated in this professional reality. It has been both influenced by and influential in the dialogue of conflict between proponents of "the one true way" and those who view knowledge as tentative.
7. Finally, we need to move past the conflicts.

Our collective effort to generate a body of knowledge that we can name nursing science (what Einstein calls "the most precious thing we have") is an enterprise fraught with risks, missed opportunities, failures, and moments of insight and triumph. We can, collectively, either succumb to the dangers or conquer the risks. One seemingly obvious asset that we have is the history of nursing and science.

Several realities of nursing history are relevant. We have emerged in this century from a system that Ashley (1976) has labeled paternalistic. That has made us often, to our detriment, either passive or petulant about our fate. Reclaiming our profession has consequently made us seem more like victims becoming whole rather than scholars becoming wise. We still long for perfect answers, total solutions, final dogma that will prove us once and for all adequate.

We began as doers, moved suspiciously toward becoming thinkers, and then initiated conflicts between our doers and our thinkers. That has left us willing to view the nurse theorist either as too abstract or as infallible. Neither view serves us well.

We have only recently come to science, and we are variously awed or irritated by its demands. We are just beginning to recognize its potential to advise us. It seems feasible that, while a young science, we are particularly fortunate to be able to study our predecessors in the basic sciences.

To elucidate, I will trace in record time the history of one such science, the science of matter—chemistry. In the Western hemisphere, chemistry's earliest classification system, generated by the Greek philosophers, had four entities: fire, air, water, and earth. China, being more economical, had two: yin and yang. The seminal efforts of the Greeks, however, degenerated in time to alchemy, the effort to change base metals to gold. Chemistry began to emerge gradually, beginning in the thirteenth century with Roger Bacon and culminating in the scientific revolution of the sixteenth century, with the contributions of Francis Bacon. By the end of the seventeenth century, chemistry was dominated by the German school, which argued that substances contained three essences or principles:

1. Sulfur: the principle of inflammability
2. Mercury: the principle of fluidity and volatility
3. Salt: the principle of fixity and inertness

Phlogiston, the motion of fire, was considered the source of change in matter (Mason, 1962). The marked empiricism of the eighteenth century chemists led to increased theoretic empiricism. Lavoisier, describing the work of his contemporary, Priestly, said he engaged in "a web of experiments almost uninterrupted by any kind of reasoning" (Mason, 1962, p. 306). But because of this empiricism, chemists began to systematically describe the properties of forms of matter, for example, their color, hardness, solubility, odor, density, and boiling point. By the nineteenth century, rigorous, systematic observation made simplification by classification possible. The result was the periodic table of the elements (Figure 1). The periodic table, elegant in its simplicity, unearths, however, a disturbing fact. This taxonomy has

Element	Symbol	Valence	Atomic number	Atomic weight[*]	Element	Symbol	Valence	Atomic number	Atomic weight[*]
Actinium	Ac	3	89	(227.0278)	Mendelevium	Md		101	(257.0956)
Aluminum	Al	3	13	26.98154	Mercury	Hg	1,2	80	200.59
Americium	Am	3,4,5,6	95	(243.0614)	Molybdenum	Mo	3,4,6	42	95.94
Antimony	Sb	3,5	51	121.75	Neodymium	Nd	3	60	144.24
Argon	Ar	0	18	39.948	Neon	Ne	0	10	20.179
Arsenic	As	3,5	33	74.9216	Neptunium	Np	4,5,6	93	237.0482
Astatine	At	1,3,5,7	85	(209.987)	Nickel	Ni	2,3	28	58.70
Barium	Ba	2	56	137.34	Niobium	Nb	3,5	41	92.9064
Berkelium	Bk	3,4	97	(247.0703)	Nitrogen	N	3,5	7	14.0067
Beryllium	Be	2	4	9.01218	Nobelium	No		102	(255.0933)
Bismuth	Bi	3,5	83	208.9804	Osmium	Os	2,3,4,8	76	190.2
Boron	B	3	5	10.81	Oxygen	O	2	8	15.9994
Bromine	Br	1,3,5,7	35	79.904	Palladium	Pd	2,4,6	46	106.4
Cadmium	Cd	2	48	112.40	Phosphorus	P	3,5	15	30.98376
Calcium	Ca	2	20	40.08	Platinum	Pt	2,4	78	195.09
Californium	Cf	3	98	(251.0796)	Plutonium	Pu	3,4,5,6	94	(244.0642)
Carbon	C	2,4	6	12.011	Polonium	Po	2,4	84	(208.9824)
Cerium	Ce	3,4	58	140.12	Potassium	K	1	19	39.098
Cesium	Cs	1	55	132.9054	Praseodymium	Pr	3	59	140.9077
Chlorine	Cl	1,3,5,7	17	35.453	Promethium	Pm	3	61	(144.9128)
Chromium	Cr	2,3,6	24	51.996	Protactinium	Pa		91	(231.0359)
Cobalt	Co	2,3	27	58.9332	Radium	Ra	2	88	(226.0254)
Columbium	See:	Niobium			Radon	Rn	0	86	(222.0176)
Copper	Cu	1,2	29	63.546	Rhenium	Re		75	186.207
Curium	Cm	3	96	(247.0704)	Rhodium	Rh	3	45	102.9055
Dysprosium	Dy	3	66	162.50	Rubidium	Rb	1	37	85.4678
Einsteinium	Es		99	(254.0881)	Ruthenium	Ru	3,4,6,8	44	101.07
Erbium	Er	3	68	167.26	Samarium	Sm	2,3	62	150.4
Europium	Eu	2,3	63	151.96	Scandium	Sc	3	21	44.9559
Fermium	Fm		100	(257.0951)	Selenium	Se	2,4,6	34	78.96
Fluorine	F	1	9	18.9984	Silicon	Si	4	14	28.086
Francium	Fr	1	87	(223.0198)	Silver	Ag	1	47	107.868
Gadolinium	Gd	3	64	157.25	Sodium	Na	1	11	22.98977
Gallium	Ga	2,3	31	69.72	Strontium	Sr	2	38	87.62
Germanium	Ge	4	32	72.59	Sulfur	S	2,4,6	16	32.06
Glucinum	See:	Beryllium			Tantalum	Ta	5	73	180.9479
Gold	Au	1,3	79	196.9665	Technetium	Tc	6,7	43	96.9062
Hafnium	Hf	4	72	178.49	Tellurium	Te	2,4,6	52	127.60
Helium	He	0	2	4.0026	Terbium	Tb	3	65	158.9254
Holmium	Ho	3	67	164.9304	Thallium	Tl	1,3	81	204.37
Hydrogen	H	1	1	1.0079	Thorium	Th	4	90	232.0381
Indium	In	3	49	114.82	Thulium	Tm	3	69	168.9342
Iodine	I	1,3,5,7	53	126.9045	Tin	Sn	2,4	50	118.69
Iridium	Ir	3,4	77	192.22	Titanium	Ti	3,4	22	47.90
Iron	Fe	2,3	26	55.847	Tungsten	W	6	74	183.85
Krypton	Kr	0	36	83.30	Uranium	U	4,6	92	238.029
Lanthanum	La	3	57	138.9055	Vanadium	V	3,5	23	50.9414
Lawrencium	Lw		103	(256.0986)	Xenon	Xe	0	54	131.30
Lead	Pb	2,4	82	207.2	Ytterbium	Yb	2,3	70	173.04
Lithium	Li	1	3	6.941	Yttrium	Y	3	39	88.9059
Lutetium	Lu	3	71	174.97	Zinc	Zn	2	30	65.38
Magnesium	Mg	2	12	24.305	Zirconium	Zr	4	40	91.22
Manganese	Mn	2,3,4,6,7	25	54.938					

[*]Based on Carbon-12. Figures enclosed in parentheses represent the mass number of the most stable isotope.

FIGURE 1   Periodic table of the elements.

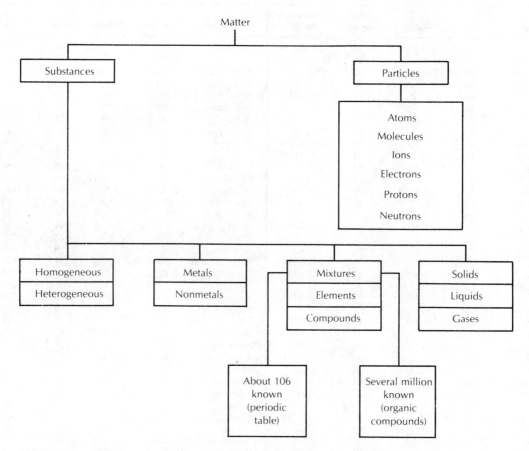

FIGURE 2   Schematic summary of periodic table of the elements.

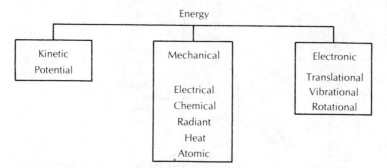

FIGURE 3   Schematic summary of the classification principles of physics.

numerous organizing principles. This diverse array can be schematically summarized as shown in Figure 2.

A seemingly independent discipline, physics, was concurrently developing. Just as chemistry explored the world of matter, physics explored the world of energy. The classification principles of physics can be summarized (Figure 3) much as we summarized those of chemistry. The simple elegance of each system was thrown into irrevocable disruption with one simple formula: $e = mc^2$. Matter and energy, seemingly so separate when classified, were found to be intimately related. As Durant (1953, p. 43) describes it, "the atom, it seems, is born, develops, loses its vitality, and dies."

This historic digression, is of course, deliberate and is intended to set the stage for an analysis of nursing diagnosis classification systems. If indeed we can go from three elements, to several, to 106 (systematically ordered on a periodic table with multiple classification principles) only to be thrown into disarray by energy "c squaring" our collective world of matter, we may wish to approach the task of nursing diagnosis classification with the tentativeness, doubt, respect, and humility befitting the scientist.

Classification is the systematic arrangement of entities into groups or categories according to their relevant features or properties. It assumes the recognition of similarities as a basis for grouping or clustering and assigning entities into categories. According to Sokal (1974), classification enables us to delineate natural systems and to achieve economy of memory and ease of handling, making it possible for us to organize, characterize, and assimilate what is known. The primary purpose of classification is the description of the structure and relationships of groups of similar objects. Each group and its properties can then be studied in detail or related to other groups or properties. While such classification work often has applied practical goals, successful classifications are a source of scientific hypotheses. Recent developments that argue for classification based on many, equally weighted characteristics have created a major conceptual advance. Computer technology has enabled us to enhance classification across a broad range of disciplines using techniques such as cluster or discriminant analysis. Such technology while enhancing objectivity, cannot eliminate subjective and cultural biases and prejudices. These systematic prejudices and biases are the key issues facing those who wish to classify nursing diagnoses.

"Nursing is the diagnosis and treatment of human responses to actual or potential health problems" (ANA, 1980, p. 9). This definition of nursing forms the base of ANA's most comprehensive policy statement to date. Diagnoses, in this sense, are nursing's phenomena of concern, that is, human responses to actual or potential health problems. These human responses are the core of our nursing diagnoses classification systems, the entities to be clustered or grouped. It is here, then, that we must look to discover our systematic prejudices and do so in the spirit of the humble scientist.

Popper (1953, p. 364) notes that Einstein showed us that in the light of experience "we may question and revise our presuppositions regarding even space and time, ideas which had been held to be necessary presuppositions of all science." It is Popper's contention (1953, p. 364) that Einstein demonstrated that "the empirical method has proved to be quite capable of taking care of itself. It does so, he contends, by taking care of our prejudices, not all at once, but one by one. However, we discover the fact that we have such a prejudice only after having gotten rid of it. We criticize existing prejudices through public discourse guided by scientific objectivity.

Science asks that we engage in four tasks fundamental to all sciences—observation, classification, theorizing, and testing. This is a trial and error, piecemeal, essentially practical approach. Francis Bacon argued this by proposing that one must interconnect theory and experiments so that one checked the other. He argued for exploring all possible hypotheses when critiquing existing principles. We need both inductive inferences and systematic testing on an ongoing basis. We need not only to focus on hypotheses we can support, but also to disprove the diverse alternative hypotheses.

I would argue that the time is now for some concerted analytic scrutiny of the several existing principles of the classification of nursing diagnoses. Great synthesizers of knowledge are needed. Platt (1964), discussing strong inference in science, noted that small studies that add another brick to the temple of science often are bricks that just lie around the brickyard. We need to synthesize—to include and to exclude. In particular, we must address old prejudices and biases.

Einstein's scientific struggles were always driven by his belief that nature was simple. For him, complexity indicated error, undiscarded prejudices. A common expression of his was "This is so simple God could not have passed it up" (Hoffman, 1972, p. 228). Scientific gains are made by building on that which one is replacing. To begin to make such gains, I would propose that we need to know well what we might replace. We need to understand our current ideas well and unearth their principles and their prejudices.

The next task in the classification of nursing diagnoses is an in-depth analysis of existing classification systems. Although it is clearly beyond the scope of this presentation to exhaust this task, it is introduced and outlined here. Popper (1953, p. 365) argues that "practice is not the enemy of theoretical knowledge, but the most valuable incentive to it." He argues that we must stay in touch with practice or risk irrelevance. He notes that those who are most convinced of having gotten rid of prejudices are most prejudiced.

With this in mind, I will briefly review diverse classification systems from diverse sources designed for diverse purposes. I wish, however, to first present a disclaimer. The following examples represent no underlying attraction or repulsion on my part. Many alternate examples are available. My goal is merely to be somewhat representative in an effort to demonstrate both our differences and our areas of consensus. An effort was made to exemplify the state of the art, not the one best system, which I believe I have already dismissed as a myth.

It seems only appropriate to begin with this conference group's classification schema, which is predicated on the patterns of unitary man. This schema is somewhat unique because it was generated by a group. It involved many leading nurse theorists, it deliberately sought to articulate an organizing principle, and it has been affiliated with this group's collective efforts and discourse. Thus a framework is generated based on this relatively familiar conceptual schema (Box 1).

This conceptual schema includes the nine identified patterns of unitary man and the three major categories of interaction, action, and awareness. To draw an analogy from my earlier remarks, these three categories may function in a developmental sense comparable to the chemical categories of liquids, solids, and gases—a very basic classification principle of the natural state. One imagines, too, that chemists collectively did not view this primitive tripartite distinction as particularly useful. It did have a more concrete quality, however, than the categories of patterns. I think it is useful to compare this category set with the category set generated by Jones and Jakob (1977), who identify action, reaction, and interaction categories of nursing diagnoses (Box 2). Note the similarities and the differences of Box 1 and Box 2.

BOX 1 **Characteristics of unitary man***

Interaction	Action	Awareness
Exchanging	Valuing	Waking
Communicating	Choosing	Feeling
Relating	Moving	Knowing

---

*From Kim, M.J., and Moritz, D.A.: Classification of nursing diagnoses: proceedings of the third and fourth national conferences, New York, 1982, McGraw-Hill Book Co.

BOX 2 **Nursing diagnoses classified***

Action diagnoses: Inability to meet self-care needs
Reaction diagnoses: Individual's response
Interaction diagnoses: Reciprocal action of self and systems

---

*From Jones, P.E., and Jakob, D.F.: An investigation of the definition of nursing diagnoses: report of phase 1, Toronto, 1977, University of Toronto.

BOX 3   **Typology of eleven functional health patterns***

Health perception—health management   Self-perception—self-concept
Nutritional—metabolic   Role relationship
Elimination   Sexuality—reproductive
Activity—exercise   Caring—stress—tolerance
Sleep—rest   Value—belief
Cognitive—perceptual

---

*From Gordon, M.: Nursing diagnosis: process and application, New York, 1982, McGraw-Hill Book Co.

BOX 4   **Patterns of functioning***

Respiratory   Personal hygiene
Circulation   Pain/discomfort
Foods and fluids   Communication (speech, hearing, sight)
Elimination   Spiritual care
Rest/sleep   Family
Activity (locomotion)

---

*From Matthew, D.: Patterns of functioning: Wichita State University Curriculum Design, Poster presented at the Midwest Alliance in Nursing Fifth Annual Meeting, Wichita, Kan., 1982.

Going a step further, it is interesting to contrast these two category sets with the work of one of the individual theorists. Sister Callista Roy, who headed the initial Theorist Group efforts of this conference group, identifies four adaptation modes: physiologic, self-concept, role function, and interdependence modes (Roy and Roberts, 1981). One immediately wonders, in this instance, about the distinction or overlap between the interdependence adaptation mode of Sister Callista Roy and the interaction classification of Jones and Jakob (1977). Perhaps more troublesome, do they flow from a common organizing principle? Do entities that cluster in one also cluster in the other and to what degree?

Switching the focus, but strengthening the questions I've just raised, are two alternate classification systems that focus on functional health patterns and functioning patterns (Boxes 3 and 4). The two models, although different, recognize some common categories such as elimination and activity. Both these systems, although they argue the possibility of providing lists of categories for nursing diagnoses, view the categories as guides to assessment factors about patients.

BOX 5 **Medical center hospital of Vermont: patient classification system***

Diet   Behavior
Hygiene   Special emotional concerns
Mobility   Physiologic state
Medications and I.V.s

*From Roehrl, P.K.: Supervisor Nurse **10**(2):22, 1979.

BOX 6 **St. Michael's Hospital—Milwaukee, Wisconsin: patient classification system: four levels of acuity***

General health   Treatments
Eating   Medication
Grooming   Teaching
Excretion   Emotional support
Comfort

*From St. Michael's Hospital: Patient classification at St. Michael's Hospital, Unpublished hospital descriptive manuscript, Milwaukee, 1982.

I reviewed diverse extant patient classification systems because they show a remarkable degree of overlap with extant nursing diagnosis classification systems in terms of shared terminology. Patient classification systems were designed to identify patient needs and nursing care requirements to measure nursing care work load variables and appropriate nursing staffing patterns. They tell us, essentially, how to efficiently plan nursing care work load and are thus practical and familiar in terminology. Keeping in mind category systems already presented, the overlap of categories is striking. One of the first such systems by Giovanetti (1970) illustrates the early developmental stage of this process. It identified four major categories: personal care, feeding, observation, and ambulation. Given the labels alone, one is confronted immediately with the question: Do these entities describe both patient patterns and activities or nurse patterns and activities? The next two examples, both from acute care settings, reflect some commonalities between themselves and with previous schema (Boxes 5 and 6). A third example (Box 7) is very similar to the patient classification system lists but is actually a set of categories devised by a hospital to organize their nursing diagnoses list of labels.

BOX 7   **Methodist Hospital—Madison, Wisconsin nursing diagnoses categories***

Intake   Relating to self
Elimination   Relating with environment
Mobility   Regulatory mechanisms
Relating to others

*From Methodist Hospital: Nursing diagnosis categories: Methodist Hospital, Unpublished hospital descriptive manuscript, Madison, Wis., 1981.

BOX 8   **VNA of Omaha classification scheme: client problems***

Domains
  Environment
  Psychosocial
  Physiological
  Health behaviors

*From Simmons, D.A.: A classification scheme for client problems in community health nursing, DHHS, PHS, MRA, BHP, DN Pub. No. HRP-0501501, Hyattsville, Md., 1980.

BOX 9   **Assessment elements/indicators to classify chronically ill patients***

Patient-oriented indicators
  Demographic characteristics
    Physical status
      Extent of impairment
      Extent of diagnosed health problem
    Psychosocial status
      Level of mental functioning
      Personal adaptability
      Social adaptability
      Quality of life-style
    Self-care practices
      Activities of daily living
      Therapeutic
Social and environmental factors
  Characteristics of family and friends
  Program of care
  Location

*From Leatt, P., Bay, K.J., and Stinson, S.M.: Nurs. Res. **30**(3):146, 1981.

The overlap of the two classification systems (patient classification and nursing diagnosis) becomes clear at this point. Indeed, it is interesting how three words, one from each acute care setting, reflect a comparable focus: eating, intake, and diet.

The next two examples (Boxes 8 and 9) are from community health and long-term care settings. Note the deliberate focus on environment, highlighting the shift from the acute care setting. In addition, the distinction between physiologic and psychologic phenomena is noteworthy. One begins to get a sense of specialties having an interest in specific categories. A sense of blurred categories is also evident.

Returning to the issue of assessment data, if one scrutinizes the health status data factors identified in the ANA Generic Standards of Practice, Standard 1 (Box 10), the list seems strangely reminiscent of previously illustrated category systems. Here we find interaction patterns, health status satisfaction, emotional status, and patterns of coping. This blurring of assessment categories and nursing diagnosis or patient classification system categories is noteworthy. The ANA Social Policy Statement (1980) diagrammatically demonstrates this conceptual overlap by paralleling the phenomena of concern of nursing to the assessment stage of the nursing process. Yet the statement clearly takes the position that nurses diagnose human responses to actual or potential health problems and calls these the phenomena of concern.

Interestingly, the examples of human responses (phenomena) that the ANA document lists (Box 11) are closer to this conference group's nursing diagnoses list than to the ANA standard assessment categories, which is, a

---

BOX 10   **ANA generic standards of nursing practice: standard 1***

Assessment factors
  Health status data include
    Growth and development
    Biophysical status
    Emotional status
    Cultural, religious, socioeconomic background
    Performance of activities of daily living
    Patterns of coping
    Interaction patterns
    Client's/patient's perception of and satisfaction with his health status
    Client/patient health goals
    Environment (physical, social, emotional, ecological)
    Available and accessible human and material resources

---

*From American Nurses' Association: Standards of nursing practice, Kansas City, Mo., 1973, The Association. Reprinted with permission of ANA.

BOX 11 **Human responses that are the focus for nursing intervention: ANA social policy statement***

1. Self-care limitations
2. Impaired functioning in areas such as rest, sleep, ventilation, circulation, activity, nutrition, elimination, skin, sexuality
3. Pain and discomfort
4. Emotional problems related to illness and treatment, life-threatening events, or daily experiences such as anxiety, loss, loneliness, and grief
5. Distortion of symbolic functions, reflected in interpersonal and intellectual processes, such as hallucinations
6. Deficiencies in decision making and ability to make personal choices
7. Self-image changes required by health status
8. Dysfunctional perceptual orientations to health
9. Strains related to life processes such as birth, growth and development, and death
10. Problematic affiliative relationships

*From American Nurses' Association: Nursing: a social policy statement, Kansas City, Mo., 1980, The Association. Reprinted with permission of ANA.

BOX 12 **Proposed changes in NGCND classification schema***

Activity/rest
Comfort
Communication
Coping
Elimination
Growth and development
Independence/dependence
Learning
Life-style
Management of health
Management of illness
Nutrition
Oxygenation
Parenting
Protection
Relationships
Self-concept
Sleep/wake
Thought

Focus:
Intrapersonal
Changes or
deficits in
Function
Structure
Interpersonal
Changes or deficits in
Function
Structure
Nonpersonal factors

Qualifiers:
Alteration in
Potential, alteration in
Dysfunction in

*From Lunney, M.: Am. J. Nurs. **82**(3):457, 1982.

critical conceptual limitation that the profession may wish to review. It may, in part, explain our collective difficulty in defining principles of categorization. Are the traits, characteristics, or properties we assess identical to the judgments we make? I think not, given the enormous inferential and multivariate task that drawing such a judgment assumes.

Lunney (1982) wrote one of the most useful critiques of this conference's current classification system. Returning to the earlier argument that we need to go to practice to study what is real, Lunney's suggestions are practical solutions resulting from practice realities. Lunney's list (Box 12) is "modified conference group." She eliminates the distinction of pattern and process, arguing that her labels fit both. She limits qualifiers from the current conference list, arguing that her three are exhaustive. The second half of her diagnostic statement does not provide "etiology" as this group discusses but identifies a clear focus of realistically possible nursing action. Her categories are a classification system in themselves and are similar to some previous systems.

From these examples one gets a sense of several emerging principles of classification characterized by various levels of consensus. Some of these principles of classification are listed in Box 13.

The complexity and diversity of these principles is self-evident. Box 14 shows some persistent sources of bias, prejudice, or conceptual inconsistency in classification efforts.

BOX 13   **Potential problems of classification**

Potential—actual

Alteration—dysfunction

Pattern—process

Developmental stage of client

Levels of acuity

Levels of risk

Levels of response potentiation

Rate of change

Weight given response by client

Weight given response by context

Health—illness

BOX 14   **Persistent sources of classification bias/prejudice/inconsistency**

Nursing specialty language

Hospital/agency unit language

Basic sciences organization

Nursing assessment data

Nurse behaviors/treatments

Returning to the initial commitment to raise useful questions rather than propose implacable answers, the following observations are offered.

First, we must begin to identify the common denominators in diverse nursing diagnoses classification schema and the taxonomic principles that are reflected or absent. We must assess what appears to be popular—familiar and understandable to practicing nurses—and find out why. If our groups' efforts are deterrents to practice implementation, we need to know why.

Second, the question of the differentiation between cues, signs and symptoms, defining characteristics, or syntheses of these and the idea of an actual distinct entity or group of entities called nursing diagnoses needs to be addressed. Are there differences, and if so, what are they? What characteristics, traits, or variables guide members in various classification categories? I believe that the ANA Social Policy Statement provides some useful guidelines for the quandaries we face. The examples shown in Box 15 demonstrate some of these inherent practice quandaries.

Third, I would propose that on one hand arguing for holistic nursing care and on the other willingly splitting persons into minds and bodies is at best dysfunctional and at worst internally contradictory. In other words, is fear or anxiety ever not physiologic? Is impaired gas exchange ever free of psychologic phenomena? Previous taxonomic principles may require review and revision. They may not only be inelegant, but regressive, limiting nursing care potentials.

Fourth, although we are currently confined by the classification systems (and their accompanying biases) of our foundation sciences, we must move toward discovery of some principles of synthesis, to discover the organizing concepts that explain the phenomena of concern of nursing. We must free ourselves systematically from the constrictive values and prejudices of these underlying systems. For example, manipulation is a concept borrowed from psychiatry. What values and prejudices have we also borrowed in adopting this label?

BOX 15	**Sample categories of "nursing diagnosis" labels: what nurses record***

Somatic dysfunctions	Side effects
Etiologies	Equipment
Interventions	Diagnostic tests
Risk factors	

---

*From Silver, S., and others: The identification of clinically recorded nursing diagnoses and indicators, Paper presented at the Fifth National Conference for the Classification of Nursing Diagnoses, St. Louis, April 14-17, 1982. See Chapter 4 for the complete paper.

I would also, somewhat cautiously, offer a few suggestions. We must analyze extant classification systems to identify not only their common organizing principles but also their real world utility and, where present, the reasons for their development. We must adopt or develop research designs that address classification issues, generating information about the current levels of professional practice consensus. Consensus should be used to identify current research priorities. Current classification schema must be explained in terms of their classification structure, presenting not only models, but also narrative explanations of these models. Finally, I would, somewhat less cautiously, argue that we need to devise ways to enhance our understanding of human responses to actual or potential problems by asking responding humans to teach us. Our clients may better inform our thinking about classification issues than we realize.

Since Albert Einstein has been an abiding presence in my presentation, I wish to close with a final thought from his visionary perspective: "You imagine that I look back on my life's work with calm satisfaction. But from nearby it looks quite different. There is not a single concept of which I am convinced that it will stand firm, and I feel uncertain whether I am in general on the right track" (Hoffman, 1972, p. 257; letter to Solovine, 1949 on the occasion of Einstein's seventieth birthday).

All of which is to say, perhaps, that I end where I began—with a plea for systematic critical thinking, tentativeness of spirit, and the scholarship of the scientist. I encourage us collectively to avoid premature foreclosure, dogmatism, or the myth of the one best way. We must assess the state of the art in classification in a systematic fashion, which will enable us to know today's assumptions or theories honestly, so that our intellectual curiosity can demand that we question them critically and alter, embrace, or abandon them as appropriate.

REFERENCES

American Nurses' Association: Standards of nursing practice, Kansas City, Mo., 1973, The Association.

American Nurses' Association: Nursing: a social policy statement, Kansas City, Mo., 1980, The Association.

Ashley, J.A.: Hospitals, paternalism and the role of the nurse, New York, 1976, Teachers College Press.

Durant, W.: The pleasures of philosphy, New York, 1953, Simon & Schuster, Inc.

Giovanetti, P.: Measurement of patients' requirements for nursing services, research on nurse staffing in hospitals: report of the conference, DHHS, PHS, HRA, BHP, DN Pub. No. 73-434 (NIH), Hyattsville, M., 1970.

Gordon, M.: Nursing diagnosis: process and application, New York, 1982, McGraw-Hill Book Co.

Hoffman, B.: Albert Einstein: creator and rebel, New York, 1972, The New American Library Inc.

Jones, P.E., and Jakob, D.F.: An investigation of the definition of nursing diagnoses: report of phase I, Toronto, 1977, University of Toronto.

Kim, M., and Moritz, D.A.: Classification of nursing diagnoses: proceedings of the third and fourth national conferences, New York, 1982, McGraw-Hill Book Co.

Leatt, P., Bay, K.J., and Stinson, S.M.: An instrument for assessing and classifying patients by type of care, Nurs. Res. **30**(3):145, 1981.

Lipponcott, W.T., Garnett, A.B., and Verhoek, F.H.: A study of matter, New York, 1977, John Wiley & Sons, Inc.

Lunney, M.: Nursing diagnosis: refining the system, Am. J. Nurs. **82**(3):456, 1982.

Mason, S.F.: A history of the sciences, New York, 1962, MacMillan Publishing Co., Inc.

Matthew, D.: Patterns of functioning: Wichita State University Curriculum Design, Poster presented at the Midwest Alliance in Nursing Fifth Annual Meeting, Wichita, Kan., 1982.

Methodist Hospital: Nursing diagnosis categories: Methodist Hospital, Unpublished hospital descriptive manuscript, Madison Wis., 1981.

Platt, J.R.: Strong inference, Science **146**(3642):347, 1964.

Popper, K.R.: The sociology of knowledge. In Wiener, P.P., ed., Readings in the philosophy of science, New York, 1953, Charles Scribner's Sons.

Roehrl, P.K.: Patient classification: a pilot test, Supervisor Nurse, **10**(2):1, 1979.

Roy, Sister C., and Roberts, S.L.: Theory construction in nursing: an adaptation model, Englewood Cliffs, N.J., 1981, Prentice-Hall, Inc.

St. Michael's Hospital: Patient classification at St. Michael's Hospital, Unpublished hospital descriptive manuscript, Milwaukee, 1982.

Silver, S., and others: The identification of clinically recorded nursing diagnoses and indicators, Paper presented at the Fifth National Conference for the Classification of Nursing Diagnosis, St. Louis, April 14-17, 1982.

Simmons, D.A.: A classification scheme for client problems in community health nursing, DHHS, PHS, HRA, BHP, DN Pub. No. HRP-0501501, Hyattsville, Md., 1980.

Sokal, R.R.: Classification: purposes, principles, progress, prospects, Science **185**(4157):1115, 1974.

Discussion

Imogene King: Your synthesis is very good. But when I looked at that particular set of classification systems, do you know what first came to my mind?—variable and continuous variables and linear concepts that are found in a lot of previous research and that was talked about in chemistry. But my question to you is, Is that what is synthesized out of all the things that you are talking about? If so, we really do have a problem.

Phyllis Kritek: Well, I do not know if we have a problem or not. I do not think what I have developed is exhaustive. I have apprehensions about linear thinking also for I find myself engaging in it very frequently. More interestingly, I find my colleagues in the practice setting, whom I attend to as carefully as I can, being very linear. I am not prepared to describe the way they approach and organize their world until I understand it better. If I need to use all those principles to organize a set of classification systems that I can then interpret and understand, I can then challenge them. But I do not think we have it put together with enough deliberateness. We tend, I think, to either discard summarily classification systems that we find inelegant and/or try to force ourselves collectively to adopt ones that, although they appear elegant, are deficient conceptually. I guess my bias increasingly is to say; Let us look at everything out there, see what seems to be our propensity, generate some consensus statements, and figure out what we are saying to ourselves. Once we know that, then we may be prepared to discard it, if that is appropriate; or embrace it, if that is appropriate; or change it. But I am not prepared to do it permaturely. These were trends that I kept finding, some of them much more pronounced, like the potential/actual distinction. Some nurses are very animated about that, and some others less so. "Levels of risk" is a big issue for certain specialties of nursing. What I would like to do with it first is to see if I can collect data somewhat more systematically, even with a convenience sample. What this does for me is reinforce the complexity and diversity of the world of nursing's work. That is where I think we can identify our problems, because we are in such diverse settings. The work nurses do is diverse. I always think that if we read the definition of nursing seriously and think it through, the complexity of nursing becomes evident. For example, take the Social Policy Statement as the base of agreement for the discipline of nursing in the United States. As I read that now, what we are going to do is go out there with those assessment skills that we utilize, gather all that information, go in a room and make inferences, and take action on human responses. There are entire disciplines that are just trying to figure out one piece of this entire process. Yet we are saying that we are going to look at nursing and see how it impacts on the economic, physiologic, and psychologic, and anthropologic aspects.

Reimbursement mechanism based on nursing diagnosis

ROSALINDA M. TOTH, R.N., M.A.

It is a simple fact of life that money is power; the power to control, the power to bargain, the power to create change, the power to design and implement new ideas, the power for self-actualization. Aristotle (Brussell, 1970, p. 379) once said that money is "a guarantee that we may have what we want in the future. Though we need nothing at the moment, it insures the possibility of satisfying a necessary desire when it arises."

Not one of us in nursing today can deny the tremendous power physicians hold over the administration of our health care delivery system. It is my firm belief that this power will continue and will continue unchallenged as long as physicians supply that system with dollars.

A hospital exists by the admission of patients. This is how a hospital raises money. Even though many institutions are not for profit, the income generated by patients and collected through third-party payers is the basis for operation. Admission practices are currently controlled by physicians who are the primary health care providers to those institutions. So it is both logical and understandable that administration allows physicians to control policies and practices within health care institutions. At least this is true at present. Health care costs in the United States, however, have become prohibitive for the consumer who is finally demanding that an adjustment be made in the system itself.

In 18 states, the reimbursement system of hospitals is being drastically changed. Although the new programs do not diminish the power of the admitting physicians, they now give power to nurses not only in the care provided but in the actual reimbursement rate of the hospital. Once nurses recognize that this power exists for them and they take advantage of it, they will be able to change the entire health care delivery system. Nurses, however, must familiarize themselves with financial management within this new milieu and universally coordinate their efforts to create a revolution that has been unprecedented within our ranks.

The purpose of this paper is to provide an overview of the new reimbursement system in New Jersey, which is being examined as a possible basis for a national reimbursement system, and to explore the importance of nursing diagnosis and a taxonomy of nursing diagnoses within this reimbursement system.

For the past 2 years, several N.J. hospitals have participated in a reimbursement system by which patients are billed according to their medical diagnosis and other variables as determined by the N.J. State Department of Health. These rates are established by the Diagnosis-Related Groupings (DRGs)—a classification system developed by the Center for Health Service Research at Yale University (Michelette and Toth, 1981). DRGs are a method of clustering patients using the medical model and are based on shared clinical characteristics and the diverse utilization of clinical and technical resources (N.J. State Department of Health, 1978). Within this system patients are categorized by their primary and secondary medical diagnoses, age, and absence or presence of surgery. The system was created by a registered nurse to evaluate quality and utilization in hospitals. The system is excellent for predicting lengths of patient stays so that utilization review can concentrate on the atypical patient (Bentley and Butler, 1980).

The system develops an "average" patient for the state. For example, every patient who enters an N.J. hospital for coronary bypass surgery (DRG 106 or 107) is reviewed. Then an average reimbursement rate based on the average costs of all like hospitals is determined. In the same manner, an average length of stay for this patient based on the average length of stay in all like hospitals is established. The system classifies hospitals as urban, suburban, rural, major teaching, minor teaching, and nonteaching. Only like hospitals are compared. Obviously the length of stay and costs would be very different if you compared a patient in a major teaching urban hospital with a patient in a nonteaching rural hospital.

The system includes 467 DRGs in 23 major diagnostic categories (MDCs). DRGs provide a measure of output so that all direct patient care costs for any given DRG can be identified and apportioned for each patient relative to the total cost of care for all patients in that DRG in a given hospital. This apportionment includes the costs for ancillary, hotel, and nursing services.

The current system for reimbursing nursing services in most U.S. hospitals is based on a per diem or patient day rate. That is, the costs of all nursing services are divided by the number of patient days spent in the hospital and an average rate is determined. The resulting per diem rate is then multiplied by the average length of stay to determine the total cost (Figure 1). Therefore the patient who undergoes an appendectomy is charged the same daily rate as the patient who undergoes open heart surgery, and third-party payers pay the same rate. This system is completely insensitive to patient needs, patient utilization of services, and especially the type and mix of nursing services provided.

Early in the development of the DRG system in New Jersey, nursing leaders recognized the importance of these changes. Through the state nurses association, they had major input into the entire system and convinced the state Department of Health to seek separate federal funding for the Case-Mix Nursing Performance Study. Of the 18 states that use a prospective reimbursement system based on diagnosis, New Jersey is the only state with this

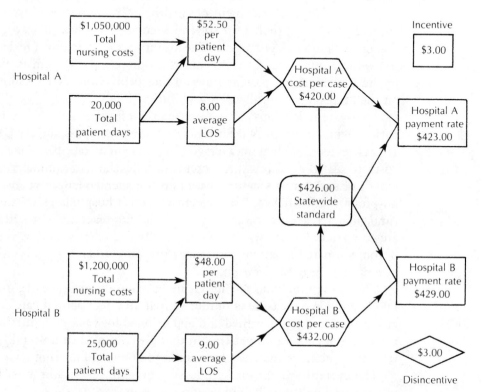

FIGURE 1   Per diem allocation: nursing cost component of direct patient care costs for DRG "X." Whereas the illustration deals with nursing care costs only, the statewide average actually deals with all direct patient care costs. The payment rate is determined by the homogeneity of the DRG's resource use and is expressed as a percentage. In this example, 50% of the hospitals average cost per case and 50% of the statewide average cost per case are used to blend a payment rate for each hospital as incentive-based reimbursement. (See Figure 2 for a comparison with RIM allocation.)

extensive nursing involvement and a separate nursing component. The goals of the Case-Mix Nursing Performance Study were to:

1. Design a more accurate alternative to the patient day for allocating nursing costs by using patient type instead of patient day as the unit of analysis
2. Generate management reports that should provide an expanded information system to facilitate the ability of nursing and hospital administration to assess an institution's activities and cost performance within the context of the incentive and efficiency standards

In this study the Department of Health, through its nursing consultants, conducted a patient classification system acuity study to develop a method for allocating nursing costs. This system is based on nursing intervention in five areas: (1) assessment of or planning with patient and/or significant others, (2) health teaching and information giving, (3) emotional support and counseling, (4) medication, treatments, and special care associated with the medical regimen, and (5) intervention for physical functioning. The first three numbers and last areas account for independent nursing interventions, and the fourth area accounts for dependent functions (Table 1). Each of the five areas is further broken down into levels of intensity—I minimum, II subacute, III acute, and IV intensive. (This last level does not connote patients who are in intensive care units.) Each patient on each shift is categorized

TABLE 1   Patient classification system acuity instrument continuum of patient needs

Nursing intervention dimensions	I Minimum	II Subacute	III Acute	IV Intensive	Direct patient care concerns
Assessment of or planning with patient and/or significant others					
Health teaching and information giving					
Emotional support and counseling					
Medication, treatments, and special care associated with medical regimen					
Intervention for physical functioning					

From a perspective reimbursement system based on case mix for New Jersey Hospital, 1976-1978: patient classification system/acuity instrument pretest instruction manual, New Jersey State Dept. of Health, Trenton, N.J., July 1977, p. 7.

TABLE 2   Second nursing intervention dimension: health teaching and information giving

I Minimum	II Subacute	III Acute	IV Intensive
Orientation: to unit, personnel, and policies Nursing interventions: to meet patient needs will *vary* based on patient's hospital experiences (admission or readmission to this or any hospital), anxiety level, personality factors, etc. Examples: explanation of procedures: admission process; routine diagnostic tests; review of discharge instructions	Routine: medical, preoperative and postoperative teaching Nursing interventions: to meet patient needs will *vary* based on prior experiences, anxiety level, personality factors, etc. Examples: deep-breathing exercises (short-term); explanation of diagnostic tests; explanation of treatments; explanation of medications to be administered by hospital personnel	Review: of initial health teaching to evaluate learning and/or retention; follow-up and return demonstration (when appropriate) Nursing interventions: to meet patient needs will *vary* based on acceptance of illness, ability and/or willingness to learn, language and socioeconomic factors; consultation with appropriate resource persons is necessary Examples: reinforce teaching urine testing for sugar; reinforce self-administration of insulin; utilize an interpreter to aid in teaching	Preliminary education: of patient and/or significant others in *health maintenance* where *changes in life style* caused by health problems are *anticipated after discharge* Education: of patients and/or significant others when there is a history of and/or demonstrated noncompliance Nursing interventions: to meet patient needs will *vary* based on degree of integrity of adaptive processes, family support, etc.; referral to appropriate resource persons is necessary Examples: teaching urine testing for sugar; teaching self-administration of insulin; motivating patient to adhere to medical regimen

From a perspective reimbursement system based on case mix for New Jersey Hospital, 1976-1978: patient classification system/acuity instrument pretest instruction manual, New Jersey State Dept. of Health, Trenton, N.J., July 1977, p. 11.

according to these dimensions. For example, if a patient needed only an orientation to the unit, an explanation of the admission procedure, routine diagnostic tests, and a beginning review of discharge instructions, he would be classified in the second category, health teaching, as minimum care or intensity I. If, however, he also required teaching urine testing, self-administration of insulin, diabetic care, and ways to adhere to the medical regimen, he would be classified in this same category, but as an intensity IV (Table 2).

Nursing activity data from these studies were used to develop relative intensity measures (RIMs). RIMs do not indicate what should be, but what is. RIMs are an allocation statistic that can distribute nursing costs based on the relationship between the intensity of nursing care and the actual nursing costs (Figure 2). We found, using a multiple regression analysis, that length

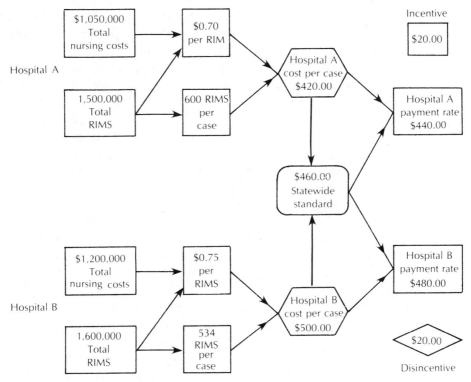

FIGURE 2 RIM allocation: nursing cost component of direct patient care costs for DRG "X." Whereas the illustration deals with nursing care costs only, the statewide average actually deals with all direct patient care costs. The payment rate is determined by the homogeneity of the DRG's resource use and is expressed as a percentage. In this example, 50% of the hospitals average cost per case and 50% of the statewide average cost per case are used to blend a payment rate for each hospital as incentive-based reimbursement. (See Figure 1 for a comparison with per diem allocation.)

of stay, age, and surgical intervention were the most significant predictors of nursing intensity. The medical diagnosis, as one might suppose, had very little significance (N.J. State Department of Health, 1978).

RIMs not only provided nursing service administrators with the first real management tool they ever had to truly predict budget and staffing requirements but also the first comprehensive statistical data base that could be used to develop nursing into a revenue-producing cost center. And herein lies the challenge. Nursing is traditionally 40% to 65% of a hospital's budget. If we can generate income by creative management and quality outcomes, our financial base will become the power needed to make the changes we all talk about. We can have the control and autonomy so often afforded only to our physician colleagues.

One of the last components of the Case-Mix Nursing Performance Study was Task 17. Unfortunately, funding was not provided to complete this component. However, many nurses in New Jersey are interested enough to seek outside funding and complete Task 17 as a private research project. Task 17 involved the collection of nursing diagnoses from the medical abstracts to assess the quality of nursing care in terms of process and to provide a framework for examining nursing costs (N.J. State Department of Health, 1978). This project is highly innovative and controversial, especially since it relates nursing diagnosis to medical diagnosis. In Task 17, we used twenty-eight nursing diagnoses, identified by the First and Second National Conferences on the Classification of Nursing Diagnoses.

Since most patient classification systems have been based on a task-oriented approach, using nursing diagnoses represented a departure by emphasizing the professionalism of nursing as advocated in the N.J. Nursing Practice Act (1979, p. 13) which charges us with "diagnosing and treating human responses to actual or potential physical and emotional health problems, through such services as case-finding, health teaching, health counseling and provision of care supportive to or restorative of life and well-being, and executing medical regimens."

The responsible registered nurse establishes nursing interventions to be used by all staff members as a basis for administering individualized patient care by daily monitoring patients' responses to the prescribed interventions and by maintaining interventions that are timely. Using the system, a registered nurse can map patients' progress as they move along the health care continuum during hospitalization (N.J. State Department of Health, 1977).

I believe that certain nursing diagnoses will cluster around certain medical diagnoses. If this is true, the DRG reports could include the DRG number, patient age, primary and secondary medical diagnoses, absence or presence of surgery, and primary and secondary nursing diagnoses. With this combination we could realistically project not only length of stay, but also intensity and level of nursing care required (RN, LPN, nursing assistant) and, therefore, the actual cost of services. It would truly be the first prospective management tool available to nurse managers.

There is one major common denominator in the current DRG system and the Case-Mix Nursing Performance Study—length of stay as a predictive variable. Physicians can have an impact on the system by medical diagnosis or by prescribing surgery. Nurses can have an impact on neither; but we can and should have an impact on the length of stay. If the care we provide is effective, the patient receives concentrated or high intensive comprehensive care over a short period. Patients are discharged because they no longer need nursing care. Since length of stay also determines the rate of reimbursement for a hospital, nurses have a great influence.

Table 3 is a partial listing of MDC #5, Diseases and Disorders of the

TABLE 3   **Major diagnostic category 5: diseases and disorders of the circulatory system**

DRG number	Definition	Outlier trim point Low	High
(103)	Heart transplant	1	99
(104)	Valve O.R. procedure with pump, w cardiac catheterization	12	28
(105)	Valve O.R. procedure with pump, wo cardiac catheterization	10	27
(106)	Coronary bypass, w cardiac catheterization	13	31
(107)	Coronary bypass, wo cardiac catheterization	9	23
(108)	Other cardio-thoracic O.R. procedure with pump	8	19
(109)	Other cardio-thoracic O.R. procedure without pump	3	32
(110)	Vascular O.R. procedure, w major reconstruction, w age 70 cc	7	38
(111)	Vascular O.R. procedure, w major reconstruction, wo age 70 cc	7	22
(112)	Vascular O.R. procedure, except major reconstruction	3	25
(113)	Amputation, except upper limb and/or toe	8	31
(114)	Amputation, upper limb and/or toe	8	31
(115)	Permanent pacemaker implantation, w principal diagnosis of AMI or CHF	7	31
(116)	Permanent pacemaker implantation, wo principal diagnosis of AMI or CHF	4	25
(117)	Pacemaker replacement and/or revision, wo pulse generator	2	19
(118)	Pacemaker replacement and/or revision, w pulse generator	2	10
(119)	Vein ligation and stripping	3	11
(120)	Other circulatory system O.R. procedure	4	42
(121)	Circulatory disorder with acute myocardial infarction, discharged alive, with cardiovascular complications, medical	9	28
(122)	Circulatory disorder with acute myocardial infarction, discharged alive, wo cardiovascular complications, medical	7	22
(123)	Circulatory disorder with acute myocardial infarction, discharged dead, medical	1	10
(124)	Circulatory disorder wo acute myocardial infarction, w cardiac catheterization, w complex diagnoses, medical	2	23
(125)	Circulatory disorder wo acute myocardial infarction, w cardiac catheterization, wo complex diagnoses, medical	2	5
(126)	Acute and/or subacute endocarditis, medical	6	70
(127)	Heart failure and/or shock, medical	4	17
(128)	Deep vein thrombophlebitis, medical	5	21
(129)	Cardiac arrest, medical	1	20

From DRG list regulation, New Jersey State Dept. of Health, Trenton, N.J., Jan. 7, 1982, p. 8.

Circulatory System. The MDC contains eighty-seven DRGs, of which twenty-seven are listed in Table 3. The left-hand column is the DRG number with a descriptive definition. The two right-hand columns indicate the standard or average length of stay for N.J. hospitals. Each length of stay is a range from the least number of inpatient days to the maximum number of inpatient days. If a patient is discharged from the hospital within the range, a hospital receives the full DRG rate. The rate usually reflects the median cost plus an equalization factor. Therefore if the range is 1 to 99 days, as shown for DRG 103, the hospital receives a rate that is commensurate with the cost of 49 to 50 inpatient days plus the equalization factor. Obviously then a hospital can make a net gain or an "incentive" if the patient is discharged at the lower end of the range. If the patient is discharged outside the range, either on the lower or upper end, the hospital is reimbursed a direct cost that is based on the per diem rate. There is no chance to create any incentive, and the hospital actually loses money on the cases. Therefore the goal is to discharge the patient within the range, but at the lower end. Additionally, the sooner one patient can be discharged, the sooner another patient can be admitted, thereby ensuring a higher rate of occupancy. Since the system is prospective, one can predict from 1 year to another the occupancy rate and the mix or types of DRGs that will be in a facility. From the projection, the costs for the next fiscal year can be determined. Should there be a change in occupancy rate or the DRG mix, provision is made for the fluctuations.

Now let us look at the effect of nursing diagnosis on this system. Gordon's concept of nursing diagnosis (1978) contains three components: (1) a concise description of the state of the patient—the problem, (2) the probable etiology of the problem, and (3) the defining signs and symptoms. Identifying all three components assists in identifying the appropriate and specific therapy required to correct a problem. When properly used, the model not only suggests the necessary intervention but the proposed goal or outcome of the intervention. Likewise, DRGs are measures of outcomes. We can assess a patient's needs at point A, admission, and formulate the appropriate nursing diagnosis to get him to point B, discharge. The interventions are then implemented to move the patient from point A to point B. If we want the patient to reach point B within the standard length of stay, we can plan the intensity of the interventions necessary to do this within the timeframe and which nursing personnel are necessary to provide that intensity. The system now provides for planned professional therapy rather than routine hospital tasks based on traditional timeframes and services. It is no longer crisis intervention but a planned, goal-oriented approach. If the patient does not reach point B within the given timeframe, we must reexamine our assessments, treatments, and any other variables that may have affected the plan. Most often, however, therapeutic plans can be predicted to their final outcome. We can literally plot a patient's course of care across a continuum just as we can plot management or educational objectives and goals.

The obvious argument is that patients are people and therefore unpredictable in circumstances in which their integrity is jeopardized. That is true. It simply means, however, that nurses must become expert at assessing patient needs and at diagnosing based on the assessment and not on any prejudged criteria. We can no longer assume that a patient who is dying is fearful or that a patient who has learned to give his own insulin understands his diabetic regimen. We cannot assume anything; we must know for sure. It also means that we cannot set goals that are our goals or that we think the patient should achieve. We must set mutual goals. Point B must be the outcome the patient desires.

The entire DRG concept provides a tool not only for planning staffing but also for evaluating the quality of care given. For example, if a nurse's patients never reach point B within the prescribed time, it may indicate that the nurse is a poor assessor or planner or is weak in implementation. If the problem involves only one DRG, it may indicate a weakness in one clinical area and a need for additional education in that area. Once nurses learn to accurately predict point B or length of stay, they can have an impact on the reimbursement system equal to that of physicians.

Remember that each time you discharge a patient at the lower end of the length of stay range, the hospital receives an incentive. If nurses could effectively get every patient in every DRG discharged at the lower end of the spectrum, they would realize for their institutions a tremendous monetary gain over costs, thereby becoming a revenue-producing cost center. It would be the first time in history that this ever occurred.

To become this effective, one other component is paramount and was validated in the Case-Mix Nursing Performance Study. In New Jersey an average of 36% of the nurse's day is spent in nonnursing activities. Historically we have all known that, but now it has been demonstrated. To provide the intensity necessary to become revenue generating, we must relinquish *all* non-nursing activities to other hospital departments. We cannot afford to empty the trash on the 11 PM to 7 AM shift, wrap bedpans for central supply, clean stretchers for housekeeping, do medication inventories for pharmacy, serve trays for dietary, or transport patients for other ancillary departments unless indicated for nursing reasons. We must give up the traditional handmaiden tasks to free us to do nursing care only. Anyone who is not willing to fight to relinquish nonnursing tasks does not belong in nursing management today. For it will be a fight and a hard one. It is very difficult to convince hospital administrators that although we have done these tasks for many years we cannot afford to do them anymore. It is always possible to change an opinion when you can show a less expensive way of getting the same task accomplished. My philosophy has always been that nothing is impossible, it just takes a little longer.

Since most U.S. hospitals do not use a prospective reimbursement system, how can they use nursing diagnosis for budgetary purposes? Once again, since nursing diagnoses are outcome predictors, they can help any nursing department to plan staffing needs. Since a nursing department's budget is labor intensive and also based on outcome criteria, it follows that one can assist in predicting the other. For example, if you know that patients in a given DRG generally have a given nursing diagnosis that requires an RN rather than an LPN for a given number of days and if you also know that this year you had 100 such patients in your facility, you can predict how many RNs and how many days will be needed to care for the patients next year provided all other variables remain constant. If a hospital does not use the DRG system, patients can be manually classified, solely by nursing diagnosis and standard lengths of stay in the hospital. Length of stay can be manually calculated from current medical abstracts.

If a universal taxonomy of nursing diagnoses existed, nurses in one hospital could call another hospital and make comparisons. How many days do your acute diabetic patients who are noncompliant with therapy because of a knowledge deficit stay in your hospital as compared with mine? Is your length of stay shorter because you assign a clinical nurse specialist to that patient for the first 2 days? We can learn from our colleagues in medicine in this regard. I hope that the outcome of the national conferences will provide our profession with a standardized set of labels for describing not only what we assess, but what we do.

A universal taxonomy could also make direct third-party reimbursement easier to achieve. Just as there is now a "reasonable" rate prescribed for a medical diagnosis, the same could be true for a nursing diagnosis that is a descriptor of service mix and service intensity. Certainly reimbursement should not be based on wage and salary guides or "going-rate" criteria but on actual cost to a patient based on a need/response analysis, which nursing diagnoses describe very adequately.

Most hospitals today are also using some form of patient classification system to determine staffing requirements. If a patient classification system were based on nursing diagnoses, several forms of data would be generated by one collection tool. Nursing diagnoses provide a true picture of a patient because they classify a set or sets of responses by a patient to a condition and treatment. Nursing diagnoses are much more sensitive and therefore more comprehensive than medical diagnoses. For example, a myocardial infarction medically is a myocardial infarction. But a myocardial infarction from a nursing perspective is not just another myocardial infarction. To distinguish one from the other you must use nursing diagnoses. The nursing diagnostic labels then can justify or substantiate the category within which a nurse places a patient. They provide a natural check and balance system that can become the basis for budget appeals. You can demonstrate statistically to your administrators that the types of myocardial infarction are either different from the types treated in the other hospitals in your area or that your staff members treat patients differently in your hospital (and be prepared to justify why), which also explains your uniqueness. Care plans and classification systems based on nursing diagnoses can identify the uniqueness unequivocally.

Because of the potential power the DRG system gives nursing, there is a great deal of opposition to it from the hospital industry. Unfortunately, nurses are more likely to hear the words of anyone other than nursing peers. Because the nursing budget is such a substantial part of a hospital's budget and because nursing care can have such a major impact on that budget by means of length of stay and revenue production, few nurses are willing to confront the industry. Armed with financial management sophistication and a national effort, we could either generate millions of dollars or bankrupt the entire system. The status quo services the industry and nurses who are afraid of change or unwilling to accept true professional autonomy. The status quo does not, however, service the consumer, of whom we say we are advocates, nor our profession.

Opponents say that the system will actually force hospital administrators to cut staff. It is true that the system forces management to become more efficient, but staffing cannot be cut if it can be demonstrated that registered nurses are indispensable and necessary for the efficiency management is trying to achieve. Nursing has not until now had the tools to do that.

Opponents say that you cannot measure what a nurse does because too many variables are involved. Is it just possible that the variables have been within our reach to control and we just have not had the knowledge or courage to stretch out and grab hold?

The nursing profession is just becoming aware of its potential power through collective bargaining. If we suddenly came to the realization that we could also control the very reimbursement system from which we are desperately trying to gain more, we would become a force that would shake the very foundation of every health care institution in the country. Karenga was quoted as saying that a revolution is merely "the creation of an alternative" (Brussell, 1970, p. 496). Isn't it time for an alternative? Patients cannot afford the current system. Hospitals and physicians gain money and prestige on the sweat of nurses, and nurses remain overworked, underpaid, inappropriately used, and told to like it because it is a "calling." We perpetuate this lopsided system by refusing to change, disagreeing among ourselves, refusing to trust our peers, downgrading education, objecting to involvement in fiduciary and management principles because "it isn't nursing, it isn't taking care of patients," and in continuing to believe that we are powerless.

When nursing service directors, through creative management, can make

$20.00 on a DRG and keep that in their cost centers to be used for nursing as they see fit, that is power to control. When nursing service directors can demonstrate statistically that patients can be treated effectively and discharged within 7 days instead of 10 days, that is power to bargain. When they can prove that an all-RN staff can lower the length of stay, that is power to create change. All of these powers are for self-actualization. We must take this power. We must earn it, and we can by using nursing diagnoses for financial management purposes. With self-actualization comes self-satisfaction, and that leads to a final quotation from Henry Labouchere, who said that self-satisfaction is "believing that the ace of trumps is up your sleeve and that God Almighty put it there" (Brussell, 1970, p. 520). Who am I to reject a gift from up above.

REFERENCES

Bentley, J., and Butler, P.: Case-mix reimbursement: measures, applications, experiments, Hosp. Finan. Manage. **10**(2):24-35, 1980.

Brussell, E.E., ed.: Dictionary of quotable definitions, Englewood Cliffs, N.J., 1970, Prentice-Hall, Inc.

Gordon, M.: Classification of nursing diagnosis, J. NY State Nurs. Assoc. **9**:5, 1978.

Michlette, J., and Toth, R.: Diagnosis-related groups: impact and implications, Supervisor Nurse **12**:33, 1981.

New Jersey State Department of Health: Nursing practice act, P.L. 1947, c. 262, as amended, Newark, 1979, New Jersey Board of Nursing.

New Jersey State Department of Health: A prospective reimbursement system based on patient case-mix for New Jersey hospitals 1976-1978, Nursing diagnosis instrument pretest instruction manual, Trenton, N.J., 1977, The Department.

New Jersey State Department of Health: A prospective reimbursement system based on patient case-mix for New Jersey hospitals 1976-1983, Second annual report, vol. 1, Trenton, N.J., 1978, The Department.

New Jersey State Department of Health: A prospective reimbursement system based on patient case-mix for New Jersey Hospitals 1976-1983, Case-mix reimbursement and DRG nursing cost allocation, Trenton, N.J., 1980, The Department.

CHAPTER 4

Research

Abstracts submitted for possible presentation at the conference were processed by a blind review process, and each selected paper was assigned to the formal, poster, or small group session to maximize the information disseminated. Research papers are at different levels of sophistication in terms of study design, data analysis, and interpretation of data. Selections based solely on the quality of abstracts may have had some bearing on this phenomenon. Research studies in progress were included only to indicate our commitment to research endeavors on nursing diagnoses and to highlight different methodologies that may prove useful for further studies.

Questions raised by the investigators and the ways in which the investigators conducted the research varied. Many studies lacked sufficient sample size and external validity, while some researchers demonstrated significant findings that will have an impact on future studies. Numerous retrospective studies indicate the need for descriptive data. Some evaluation data on the use of nursing diagnoses in clinical settings clearly indicate that the nursing practice indeed can be improved when nursing diagnoses actualize the nursing process. New nursing diagnoses that were generated from these studies need to be examined at the Sixth National Conference so that nurses can gain access to the diagnoses for discussion and approval.

| Section I | **Formal presentation** |

Essential features of a nursing diagnosis

JOYCE K. SHOEMAKER, R.N., Ed.D.

This paper gives the highlights of a research study recently completed in partial fulfillment of my doctoral requirements at Teachers College, Columbia University. The project was quite extensive; therefore, my presentation will be limited to a brief discussion of the purpose, rationale, and method of the study and some of the most interesting findings.

PURPOSE

The primary purpose of the study was to come to a clearer understanding of the meaning of the term *nursing diagnosis.* Specifically, the purpose was to determine whether consensus could be reached on the following:
1. Essential characteristics of a nursing diagnosis
2. Features that are not essential to the use of the term but that help to explain its meaning
3. Features that are not appropriate to its use
4. The context conditions that govern the use of the term

Secondary purposes were related to identification of similarities and differences between nursing and medical diagnoses and to a determination of whether clinical practice and functional roles have any bearing on a nurse's definition and use of the term. However, this report will be confined to the characteristics of a nursing diagnosis.

RATIONALE

As a member of a graduate faculty some years ago, I perceived a common concern on the part of all instructional staff members for ensuring that the graduate nursing students were competent to provide nursing care within a framework of the nursing process. My own interactions with students provided ample evidence of their acquaintance with the nursing process as a result of their baccalaureate preparation. However, without exception, students assessed, planned, implemented, and occasionally evaluated without ever having stated a nursing diagnosis. In discussions with colleagues, we

☐Paper based on Shoemaker, J.K.: The concept of nursing diagnoses, unpublished doctoral dissertation, New York, 1982, Teachers College, Columbia University.

agreed that this element seemed to be generally overlooked on the baccalaureate level and needed to be dealt with early in the graduate curriculum. Students in this program were recruited from baccalaureate programs throughout the United States; therefore, my hunch was that nursing diagnosis was not included as an essential component of the nursing process in most undergraduate curricula.

Further discussions with colleagues revealed a more fundamental concern—the lack of agreement about the nature of a nursing diagnosis. Small wonder, then, that the students had difficulty understanding the concept. This fact convinced me to do a review of the literature with the intent of convincing my colleagues that my definition was valid. What I found, however, was that no definition was acceptable to everyone. This finding was further reinforced through my attendance at the Second National Conference on the Classification of Nursing Diagnosis in which I had the opportunity to work with a group of highly committed individuals on the refinement of a label. The completion of the task was significantly hampered by a multiplicity of variations within the group on a basic understanding of the meaning of the term. Intuitively, then, I believed that the work of the National Group on the Classification of Nursing Diagnoses could be facilitated if we could agree on the characteristics of a nursing diagnosis.

METHOD

The Soltis paradigm for analysis of concepts was selected as a framework for the study (Soltis, 1978). This method consists of strategies for identifying generic, differentiation, and conditions features of a concept.

The premise of a generic analysis is that some model cases of a concept are accepted as such; however, the generic features of the concept are not clearly understood. The prior question is, what features must x have to be called an X? To illustrate the application of generic analysis, one can use the concept of a square. The prior question is, what features must a two-dimensional figure have to be called a square? By thinking of standard uses of the term, one determines that a necessary feature is that it must have four sides. One then asks the question, is it possible to draw a square that does not have four sides? If not, then four sides is a necessary feature of a square. But can one draw a four-sided figure that is not a square? Using contrary cases, one determines that there are four-sided figures that are not squares, the implication being that four sides is a necessary but not sufficient feature. Through continued use of model cases and contrary cases, one finally concludes that the essential features—those that are both necessary and sufficient for clarification of the term—include four equal sides with internal angles being right angles.

The premise of a differentiation analysis is that a concept has more than one meaning and that these meanings and the bases for them are not clear. The prior question is, what are the basic (different) meanings of *X*? The strategy, then, consists of searching for standard uses of the concept, classifying them, and, if possible, searching for distinguishing characteristics of each type. Examples are used to test the typology. The intended result of this strategy is to arrive at "a clearer idea of the logical terrain covered by different meanings of a concept" (Soltis, 1978, p. 102).

To illustrate the application of differentiation analysis, one can use the concept of *material object*. Generic analysis reveals that features of a material object include having visible form, mass, and capability of being perceived through the senses. But if the analysis stops there, then all material objects are lumped together and the term remains vague. The prior question, therefore, is, what are the different basic meanings of the term *material object*? Examples of intuitive uses of the term suggest that material objects can be classified as animal, vegetable, or mineral. The range and adequacy of this classification are tested through examples, and then the key characteristics of each category are identified. Differentiation analysis, therefore, is a means of determining the use of the term as it applies to different kinds of things.

Conditions analysis is based on the premise that undisputed model cases are not available and that standard uses of a concept are altered by the context in which they are used. The prior question is, what context conditions govern the *use* of X? The strategy begins with identifying a necessary condition for the concept of X; altering the context and looking for examples in which condition holds, but the concept is not present; examining other contexts and their conditions; and testing the necessity and sufficiency of the identified conditions. The intended result is to develop a clearer understanding of the various contexts in which a concept is used.

Using the example of the term *seeing*, one asks the prior question, what are the logical conditions for properly using the term *seeing*? Clearly, the presence of eyes that are functional and open is a fundamental condition. Further analysis reveals that a material object must be within the visual field and the subject must be able to discriminate that object. These conditions are identified by the use of examples and contrary examples of context conditions that test for necessity and sufficiency.

The seventy variables related to nursing diagnosis that were identified from the literature were categorized into generic, differentiation, and conditions features, consistent with the Soltis technique for analysis.

A Delphi study was then conducted. A Delphi study is a method of seeking group consensus through a series of mailed questionnaires. This method is characterized by the following features:

1. A panel of experts or informed individuals is identified.
2. The membership of the panel and their individual responses remain anonymous throughout the study.

3. The questionnaires provide feedback from previous rounds regarding positions taken by the panel and the reasons for these positions. This feedback provides opportunities for panelists to change their positions as more thought is given to the question.

An obvious advantage of the Delphi study is that it permits individuals residing in remote locations to work together on a problem. In addition, it avoids domination of outspoken individuals in the group process, unwillingness of individuals to take a stand on an issue before the position of the majority is known, and public contradiction of participants in higher positions. It also facilitates discarding a position once it has been taken, and it encourages initiation of ideas without loss of face.

The study panel consisted of 111 nurses throughout the United States and Canada, all of whom had a minimum of a master's degree with a nursing major. Doctorate degrees had been earned by 22% of the panel members. All the panelists had identifiable knowledge of nursing diagnosis through research, publications, or workshop leadership.

In the first round of the Delphi study, panelists were asked to rank each of the variables as essential, important but not essential, useful for explaining the term, or reject because not appropriate. They were also asked to give reasons for their rankings. The responses and reasons were then collated, and the second round of the Delphi study was prepared. It included the original seventy variables with statistics, including the median and interquartile range for each response. It also included a collation of the reasons given for each response and the individual panelist's original position on each variable. Panelists were asked to reconsider positions on the basis of the new data. The third round of the Delphi study consisted only of variables that needed further clarification by the panel. In addition, the panel was asked to rank key phrases in an effort to construct a general definition of nursing diagnosis using nomenclature acceptable to the majority of the participants.

This discussion of the findings of the Delphi study is confined to those variables that were identified as essential and those that were rejected. It is important to note that no one feature that was identified can stand alone. Only collectively can these features be considered both necessary and sufficient.

Generic features considered essential are as follows:

1. A nursing diagnosis is a statement of a patient-client problem.
2. A nursing diagnosis refers to a health state.
3. A nursing diagnosis refers to a potential health problem.
4. A nursing diagnosis is a conclusion resulting from identification of a pattern or cluster of signs and symptoms.
5. A nursing diagnosis is based on subjective and/or objective data that can be confirmed.

Differentiation features considered essential are as follows:
1. A nursing diagnosis is a statement of a *nursing* judgment.
2. A nursing diagnosis refers to a condition that nurses are licensed to treat.
3. A nursing diagnosis refers to physical, psychologic, sociocultural, and spiritual conditions.
4. A nursing diagnosis is a short, concise statement.
5. A nursing diagnosis is a two-part statement that includes the etiology when known.

Conditions features considered essential are as follows:
1. A nursing diagnosis refers to conditions that can be treated independently by a nurse.
2. Nurse practitioners who function in expanded roles should clearly differentiate between the nursing and the medical diagnoses they make.
3. A nursing diagnosis should be validated with the client whenever possible.
4. Diagnosing is an independent nursing function.

Variables that were rejected are as follows:
1. A nursing diagnosis is a statement of a nursing problem.
2. A nursing diagnosis is a statement of a nursing concern.
3. A nursing diagnosis is a statement of a patient-client need.
4. A nursing diagnosis is a statement of a potential health problem only if it is immediate in nature.
5. A nursing diagnosis is a conclusion based on a single sign or symptom.
6. A nursing diagnosis is a statement reflecting a diagnostic procedure, a medical regimen, equipment used in a medical regimen, or a nursing activity.
7. A nursing diagnosis is a statement of an interpersonal problem the nurse has with the client.
8. A nursing diagnosis is a statement that no problems exist that require nursing intervention.
9. A nursing diagnosis is a statement that includes the care required by the individual.
10. A nursing diagnosis is a statement that expresses a value judgment of a nurse.
11. A nursing diagnosis is the same as the medical diagnosis.
12. A nursing diagnosis is stated in a summarizing paragraph.
13. A confirmed medical diagnosis is necessary to the determination of a nursing diagnosis.
14. A nursing diagnosis is valid only if corroborated with the physician.

15. A nursing diagnosis must be congruent with the diagnoses of all other professionals caring for the patient.
16. Nursing diagnoses are limited to those conditions that any nurse can recognize and treat in any setting.

DISCUSSION OF FINDINGS

First, my definition of a nursing diagnosis is presented. This definition is consistent with the essential characteristics agreed on by the panel and uses terminology agreed on in the third round of the Delphi study. The definition is as follows: *a nursing diagnosis is a clinical judgment about an individual, family, or community that is derived through a deliberate, systematic process of data collection and analysis. It provides the basis for prescriptions for definitive therapy for which the nurse is accountable. It is expressed concisely and includes the etiology of the condition when known.*

A review of the data from the second and third rounds of the Delphi study suggests some interesing findings in relation to several of the variables. At the conclusion of the second round, there was a strong trend toward consensus relative to several features, although the 50th percentile was not reached. For example, 44% of the panel considered "a nursing impression" as a useful but not important feature and 43% rejected it. By collapsing those two categories, one can postulate that as a characteristic it is not worthy of further consideration. Similarly, "a statement that includes the client's strengths," "a statement that describes a patient-client behavior," "a statement that includes signs and symptoms," and "a statement that describes a healthy response that may require reinforcing" might be considered in the same way, since the majority of the panelists ranked them in the useful or reject categories. On the other hand, "a statement that includes modifiers describing degrees of intensity" was rated as essential by 40% of the panel and as important by 44%. Though consensus was not reached at the 50th percentile, collapsing of those categories leads one to believe that a significant percentage of the panel viewed this characteristic favorably. A major reason for lack of consensus was that panelists believed that degrees of intensity had not been well defined, which suggests an area for further investigation.

The statement, "Nursing diagnoses must be based on a standardized nomenclature," was ranked in the essential category by 42% of the panel and as important by 31%. Again, these data imply that this is a characteristic with substantial support. Opposition to the characteristic was related to concern that standardization would not take into consideration nomenclature that is consistent with the variety of practice models that are currently used, which suggests a position that should be of concern to the National Group on the Classification of Nursing Diagnoses as it continues its deliberations.

The data from the third round in which panelists were given a choice of statements with similar meanings revealed some results worthy of mention. The statement, "A nursing diagnosis refers to a client's response to an illness," had previously reached consensus in the important category. Rewording to state, "A nursing diagnosis refers to a client's response to an unfavorable health state," resulted in 48% of the panel ranking it essential and 34% ranking it important. Though consensus was not reached, a significant percentage of the panel rated it as an essential or important feature because the reference to illness had been deleted. In my opinion, had that referent not been used at the outset of the study, this variable might have reached consensus in the essential category. Similarly, the statement, "A nursing diagnosis refers to health conditions of populations of people as well as individuals," did not reach consensus in the second round although 82% of the panel considered it either essential or important. Changing the referents in the third round to "individuals, families, groups, or communities" resulted in 80% of the panel considering it essential or important. This change clearly suggests that the majority of the panel supported the idea that a generic feature of a nursing diagnosis (worthy of further investigation) is the fact that the referent is not limited to the individual. This conclusion was further supported by the panel's preference for referents other than an individual when asked, in the third round, to rate the terminology they preferred to use in the definition.

In the first two rounds, a statement referring to environmental needs did not reach consensus. In the third round, the statement, "A nursing diagnosis refers to conditions affecting the client within the context of the environment," was considered essential by 47% of the panel and important by 49%. Though the results are not conclusive, based on the concern of some of the panelists that diagnoses should refer to the client rather than conditions affecting the client, it is my opinion that this variable should be investigated further.

Of particular interest is that some of the statements for which there was consensus included some implied philosophic beliefs about nursing. First, an essential feature of a nursing diagnosis is that it refers to a condition that nurses may legally treat. This feature demonstrates recognition of the legal basis for professional nursing practice, which no longer permits the nurse to rely solely on medical orders and judgments as a basis for nursing intervention. Second, there was recognition of the independence of professional nursing decisions while valuing the collaborative role of the nurse in relation to other health care providers. This independence was demonstrated by consensus of the panel that an essential condition for a nursing diagnosis is that it is an independent nursing function and that an important condition is consultation with other health care providers. This independence was also demonstrated when the panel rejected as conditions corroboration by the physician and congruency between the nursing diagnosis and diagnoses made by other health professionals.

Throughout this study there was a clearly implied value placed on health maintenance and health surveillance as a focus of nursing. This value was demonstrated by consensus of the panel that a potential problem is an essential feature of a nursing diagnosis and by their rejecting as a feature a potential problem only if it is immediate in nature, since immediacy limits health surveillance activities. Furthermore, the panel consistently had difficulty with statements that included references to "illness" or "problem," since use of those terms seemed to be in conflict with a health orientation.

In the third round of the study, the panel included spiritual conditions as a component of the assessment parameters that are essential considerations for nurses in making diagnoses. In the same round, there was no consensus on whether a diagnosis may apply to a state of the client for which the appropriate action is referral. However, there was consensus that an essential feature is that a nursing diagnosis refers to conditions that can be treated independently by a nurse. In view of this, there is a need to investigate the extent to which nurses feel competent to treat and do treat spiritual conditions without resorting to referrals. The panel's position with regard to spiritual conditions may be an outcome of the historic foundations of nursing in religious orders and not consistent with current practice.

There was no consensus by the panel regarding the condition that a nursing diagnosis is valid only if made by a professional nurse, that is, RN with BSN preparation. A major reason for lack of agreement was that data were not available to support this as a condition, which is consistent with the current controversy in nursing related to the educational preparation required for entry into professional nursing practice. An investigation of the relationship between the various basic levels of educational preparation for nursing and the ability to derive nursing diagnoses from clinical data would serve two purposes. First, it would confirm whether there is a basis for consideration of an academic degree as an essential condition for assuming responsibility for a nursing diagnosis. From a broader perspective, it would also identify one criterion for consideration in the confusion regarding differences between technical and professional nursing practice.

There was no agreement by the panel in response to two questions posed in the third round referring to relationships between the various practice models used in nursing and the types of diagnoses made and the terminology used in stating diagnoses. Because these two variables were introduced in the final round of the study, the panel did not have the advantage of reconsidering their positions on the basis of previous data. A study aimed at clarification of these points would have significant implications for the continuing development of a system for classification of nursing diagnoses. In my opinion the National Group on the Classification of Nursing Diagnoses must recognize the existence of multiple variations in conceptual models for practice that are reflective of the present state of the art in nursing. If a relationship exists between conceptual models and the types of diagnoses that are made and the terminology that is used, ignoring these variables or attempting to "force a fit" may result in resistance on the part of nurses to use the system that is finally developed.

Finally, the Soltis framework for analysis of concepts and the Delphi study were successful in producing group consensus in relation to essential and variant features of a nursing diagnoses. Many of the panelists found the framework for the study and the approach to be both stimulating and valuable as evidenced by the personal communications with me throughout the study. The Soltis framework and the Delphi method are recommended for additional investigation of some of the areas identified.

Many of you seated here were members of my panel. I want to thank you for your participation and for your thoughtful responses and thought-provoking comments throughout the study. Of the 111 panelists who began the study, 102 completed all three rounds. This represented an almost unheard of 92% return.

REFERENCES

Linstone, H.A., and Teroff, M., eds.: The Delphi method: techniques and applications, Reading, Mass., 1975, ed. 2, Addison-Wesley Publishing Co., Inc.

Shoemaker, J.K.: The concept of nursing diagnosis, unpublished doctoral dissertation, New York, 1982, Teachers College, Columbia University.

Soltis, J.F.: An introduction to the analysis of educational concepts, ed. 2, Reading, Mass., 1978, Addison-Wesley Publishing Co., Inc.

Strauss, H.J., and Zeigler, H.L.: The Delphi technique and its uses in social science research, J. Creat. Behav. 9:253, 1975.

Wilson, J.: Thinking with concepts, London, 1963, Cambridge University Press.

Discussion

Lois Hoskins: I am interested in a time relationship. Had the ANA's Social Policy Statement been published yet, and did you use it as a source for some of your variables?

Joyce Shoemaker: I did not.

Leona Parscenzo: Since your panel group did involve so many of the participants of this group, do you have any concern about generalizing your results to all nurses?

Joyce Shoemaker: Yes, I had some concern about that, but I think it was outweighed by the fact that I needed to identify informed individuals who were to participate in this study. It was clear, however, that there were some people on the panel, at least initially, who were not informed. They told me through personal communication that they had to put a great deal of thought into some of these variables and that they had learned a great deal through this study. One of the characteristics of the Delphi study is that opinions continue to change because there is always, on the part of the panel, an opportunity to exchange information with each other. But I was not able to identify another population that I felt in general would have been better subjects for the study.

Imogene King: I want to be sure that I heard one of your recommendations correctly and then ask a question. Did you, in fact, say that a recommendation from your study was to be sure not to bring any closure on some kind of conceptual framework to fit with the National Conference Group?

Joyce Shoemaker: That is my recommendation.

Imogene King: Did that flow from your data, or is that your personal recommendation?

Joyce Shoemaker: That is my personal recommendation.

Imogene King: All right. Then I guess I stand here as a member of that Theory Group and want to know why we were convened a few years ago and why we worked so hard to try to put something together which really came out of the initial diagnostic categories, not necessarily out of our own personal conceptual frameworks?

Joyce Shoemaker: I asked exactly the same question. In fact, at the Second National Conference (those of you who recall that conference), the conference participants were aware that there were theorists who were working very, very hard throughout that conference. We had relatively little contact with that group of theorists until the last day. During that period the other conference participants had been working in our small group sessions on various diagnostic labels. Then on the very last day, the Theorist Group presented their report, and we were then asked to go back to our small groups and rework our diagnostic labels within the framework of the Theory Group's conceptual framework that was presented to us, and I do not think it was done very successfully. Now I will admit that I purposely did not attend the next two national conferences while I was engaged in my study because I wanted to confine my discussions of nursing diagnosis to the Delphi study. But I have continually had some concern that there may very well be some resistance on the part of a significant population of nurses to attempt to force a fit. Now, if we can identify a framework that is general enough, that takes into consideration the various practice models that are being used with the conceptual frameworks that are being used, I would support that wholeheartedly. I do think we need to be very carful about the direction we move.

Sister Callista Roy: I appreciate bringing this issue back to the floor and would like first of all to make an historic clarification. The theorists first met at the Third National Conference. The idea of why we convened that year was because the National Group on the Classification of Nursing Diagnoses had not acted on a framework. I, as an individual, with the feeling similar to some of my colleagues about the need for something to hang this together, wrote a proposal to the Task Force and presented the notion of convening group to be of service and try to develop a framework out of what you were doing. The theorists were people who were invited. They were told that their skills in conceptualization, not their frameworks, were needed. So that was the basis on which we came together. We did homework, and so we were founded in 1977 after a Task Force meeting and worked by mail up until the Third National Conference. That was the first time we met face to face, and that is why we were meeting parallel with the total conference group. I also would like very much to reinforce Imogene's point that, yes, while there is some terminology that comes from one particular framework, the top section of the framework handout are assumptions about unitary man. And I do believe (without getting caught up with some of the terminology) that at this point, one survey shows that 50% of baccalaureate schools of nursing are now using systems frameworks, some kind of open systems framework. Nursing historically believed in holism long before holistic health came along. So, if you look at those assumptions and try not to get too hung up with the terminology and say "that is what we believe about people and health," the next section is called the framework, which is the nine patterns. Now we are asking the National Conference Group, "Do these nine patterns present a framework that can hang this thing together?" Only you can answer that question. So I agree with Joyce's concern about trying not to force a fit of one framework. But I also want you to clearly understand that that is not what we were trying to do. So, reread that sheet. Look at the assumptions and say, "Ah, there is really nothing there that we want to throw out." Except we do not want to create confusion by using words that do not have a clear meaning for everyone. I appreciate Joyce's study from the perspective of clarifying the concept of nursing diagnosis, and I appreciate this chance to respond to your recommendation.

Imogene King: I would like to stimulate your minds a little bit on this issue. We did discuss this in our Theorist Group. For all of you here who are concerned and resisting the term *unitary man,* let me give you some historic knowledge about that term. It came from the Greek philosophers, beginning probably with Aristotle or pre-Aristotelin philosophy when they debated philosophically for centuries whether the human being was composed of a body, or a mind, or a body and a mind. Centuries of debate in philosophic circles resulted in the fact that the human being is a combination of at least these two elements. The philosophers centuries ago coined the term *unitary man* when they came to grips with trying to answer this philosophic problem. If you really want to read about unitary man philosophically, there is a good book called *The Philosophy of Knowing.** So I would like for you (if you are resisting that term because you think it belongs to someones framework) to try and think of it in terms of a philosophic historic perspective. That is exactly how I think some of us in the Theorist Group thought of it. As Sister Callista Roy said, what came out of the group was really an analysis of the diagnostic categories. Out of that, we began to conceptualize what we presented at this conference. Now, I am going to inform you about two more things. When we did homework for this Theory Group meeting and I looked at the human interaction as part of that model, I went back to my theory book in which I have developed some concepts that I think are absolutely essential for professional nursing practice. One of the concepts is human interaction. I found that the nine terms resulting from the group process also relate to characteristics in my published work on the concept of human interaction. So there is some validation there. I have just finished a report of a study I conducted 2 years ago, called "A National Survey of Philosophies of Nursing Education." This study has findings generalizable to this nation. No one can fault the representative sample of the schools in this country—diploma, associated degree, and baccalaureate I do not think they can fault my research design. Since it is a representative sample from which I can generalize to this country, the major terms that were identified in the schools' philosophies that guide our educational programs should become the domain of nursing. The study shows that we should recognize that we do in fact need a common conceptual framework for our field. We need multiple theories but a common conceptual framework.

---

*Hassett, J.D., S.J., Mitchell, R.A., S.J., and Monan, J.D., S.J.: The philosophy of human knowing; Westminster, Md., 1955, The Newman Press.

Barbara Burke: I believe the purpose of all this is to provide something useful for practicing nurses. The term *unitary man* is one that we all understand and can embrace. Practicing nurses do not have that philosophic background, and I believe that that term may turn them off when they hear it.

Joyce Shoemaker: I am not going to comment on that except to say that I have accomplished my objective and that I wanted some discussion on it. In fact, I was absolutely certain that that statement would not go unchallenged.

Virginia Luetje: In the Delphi study, the first questionnaire that you used was long. Therefore I am wondering whether you thought that there was any kind of a fatigue factor operating in trying to make comments to your questions?

Joyce Shoemaker: It was long. Interestingly, it had been pilot tested with two different groups before using it. As part of the pilot, I asked those individuals to comment on how long it took them to complete. The average length of time was 30 minutes. When I received the results from the first round, some individuals told me, "I have worked on this for 3 hours." For the most part, my sense is that perhaps the difference was that part of the group did not perceive themselves as participating in the research as such and perhaps did not give as much thought to the questions. One of the things that I found so impressive was that 102 of the panelists hung in there through the whole thing despite having had such a long questionnaire.

Virginia Luetje: I think it is a fascinating approach to trying to find some consensus. I just want to applaud you on the effort.

Question: Were the research subjects using nursing diagnosis in clinical practice?

Joyce Shoemaker: The panel was made up of a representative sample of nurses who were educators, clinicians, researchers, and administrators. The largest group were educators, but very close behind that group were clinicians. All of the clinicians indicated to me that they were using nursing diagnoses in their clinical practice.

Lynda Carpenito: Since the inception of this group we have talked about the "professional nurse" and until a change occurs, the "professional nurse" is an AD, a diploma, or a baccalaureate prepared nurse. I am very concerned that we not give an impression to the nurses with an A.D. or diploma education that they cannot formulate a nursing diagnosis. Perhaps yes, indeed, that is where we are going, but it certainly would not affect any practicing nurse today.

Joyce Shoemaker: I think that was the basis for that variable being rejected.

Development and validation of a diagnostic label: powerlessness

JUDITH FITZGERALD MILLER, R.N., M.S.N.

Nurses are challenged to make accurate nursing diagnoses and to develop new diagnostic categories for behavior patterns previously unlabeled and unclassified. In developing new categories, the subject matter of the discipline of nursing is shaped. A systematic method (possibly scientific rigor) must be used in the process of diagnostic category development to ensure that the generated diagnostic category is appropriate for nursing and is within the domain of nursing practice. Appropriate for nursing means that the diagnostic category is compatible with the existing nursing frameworks. Nurses must also have the skills to identify, validate, and treat the diagnosis and to evaluate the effectiveness of treatment. Comparing nursing to other health disciplines involved in the patient's care, nursing should be the discipline best prepared and uniquely suited to alleviate the unhealthy response pattern (nursing diagnosis).

The diagnostic category's compatibility with nursing frameworks can be studied by examining methods of treating the diagnosis and the goal of nursing or the nature of nursing acts for the various frameworks. If the nursing treatment for the diagnosis does not contribute to the overall goal of nursing as shown by the framework (for example, promote adaptation, enhance self-care agency, stabilize behavioral system balance), the diagnosis may need to be examined because it may not be within the domain of nursing practice in its autonomous sense, but may be a delegated function that is included in the nurse's work, or it may not be appropriate for nursing at all. A specifically defined process must be used to develop appropriate nursing diagnostic categories.

Specific procedures for concept analysis have been proposed by Wilson (1970). Direct application of these procedures to nursing have been discussed by Chinn and Jacobs (1978). Forsyth's analysis of empathy (1980) is a good example of Wilson's concept analysis format. The process of analyzing concepts results in deep insights about the essence of the concept, that is, understanding the explicit and implicit nature of the concept. Wilson (1970) describes the process of concept analysis as developing a model case of the concept, that is, creating a description that most accurately represents the concept; developing an alternate case example, that is, the contrary case that does not in any way represent the concept; then developing a variety of cases, that is, borderline and related cases. Literature is used to delineate implications of the concept. Provisional criteria are identified that are indicators or features of the concept. Critical indicators are those criteria that definitely must be observed to confidently state that the concept exists in this setting. This seemingly abstract procedure does provide some direction for nursing's development of diagnostic categories.

For purposes of this paper the phases of concept development used to develop the diagnostic category, powerlessness, include:

1. Developing a commitment to study the concept, having identified a need in clinical nursing practice.
2. Posing an initial working definition of the concept.
3. Developing theoretic propositions and practice speculations from a thorough literature review.
4. Making field observations to confirm the relevance of the concept to nursing.
5. Designing specific studies.
6. Drawing conclusions from personal and other nursing research about the concept (Miller, 1983).

This process of concept development provides direction for this paper. Examples of work for each of the phases are discussed. Miller (1983) provides a complete development of the content on the concept, *powerlessness.*

Using the six phases just listed ensures that the category is within the realm of nursing. The idea of studying the phenomena in clinical practice is a powerful force motivating continued study. The response pattern is observed and is deemed potentially unhealthy, thereby needing resolution. Thus study of the phenomena is initiated.

Examination of nursing phenomena through inductive, qualitative approaches is the first step in developing diagnostic categories. Studying phenomena in the field confirms or challenges the relevance of the concept for nursing. Once the model case is completed with the empirical referents verified, psychometric tools can be designed to carry out quantitative studies of the concept.

Dubin (1978) distinguishes between descriptive research and hypothesis testing research. Descriptive research is the questioning aspect, the building of level one of theory—isolating facts, describing facts, and clustering and categorizing defining characteristics of the phenomenon studied. Hypothesis testing is the theory testing aspect of research whereby predictive and prescriptive theories are built. Development and validation of the label as described in this paper are confined to the descriptive phase of research.

PHASE 1: DEVELOPING A COMMITMENT TO STUDY THE CONCEPT

Nurses may feel challenged or perplexed or have their curiosity piqued as a result of observations of patients' responses. This interest is stimulus arising from grounded data (behaviors of subjects in their own settings) versus data deduced from an abstract paradigm. I was compelled to learn more about the concept of powerlessness because I felt challenged and at times overwhelmed as I became involved with chronically ill patients. For some patients, despite the most current therapies and strict adherence to regimens, their physical condition continued to worsen. Some patients manifested psychologic resiliency and hope whereas others were filled with despair, hopelessness, and depression. Was perceived powerlessness a factor that differentiated between the two types of patient responses to the dilemma of being chronically ill?

PHASE 2: POSING AN INITIAL WORKING DEFINITION OF THE CONCEPT

Powerlessness is the perception of the individual that one's own actions will not significantly affect an outcome. Powerlessness is a perceived lack of control over a current situation or immediate happening (Miller, 1983). Unlike locus of control, which is a rather stable personality trait, powerlessness is situationally determined. To understand powerlessness, a contrasting case of patient power resources (powerfulness) is constructed. Patient power resources consist of physical strength and reserve, psychologic stamina, positive self-concept (specifically self-esteem), energy, knowledge, motivation and belief system—hope (Miller, 1983). When the power resources are intact, powerlessness is not a problem; rather, the patient may have a perceived sense of control. A patient's unique and varied coping strategies compensate for deficit resources and enhance remaining intact resources, such as hope or positive self-esteem.

PHASE 3: DEVELOPING THEORETIC PROPOSITIONS AND PRACTICE SPECULATIONS FROM A LITERATURE REVIEW

After reviewing the literature on powerlessness and locus of control, the following categories were established:
1. Powerlessness and learning
2. Individual's beliefs or illusion and control
3. Effects of no control on animals
4. Effects of no control on human beings' physiologic responses
5. Effects of no control on children and the elderly
6. Control in selected health-illness situations
7. Powerlessness as a precipitant of death (Miller, 1982)

Theoretic propositions and practice speculations were drawn from each category of literature. Theoretic propositions are translations and conclusions drawn from research findings (Newman, 1979). Findings from several research studies can be generalized into one theoretic proposition. To develop practice speculations, the nurse must determine whether or not there is any relevance (clinical merit) in the research for nursing (Haller, Reynolds, and Horsley,

TABLE 1   **Powerlessness and learning**

Theoretic propositions	Practice speculations
Perceived powerlessness leads to poor learning of control relevant information (Seeman, 1962, 1963, 1972).	Before beginning patient teaching, determine the patient's feelings of powerlessness.
Involving learners in decision making regarding content to be learned enhances learning (Stotland and Blumenthal, 1964; Perlmuter and Monty, 1973).	Patients with an internal locus of control need emphasis on that information which gives them a sense of control.
The personality trait, locus of control, influences ability to utilize control relevant information (Phares, 1968; Phares, Ritchie, and Davis, 1968).	High powerless patients may need structured approaches, teaching self-care in small increments so patients can feel a sense of control without being overwhelmed with care demands.
	Involve patients by having them determine what aspects of care they are ready to learn and when they want to learn them.

From Miller, J.F.: Coping with chronic illness: overcoming powerlessness, Philadelphia, 1983, F.A. Davis Co.

1979). The theoretic propositions and practice speculations for the category powerlessness and learning, are shown in Table 1.

Although all the items in Table 1 deserve elaboration, discussion in this paper is confined to the process of concept analysis and in this instance to the examination of the literature for relevance for practice. Further speculation on the practice-related items could be made. For low powerlessness patients, many teaching aides may be needed to present multiple avenues of content. They may benefit from comparing methods of self-care, questioning rationale for care practices, or pursuing alternate ways of meeting self-care needs. The person's sense of control may be enhanced by explicit verbalizations when information is given; for example, "Knowing this will give you the ability to be in control."

Although only one category summary is presented here, a thorough literature review was conducted and theoretic propositions and practice speculations were developed for all seven categories of literature (Miller, 1983). This review of literature revealed that powerlessness has devastating effects on a person's physical and emotional states. Unrelieved states of powerlessness may lead to hopelessness and eventually may affect survival (Engel, 1968, 1971; and Lefcourt, 1973; Miller and Oertel, 1983; Seligman, 1975). The practice speculations derived from a research base confirm the relevance of powerlessness as a concept for nursing. At this point in the development of the diagnostic category, the diagnosis seems to be not only amenable to nursing for alleviation but also unique to nursing practice for treatment.

PHASE 4: MAKING FIELD OBSERVATIONS TO CONFIRM THE RELEVANCE OF THE CONCEPT TO NURSING

Determining real world relevance of the concept is essential. A participant observation method was used to determine factors in the hospital environment and in the actions of health care providers that could increase or decrease control in patients who had chronic renal failure. Observations were made at varying times during the day for 6 weeks. Averill's categories (1973) of behavioral, cognitive, and decisional control were used as a guide to categorize the factors. Behavioral control is the availability of a response that may influence or modify the threatening event. Cognitive control is the way an event is interpreted. Decisional control is the opportunity to choose among various alternatives (Averill, 1973). Examples of these observations appear in Tables 2 and 3. These field observations lend further support for the need to develop and validate the nursing diagnostic category *powerlessness* (Miller, 1983).

PHASE 5: DESIGNING SPECIFIC STUDIES

The next phase in developing the diagnostic category *powerlessness* was refining a list of critical indicators of the diagnosis. Nurses must have the critical indicators identified and verified through replicated study so that when patients manifest a set of behaviors that seem to create a pattern, clinical judgments can be made with confidence; that is, the diagnosis is made with accuracy.

Data were collected by 27 graduate students enrolled in a clinical nursing course who made nursing diagnoses of powerlessness on 81 chronically ill patients in their case loads. Data were collected using the Impact of Chronic Illness Inventory (Miller, 1980), which was designed to enhance the students' insight into the world of the chronically ill and to generate data about nursing diagnoses. Content on powerlessness as it existed in the literature was part of the course content. The graduate students recorded the indicators that led them to believe that powerlessness was a problem for their patients. The indicators were clustered into 16 categories. These broad indicators were then rated by a panel of 24 experts (2 graduate nursing faculty members and 22 advanced standing graduate students) to determine if the characteristics indicated severe, moderate, low, or no powerlessness. Those characteristics that were classified as severe were labeled critical indictors or referents; that is, when these indicators are present, nurses can conclude with confidence that powerlessness exists (Table 4).

These provisional criteria must be studied systematically so that valid and reliable tools for measuring powerlessness can be made available.

After the indicators of powerlessness were rated by the panel of experts, patient data on help seeking and powerlessness were analyzed. Descriptive

TABLE 2 Factors decreasing behavioral, cognitive, and decisional control in hospitalized chronically ill patients

Behavioral control	Cognitive control	Decisional control
Blind patient was left in a wheelchair in the center of the waiting room—was not told where she was or how long she must wait.	Patient was reprimanded for leaving waiting room to go to restroom after waiting 2 hours. "If you aren't here when we call you, you will miss your turn."	Appointment scheduled in ambulatory care department without asking patient if date and time are convenient.
Patient was left alone in x-ray room—on hard table, in cold room, only partially covered.	Patient was not informed of his daily lab values, although he had requested that this be done.	Patient in x-ray department told to "try to hold it" when he asked location of bathroom.
	Health care personnel more knowledgeable about patient' illness and treatment than he is.	Diagnostic and treatment procedures scheduled without asking patient or explaining why they were being done.
	Health care personnel walk into patient's room without knocking.	Patient has little or no choice about who will share room.
	Health care personnel talking "over" patient about their personal activities.	Little choice over scheduling activities—eating, sleeping, bathing, and treatments.
	Health care personnel not wearing name tags.	

From Miller, J.F.: Coping with chronic illness: overcoming powerlessness, Philadelphia, 1983, F.A. Davis Co.

TABLE 3 Factors increasing behavioral, cognitive, and decisional control in hospitalized chronically ill patients

Behavioral control	Cognitive control	Decisional control
Nursing care plan: allow patient to sleep until breakfast trays arrive—do not awaken for TPR.	Patient informed of his weight, blood pressure, lab values.	Patient given access to refrigerator to get his own soft drinks.
Patient moved to another room at her request because roommate smoked.	Patient taught about medications.	Patient given list of all U.S. dialysis centers, given full responsibility for making own vacation arrangements.
Patient in x-ray room was told: "We can see you through the window. Hold up your hand if you need something."	Nursing care plan: detailed description of how to do patient's dressing change had been worked out with the patient.	Medications left at bedside for patient to take when ready.
After patients were taught specific procedures, expectation given for them to take full responsibility—catheter care, urine testing, dressing change, shunt care.	Patients given feedback about lab values, taught how to record results on a flow sheet.	

From Miller, J.F.: Coping with chronic illness: overcoming powerlessness, Philadelphia, 1983, F.A. Davis Co.

TABLE 4   **Defining characteristics of powerlessness**

Severe	Moderate	Low
Verbal expressions of having no control or influence over situations	Nonparticipation in care or decision making when opportunities are provided	Expressions of uncertainty about fluctuating energy levels
Verbal expressions of having no control or influence over outcomes	Expressions of dissatisfaction and frustration over inability to perform previous tasks and/or activities	
Verbal expressions of having no control or influence over self-care	Expressions of uncertainty about treatment outcomes	
Depression over physical deterioration which occurs despite patient compliance with regimens	Dependence on others that may result in irritability, resentment, anger, and guilt	
Passivity	Does not seek information regarding self-care	
	Does not monitor progress	
	Does not defend self-care practices when challenged	
	Hesitant to plan for future, set goals	
	Expressions of doubt regarding role performance	
	Reluctance to express true feelings, fearing alienation of self from care givers	

From Miller, J.F.: Coping with chronic illness: overcoming powerlessness, Philadelphia, 1983, F.A. Davis Co.

help-seeking data were recorded on the Impact of Chronic Illness Inventory for 81 patients. Based on the descriptive examples, help seeking was classified as:

1. Did not seek help or delayed seeking help
2. Sought help when situation was interpreted by the patient as a crisis such as pain or symptoms that were limiting activity
3. Actively sought help for various needs, problem solving, and preventive care

As expected, persons who experienced severe powerlessness did not seek help. They were reluctant to initiate contact with the health care system; for example, patients who needed more medicine waited until their next clinic visit to obtain it. One patient who had arthritis called her physician to obtain pain relief medicine. When the doctor did not return her call, she made no more attempts to obtain the medicine. Patients expressed being uncertain about criteria to use in making a decision to call the physician. It seemed easier to wait until their next appointment. Data on moderate and low powerlessness patients were inadequate to make any statements about patient help seeking.

PHASE 6: DRAWING CONCLUSIONS FROM PERSONAL AND OTHER NURSING RESEARCH

Scholarly activity of reviewing related research is a continuous effort in validating the diagnostic label and in generating new insights about the concepts. Studies have been conducted on powerlessness and patients with specific health problems, for example, chronic renal failure (Stapleton, 1978) and diabetes (Gotch, 1983; Pfister-Minogue, 1983); on children (Baumann, 1983); and on the elderly (Miller and Oertel, 1983). These studies have led to developing nursing interventions to alleviate powerlessness.

Stapleton (1978) used a participant observation method to identify stimuli causing powerlessness in patients with chronic renal failure. The categories of stimuli identified were as follows:

1. Patient-staff relationships
2. Disease process
3. Family relationships
4. Hospitalization
5. Finances
6. Employment
7. Dialysis procedure
8. Medical regimen

Specific stimuli and patient behavioral responses were classified for each category. Nursing strategies to alleviate powerlessness for each category were developed.

A behavioral assessment tool (Figure 1) was developed based on the previously described efforts to identify indicators of powerlessness and case studies of elderly patients who displayed powerlessness (Miller and Oertel, 1983). The tool contains four categories of behavioral assessment data: verbal responses, emotional responses, participation in activities of daily living, and involvement in learning about care responsibilities. Consistent scores of three or more on one or two items from each category alert the nurse to the potential diagnosis of powerlessness.

Continuing study of powerlessness must include critical review works such as Arakelian (1980), Lowery (1981), and others who have studied determinants of powerlessness. For example, Weisman's studies (1979) on coping reveal that noncoping results in powerlessness and depression that eventually can lead to despair (Figure 2). These devastating consequences can be averted by astute nursing in terms of a prompt, accurate nursing diagnosis and appro-

	Percentage of cases	Nurse ratings of behaviors			
		1 Never	2 Occasionally	3 Frequently	4 Always
Verbal response	Verbal expressions or lack of control over what is happening.				
Verbal response	Verbal expressions of doubt that self-care measures can affect outcome.				
Verbal response	Verbal expressions of giving up.				
Verbal response	Verbal expressions of fatalism.				
Emotional response	Withdrawal.				
Emotional response	Pessimism.				
Emotional response	Undifferentiated anger.				
Emotional response	Diminished patient-initiated interaction.				
Emotional response	Submissiveness.				
Participation in activities of daily living	Non-participation in daily personal hygiene.				
Participation in activities of daily living	Non-interest in treatments.				
Participation in activities of daily living	Refusal to take food or fluids.				
Participation in activities of daily living	Inability to set goals.				
Participation in activities of daily living	Lack of decision-making when opportunities are provided.				
Participation in activities of daily living	Dependency on others for activities of daily living.				

FIGURE 1 Powerlessness behavioral assessment tool.

From Miller, J. F., and Oertel, C.B.: Powerlessness in the elderly: preventing hopelessness. In Miller, J.F., ed.: Coping with chronic illness: overcoming powerlessness, Philadelphia, 1983, F.A. Davis Co.

Percentage of cases	Nurse ratings of behaviors			
	1 Never	2 Occasionally	3 Frequently	4 Always
Involvement in learning about care responsibilities				
Lack of questioning concerning illness.				
Low level of knowledge of illness after being given information.				
Lack of knowledge related to treatment.				
Lack of motivation to learn.				

FIGURE 1, cont'd   For legend see opposite page.

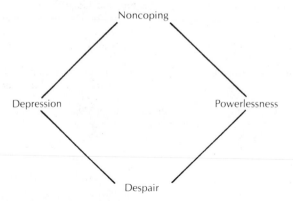

FIGURE 2   Consequences of noncoping.

priate intervention to facilitate coping and alleviate powerlessness and depression.

Phases of developing the diagnosis of powerlessness reviewed in this paper included uncovering a behavior pattern in the clinical setting that results in a commitment to study the behavior, defining the concept, developing theoretic propositions and practice speculations through a review of the literature, confirming relevance of the concept to nursing, designing studies, and drawing conclusions from ongoing research to continue discovering insights about the concept. The next phases of development include development of a psychometric tool and research to test nursing interventions.

REFERENCES

Arakelian, M.: An assessment and nursing application of the concept of locus of control, Adv. Nurs. Sci. **3**:25 1980.

Averill, J.: Personal control over aversive stimuli and its relationships to stress, Psychol. Bull. **80**:286, 1973.

Baumann, D.R.: Coping behavior of children experiencing powerlessness from loss of mobility. In Miller, J.F., ed.: Coping with chronic illness: overcoming powerlessness, Philadelphia, 1983 F.A. Davis Co.

Chinn, P., and Jacobs, M.: A model for theory development in nursing, Adv. Nurs. Sci. **1**:1, 1978.

Dubin, R.: Theory building, New York, 1978, The Free Press.

Engel, G.: A life setting conducive to illness: the giving up-given up complex, Ann. Intern. Med. **69**:293, 1968.

Forsyth, G.: Analysis of the concept of empathy: illustration of one approach, Adv. Nurs. Sci. **2**:33, 1980.

Gotch, P.M.: Locus of control and implementation of health regimens in adults with insulin-dependent diabetes. In Miller, J.F., ed.: Coping with chronic illness: overcoming powerlessness, Philadelphia, 1983, F.A. Davis, Co.

Haller, K., Reynolds, M., and Horsley, J.: Developing research-based innovation protocols: process, criteria, and issues, Res. Nurs. Health **2**:45, 1979.

Lefcourt, H.: The function of the illusions of control and freedom, Am. Psychol. **28**:417, 1973.

Lowery, B.: Misconceptions and limitations of locus of control and the I-E scale, Nurs. Res. **30**:294, 1981.

Miller, J.F.: A practitioner/teacher role for graduate program faculty, In Machan, L., ed.: The practitioner-teacher role: practice what you teach, Wakefield, Mass., 1980, Nursing Resources.

Miller, J.F., ed.: Coping with chronic illness: overcoming powerlessness, Philadelphia, 1983, F.A. Davis Co.

Miller, J.F., and Oertel, C.B.: Powerlessness in the elderly: preventing hopelessness. In Miller, J.F., ed.: Coping with chronic illness: overcoming powerlessness, Philadelphia, 1983, F.A. Davis Co.

Newman, M.: Theory development in nursing, Philadelphia, 1979, F.A. Davis Co.

Perlmuter, L.C., and Monty, R.A.: Effect of choice of stimulus on paired associate learning, J. Exper. Psychol. **99**:120, 1973.

Pfister-Minogue, K.: Enabling strategies. In Miller, J.F., ed.: Coping with chronic illness: overcoming powerlessness, Philadelphia, 1983, F.A. Davis Co.

Phares, E.: Differential utilization of information as a function of internal-external control, J. Pers. **36**:649, 1968.

Phares, E., Ritchie, D., and Davis, W.: Internal-external control and reaction to threat, J. Pers. Soc. Psychol. **10**:402, 1968.

Seeman, M.: Alienation and learning in a hospital setting, Am. Sociol. Rev. **27**:772, 1962.

Seeman, M.: Alienation and social learning in a reformatory, Am. J. Sociol. **69**:270, 1963.

Seeman M.: Alienation and knowledge-seeking: a note on attitude and action, Soc. Prob. **20**:3, 1972.

Seligman, M.: Helplessness: on depression, development, and death, San Francisco, 1975, W.H. Freeman and Co. Publishers.

Stapleton, S.R.: Powerlessness in individuals with chronic renal failure, master's essay, Milwaukee, 1978, Marquette University.

Stotland, E., and Blumenthal, A.: The reduction of anxiety as a result of the expectation of making a choice, Can. J. Psychol. **18**:139, 1964.

Weisman, A.: Coping with cancer, New York, 1979, McGraw-Hill Book Co.

Wilson, J.: Thinking with concepts, London, 1970, Cambridge University Press.

Discussion

Comments: Under your defining characteristics, there were many verbal expressions about the feeling of loss or power. We find in our patients with acute illness some nonverbal behaviors that might indicate powerlessness. We cannot check these out verbally with the patient many times; that is, what they are feeling. What are your thoughts on nonverbal behaviors as indicators of powerlessness?

Judith Miller: My focus has been on patients who were able to respond, so I have been able to validate my impressions with them. Nonverbal behaviors are a little more nebulous, and so I have been more hesitant to use them. But I think we really need to work on them.

Clinical validation of cardiovascular nursing diagnoses

MI JA KIM, R.N., Ph.D., F.A.A.N.
RUBY AMOROSO-SERITELLA, R.N., M.S.N, F.A.A.N.
MEG GULANICK, R.N., M.S.N.
KAREN MOYER, R.N., M.S.N.
ELINOR PARSONS, R.N., M.S.N.
JANET SCHERBEL, R.N., M.S.N.
MARGARET J. STAFFORD, R.N., M.S.N., F.A.A.N.
ROSEMARIE SUHAYDA, R.N., M.S.N.
CAROLYN YOCOM, R.N., M.S.N.

Although nursing diagnoses have become an integral part of the definition of nursing (ANA, 1980) and numerous books and articles about nursing diagnoses have been published in various journals (Kim and Moritz 1982), since the Fourth National Conference on the Classification of Nursing Diagnoses in 1980, only limited research studies have been published that validate nursing diagnoses in the clinical setting. Until the validity and clinical relevance of these nursing diagnoses are established and demonstrated, the diagnoses will have limited value as valid nomenclature for nursing. The purpose of this study was to establish content and face validity of nursing diagnoses and the associated defining characteristics and to document clinical relevance of nursing diagnoses by an empirical research method.

METHODS

The measures and procedure of this study are similar to those reported by Kim and Moritz (1980). Four cardiovascular clinical specialists (nurse experts) and 18 staff nurses from two metropolitan teaching hospitals participated in the study. Staff nurses were randomly selected from a group of 100. All the clinical specialists had a master's degree and a minimum of 1 year's experience as a clinical specialist. Staff nurses had either a diploma or a baccalaureate degree and had a minimum of 1 year's experience in identifying and using nursing diagnoses. Staff nurses randomly selected 158 patients who had cardiovascular disorders from critical care and general medical-surgical populations. The sample of patients contained 138 men and 22 women with a mean age of 59.87 years (SD = 10.74; range: 20 to 90 years of age). Major medical diagnoses for these patients were coronary artery disease, congestive heart failure, myocardial infarction, cardiomyopathy, and valve disease.

Written consent from both the patients and the nurses was obtained before inclusion in the study. To standardize the procedures, a 70-minute videotaped orientation to the study was presented to participating staff nurses before data collection. The tape was developed and presented by the clinical specialists and medical-surgical nursing faculty. It included an overview of study purposes and procedure, instruction on basic techniques of data collection and physical assessment, and an explanation of nursing diagnosis and the diagnostic process.

For purposes of this study, nursing diagnosis was defined as a statement of a problem derived from a nursing assessment that points to specific interventions and outcomes. Its description contained both the conceptual and structural components of a problem statement, etiology, and signs and symptoms. Staff nurses received a list of 45 nursing diagnoses approved by the Third National Conference in 1978 and selected by clinical specialists as representative of patients who have cardiovascular disorders. Nurses were instructed to use the list as a guide whenever appropriate.

The patient assessment guide used by both the staff nurses and the clinical specialists was developed by the clinical specialists and participating medical-surgical nursing faculty. The assessment guide included relevant physical and psychologic data, items pertaining to patterns of daily living and health management, and parameters of physical assessment.

Following the orientation, staff nurses participated in a 1-hour practice session in which they examined two case studies and identified relevant nursing diagnoses. The same case studies had been used to determine interrater agreement in the identification of nursing diagnoses among four clinical specialists; the agreement was 97%.

Data collection spanned 4 months. Each nurse and clinical specialist received one coded packet for every patient assessed. The packet contained patient assessment guide, list of approved nursing diagnoses, and several worksheets used to record the nursing diagnosis, etiology, signs and symptoms, and nursing order and/or interventions. Each nursing diagnoses list included a question about the clinical relevance of the identified nursing diagnosis.

Staff nurses randomly selected patients with cardiovascular disorders from their respective units. Each nurse used the assessment guide to obtain and record patient data. Based on analysis of assessment data, each nurse identified and recorded nursing diagnoses, etiology, signs and symptoms, and nursing orders and/or interventions. Nurses were to describe how well the stated diagnoses reflected problems dealt with by nurses and how accurately the diagnostic labels reflected the patients' problems. The completed assessment guide and worksheets were placed in sealed envelopes and submitted to the project coordinator (clinical specialist) at each hospital before the end of the shift. Clinical specialists reassessed 32 patients (20% of the total sample) independently of staff nurses within a 6-hour period using the same assessment guide and research data sheets as the staff nurses used. Sealed envelopes from the clinical specialists and staff nurses were then delivered to the principal investigator.

RESULTS AND DISCUSSION

The average number of nursing diagnoses per patient listed by staff nurses was 3.76 (SD = 1.76; range: 1 to 11) and by clinical specialists, 5.32 (SD = 3.09; range: 1 to 20). There was a significant difference in the mean number of nursing diagnoses identified between staff nurses and clinical specialists (t [51.04] = -2.84; p = .006). The average number of defining characteristics per nursing diagnosis by staff nurses was 2.38 (SD = 1.39; range: 1 to 11) and by clinical specialists, 3.11 (SD = 1.84; range: 1 to 11). Again, clinical specialists identified significantly more defining characteristics than staff nurses (t [336.84] = -4.37; p < .001). Possible explanations for differences between staff nurses and clinical specialists in the number of nursing diagnoses per patient and in the number of defining characteristics per nursing diagnoses are (1) the higher education of the clinical specialists, (2) more thorough patient assessment by the clinical specialists, (3) better understanding of the concept and use of nursing diagnosis by the clinical specialists, (4) limited time and flexibility of the staff nurse's role as compared with that of the clinical specialist, (5) other demanding nursing duties of staff nurses within the 8-hour period, (6) variable levels of nursing administrative support for staff nurses to carry out the study, and (7) the lengthy study period (4 months), which might have overwhelmed the staff nurses or produced boredom.

From the total of 601 diagnoses reported by staff nurses for 158 patients, 41 different nursing diagnoses were identified. The majority of diagnoses were physiologic alterations. All nursing diagnoses were rated by staff nurses as reflecting problems dealt with by nurses and as accurate terminology usable by staff nurses at the clinical setting. Nursing diagnoses agreed on by pairs of clinical specialists and staff nurses for the same patients were reported by Kim and Moritz (1980). The 10 most frequently identified nursing diagnoses by staff nurses are given in Table 1.

Defining characteristics for each of the 10 nursing diagnoses are given in Tables 2 through 11. Only the defining characteristics that were identified more than 10 times are reported. Even with clinical assessment of 158 patients, the frequency of the defining characteristics for each diagnosis is too small to draw any conclusions, partly because so many nursing diagnoses were identified that produced a scattering of the defining characteristics, thus decreasing their occurrence per diagnosis. Three major problems were evident from this finding. First, several terminologies or words were used for the same defining characteristic, sign, or symptom, necessitating content analysis by nurse experts and comparison with standard terminologies. Second, several clusters of signs and symptoms were placed in each nursing diagnosis. To avoid a lengthy list of defining characteristics with low frequencies of occurrence, the defining characteristics of similar nature were grouped by nurse experts. For example, indicators of inadequate gas exchange were the second most frequently identified defining characteristic for the nursing diagnosis *alteration in coronary circulation* (Table 2). The indicators of inadequate gas exchange included labored breathing, Kussmaul's respirations, pulmonary congestion, adventitious breath sounds, shortness of breath/dyspnea-on exertion, shallow respirations, orthopnea, Cheyne-Stokes respirations, tachypnea, and accessory muscle use. Another defining characteristic, hemodynamic pressure changes, under the same nursing diagnosis, had the following cluster of signs and symptoms: changes in pulmonary artery pressure/

Text continued on p. 135.

TABLE 1 **The 10 most frequently identified nursing diagnoses by staff nurses for 158 cardiovascular patients**

Nursing diagnosis	Frequency	Rank
Alteration in coronary circulation	47	1
Decreased cardiac output	43	2
Alteration in comfort	42	3
Decreased activity tolerance	33	4.5
High-risk coronary artery disease	33	4.5
Alteration in respiratory function	32	6
Alteration in peripheral circulation	30	7.5
Anxiety	30	7.5
Lack of knowledge	27	9
Mobility impairment	22	10

TABLE 2 **Defining characteristics listed by staff nurses for the nursing diagnosis *alteration in coronary circulation* (N = 47)**

Defining characteristic	Frequency
Ischemic pain*	31
Indicators of inadequate gas exchange†	11
Hemodynamic pressure changes‡	10
ECG/enzyme changes§	10
History of cardiovascular disease‖	10

*Pain, angina, neck pain, hand-arm pain.
†Labored breathing, Kussmaul's respirations, pulmonary congestion, adventitious breath sounds, shortness or breath/dyspnea on exertion, shallow respirations, orthopnea, Cheyne-Stokes respirations, tachypnea, accessory muscle use.
‡Changes in pulmonary artery pressure/central venous pressure, hypotension, jugular vein distention, hypertension, intraaortic balloon pump use, papilledema.
§Arrhythmias (all), ECG changes, palpitations, abnormal heart sounds, abnormal cardiac enzymes, abnormal treadmill test results.
‖Myocardial infarction, CHF, CAD, valve disease, tamponade, ASO/ASHD, anemia.

TABLE 3 Defining characteristics listed by staff nurses for the nursing diagnosis *decreased cardiac output* (N = 43)

Defining characteristic	Frequency
Indicators of inadequate gas exchange*	21
ECG/enzyme changes†	20
Abnormal neurologic responses‡	14
Ischemic pain§	11
Hemodynamic pressure changes‖	11
Fluid shift¶	10

*Labored breathing, Kussmaul's respiration, pulmonary congestion, adventitious breath sounds, shortness of breath/dyspnea on exertion, shallow respirations, orthopnea, Cheyne-Stokes respirations, tachypnea, accessory muscle use.
†Arrhythmias (all), ECG changes, palpitations, abnormal heart sounds, abnormal cardiac enzymes, abnormal treadmill test results.
‡Syncope, vertigo/dizziness, abnormal neurologic signs, tinnitis, history of TIA, headache.
§Pain, angina, neck pain, hand-arm pain.
‖Changes in pulmonary artery pressure/central venous pressure, hypotension, jugular vein distention, hypertension, intraaortic balloon pump use, papilledema.
¶Effusion, unusual weight gain, peripheral edema, imbalanced intake and output fluid retention, vasoconstriction.

TABLE 4 Defining characteristics listed by staff nurses for the nursing diagnosis *alteration in comfort* (N = 41)

Defining characteristic	Frequency
Pain complaints*	26
Ischemic pain†	15

*Pain, headache, leg pain, arthritic pain, lumbosacral pain, abdominal pain, incisional pain, sore throat, requests pain medication, musculoskeletal pain, hand-arm pain, hip pain.
†Pain, angina, neck pain, hand-arm pain.

TABLE 5 Defining characteristics listed by staff nurses for the nursing diagnosis *decreased activity tolerance* (N = 33)

Defining characteristic	Frequency
Inability to perform activities of daily living*	21
Indicators of inadequate gas exchange†	12

*Lethargy/weakness, self-management deficit, decreased activity tolerance, requires assistance with care, requires assistance with ambulation, requires assistance with ADLs, decreased ADL performance, naps frequently.
†Labored breathing, Kussmaul's respirations, pulmonary congestion, adventitious breath sounds, shortness of breath/dyspnea on exertion, shallow respirations, orthopnea, Cheyne-Stokes respirations, tachypnea, accessory muscle use.

TABLE 6   Defining characteristics listed by staff nurses for the nursing diagnosis *high-risk coronary artery disease* (N = 33)

Defining characteristic	Frequency
Ischemic pain*	19
History of CAD: risk factors†	15

*Pain, angina, neck pain, hand-arm pain.
†Risk factors: CAD, smoking history, overweight, history of CVA, hypertension.

TABLE 7   Defining characteristics listed by staff nurses for the nursing diagnosis *alteration in respiratory function* (N = 32)

Defining characteristic	Frequency
Indicators of inadequate gas exchange*	34
Cough†	15
Indicators of abnormal pulmonary function‡	11

*Labored breathing, Kussmaul's respirations, pulmonary congestion, adventitious breath sounds, shortness of breath/dyspnea on exertion, shallow respirations, orthopnea, Cheyne-Stokes respirations, tachypnea, accessory muscle use.
†Cough, productive cough, nonproductive cough, poor cough, smoking history.
‡Abnormal pulmonary function test results, abnormal ABGs, marginal ABGs, x-ray changes.

TABLE 8   Defining characteristics listed by staff nurses for the nursing diagnosis *alteration in peripheral circulation* (N = 30)

Defining characteristic	Frequency
Signs of peripheral vascular dysfunction*	37
Indicators of hypothermia†	18

*Circulatory impairment, decreased peripheral pulses, leg ulcer, previous arterial surgery, intermittent claudication, altered peripheral circulation, vein grafts for CABG, amputee, sensory impairment.
†Pallor, cool skin, decreased body temperature, change in body temperature, skin temperature change, skin color change.

TABLE 9   Defining characteristics listed by staff nurses for the nursing diagnosis *anxiety* (N = 30)

Defining characteristic	Frequency
Psychosocial indicators of stress*	32
Concern about life events†	13

*Anxiety, tense, restless, tranquilizer use, hyperalert, nervous mannerisms, hyperkinetic, questioning, depressed.
†Concern about illness, future, family, finances/job.

TABLE 10   **Defining characteristics listed by staff nurses for the nursing diagnosis** *lack of knowledge* **(N = 27)**

Defining characteristic	Frequency
Lack of understanding about therapy*	22
Nonadherence to therapeutic regiment	19

*Unable to state medications, treatments, and the like; has questions about medications, treatments, and the like; misconceptions about disease.
†Noncompliance not following medication, diet, activity restrictions, and/or instructions.

TABLE 11   **Defining characteristic listed by staff nurses for the nursing diagnosis: mobility impairment (N = 22)**

Defining characteristic	Frequency
Indicators of physical/mechanical limitations to movement*	14

*Use of ambulatory aids, equipment restrictions, Foley catheter, presence of chest tubes, bed rest, commode use, restricted activity, activity restrictions at home.

TABLE 12   **The 10 most frequently identified etiologies by staff nurses for 41 nursing diagnoses**

Etiology	Frequency	Percentage of responses*	Percentage of cases†
CAD, ASHD, ASO, ischemic heart disease, heart disease	110	10.9	18.4
Surgery: coronary artery bypass graft	63	6.3	10.6
Congestive heart failure	52	5.2	8.7
Risk factors: CAD	38	3.8	6.4
Myocardial infarction, r/o myocardial infarction	30	3.0	5.0
Hypertension	28	2.8	4.7
Inactivity, immobility, disabled	26	2.6	4.4
COPD, emphysema, asthma, airway disease	26	2.6	4.4
Surgery: nonspecific, postop, postcardiac catheterization	23	2.3	3.9
Arrhythmias	20	2.0	3.4

*Total responses = 1004.
†Total cases = 597.

central venous pressure, hypotension, jugular vein distention, hypertension, IABP use, and papilledema. These two defining characteristics and defining clusters clearly indicate that this diagnosis has two different domains that may need further delineation. Third, the same defining characteristic was found under several nursing diagnoses. For example, ischemic chest pain was identified for alteration in coronary circulation, decreased cardiac output, high-risk coronary artery disease, and alteration in comfort. In addition, some nursing diagnoses were used as defining characteristics; for example, impaired gas exchange was used as a defining characteristic for the nursing diagnosis *alteration in coronary circulation*.

Twenty-five etiologies, reported 10 or more times by staff nurses, were found related to the 41 nursing diagnoses; the majority were medical diagnoses. The 10 most commonly identified etiologies are given in Table 12, which also describes the frequency of the etiology selection, the percentage

TABLE 13 **Staff nurses' ratings of the 10 most commonly identified nursing diagnoses as reflecting problems dealt with by nurses**

Nursing diagnosis	Rating scale				
	Strongly agree	Agree	Disagree	Strongly disagree	Don't know
Alteration in coronary circulation	15	22	4	0	1
Decreased cardiac output	9	25	6	1	0
Alteration in comfort	19	17	1	1	0
Decreased activity tolerance	12	17	1	1	0
High risk: CAD	9	19	3	0	1
Alteration in respiratory function	18	11	0	0	0
Alteration in peripheral circulation	20	6	1	1	0
Anxiety	14	11	1	0	1
Lack of knowledge	9	13	0	1	0
Mobility impairment	11	8	0	1	0
TOTALS	136*	149	17	6	3
	43.7%†	47.9%	5.5%	1.6%	1.3%

*Frequency of response.
†Percentage of responses for the 10 nursing diagnoses.

of the total responses (1004 etiologies were identified) represented by the etiology, and the percentage of times each etiology appeared in 597 patient cases. The preponderance of medical diagnoses as etiologies reflects the developmental stage of our diagnostic conceptualization and the clinical reality. It appears that staff nurses, when incorporating nursing diagnosis in their practice setting, needed some bridge to the medical diagnosis. With further development of the theories and rationale for having nursing-based etiologies, we expect that this situation will change. Nursing interventions are intended to treat (ameliorate, modify, and so forth) the etiology so that the patients' problems can be corrected. From this logic it follows that etiologies should be something for which nurses can intervene; hence, they cannot be medical diagnoses.

Using a 5-point rating scale, staff nurses were asked to rate whether the 41 individual diagnoses reflected problems dealt with by nurses. Almost half the subjects (45%) strongly agreed, and 46.5% agreed with the clinical rele-

TABLE 14   **Staff nurses' ratings of the wording accuracy of the 10 most commonly identified nursing diagnoses for reflecting patient problems**

Nursing diagnosis	Rating scale				
	Strongly agree	Agree	Disagree	Strongly disagree	Don't know
Alteration in coronary circulation	11	23	6	1	1
Decreased cardiac output	6	25	7	2	0
Alteration in comfort	16	14	4	2	2
Decreased activity tolerance	10	18	2	0	1
High risk: CAD	8	17	5	2	0
Alteration in respiratory function	16	8	4	1	1
Alteration in peripheral circulation	19	6	2	1	0
Anxiety	13	12	1	1	0
Lack of knowledge	6	16	0	0	1
Mobility impairment	10	8	1	0	1
TOTALS	115*	147	32	10	7
	37.0%†	47.3%	10.3%	3.2%	2.2%

*Frequency.
†Percentage of responses for the 10 nursing diagnoses.

vance of the diagnoses. A few subjects disagreed (5%) or strongly disagreed (1.6%), and a few chose the "don't know" option (1.6%). Staff nurses' responses for the 10 most frequently identified diagnoses also reflect the high degree of relevance that nurses stated the diagnoses have for clinical practice. In addition, the nurses were asked if the wording of the 41 diagnoses (diagnostic labels) were accurate for use as nursing diagnoses and reflected patient problems. Using the same 5-point rating scale, the nurses again responded in agreement: 38.7% strongly agreed, 45.9% agreed, 9.0% disagreed, 3.6% strongly disagreed, and 2.9% didn't know. Wording ratings for the 10 most frequently identified nursing diagnoses are listed in Table 14.

In summary, this study has shown that the 10 most frequently identified nursing diagnoses appear to have content and face validity as judged by nurse experts and staff nurses who used them in daily practice for 4 months. The high level of the clinical relevance ratings of predominantly physiologic nursing diagnoses suggests that these are clearly part of the domain of nursing practice. Defining characteristics for each nursing diagnosis need further validation, since the frequency of occurrence was not large enough for meaningful interpretations. To identify critical defining characteristics, the sample size of patients and nurses should be considerably larger in future studies. Finally, the need for clarification of the concept and use of etiologies for nursing diagnoses is apparent and should be studied further.

REFERENCES

American Nurses' Association: Nursing: a social policy statement, Kansas City, Mo., 1980, The Association.

Kim, M.J., and Moritz, D.A.: Classification of nursing diagnoses: proceedings of the third and fourth national conferences, New York, 1982, McGraw-Hill Book Co.

Discussion

Carol Hayes: My question is about the nurses who are practicing in your CCU. They have to say that what they are doing is relevant to nursing practice because if they say it is not relevant, what are they doing there? I wonder how you can say because they say it is relevant, that it is relevant? And, for instance, does the nurse really start an intraaortic balloon pump? Does she put it in? Does she alter its rate? I know interdependent practice, and I have no problem with nurses monitoring and referring problems to physicians. But you do really see it as independent nursing. It can still be nursing, but I do not see it as a nursing diagnosis as such.

Mi Ja Kim: Your first comment was about clinical relevancy. Maybe you are right that we really did not have to ask that question. However, I want to remind you that these nurses had a choice to use any diagnosis to begin with and the clinical relevancy rating was graded such a way to express the range of their opinions. What we have done here is document that it is indeed clinically relevant and is indeed within nursing because it has been questioned. Your second comment was about the concept of nursing diagnosis and its relationship to independent and interdependent functions. We have been struggling with this controversial issue, and I am not pretending that I have the answer. There are many interdependent nursing functions not only in critical care nursing but also in acute care nursing. Many of these interdependent nursing functions have been traditionally subsumed under medicine and the contributions that nurses make in the clinical setting have not been properly credited. So the real question is, how can we get proper credit for our judgment and decisions that are integral for the problem-solving process? We are trying to sort out physiologic concepts from the medical diagnosis or disease entity so that we can describe those physiologic concepts for which nurses intervene. I guess what I am saying is that nursing diagnoses should describe patient problems for which nurses intervene interdependently as well as independently.

Nursing diagnoses associated with heart failure in critical care nursing

KATHRYN HUBALIK, R.N., M.S.N.
MI JA KIM, R.N., Ph.D., F.A.A.N.

Nursing practice has advanced rapidly in the past few decades. This advancement is particularly notable in critical care, where nurses have assumed more responsibility in clinical judgment and decision making. Nursing diagnosis, a concept described in the literature since the 1950s, is synonymous with nursing clinical judgment. With the evolution of a nursing diagnosis taxonomy, nurses have begun describing their scope of practice. However, the lag in use of nursing diagnoses in all phases of practice is still evident.

Even with role expansion, some nursing leaders are narrowing the focus and scope of nursing judgments and decisions. For example, some strong supporters of nursing diagnoses insist that nurses must be able to treat these entities independently. Gordon (1976, p. 1299) stated that her definition "excludes health problems for which the accepted mode of therapy is prescription drugs, surgery, radiation, and other treatments that are defined legally as the practice of medicine." The American Medical Association (AMA), on the other hand, in its 1970 position on the extended scope of nursing practice, broadens the concept of nursing judgment by the statement, "An identical act or procedure may be the practice of medicine when carried out by a physician and the practice of nursing when carried out by a nurse" (Campbell, 1978, p. 13). It is curious that this nonnursing organization is less restrictive in its definition of nursing than is nursing itself. It is crucial that nursing defines its independent boundaries. It is, however, just as critical that nursing retains within its scope those judgments that require nursing decisions in the institution and implementation of medical therapies. This interdependent domain of nursing must be recognized by all health professionals.

Nursing diagnosis literature does not address the interdependent domain of nursing care, since nursing judgments are defined as being purely independent of medical intervention. This limited definition does not support nursing as it is practiced in critical care where, for example, many judgments are based on acute hemodynamic alterations, and the delineation between nursing and medical practice is ill-defined. Although medical therapies are required for critical care patients, institution of the therapies depends on nursing judgments and nursing decisions. Judgments that reflect interdependent health problems must be incorporated into the scope of nursing practice. The ANA has already accepted this fact in their position on the scope of nursing.

To be encompassing, a nursing diagnosis taxonomy must also reflect interdependent actions to define and direct critical care nursing practice.

This study was undertaken to provide data that the criteria for accepting nursing diagnoses may need to be expanded to include those judgments that require nursing decision in the institution and implementation of medical therapy. The purposes of this study were to (1) identify nursing diagnostic terms associated with those interventions that are independent and those that are interdependent, (2) identify which of the nursing diagnostic labels and associated interventions are within the scope of nursing practice, and (3) identify the level of clinical relevancy for nursing practice of the nursing diagnostic labels and associated interventions.

In this study, nursing diagnosis was defined as a statement of a problem derived from a nursing assessment that points to a specific intervention and outcome (Gebbie and Lavin, 1973). An independent nursing intervention was defined as a therapeutic action initiated by a nurse without consultation from other professionals, including physicians. An interdependent nursing intervention was defined as a therapeutic action performed by a nurse with a reciprocal dependence on a physician or other health professional for prescription or regulation of that action, including nursing judgments made when carrying out physicians' orders. Interdependent nursing interventions are within the scope of nursing practice (ANA, 1980).

METHODS

Surveys presenting a congestive heart failure situation defined by specific etiologies, defining characteristics, and interventions were distributed to critical care nurses. A congestive heart failure situation was used in this study because many patients in critical care units have this problem (Kim and co-workers, 1981). The interventions were varied in each survey group—only independent (Group A) and only interdependent (Group B). The nurses were asked to identify nursing diagnostic labels based on the situation and the interventions presented. They were also asked if the labels and interventions are within the scope of nursing practice and if use of the labels is clinically relevant.

Data collection was accomplished in three phases. In Phase I 15 experts, critical care clinical specialists or clinical nursing instructors, identified labels for the patient situation. These labels were incorporated into the survey as choices for the nurses. The experts also answered questions about the scope of practice and clinical relevancy of the labels they identified.

After completing a preliminary survey with 14 acute care nurses to test possible semantic problems with the surveys, Phase II was begun. In this phase, either the Group A survey or the Group B survey was given at random to 225 critical care staff nurses. Respondents were asked to choose nursing diagnostic labels appropriate to the patient situation and then answer questions about the scope of practice and clinical relevancy of the labels. Of the 225 nurses, 185 were not familiar with nursing diagnoses and 40 were familiar with nursing diagnoses. Nurses in this phase had to be currently licensed as a registered nurse in one or more states and practicing in a medical-surgical critical care unit for at least 1 year.

Phase III of the study involved the experts again to bring credibility and validity to the findings of the staff nurses. The experts completed another survey that incorporated the results of Phase II. Verification of the interventions was established, and nursing diagnostic labels appropriate to the patient situation were chosen. The experts were also asked about the clinical relevancy of a system of diagnostic terminology for patients with congestive heart failure.

Phase I and Phase III data were collected from the experts at their places of employment. They were telephoned and an appointment was made with the investigator, during which the survey was completed. Phase II data were collected from critical care nurses from three metropolitan hospitals after approval from the directors of nursing. Surveys were delivered to the unit by the investigator, and staff nurses completed the surveys on a voluntary basis. A cover letter provided the staff nurses with specific information about the purpose of the study and possible benefits for the nursing profession and explained how they were chosen to participate. The completed surveys were picked up by the investigator 1 to 2 weeks after they were delivered to the units. From the beginning of Phase I to the end of Phase III approximately 3 months elapsed.

The surveys consisted of two parts—an example of a patient problem and scales of opinion about the clinical relevancy of labels used to describe the problem. Content validity of the selected patient situation was established by a review of the literature involving congestive heart failure and by clinical specialists. The literature served as a theoretic basis for the etiologies, defining characteristics, and interventions. Content validity of the questions about the clinical relevancy was established by a review of the literature on the value of nursing diagnoses. The clinical specialists and instructors were considered experts and established the reliability and validity of the surveys. They consistently agreed that the listed etiologies, defining characteristics, and interventions were complete and representative of a person with congestive heart failure.

RESULTS
Phase I

A total of 61 labels were identified by the clinical specialists in Phase I of this study. Each label was placed in one of 11 problem categories. Table 1

TABLE 1   Nursing diagnostic labels identified by experts—Phase 1

Nursing diagnostic labels	Frequency	Problem categories	Frequency
Congestive heart failure	5	Circulation	15
Alteration in circulation	6		
Decreased cardiac output	4		
Anxiety	9	Emotion	11
Emotional stress	2		
Alteration in respiration	5	Respiration	6
Impaired gas exchange	1		
Fluid overload	2	Fluid volume	5
Fluid volume excess	3		
Decreased activity tolerance	2	Activity	5
Fatigue	3		
Impaired skin integrity, potential	2	Integument	4
Potential tissue breakdown	2		
Electrolyte imbalance, potential	1	Electrolytes	4
Disturbance in H_2O/electrolyte balance	3		
Alteration in nutrition	2	Nutrition	4
Poor appetite	2		
Knowledge deficit	1	Cognition	3
Lack of knowledge	2		
Potential independency/dependency conflict	1	Self-concept	3
Ineffective patient coping	2		
Disturbance in rhythm	1	Electrophysiology	1
TOTALS	61	11	61

lists the nursing diagnostic labels that were identified (23), the frequency of identification, the problem category in which they were placed during data analysis, and the frequency of placement. The following problem categories were chosen to be included in the Phase II survey: circulation, fluid volume, activity, emotion, cognition, and integument.

Data about the scope of practice of each label identified were gathered by use of a continuum of nursing and medicine practice. Respondents decided where the scope of practice fell for each of their labels and placed an *x* on a blank continuum. The "*x*'s" were then transformed into numeric data that described the label as being within the nursing scope (1.0 to 3.9), the medicine scope (5.1 to 8.0), or the interdependent (nursing and medicine) scope (4.0 to 5.0). Figure 1 illustrates the continuum and scale used. Analysis of the scope of practice of the labels identified in Phase I revealed that most of the experts placed the diagnostic labels within either the scope of nursing or the interdependent scope. The average scope of practice of all the labels identified in Phase I was 3.17, which falls within the scope of nursing according to the scale used.

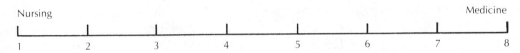

FIGURE 1   Scope of practice continuum and scale.

Clinical relevancy of each diagnostic label identified was determined by a response to four statements about the clinical usefulness of nursing diagnoses. A mean value for all four responses was computed for each label. A value between 1.0 and 2.9 was considered disagreement with the statements, or clinical irrelevancy of the nursing diagnostic label. A value between 3.0 and 4.0 was considered agreement with the statements, or clinical relevancy of the nursing diagnostic label. Data analysis revealed that the experts rated their diagnostic labels as clinically relevant. The average clinical relevancy rating for all the labels identified in Phase I was 3.47.

Preliminary survey

Surveys were completed by 14 staff nurses who were not involved in this study. Semantic problems with directions were resolved based on information given by the respondents. Because few of the respondents chose *emotional stress* (2 out of 14) and some expressed verbal disagreement with the label, this diagnostic term was replaced by *fear* for the Phase II survey.

Phase II

Of the 225 critical care nurses given a survey to complete, 100 responded and met the sample criteria, for a response rate of 49%. Based on the data collected in Phase I, staff nurses were asked to choose nursing diagnostic labels appropriate for the same patient situation as given in Phase I. The most frequently chosen nursing diagnostic labels in Phase II from both the Group A and Group B survey groups were *congestive heart failure, fluid overload, decreased activity tolerance, anxiety, lack of knowledge,* and *potential tissue breakdown.* The chi-square statistic demonstrated that the association between label frequency and survey group was not statistically significant ($p > .05$). Staff nurses at one institution were given the opportunity to identify an alternate label. Two nurses did identify alternate labels for the cognition category—*learning need* and *inadequate knowledge.*

Analysis of the scope of practice continuum in Phase II revealed that most of the staff nurses placed the diagnostic labels in the scope of nursing or in the interdependent scope. Only *congestive heart failure* and *fluid volume excess* were placed in the interdependent scope. No labels were placed in the medicine scope. The average scope of practice rating for all labels in Phase II was 2.93. The results of a *t*-test determined that there was no significant difference ($p > .05$) between the scope of practice ratings given by the Group

A and Group B survey groups. Results of chi-square tests determined that there was no statistically significant association ($p > .05$) between the nursing diagnostic labels in each problem category and the scope of practice rating, regardless of the differences in the two survey groups.

The staff nurses rated their level of agreement with four statements about each nursing diagnostic label to determine clinical relevancy. Analysis of the data shows that the staff nurses rated the diagnostic labels they chose as clinically relevant. The average numeric value for clinical relevancy of all the diagnostic labels in Phase II was 3.215. Results of t-test determined that there was no significant difference ($p > .05$) between the mean clinical relevancies in the Group A and Group B survey groups. Chi-square tests were used to determine if there was an association between the nursing diagnostic labels in each problem category and their clinical relevancies, rgardless of the differences between the two survey groups. Results showed that there was a significant association between the nursing diagnostic labels and their clinical relevancies in two problem categories—emotion ($x^2(1) = 7.419; p < .05$) and *activity* ($x^2(1) = 6.652; p < .05$). Application of analysis of variance then determined that there was no statistical significance ($p > .05$) between the nursing diagnostic labels in each category and their clinical relevancies, regardless of the differences in survey groups.

Phase III

The most frequently chosen labels in Phase III were *fluid overload, decreased activity tolerance, anxiety, knowledge deficit,* and *potential impaired skin integrity.* There was no consensus by the experts in the circulation problem category. The experts agreed that all the labels they chose, along with the interventions, are the scope of nursing practice.

Clinical relevancy of a diagnostic terminology system was rated by the experts in Phase III. Most of them believed a diagnostic terminology system would be helpful for the following reasons: it would gear thinking toward nursing interventions, it would make interventions more specific, it would improve documentation, it would foster accountability, it would simplify the study of nursing problems, and it would be a good teaching tool. Negative reactions included the following reasons: it would force nurses to memorize labels, there is no need for nurses to have their own labels, it would hinder communication and be confusing with Problem-Oriented Medical Records (POMR), and the majority of the profession would not be able to integrate the use of a terminology system. Eight experts were positive about a diagnostic terminology system, four were negative, and three had both positive and negative reactions.

To determine which of the nursing diagnostic labels used for choices in the Phase II and Phase III surveys were the most appropriate for patients with

TABLE 2   Consensus values of nursing diagnostic labels—Phases II and III

Nursing diagnostic labels	Mean frequency/SD, phases II and III	Mean scope/SD, phase II	Mean scope code	Mean clinical relevancy/SD, phase II	Consensus values
Alteration in circulation	13.89-2.78	3.27-1.31	3	3.12-.755	130.01
Congestive heart failure	24.50-5.67	4.46-1.34	2	3.11-.539	152.39
Decreased cardiac output	11.50-3.89	3.89-.657	3	3.32-.680	114.54
Fluid overload	28.89-2.26	3.69-1.26	3	3.09-.560	267.81
Fluid volume excess	19.67-1.25	3.92-1.58	3	3.16-.678	186.47
Decreased activity tolerance	33.67-2.87	2.09-1.10	3	3.37-.639	340.40
Fatigue	16.33-2.62	2.55-1.16	3	3.01-.565	147.75
Anxiety	46.00-3.27	2.65-1.96	3	3.24-.594	447.12
Fear	3.33-2.49	2.29-1.33	3	3.11-.954	31.07
Knowledge deficit	19.56-5.03	2.35-1.31	3	3.32-.614	194.82
Lack of knowledge	27.78-3.14	2.62-1.35	3	3.29-.630	274.19
Impaired skin integrity, potential	24.22-8.84	2.21-1.11	3	3.33-.550	241.96
Potential tissue breakdown	24.44-8.03	2.12-1.14	3	3.40-.626	249.29

congestive heart failure, a consensus formula was devised. The mean frequency, scope of practice rating, and clinical relevancy rating were determined for each label, using Phase II and Phase III data. A coding system was devised for the scope of practice mean, because a low numeric value correlated with nursing practice. A consensus value was then computed for each nursing diagnostic label. This value was a cross-product of the mean nursing diagnostic label frequency, the mean scope of practice code, and the mean clinical relevancy rating. Table 2 lists the mean frequencies, mean scope, scope of practice code, mean clinical relevancy rating, and consensus value for each nursing diagnostic label. The nursing diagnostic labels with the highest consensus value from each problem category were *congestive heart failure, fluid overload, decreased activity tolerance, anxiety, lack of knowledge,* and *potential tissue breakdown.*

DISCUSSION
Diagnostic labels

In Phase I of this study, clinical specialists identified problems associated with congestive heart failure, a condition seen commonly in critical care. It is notable that one medical diagnosis propagated 11 problem categories, a fact that supports an important distinction made between medical and nursing diagnoses. Nursing diagnoses encompass all dimensions of man and describe many responses to illness. Medical diagnoses are more limited in their focus.

In the 11 categories, the labels most frequently identified were physiologically oriented. One might infer that critical care nursing centers frequently on a patient's physiologic status. This belief is congruent with Maslow's hierarchy of basic human needs, the first being the physiologic needs of survival and stimulation (Luckmann and Sorensen, 1980). The current nursing diagnostic classification system is deficient in describing physiologically oriented nursing diagnoses. These types of diagnoses raise controversies in discussions of the nurse's role. It is evident that patients in critical care suffer from acute, life-threatening, physiologic disturbances. These problems are often recognized and treated by nurses who use sophisticated judgment and decision making in implementation of medical protocol. To withhold description of these problems from a nursing taxonomy minimizes the significant contributions of critical care nursing to the advancement of the profession.

It is curious, but not surprising, that in the category *circulation* the most frequently selected label was *congestive heart failure*, which is a clinical syndrome familiar to and readily recognized by most staff nurses. The frequent selection of *congestive heart failure* might be attributed to the orientation of nursing programs. Many nursing curricula mold thought processes conforming with the medical model of disease recognition and present nursing interventions relevant to medical diagnoses. A challenge to educators is the development of nursing curricula congruent with the concept of nursing diagnoses, which is antecedent to uniformity in practice.

Antecedent also is the education of practicing nurses in the diagnostic process (Aspinall, 1976; Matthews and Gaul, 1979). Nurses must become familiar not only with the concept of nursing diagnosis, but also with the accepted terminology. It is notable that *alteration in circulation* and *decreased cardiac output* were selected in 43% of the cases in Phase II. Both are labels approved by the national conference. Another approved label, *decreased activity tolerance*, was selected most frequently from the activity category. These results are interesting because 82% of the staff nurses were not exposed to nursing diagnoses. One might infer that the approved labels do hold relevance for practicing nurses.

In the category *cognition*, two staff nurses identified the alternate labels *learning need* and *inadequate knowledge*. The experts, when asked about the appropriateness of the labels, indicated that *learning need* conveyed a more positive meaning than knowledge deficit or lack of knowledge. The connotation of a label is an interesting point to consider in the development and approval of terminology.

Data results revealed that, in most instances, the experts and the staff nurses agreed in their selection of nursing diagnostic labels. However, a high standard deviation score for *congestive heart failure* indicates some variability of the frequency with which it was chosen. Congestive heart failure was selected by 33% of the experts compared with 57% of the staff nurses. The high standard deviation scores for both labels in the integument category indicate that most clinical specialists selected *potential impaired skin integrity* and most staff nurses chose *potential tissue breakdown*. One might agree that clinical specialists view patient problems at higher levels of abstraction. Whereas both groups of nurses are essential for development of a nursing taxonomy, perhaps clinical specialists should be the subjects in primary testing of labels.

Scope of practice

The experts and staff nurses in Phases I and II rated most of their diagnostic labels in the independent or interdependent scope of nursing practice. The *t*-test result from Phase II demonstrated no significant difference between the scope of practice and the independent and interdependent survey groups. This result supports one of the assumptions of this study—interdependent interventions, reflecting interdependent nursing judgment, are within the scope of nursing practice. It is evident that critical care nurses view their clinical judgments within the scope of nursing, even when such judgments require decisions involving medical treatment.

Clinical relevancy

Statements about clinical relevancy of the nursing diagnostic labels were rated by experts and staff nurses. The mean clinical relevancies of the labels from both experts and staff nurse responses were high, supporting the results obtained by Jones (1981) in studying the usefulness of nursing diagnoses.

It is interesting to note that some currently approved nursing diagnostic labels had higher clinical relevancy ratings than did alternate labels from the same problem category. *Decreased cardiac output*, for example, had a higher clinical relevancy rating than *congestive heart failure; fluid volume excess* had a higher clinical relevancy rating than *fluid overload*. This may indicate that the labels are more directive of nursing actions than are the alternate labels.

Results of chi-square tests indicated a statistically significant association between the nursing diagnostic labels and their clinical relevancies in the problem categories of *activity* and *emotion*. These results may indicate that the nursing diagnosis, *decreased activity tolerance*, has a higher level of clinical relevancy than *fatigue* and that *anxiety* has a higher level of clinical relevancy than *fear*. One might surmise that *decreased activity tolerance* is more explicit in directing nursing care than *fatigue*. *Anxiety* may be more clinically relevant because it is more familiar to the staff nurses than the new nursing diagnosis approved by the national conference, *fear*.

Although most of the comments from the experts about a diagnostic terminology system were positive, some showed resistance to the concept. These experts believed that a new terminology system may confuse communication among health professionals by the use of various labels when recording patient behavior. Confusion may exist, for example, if *congestive heart failure* and *decreased cardiac output* were used to describe a patient's response in the POMR format. These problems need to be addressed. Implications for supporters of the nursing diagnosis concept include conducting validation research on the nursing diagnostic labels to determine which of these labels are the most appropriate and the most clinically useful. Those nurses who clinically implement nursing diagnoses must be alert to these reactions and must base the use of nursing diagnoses on sound research.

Future research

The following recommendations have evolved from this study:
1. Replication of this study, using a larger sample size and randomization, which would determine invariance of response across many settings, involving many types of nurses.
2. Testing and validation of the labels described in this study, focusing on those labels of a physiologic nature. By testing these labels within the clinical setting, their relevancy can be further determined.
3. Replication of the same methodology of this study to describe nursing diagnostic labels for other patient situations.

SUMMARY

Surveys were used to identify nursing diagnostic labels for patients with congestive heart failure. The scope of practice and the clinical relevancy of each of these labels were also described. The following nursing diagnostic labels were identified as the most appropriate for patients with congestive heart failure: *heart failure, fluid overload, decreased activity tolerance, anxiety, lack of knowledge,* and *potential tissue breakdown.* The participants in this study indicated that physiologically oriented nursing diagnostic labels are within the scope of nursing practice and are clinically relevant. The concept of interdependent functions in critical care nursing is also supported. The result of this study suggest the importance of addressing interdependent nursing function in a nursing diagnosis taxonomy.

REFERENCES

American Nurses' Association: Nursing: a social policy statement, Kansas City, Mo., 1980, The Association.

Aspinall, N.J.: Nursing diagnosis—the weak link, Nurs. Outlook **24**(7):443, 1976.

Campbell, C.: Nursing diagnosis and Intervention in Nursing Practice, New York, 1978, John Wiley & Sons, Inc.

Gebbie, K., and Lavin, M.A.: Classifying nursing diagnoses, Mo. Nurs. **42**:10, 1973.

Gordon, M.: Nursing diagnosis and the diagnostic process, Am. J. Nurs. **76**(8):1298, 1976.

Jones, P.E.: The revision of nursing diagnostic terms. In Kim. M. I., and Moritz, D.A., eds.: Classification of nursing diagnoses: proceedings of the third and fourth national conferences, New York, 1982, McGraw-Hill Book Co.

Kim, M.J., and others: nursing diagnosis in cardiovascular Nursing. In Kim, M.J., and Moritz, D.A., eds.: Classification of nursing diagnoses: proceedings of the third and fourth national conference, New York, 1982, McGraw-Hill Book Co.

Luckmann, J., and Sorensen, K.: Medical-surgical nursing, Philadelphia, 1980, W.B. Saunders Co.

Matthews, C.A., and Gaul, A.L.: Nursing diagnosis from the perspective of concept attainment and critical thinking, Adv. Nurs. Sci. **2**(1):17, 1979.

The influence of amounts and relevance of data on identifying health problems

KENNETH L. CIANFRANI, R.N., Ph.D.

INTRODUCTION

During the nursing process, nurses collect data about a patient's condition (Yura and Walsh, 1973). What do nurses do with the data? Identification of problems is also a step of the nursing process, or it may be included in the step of collecting data (Gordon, 1979). Nurses have been identified as problem solvers, with problems defined as health disorders (Abdellah and others, 1960). Identifying a health problem is making a judgment based on data gathered about the condition of the patient. For this reason, Kelly (1964) and Hammond (1964) referred to problem identification as an inference task. The task also was described by Matthews and Gaul (1980) and Gordon (1973; 1980) as concept identification. Studies in psychology have shown that amounts and relevance of data influence the identification of concepts (Bourne and Dominowski, 1972). Do amounts and relevance of data influence identifying health problems? The influence of information received by nurses about a patient's condition on identifying health problems has not been studied. The purpose of this study is to answer the questions: What do nurses do with data they receive? Do amounts and relevance of data influence identifying health problems by nurses? The objectives of this study were to clarify the nursing task of concept identification and to describe the influence of amounts and relevance of data on the cognitive aspect of the nursing process.

Because of a lack of research about the influences on processing information in nursing, formal hypotheses could not be developed. From results of studies on concept identification, the following expectations guided this investigation:

1. With an increase in amounts of data, it is expected that there will be a decrease in accuracy.
2. With an increase in amounts of data, it is expected that there will be an increase in the number of health problems hypothesized.
3. With an increase in amounts of data, it is expected that there will be an increase in errors.
4. With an increase in amounts of data, it is expected that there will be an increase in the amount of time subjects take to identify the health problem.

□Research done in partial fulfillment of the requirements for Doctor of Philosophy degree.

5. With low relevant data, it is expected that there will be a decrease in accuracy.
6. With low relevant data, it is expected that there will be an increase in health problems hypothesized.
7. With low relevant data, it is expected that there will be an increase in errors.
8. With low relevant data, it is expected that there will be an increase in the time needed to identify the health problems.

BACKGROUND

Florence Nightingale identified observation, reflection, and action as the essence of nursing (Newton, 1949). In 1895 she stated: "Observation tells how the patient is; reflection tells what is to be done. . . . Observation tells us the fact, reflection tells us the meaning of the fact" (Nightingale, 1907, p. 225). Observation, for Nightingale, is gathering facts about the patient to learn about his condition. Nightingale gave reflection a two-pronged definition of deriving meaning from observed facts about a patient and deciding intelligently what action should be taken to relieve the patient's suffering (Nutting and Dock, 1907).

The nurse identifies a health problem by making a judgment based on observed facts regarding the patient's condition (Gordon, 1973; Hammond, 1966; Kelly, 1964). The purpose of identifying a health problem is to make decisions about nursing care (Kelly, 1964). The health problem is used to define the goals of care, to generate alternate nursing activities, and to decide which action is appropriate for the patient (Bailey and Claus, 1975; Gordon, 1979; Grier, 1976; Little and Carnevali, 1976). The inference of what is wrong with the patient is only one of many cognitive tasks the nurse must perform, but it is the basis for planning nursing care.

Nurses use strategies to collect data regarding the state of the patient (Hammond and coworkers, 1966c). Their results showed that different nurses used different strategies for different inferences. Gordon (1973, 1980) also studied strategies used to collect information for identifying health problems. Viewing the inference task from a cognitive perspective, she used Bruner's work (1956) on attainment of simple concepts as a framework for her investigation. She concluded that nurses used different strategies early in the diagnostic task and changed strategies as the task progressed. Results from concept identification are similar. A variety of strategies is used to identify concepts, and dfferent strategies may be used to identify the same concepts (Dominowski, 1974).

Hammond (1966) viewed nurses as processors of information and not "one-cue, one-response organisms." He stated that nurses make judgments about the state of the patient by weighing cues and recognizing patterns of cues about the state of the patient. He was unable, however, to identify patterns of cues that were used by nurses in the study (Hammond and others, 1966b). Cues have uncertain relationships with inferences; a cue may be present at one time but not at another time (Hammond, 1966). He concluded that inferences are probabilistic. Kelly (1964) showed that nurses used 165 cues to infer pain in 212 patients who had abdominal surgery and identified 18 nursing actions and 58 medical orders for relieving pain. Both Hammond and Kelly concluded that the inference task performed by nurses was complex. Findings from outside nursing support this conclusion.

Kleinmuntz (1968) studied the diagnostic process of neurologists in identifying neurologic disorders. He concluded that the process of diagnosing in neurology was not an all or nothing decision but a complex concept identification task in which data must be sifted, sorted, accepted, and rejected and in which hypotheses were formulated and confirmed or disproved. He also concluded that neurologists used strategies that involved long- and short-term memory.

Elstein, Shulman, and Sprafka (1978) studied the diagnostic process of physicians, emphasizing the role of memory and prior knowledge. Their findings supported the notion that performance in identifying and solving medical problems is highly specific for each problem. They stated that measures of the diagnostic process do not reflect individual consistency in defining and solving the problem. For them, problem solving in medicine depends on knowledge and experience with the content and demands of each particular problem.

FRAMEWORK

In considering the question of what nurses do with data, an information-processing approach was used to view concept identification. An information-processing approach attempts to explain cognitive performance in terms of mental operations performed on information (Newell, Shaw, and Simon, 1958). The senses provide information about present events, and memory provides information about past events (Bourne and Dominowski, 1979). The information is interpreted by a series of processes or mental operations called strategies (Bruner, Goodnow, and Austin, 1956). Concept identification, for this study, was defined as the attainment of an abstraction through the use of strategies operating on information encountered in the environment. Using memory and strategies, the person organized the inference task into the concept to be identified and the information to be processed.

The concept to be identified in nursing is the health problem. Hammond (1966) described the health problem as probabilistic because of the uncertain relationship between the cues and the problem. He concluded that this relationship contributed to the difficulty and complexity of the task. In concept identification studies, the relationship between the cues was also found to influence the difficulty of identifying concepts (Neisser and Weene, 1962). Neisser and Weene described 16 possible logical relationships between cues. Cues with affirmative relationships had less influence on the difficulty of identifying concepts than cues with more complex relationships. A simple combination of cues can be recognized as an instance of the concept and can aid concept identification (Dominowski, 1968). However, if the combination of cues is not an instance of the concept, difficulty is increased. Positive instances of the health problem can be developed by nurses.

Nurses use memory and strategies to identify health problems (Gordon, 1980). Memory has several stages with different processes (Bourne and Dominowski, 1979). Whereas sensory memory receives data from the environment, information from past experience is retrieved from long-term memory. Nurses receive information from the environment and recall past experiences to identify health problems (Gordon, 1980; Kelly, 1964; Little and Carnevali, 1976). Past knowledge that is organized is more easily retrieved and facilitates identifying concepts (Bousefield, Cohen, and Whitmarsh, 1958). Identification of health problems may be facilitated by the organization of knowledge according to a theoretic framework. Short-term memory is the working memory that processes both newly received data and recalled information. Reducing the load of information used in short-term memory leads to better use of information and to better performance in identifying concepts (Wetherick and Dominowski, 1976). In identifying concepts, information is weighed, selected, clustered, combined, and eliminated (Bruner, Goodnow, and Austin, 1956). Combinations of these basic mental operations are called *strategies*, and studies show that a variety is used to identify concepts (Dominowski, 1974).

Hammond and others (1966c) showed that nurses used ineffective strategies for gathering information. Gordon (1973; 1980) showed that nurses used multiple- and single-hypothesis testing to identify patient health problems. In multiple-hypothesis testing, many health problems are hypothesized simultaneously to confirm the patient's problem. In single-hypothesis testing, one health problem is hypothesized at a time until a diagnosis is confirmed. Another strategy identified by Bruner, Goodnow, and Austin, (1956) for identifying concepts was attribute testing, in which a list of cues that match cues received about the patient's condition is identified from long-term memory. The cues from long-term memory are associated with a particular concept. Dominowski (1969) showed that attribute testing may be related to early hypothesizing and to improved problem solving.

Nurses use strategies and memory to process information. They receive this information from a variety of sources (Kelly, 1964). Characteristics of information have been shown to influence the difficulty of identifying concepts. With an increase in the number of cues, there was an increase in difficulty of identifying concepts (Bourne and Dominowski, 1972; Walker and Bourne, 1961). Studies of increases in relevant and irrelevant cues showed that the number of errors increased. The conclusions were that subjects were less able to identify concepts with an increase in either irrelevant or relevant cues (Bowers and King, 1967; Byers and Davidson, 1968; Dominowski, 1969; Haygood and Stevenson, 1967; Keele and Archer, 1967; Walker and Bourne, 1961). The National Conference on the Classification of Nursing Diagnoses has been identifying defining characteristics that are commonly associated with nursing diagnoses (Gebbie, 1976; Gebbie and Lavin, 1975; Kim and Moritz, 1982). The defining characteristics are a beginning step in the identification of relevant cues for health problems. The influence of amounts and relevance of data on identifying health problems by nurses has not been studied.

METHOD

Using an experimental approach, the influence of amounts and relevance of data on identifying health problems was examined. A factorial design was constructed with two conditions of relevant cues and three levels of amounts of data. The two conditions of relevance consisted of high and low relevant cues. The three levels of amounts of data consisted of 4, 8, and 12 cues in each condition of relevance. To construct the three levels of amounts of data, 4 and 8 low relevant cues were added to 4 high and 4 low relevant cues. Subjects were assigned randomly to one of the six groups. They received data varying in amounts and relevance according to the group to which they were assigned. The subjects were asked to identify three separate target health problems. The influence of amounts and relevance of data on identifying health problems was determined by comparing the subjects' performance in the six groups an accuracy, number of health problems hypothesized, errors, and time taken to identify the health problems.

Subjects

Subjects for the study were 120 students in four graduate nursing programs approved by the National League of Nursing and 60 members of the American Critical Care Nurses Association in the Chicago area. The mean years experience was 7.5 with a range of 1 to 42 years. The number of subjects at each test session ranged from five to 34. Subjects were informed of the purpose of the study before they were given the data.

Instrument

The pencil-and-paper instrument consisted of five parts: a consent form, instructions, vignette, three patient information sheets of two pages each, and request for demographic information. Instructions included an explanation of the tasks, which were to record the time, list the health problem(s), and rank the problems if more than one was listed. The vignette described a hypothetic work setting. It delineated circumstances in a hospital setting in which patient health problems might be identified. The three target health problems were taken from a study by Kim and others (1982). Among the most frequently identified nursing diagnoses were *decreased cardiac output, alterations in comfort,* and *alterations in peripheral circulation. Alterations in comfort* was made more specific by choosing the most frequently identified alteration in comfort in the study by Kim and others—*chest pain.*

The high and low relevant cues were also taken from the study by Kim and others (1982). After identifying nursing diagnoses for a particular patient, the nurses listed the defining characteristics or cues used to make the diagnoses. The frequency of the defining characteristics for each diagnosis was determined. For purposes of this study, the defining characteristics with the highest frequency were assumed to have high relevance and those used less frequently were assumed to have low relevance for the same diagnosis.

Based on previous concept identification studies by Bowers and King (1967), Byers and Davidson (1968), and Dominowski (1969), a study by Phelps and Shanteau (1980), and a study by Miller (1956), 4 cues were chosen as the lowest amount and 12 cues as the highest amount of data given to the subjects. To increase the amount of data, low relevant cues were added to avoid giving redundant information (Bourne and Dominowski, 1972) and to keep identifying data consistent. The cues added to each level were the same for both conditions of relevance.

Procedure

Data were collected from groups of five to 34 subjects in a classroom or lecture hall environment. A brief explanation of the purpose of the study was given without disclosing the two variables under study. A digital clock displaying the minutes and seconds in large illuminated numbers was placed in full view of all the subjects.

One set of patient information was compiled for each target health problem. This information included data about a hypothetic patient that varied in relevance and amounts according to the six conditions for study. Before reading the cues, subjects recorded in the space provided the time displayed on the digital clock. After reading the cues, the subjects listed the health problem(s) they thought the patient was experiencing. If subjects listed more than one health problem, they ranked the problems according to those they considered most appropriate for the data presented. After listing a health problem, subjects again recorded the time; it they listed more than one health problem, they recorded the time after listing each health problem.

Analysis

Analysis of data was done using chi-square for the dichotomous data on accuracy and two-way analysis of variance for health problems hypothesized, errors, and time to determine if interactions occurred between amounts and relevance of data. Responses were considered accurate if the target health problem was listed or selected. However, subjects did not use labels similar to those chosen from the Second National Conference on the Classification of Nursing Diagnoses (Gebbie, 1976). The labels that did not match the target health problems were submitted to two nurses, a coronary care clinical specialist and a nursing instructor, who had master degrees. They independently chose from the labels identified by the subjects those labels judged similar to the target health problems used for the study. Agreement between the two raters for decreased cardiac output was .93; for alterations in comfort .93; and for alterations in peripheral circulation .89. Only those labels agreed on by the raters as being synonymous with the target health problems were considered correct.

RESULTS

Accuracy significantly decreased with low relevant data for all three health problems (decreased cardiac output: Yates' χ^2 = 36.5, df = 1, p = .00005; alterations in comfort: Yates' χ^2 = 24.21, df = 1, p = .00005; alterations in peripheral circulation: Yates' χ^2 = 32.33, df = 1, p = .00005). Accuracy decreased significantly with more data only in alterations in comfort (χ^2 = 12.86, df = 2, p = .001). Results supported the expectation for decreased accuracy with low relevant data.

Subjects often listed the correct health problem. The responses of those who listed the correct health problem were compared with the responses of those who did not list it, using the chi-square. This comparison was done to determine the influence of amounts and relevance of data on listing the correct health problem. The listing of the correct health problem significantly decreased for all three problems with low relevant data (decreased cardiac output: Yates' χ^2 = 44.95, df = 1, p = .0000; alterations in comfort: Yates' χ^2 = 37.64, df = 1, p = .0000; alterations in peripheral circulation: Yates' χ^2 = 40.53, df = 1, p = .0000). Findings showed one problem with a decrease in listing with more data (alterations in comfort χ^2 = 28.02, df = 2, p = .0000). The other two problems had decreases with more data that were not significant.

Only those subjects who listed the correct health problem could rank it as number one. Chi-square was used to compare those subjects who, after listing the correct health problem, ranked it as number one and those who did not. Alterations in peripheral circulation was the only problem in which data showed a significant decrease in ranking with increased amounts of data (χ^2 = 6.85; df = 2; p = .03). There was no significant difference in ranking the correct health problem with low relevant data even though a decrease was found in all three problems.

Results of analysis for two health problems supported the expectation that more health problems would be hypothesized with increased amounts of data (decreased cardiac output: $F_{2,174} = 2.88$, $p = .05$; alterations in comfort: $F_{2,170} = 5.22$, $p = .01$). Findings for the third problem were consistent with this but not significant (alterations in peripheral circulation: $F_{2,174} = .77$, $p = .46$). The influence of relevance on health problems hypothesized was inconsistent. For one health problem there was a significant increase in health problems hypothesized with low relevant data (alterations in peripheral circulation: $F_{1,174} = 7.68$, $p = .01$). For another problem significantly fewer health problems were hypothesized (alterations in comfort: $F_{1,170} = 8.80$, $p = .00$). Data for the third problem were in keeping with the decrease in hypotheses with low relevant data but was not significant (decreased cardiac output: $F_{1,174} = 0.72$, $p = .39$).

The results of analysis supported the expectation for errors with increased amounts of data. For two problems there was an increase in errors with increased amounts of data (decreased cardiac output: $F_{2,174} = 3.97$, $p = .02$; alterations in comfort: $F_{2,173} = 7.72$, $p = .001$). For the third problem an increase occurred but was not significant (alterations in peripheral circulation: $F_{2,174} = 1.15$, $p = .31$). The expectation of increased errors with low relevant data was also supported with significant increases in two problems (decreased cardiac output: $F_{1,174} = 3.96$, $p = .04$; alterations in peripheral circulation: $F_{1,174} = 29.15$, $p = .000$). For the third problem more errors were made with a few low relevant cues, but this was not significant (alterations in comfort: $F_{1,173} = 0.87$, $p = .35$). An interaction occurred between amounts and relevance in the same problem (alterations in comfort: $F_{2,173} = 5.08$, $p = .007$).

The expectation that more time would be taken with increased amounts of data was supported in two of the health problems, with an increase in the third that was not significant (decreased cardiac output: $F_{2,171} = 5.41$, $p = .005$; alterations in peripheral circulation: $F_{2,171} = 2.87$, $p = .05$; alterations in comfort: $F_{2,170} = 1.20$, $p = .30$). Results were inconsistent for the influence of relevance on time. A significant decrease in time rather than an increase was found for one problem (alterations in comfort: $F_{1,170} = 5.51$, $p = .02$). Time to identify the other two problems showed an increase that was not significant (decreased cardiac output: $F_{1,171} = 2.53$, $p = .11$; alterations in peripheral circulation: $F_{1,171} = .92$, $p = .33$).

SUMMARY

Findings showed that there was an increase in health problems hypothesized and in time with increased amounts of data. A decrease in accuracy for all three health problems was found with low relevant data. An increase in errors was found for both increased amounts of data and low relevant data. Variations in results among the three health problems were also found. Additional analysis showed that there was a decrease in listing the correct health problem with low relevant data but not for amounts of data. In one problem a decrease in the selection of the target health problem was found significant with increased amounts of data and decreases in the selection of the correct health problem occurred for both increased amounts and low relevant data but were not significant.

DISCUSSION

Amounts of data influenced health problems hypothesized and time. When data increased, more health problems were hypothesized and more time was taken to identify the health problems. Bruner, Goodnow, and Austin (1956) stated that cues are weighed, selected, and clustered and combined in identifying concepts. Elstein, Shulman, and Sprafka (1978) stated that more hypotheses are generated with more cues. With an increase in the number of cues, more time was needed to consider the cues and more health problems were hypothesized to make use of the cues.

Relevance of data influenced accuracy; that is, accuracy decreased with low relevant data. Elstein, Shulman, and Sprafka (1978) stated that alternative diagnoses were generated from long-term memory by association with clusters of cues. However, generating and hypothesizing the correct diagnosis did not guarantee selecting the correct alternative. With low relevant data, the cluster of cues associated with the correct health problem in long-term memory was not available. As a result the correct health problem was not hypothesized. When it was hypothesized, a decrease in selecting the correct alternative occurred, although results were not significant.

Amounts and relevance of data were both found to influence errors. With increased amounts of data and low relevant data, more errors were made because the correct health problem was less likely to be hypothesized and selected. For this study, the increase in errors may also have been a function of the definition of errors. Health problems that were hypothesized but were not the correct health problem were counted as errors; with increased amounts of data more health problems were hypothesized, which could then account for the increase in errors.

The influence of amounts and relevance varied for alterations in comfort. Differences between problems have been found in other studies and should be expected in concept identification (Newell and Simon, 1967). Elstein, Shulman, and Sprafka (1978) stated that content and the response of the problem solver to that content are specific for each problem. Variability on different problems emphasized the knowledge and experience of the individual, especially when the problem may be associated with different cues on different occasions. Differences in this problem were that amounts influenced accuracy and relevance influenced health problems hypothesized and time. With increased amounts of data, accuracy decreased as a result of failure to list or select the correct health problem. Less time was taken and fewer health problems were hypothesized as an influence of low relevant cues, which may have occurred because subjects were either satisfied with the health problems they hypothesized or were frustrated with low relevant data and ended the task early. Simon (1967) stated that cognitive processing of information can be terminated as a result of feeling that the task was done "well enough" or because attempts to accomplish the task fail. An interaction occurred between amounts and relevance of data for errors. Fewer errors were made with a small amount of high relevant cues; subjects hypothesized several problems that were synonymous with the target health problem.

This study investigated the influence of amounts and relevance of data for three health problems. The results are limited in their generalizability to all problems. Results are also limited because the study used an experimental approach. In a real situation, nurses may have more data, may select data they believe is important, and may have to identify more than one problem per patient.

Even though the study has limitations, the results have implications. Nurses with increased amounts of data and/or low relevant data take more time and are less likely to be accurate. In addition, low relevant data may discourage nurses in their attempts to make judgments about health states and result in premature termination of the task necessary for making decisions about nursing care. As accuracy decreases with increased amounts of data and low relevant data, nurses need strategies to cope with these influences.

The results of this study offer a clear indication that further research is needed to develop strategies that focus on evaluation of relevance of data and allow for limiting amounts of data to be processed by nurses in identifying health problems. Research is also needed to determine cues that are relevant for health problems treated by nurses. Another area for research is the variability of results among problems. Results of problems with similar content should be compared to determine if they are similar. Further research is indicated to determine the relationship of concepts to be identified, the use of memory and strategies by nurses, and the information to be processed.

REFERENCES

Abdellah, F.G., and others: Patient-centered approaches to nursing, New York, 1960, Macmillan Publishing Co., Inc.

Bailey, J.T., and Claus, K.F.: Decision making in nursing—tools for change, St. Louis, 1975, The C.V. Mosby Co.

Bourne, L.E., and Dominowski, R.L.: Thinking, Ann. Rev. Psychol. **24**:105, 1972.

Bourne, L.E., Dominowski, R.L., and Loftus, E.F.: Cognitive processes, Englewood Cliffs, N.J., 1979, Prentice-Hall, Inc.

Bousefield, W.A., Cohen, B.W., and Whitmarsh, G.A.: Association clustering in recall of words of different taxonomic frequencies of occurence, Psychol. Rev. **4:**39, 1958.

Bowers, A.C., and King, W.L.: The effect of number of irrelevant stimulus dimensions, verbalization, and sex on learning biconditional classification rules, Psychonom. Sci. **8:**453, 1967.

Bruner, J.S., Goodnow, J.J., and Austin, G.A.: A study of thinking, New York, 1956, John Wiley & Sons, Inc.

Byers, J.K., and Davidson, R.E.: Relevant and irrelevant information in concept attainment, J. Exper. Psychol. **76:**277, 1968.

Dominowski, R.L.: Stimulus memory in concept identification, Psychonom. Sci. **10:**359, 1968.

Dominowski, R.L.: Concept attainment as a function of instance contiguity and number of irrelevant dimensions, J. Exper. Psychol. **82:**573, 1969.

Dominowski, R.L.: How do people discover concepts? In Solso, R.L., ed.: Theories in cognitive psychology: the Loyola symposium, Washington, D.C., 1974, V.W. Winston & Sons.

Elstein, A.C. Shulman, L.S., and Sprafka, S.A.: Medical problem solving, Cambridge, Mass., 1978, Harvard University Press.

Gebbie, K.: Summary of the second national conference for the classification of nursing diagnoses, St. Louis, 1976, Clearinghouse—National Group for Classification of Nursing Diagnoses.

Gebbie, K., and Lavin, M.: Classification of nursing diagnoses: proceedings of the first national conference, St. Louis, 1975, The C.V. Mosby Co.

Gordon, M.R.: Information processing strategies in nursing diagnosis, Paper presented at the ANA Ninth Nursing Research Conference, San Antonio, March 1973.

Gordon, M.R.: The concept of nursing diagnoses, Nurs. Clin. North Am. 14:487, 1979.

Gordon, M.R.: Predictive strategies in diagnostic tasks, Nurs. Res. **29:**39, 1980.

Grier, M.R.: Decision making about patient care, Nurs. Res. **25:**105, 1976.

Hammond, K.R.: An approach to the study of clinical inference in nursing. Part II: a methodological approach, Nurs. Res. **13:**315, 1964.

Hammond, K.R.: Clinical inference in nursing. Part II: a psychologist viewpoint, Nurs. Res. **15:**27, 1966.

Hammond, K.R., and others: Clinical inference in nursing: information units used, Nurs. Res. **15:**236, 1966a.

Hammond, K.R., and others: Clinical inference in nursing: use of information-seeking strategies by nurses, Nurs. Res. **15:**330, 1966b.

Haygood, R.C., and Stevenson, M.: Effects of the number of irrelevant dimensions in nonconjunctive concept learning, J. Exper. Psychol. **74:**302, 1967.

Keele, S.W., and Archer, E.J.: A comparison of two types of information in concept identification, J. Verbal Learn. Verbal Behav. **6:**185, 1967.

Kelly, K.J.: An approach to the study of clinical inference in nursing. Part I: introduction to the study of clinical inference in nursing, Nurs. Res. **13:**314, 1964.

Kim, M.J., and Moritz, D.A., eds.: Classification of nursing diagnoses: proceedings of the third and fourth national conferences, New York, 1982, McGraw-Hill Book Co.

Kim, M.J., and others: Clinical use of nursing diagnosis in cardiovascular nursing. In Kim, M.J., and Moritz, D.A., eds.: Classification of nursing diagnoses: proceedings of the third and fourth national conferences, New York, 1982, McGraw-Hill Book Co.

Kleinmuntz, B.: The processing of clinical information by man and machine. In Kleinmutz, B., ed.: Formal representation of human judgment, New York, 1968, John Wiley & Sons, Inc.

Little, D.E., and Carnevali, D.: Nursing care planning, Philadelphia, 1976, J.B. Lippincott Co.

Matthews, C.A., and Gaul, A.L.: Nursing diagnosis from the perspective of concept attainment and critical thinking, Ad. Nurs. Sci. **2:**17, 1979.

Miller, G.A.: The magical number seven, plus or minus two: some limits on our capacity for processing information, Psychol. Rev. **63:**81, 1956.

Neisser, U., and Weene, P.: Hierarchies in concept attainment, J. Exper. Psychol. **64:**640, 1962.

Newell, A., Shaw, J.C., and Simon, H.A.: Elements of a theory of human problem solving, Psychol. Rev. **5:**151, 1958.

Newell, A., and Simon, H.A.: Overview: memory and process in concept formation. In Klein-muntz, B., ed.: Concepts and the structure of memory, New York, 1967, John Wiley & Sons, Inc.

Newton, M.: Florence Nightingale's philosophy of life and education, unpublished doctoral dissertation, San Francisco, 1949, Stanford University.

Nightingale, F.: Training of nurses. In Nutting, M.A., and Dock, L.L., eds.: History of nursing, vol. II, New York, 1907. G.P. Putnam's Sons.

Nutting, M.A., and Dock, L.L.: History of nursing, vol. II, New York, 1982, G.P. Putman's Sons.

Phelps, R.N., and Shanteaw, J.: Livestock judges: how much information can an expert use? Organiz. Behav. Human Perform. 21:209, 1978.

Simon, H.A.: Motivational and emotional control of cognition, Psychol. Rev. 74:29, 1967.

Walker, C.M., and Bourne, L.E.: The identification of concepts as a function of amounts of relevant and irrelevant information, Am. J. Psychol. 74:410, 1961.

Wetherick, N.E., and Dominowski, R.L.: How representative are concept attainment experiments? Br. J. Psychol. 67:231, 1976.

Yura, H., and Walsh, M.B.: The nursing process, New York, 1973, Appleton-Century-Crofts.

Discussion

Marjory Gordon: This is such an important area. We really need to get the process of diagnosis and the development of a taxonomy going. There are so many articles to study in terms of redundancy. Is there a program of research in the process of diagnosis?

Kenneth Cianfrani: I know there are several students who are interested in the process of diagnosis, but I am not sure exactly in what phase they are interested. My feelings are that while nurses are identified as problem solvers, we do not understand what the problem is that we are trying to solve. That issue has certainly affected all of us.

Carol Baer: Although I appreciate the fact that you primarily emphasize the process of data collection, what do you think might be the relevance of doing an experimental group–control group study in which the experimental group has learned to collect cues by a particular assessment guide versus another group that collected data by arbitrary means?

Kenneth Cianfrani: Are you asking why this study was experimental or presenting an idea for another study, that is, whether or not an experimental study should be looked at for controlling the kinds of information collected?

Carol Baer: The latter. Do you have any ideas about how the groups might look if one group of students had a structured assessment guide that they used in collecting the cues versus another group that had a variety of different methods of data collection?

Kenneth Cianfrani: No, I am sorry. The only study that I can think of is Marjory Gordon's* with the unrestricted and restricted groups. But I am not sure about the assessment. I have been concentrating on the process of diagnosing rather than the collection of data. That was why I gave my subjects data rather than let them select data. I think we might have to do studies in which nurses select data for the influence of various variables. There would certainly be some differences in the processes.

*Gordon, M.R.: Predictive strategies in diagnostic tasks, Nurs. Res. 29:39, 1980.

The identification of clinically recorded nursing diagnoses and indicators

SALLY McDONALD SILVER, R.N., M.S.N.
TERESE M. HALFMANN, R.N., M.S.N.
RUTH E. McSHANE, R.N., M.S.N.
CAROL A. HUNT, R.N., M.S.N.
CAROLYN A. NOWAK, R.N., M.S.N.

The concept of nursing diagnosis is currently recognized as a focal issue in the development of nursing as a science. This study investigated the following questions: (1) What nursing diagnoses do nurses identify clinically? (2) What are the indicators identified that substantiate the diagnoses? A list of 1344 diagnostic labels, with multiple indicators, were collected retrospectively from 377 charts. The sample was drawn from three adult medical-surgical units in a 600-bed, private, urban, teaching hospital located in the Midwest. Labels were transcribed from the patients' problem lists as recorded by staff registered nurses. For purposes of this study, labels were terms on patients' problem lists that were intended by the nurse to be nursing diagnoses. Subjective and objective data used in making the initial diagnosis were also transcribed.

The labels recorded as nursing diagnoses included those accepted by the Third National Conference on the Classification of Nursing Diagnoses as well as labels not accepted by the conferences. To explain and analyze the data, 16 major categories were developed, under which labels were placed (Table 1). Five national experts in nursing diagnosis assisted in refining the nursing diagnosis classification system.

The experts placed 25% (342) of the labels in the signs and symptoms category. *Shortness of breath* and *elevated temperature* were examples of labels in this category. The experts categorized 23% (311) of the labels as National Conference List (NCL) nursing diagnoses. Each remaining category contained from 12% to less than 1% of the 1344 labels.

Examination of the NCL nursing diagnoses category revealed that 15 of the nursing diagnoses accepted by the Third and Fourth National Conference

□The authors gratefully acknowledge the assistance of Lucy Feild, R.N., M.S.; Marjory Gordon, R.N., Ph.D., F.A.A.N.; Mi Ja Kim, R.N., Ph.D., F.A.A.N.; Phyllis Kritek, R.N., Ph.D., F.A.A.N.; and Audrey McLane, R.N., Ph.D. who served as our panel of experts. This research was supported in part by the Division of Nursing, U.S. Department of Health, Education, and Welfare Grant No. NU 00648 for research development awarded to the University of Wisconsin–Milwaukee School of Nursing and a grant from the Nurses' Foundation of Wisconsin.

TABLE 1   **Nursing diagnosis classification system**

Category	Percentage of all labels	Definition
National conference list (NCL) of nursing diagnoses	23	A label accepted at the Third and/or Fourth National Conferences on the Classification of Nursing Diagnoses
Non-NCL of nursing diagnoses	3	A label for a cluster of signs and symptoms describing an actual or potential health problem that nurses by virtue of their education and experience are capable and licensed to treat that does not appear on the Third or Fourth NCL of accepted diagnoses
Incomplete nursing diagnoses	2	A label that is a portion of a nursing diagnosis accepted at the Third and/or Fourth National Conferences on the Classification of Nursing Diagnoses
Somatic dysfunction	12	A label describing a potential or actual generalized physiologic deviation
Patient need	<1	A label describing a patient-family deficiency
Nursing problem	2	A label describing nursing responsibilities that are not directly related to patient-family care
Etiology	4	A label describing that which produces an alteration in the patient-family health status for which nursing intervention is needed to treat the effects of the alteration
Intervention	1	A label describing an action implemented to help meet a patient-family goal
Goal	<1	A label describing an intended expectation of the patient-family health status by a certain time
Sign or symptom	25	A label describing a subjective and/or objective indicator of patient-family health status
Risk factor	6	A label describing a fact, circumstance, or pattern of behavior that tends to put the patient or family at a higher than normal probability of incurring an alteration in health
Side effect/complication	<1	A label describing an actual or potential undesirable result of a therapeutic intervention
Equipment	<1	A label describing an apparatus used in the care of a patient
Diagnostic test	<1	A label describing an examination or procedure performed for the purpose of gathering information
Medical diagnoses and/or surgical procedure	11	A label appearing in the International Classification of Diseases specifically adapted for use in the hospitals of North America (H-ICDA)
Multiple title	9	A label combining two or more descriptive statements

Groups were represented. *Alteration in comfort: pain* was the most frequent nursing diagnosis in this category. This high incidence was anticipated because of the acute care setting from which the sample was drawn. Several nursing diagnoses, such as *sleep pattern disturbance* and *alterations in nutrition*, were considered significant by their absence in the same setting.

Only indicators from nurses' notes for the NCL and non-NCL diagnoses were examined. Indicators were those statements recorded by nurses in the subjective and objective sections of the initial subjective, objective, assessment, plan (SOAP) note.

Since *alteration in comfort: pain* was the most frequently occurring NCL nursing diagnoses, the indicators were analyzed separately. Subjective indicators comprised 33% of all indicators for pain and expand the NCL of verbal complaints. Objective indicators were divided into three divisions: negative indicators, positive indicators (those that describe desirable patient conditions), and general assessment data (descriptions of patient status such as blood pressure and bowel sounds).

A high incidence of positive indicators for *alteration in comfort: pain* were found and may be explained by considering its subjective nature. This diagnosis probably can be made on subjective data alone; therefore nursing's responsibility is to manage the duration, intensity, and effect on the patient's life-style. Objective data collected about pain described what a patient could or could not accomplish as a result of the pain. For instance, statements about the ability as well as the inability to sleep were frequently found. These indicators clearly outlined the problems associated with pain, not whether pain existed but how the patient was coping with it.

Increased abdominal girth and decreased bowel sounds were the indicators for *alteration in bowel elimination: constipation* that had not previously been identified on the NCL. Although the literature does not identify any one indicator as a critical parameter for making the diagnosis, frequency less than 3 times weekly was listed as an indicator in every SOAP note for *constipation.*

Indicators for the nursing diagnoses *self-care deficit* described deficits in bathing, feeding, and toileting. Self-dressing deficit was not found in the data, although it was identified on the NCL probably because of the lack of dressing as an expectation of a patient in the acute care setting.

The non-NCL nursing diagnosis category was created to analyze and evaluate the clinical usefulness of labels for problems managed by hospital nurses. Some of the titles were previously accepted diagnoses such as *anxiety.* Others, such as *altered energy level*, have never appeared on the NCL. It is hoped that the examination and presentation of the non-NCL labels and indicators will provide the impetus for developing a more complete and refined nomenclature.

One positive nursing diagnosis, *knowledge: health care regimen,* was found, for which only positive indicators were noted. Diagnoses that document the state of the patient's health rather than illness may be seen more frequently as wellness becomes a central focus for nursing.

Recommendations for nursing practice include the use of the 16-category system (Table 1) to measure nurses' diagnostic abilities. It is also recommended that nurses use possible or probable nursing diagnoses in acute care settings to eliminate the high incidence of signs and symptoms being documented as nursing diagnoses.

The developers of nursing curricula should examine nursing diagnosis as a basis for organizing concepts. High-frequency diagnoses such as *alteration in comfort: pain* and *self-care deficit* should have proportionately more time devoted to them in the study of health restoration than less frequently encountered diagnoses.

It is recommended that this study be replicated using a regional or national sample with different types of client populations in varied health care settings. Replication especially with changes in sampling would increase reliability and ability to generalize the results.

REFERENCE

Kim. M.J., and Moritz, D.A., eds.: Classification of nursing diagnoses: proceedings of the third and fourth national conferences, New York, 1982, McGraw-Hill Book Co.

Discussion

Margaret Lunney: How long had the nurses been using nursing diagnosis on the units that you chose?

Sally Silver: Three years.

Margaret Lunney: Did you look at any other variables such as continuing education?

Sally Silver: No, we did not formally look at educational preparedness as a variable. The reason we used the list of the Second and Third National Conferences was because the Fourth Conference list was not available at the time we collected our data. Nurses making diagnoses had multiple in-service classes on nursing diagnoses and multiple references, such as Campbell (1978) and the lists of the First, Second, and Third National Conferences (Gebbie, 1976; Gebbie and Lavin, 1975; Kim and Moritz, 1982).

Campbell, C.: Nursing diagnosis and intervention in nursing practice, New York, 1978, John Wiley & Sons, Inc.

Gebbie, K.M., ed.: Summary of the second national conference for the classification of nursing diagnoses, St. Louis, 1976, Clearinghouse—National Group for Classification of Nursing Diagnoses.

Gebbie, K.M., and Lavin, M.A., eds.: Proceedings of the first national conference classification of nursing diagnoses, St. Louis, 1975, The C.V. Mosby Co.

Kim, M.J., and Moritz, D.A., eds.: Classification of nursing diagnoses: proceedings of the third and fourth national conferences, New York, 1982, McGraw-Hill Book Co.

Documentation of nursing process in critical care

ROSEMARIE SUHAYDA, R.N., M.S.N.
MI JA KIM, R.N., Ph.D., F.A.A.N.

The nursing process has long been accepted as the foundation for nursing practice because it structures clinical judgments and decisions within the context of nursing theory and the scientific method. Carlson, Craft, and McGuire (1982) have identified several benefits of using the nursing process, including identifying actual and potential health problems, defining specific nursing responsibilities, communicating nursing therapies, and developing and fostering nursing autonomy and accountability.

It seems paradoxical that this process that governs cognitive processing of clinical decisions and serves as an expression of nursing's autonomy, accountability, professionalism, and worth is somehow invisible in actual documentation on the patient's permanent record. Numerous examples of documentation practices recount vast amounts of assessment data without diagnostic conclusions or related nursing decisions (Gordon, 1980). Certainly, nurses must realize that documentation provides objective data that can be used to substantiate and evaluate health care.

Critical care is an area in special need of evaluation of documentation practices. Current modes of charting allude to practice that is fragmented and technically oriented. Critical care nurses themselves have identified the need to succinctly and accurately express their nursing care within the context of the nursing process (Christopherson, 1981). The recent emphasis by the American Association of Critical Care Nurses on the integration of the nursing process into its own Standards of Care reinforces this need (AACN, 1981).

PURPOSES OF STUDY

The purposes of this study were to evaluate the documentation of the nursing process in critical care, identify the most commonly documented patient problems, and describe documented nursing actions and patient outcomes.

METHOD

A retrospective chart audit was conducted on 50 charts, 25 medical and 25 surgical, selected randomly from two medical and two surgical intensive care units in a large metropolitan teaching hospital. The units were staffed primarily by R.N.s with a 1:1 or 1:2 nurse/patient ratio. The charting format was narrative with flow sheets that became a permanent part of the patient's record. Both the charting and the flow sheets were examined. Standard care plans and standing orders were not used in the units. The average patient age was 53 years with a range of 20 to 75 years. The average length of stay within the critical care units was 3.45 days with a range of 3 to 15 days. Approximately 40% of the patients had a cardiovascular disorder on admission. The remaining 60% had a variety of medical-surgical disorders.

INSTRUMENT

The data collection tool was designed by the investigators as an open-ended form that included all components of the nursing process and pertinent demographic and medical data. Content validity of the tool was established by a panel of experts. Ten of the 50 charts (20%) were randomly selected and independently reexamined by a medical-surgical clinical specialist who used the same tool. Interrater agreement was 93%.

RESULTS
Documentation of the nursing process

Examination of nursing judgment and decision links revealed that the nursing process at best was documented as scattered fragments of an incomplete chain. In no instance could problem identification, nursing action, and patient outcome be traced in such a way as to indicate cognitive information processing and decision making. That is not to say that these processes did not take place. However, they were not evident in the documentation.

Examination of the individual components of the process revealed that patient problems were reflected in unclustered and unrelated pieces of assessment data. Inferential diagnostic statements, however, were not documented. Assessment data were recorded and often repeated every shift without indication of problem advancement or resolution. For example, there were instances in which data indicated a ventilatory problem related to inadequate clearance of pulmonary secretions. Since an inferential statement was never documented, the problem was never treated or evaluated on a consistent basis. Consequently, patients were discharged from the unit without resolution of the problem. Furthermore, no summary statement was made as to the existence of the problem, its treatment, or its course. Other instances involved much documentation of diagnostic parameters such as hemodynamic measurements, blood gas and electrolyte values, and intake and output. Interpretation of the values was not documented, however. One might infer from some of the recorded nursing actions that nurses recognized actual or potential problems and accordingly titrated IV fluids, regulated oxygen flow, or notified physicians. The inference, however, was not explicit. Furthermore, it was difficult to determine whether nursing actions were based on nursing judgment or physicians' orders. A review of physicians' orders revealed that some of the most basic types of nursing interventions were indeed ordered by physicians, for example, notification of physician of urine output less than

30 ml/hour. This situation may have been a reflection of the type of teaching institution.

Links between nursing interventions and patient problems were difficult to determine and in some instances absent. For example, interventions unrelated to any apparent problem were often documented. Oftentimes a PRN analgesic was administered without descriptive data to indicate a need for the analgesic. In other instances, problems were described but interventions were missing. One case contained repeated documentation describing the patient's inability to sleep and concern regarding an upcoming cardiac catheterization, yet the chart contained no notation of nursing interventions directed at these problems.

Patient outcomes in most instances were either not recorded or were buried in the scattered assessment data of the next shift.

Common patient problems

Since chart examination of nurses' notations revealed primarily assessment data, the patient problems identified in this paper are based on the investigators' inferences of the nurses' descriptions.

Patient problems were categorized broadly according to the list of Human Responses suggested by the ANA in its Social Policy Statement (ANA, 1980). To determine differences in the frequency of problem occurrence between clinical units, the Spearman Rho was applied and found to be insignificant at the .05 level. This result indicated that common types of problems existed in all study units.

TABLE 1   **Common patient problem categories**

Problem category	Percentage of cases
Impaired function	
Ventilation	84
Circulation	76
Fluid and electrolyte regulation	42
Elimination	34
Skin	34
Temperature regulation	24
Rest/sleep	10
Nutrition	8
Neurologic	4
Pain/discomfort	66
Behavioral/perceptual	36
Emotional	24

From American Nurses' Association: Nursing: a social policy statement, Kansas City, Mo., 1980, The Association. Reprinted with permission of ANA.

Of the problem categories, the two most frequently identified were impaired function and pain/discomfort (Table 1). In the impaired function category, ventilatory problems occurred in 84% of the cases and circulatory problems in 76% of the cases. Pain/discomfort occurred in 66% of the cases. Other assessment data described behavioral/perceptual problems, including disorientation and noncompliance, in 36% of the cases and emotional problems, including anxiety, in 24% of the cases. Mean frequency of problems per patient was 4.76, with a range of 2 to 11.

Nursing actions

Documented interventions generally followed problem categories, although they were not always clearly related. Interventions directed at ventilatory problems were noted in 68% of the cases, at circulatory problems in 54% of the cases, at pain/discomfort problems in 46% of the cases, at behavioral/perceptual problems in 8% of cases, and at emotional problems in 6% of the cases (Figure 1). On the average, nursing interventions were documented in only 81% of the cases describing patient problems.

All nursing interventions were rated by head nurses of the two units according to the degree of independence, interdependence, or dependence. *Independent* was defined as a therapeutic action initiated by a nurse without consultation from other professionals, including physicians. Interdependent was defined as a therapeutic action performed by a nurse with reciprocal dependence on a physician or other health professional for prescription or regulation of that action, including nursing judgments made when instituting physicians' orders. *Dependent* was defined as a therapeutic action initiated only by a physician or other health professional, with nursing judgment not a factor in regulation or implementation of the action. The head nurses rated 61% of the interventions as independent, 34% as interdependent, and 4% as dependent. Discrepancies, however, existed between the two units; that is, an activity considered independent in one unit was considered interdependent in another.

The only activities considered dependent in both units included adjusting or changing ventilator settings; administering specific IV solutions, for example, albumin; and performing external massage and cardioversion. Activities considered interdependent by both units included stripping chest tubes, providing explanation or reassurance regarding surgical procedures, pacemaker teaching, advising on consequences of not voiding (straight catheterization), modifying or changing activity level, applying heating and cooling mattresses, initiating diagnostic blood work, performing and interpreting ECGs, and administering medications. Activities considered independent by both units included providing tracheal hygiene; elevating head of bed; providing explanation or reassurance regarding oxygen mask, ventilator effectiveness, equipment and room, call light operation, need for NPO, hazards of

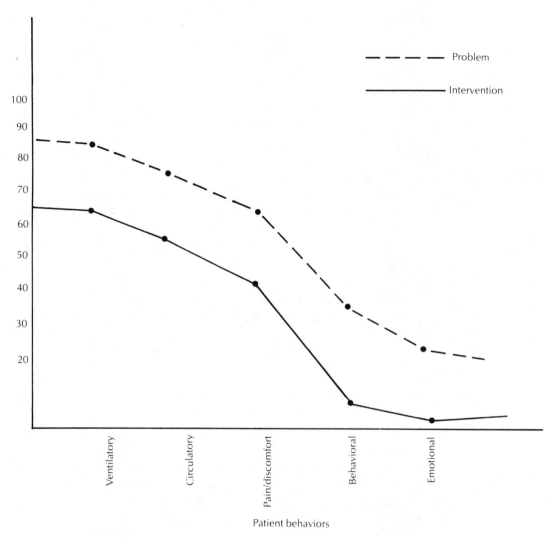

FIGURE 1   Comparison between frequency of problems and documented interventions.

smoking, and need for fluids; notifying physician of change in patient's status; providing skin and comfort measures; providing rest periods; elevating Gatch bed; observing safety precautions; administering wound and IV insertion site care; recalibrating arterial lines; administering CPR; assessing cardiovascular and respiratory status; irrigating nasogastric tubes; assessing communication skills and providing note pad; checking stools and urine for occult blood; and observing hourly intake and output. Box 1 lists the categories of nursing interventions.

BOX 1	Categories of nursing interventions

Respiratory care
Cardiac rehabilitation
Explanation/reassurance regarding therapies/condition
Skin/comfort
Activity
Safety
Temperature regulation
Nutrition
Hemodynamic/fluid monitoring
Arrhythmia monitoring
Wound care
Miscellaneous therapies/diagnostics
Notification of physician
Medication administration

DISCUSSION AND CONCLUSIONS

Findings of this study suggest grave implications for critical care nursing. Integration of the nursing process into practice as emphasized by the AACN is not evident when examining documentation practices. Lack of documentation reinforces the idea that optimal clinical proficiency among critical care nurses is not as prevalent as one would expect (Cantor, 1982). Several explanations have been offered for inadequate documentation by nurses (Barbiasz, 1981). Allen, Jackson, and Younger (1980, p. 838) suggest that nurses have been socialized into submissive roles that foster passive-aggressive communication in which nurses "disguise opinions as suggestions and circumvent conflict by withholding information or contributions that might improve patient care." Gordon (1980) and Matthews and Gaul (1979) pointed out nurses' inadequate development of inferential ability. Christopherson (1981) suggests that the charting format itself might need modification to reflect the nursing process. The narrative charting format that is used in many critical care units may not be conducive to adequate documentation. It may need to be supplemented by a format that elicits inferential diagnostic statements, related interventions, and expected and actual outcomes of actions. Other charting formats may also need to be investigated. A more effective format for documentation may reveal whether deficiencies in documenting the nursing process lie within the format of charting, within nursing practice itself or both.

The high percentage of independent nursing activities identified by head nurses in this study is contrary to conventional beliefs and suggests autonomy of nursing judgments and decisions in critical care. However, this was poorly reflected in actual documentation. Since described problems and interventions were charted in isolation of each other, without inferential statements, it was difficult to determine the relationship, if any, between problem and action.

The incongruity between critical care units within the same institution in the rating of independent and interdependent actions for the same nursing intervention raises the question of who defines the scope and boundaries of nursing practice in critical care, especially in view of the current debate surrounding the inclusion or exclusion of certain nursing diagnoses as determined by the scope of their intervention. Perhaps it is premature to discard or overlook nursing diagnoses not in the realm of current nursing practice. Nursing should maintain open boundaries and avoid closure until the changing and expanding role of nursing is more clearly defined.

REFERENCES

Allen, M.L., Jackson, D., and Younger, S.: Closing the communication gap between physicians and nurses in the intensive care setting, Heart Lung **9**:836, 1980.

American Association of Critical Care Nurses: Standards for nursing care of critically ill, Irvine, Calif. 1981, The Association.

American Nurses' Association: Nursing: a social policy statement, Kansas City, Mo., 1980, The Association.

Barbiasz, J.: Nursing documentation: a format not a form, J. Nurs. Admin. **11**(6):22, 1981.

Cantor, P.: A mandate for clinical proficiency, Focus on AACN **8**(6):16, 1982.

Carlson, J., Craft, C., and McGuire, A.: Nursing diagnosis, Philadelphia, 1982, W.B. Saunders Co.

Christopherson, D.: Implementing nursing process in ICU, Focus on AACN **8**(5):15, 1981.

Gordon, M.: The diagnostic process. In Kim, M.J., and Moritz, D.A., eds.: Classification of Nursing Diagnoses: proceedings of the third and fourth national conferences, New York, 1982, McGraw-Hill Book Co.

Matthews, C.A., and Gaul, A.L.: Nursing diagnosis from the perspective of concept attainment and critical thinking, Adv. Nurs. Sci. **2**:17, 1979.

Discussion

Jo Mary Aspinall: I have been a critical care nurse, and some people were surprised that after having written a couple of books on heart surgery, I switched to writing about the nursing process, as though the two somehow or other did not fit. I do have some kinds of questions, though, about how we are moving, and I think we need to look at that. If we say that the role of the nurse is primarily that of formulating nursing diagnoses, then to a certain extent we do exclude many of the nursing activities that have been related to the medical problem of the patient. (These nursing activities are more medically oriented or medically directed.) Yet having read some of the literature and seen some of the poster exhibits on acute care, it seem like most of the nursing actions are really monitoring, which is assessment and not really intervention. I think we need to try to clean up that because I do not think this is any place for fuzzy theory. I think assessment is assessment, and intervention is intervention. Then there are many acute patients for whom the physician as director of the team writes the orders for certain things. The nurse uses her judgment about timing and a lot of other things, but she is primarily functioning dependently. For example, there is nothing the nurse does independently as far as decreasing or increasing cardiac output. Now, the nurse may help that patient cope with the stress of the illness. But as far as the physiologic cardiac output is concerned, there is not very much the nurse can do to increase the patient's cardiac output. I think we need to look at this area. I would certainly hate to think that nursing is going to say that the primary thing a nurse does is make nursing diagnoses and leave this other extremely important area of nursing functions to someone else who would be less equipped to take care of it.

Section II   **Small group presentation**

Constipation: conceptual categories of diagnostic indicators

AUDREY M. McLANE, R.N., Ph.D.
RUTH E. McSHANE, R.N., M.S.N.*
MAXINE SLIEFERT, R.N., M.S.†

Constipation has appeared as a diagnostic label on the list of accepted diagnoses of the National Group on the Classification of Nursing Diagnoses since the First National Conference in 1973. The original label, *bowel function, irregular: constipation,* was changed to *bowel elimination, alteration in: constipation* at the Second National Conference in 1975. The label remained unchanged during succeeding conferences, (Kim and Moritz, 1982). Despite agreement of the participants of five national conferences that nurses diagnose and treat constipation and in the absence of a research base, none of the defining characteristics have been upgraded to the category of critical defining characteristic that Gordon (1982, p. 134) defines as "highly reliable, highly valid cues . . . [that] . . . increase confidence in diagnostic judgments."

This study is one of a series conducted by the researchers (McLane and McShane, 1983a; McLane, McShane, and Sliefert, 1983b) in an attempt to identify the cluster of defining characteristics for the diagnosis of constipation. Two data-gathering tools were developed—the nursing practice and constipation tool: nurse perspective and the health practices tool, elimination: client perspective.

The nurse validation model described by Gordon and Sweeney (1979) was initially selected as a guide for the study of diagnostic indicators of constipation. *The Nursing Practice and Constipation Tool: Nurse Perspective* was developed for phase one of the study to gather data from nurses who diagnose and treat constipation. Toward the end of phase one, work was begun on a tool (McLane and McShane, 1983a) that would aid in gathering data from clients themselves about the signs and symptoms, perceived causes, measures taken to relieve, and outcomes of constipation. The decision to move in a new direction was based on the researchers' conviction that more descriptive research on the phenomenon of concern, bowel elimination, was needed before further validation of the diagnostic indicators of constipation.

---

*Currently doctoral student, University of Wisconsin–Madison.
†Currently doctoral student, University of Illinois.

The new instrument, *Health Practices Tool, Elimination: Client Perspective*, is currently being used to collect data from 300 healthy subjects in three broad age categories. Data from that study will be used to further validate and extend the categories of diagnostic indicators of constipation and to provide descriptive information about bowel elimmination health practices of adults.

LITERATURE

The literature contains numerous examples of variables believed to influence the presence or absence of constipation, but there is a paucity of research to support the effect of most of the variables on patterns of bowel elimination. Therefore, there are few empirical data to support the published list of defining characteristics and etiologies for the diagnosis of constipation (Kim and Moritz 1982). Although early studies of the frequency of constipation, including the report on the variation of bowel habits in two populations (Connell and others, 1965), have been called into question, they are still cited. A long list of causes of constipation is enumerated in medical and nursing textbooks and in the periodic literature, but there is an absence of empirical data to support even such often purported causes of constipation as insufficient activity and inadequate fluid intake.

In a recent study the relationship between constipation behaviors and health beliefs was studied by Hahn (1981), who reported that persons taking action to prevent or treat constipation had significantly ($p < .05$) higher scores on perceived severity and cues, with benefits the most frequently cited reason for choosing a particular health practice.

The primary focus of constipation research during the last decade has been on fiber and its affect on gut physiology. Most fiber-related clinical studies were designed to study the effects of increased fiber on groups of institutionalized persons, nursing home residents, persons with diverticular disease, patients with spinal cord injuries, psychiatric patients, and boys in a boarding school. An excellent review article on the status of fiber research is that by Godding (1980), who called for the development of physiologic yardsticks, in numerical terms, to measure bowel function.

PURPOSE

The purpose of this study was to provide some initial evidence of construct validity for an instrument, *Health Practices Tool, Elimination: Client Perspective*, which purports to assess factors indicative of constipation. The investigators hoped to demonstrate that the domain of observables, defining characteristics, and etiologies delineated in the instrument was the same or similar to that identified by clients for whom constipation was a phenomenon of concern. This approach operationalized the first step of construct validation outlined by Nunnally (1978), which specified the domain of observables related to the construct.

The research question that guided the study was: What factors do older adults identify as indicative of constipation? A factor was defined as any element, condition, or circumstance that indicates constipation. Older adults were defined as persons 50 years of age or older. Constipation was defined as decreased frequency of bowel elimination or difficulty passing stools.

THE CONSTRUCT

The construct of constipation is a physiologic condition that is observable and more amenable to measurement than more abstract constructs. However, variation in individual perception of cues or factors that indicate constipation or that contribute to its development blur the boundaries of the domain and hinder valid and reliable measurement of the phenomenon. Moreover, constipation may not be a unitary phenomenon. That is, the phenomenon observed in elderly nursing home residents differs considerably from the phenomenon observed in clients with mental disability and from the alteration in bowel elimination precipitated by abdominal surgery.

METHODOLOGY
Sample

A convenience sample of 20 subjects, 10 male and 10 female, was obtained from a senior citizen apartment building. Subjects ranged from 50 to 89 years of age, with a mean age of 74.6. Seventeen subjects were white, and three were black. All subjects were widowed or divorced and lived alone, had experienced constipation, and had chronic health problems such as arthritis or diabetes that required monitoring by health care professionals.

Interview guide

Subjects were interviewed using a set of three open-ended questions with probes:
1. What does the word *constipation* mean to you?
2. How do you recognize constipation when it is present?
   a. Any specific bodily feelings?
   b. Any bodily changes?
   c. Any changes in stool?
   d. Any changes in gas?
   e. Any changes in routine?
3. What factors do you think contribute to your constipation?
   a. Any foods you eat?
   b. Any foods you do not eat?
   c. Any fluids?

    d. Any activity change?

    e. Any changes in routine?

    f. Any medications?

    g. Any diseases?

    h. Any other factors?

Conduct of the interviews

The interviews were conducted by two researchers, following one 3-hour training session. A handout summarizing interviewing strategies and techniques was used to provide a common base. There was no attempt to establish stringent interviewer reliability, since the rationale for qualitative interviewing was to build categories from the subjects' understanding of phenomena and not to test the construct.

Interviews were generally conducted in the subject's room or a lounge area of the apartment building. The questions were not followed in a strict sequence, although both interviewers attempted to use the precise wording of the main questions. More flexibility was permitted with probing. A written consent to participate in the study was obtained from each subject. Responses to the open-ended questions were tape-recorded and then transcribed to facilitate content analysis.

Data analysis

A panel of five nurse experts, including the three researchers, independently analyzed a random sample of five of the interviews to derive initial conceptual categories for the diagnostic indicators of constipation. Definitions for the categories and subcategories were developed and refined on two occasions, with subsequent recategorization of the interview data by the five nurse experts following each refinement. Finally, the data from all interviews (N = 20) were reviewed to verify the final categories, subcategories, and definitions.

Findings

Five final categories and eight subcategories with definitions were established and compared with categories included in the previously developed instrument, *Health Practices Tool, Elimination: Client Perspective.* All categories and subcategories of diagnostic indicators developed from client data were represented in the instrument; that is, each item could be placed in one of the categories or subcategories. Placement of the items in the categories and subcategories was done independently by two research assistants and jointly by two of the researchers.

Whereas the original instrument was developed in the framework of three categories—signs and symptoms, etiologic factors, and patterning (each with

BOX 1   **Bowel elimination, alteration in: constipation—conceptual categories of diagnostic indicators**

I. Signs and symptoms
   A. Description of constipated stool:
      1. Character: qualities of the stool, for example, color or consistency
      2. Amount: amount of stool
      3. Frequency: lapse of time between stools
   B. Feelings and sensations: physical feelings and sensations associated with constipation, for example, stomach ache and bloating
II. Etiology: contributing factors, for example, diet, fluids, inadequate exercise, medications, and change in routine
III. Attending behaviors: consistent use of measures for the expressed purpose of alleviating or preventing constipation
   A. Treatment: measures taken to relieve constipation
   B. Prevention: measures taken to avoid an occurrence of constipation (action oriented)
IV. Health behaviors: health behaviors influencing normal elimination, for example, diet, fluid, and exercise
V. Patterning: behaviors related to the production of a bowel movement, including toilet routine
   A. Expected frequency: perception of normal frequency
   B. Timing
      1. Actual frequency of bowel movement(s)
      2. Time of day of bowel movement(s)
   C. Stimulus behaviors:
      1. Actions taken to stimulate a bowel movement, short-term, within the hour, for example, drink hot water
      2. Actions part of a daily routine that result in a bowel movement, for example, breakfast
   D. Response to reflexes: behaviors in response to the urge to defecate

---

subcategories)—the final schema consisted of five major categories with subcategories (Box 1). The procedures used to reconceptualize and redefine the categories and subcategories contributed to conceptual specificity and reduced the overlap between groupings, thus decreasing "fuzziness" and increasing the clarity of the classification schema.

In summary, content analysis of data obtained from 20 interviews of a self-selected sample of older adults, 50 years of age or older, provided some initial evidence for a classification schema of diagnostic indicators for the nursing diagnosis of *bowel elimination, alteration in: constipation* and for the inclusion of the variables in categories and subcategories. The task for the future includes further validation and extension of the categories and subcategories with other age-related populations; delineation of patterns of bowel elimination and associated health behaviors for various age-related and/or condition-related groups; and development and testing of interventions to influence alterations in bowel elimination.

REFERENCES

Connell, A.M., and others: Variation of bowel habit in two population samples, Br. Med. J. **2**:1095, 1965.

Godding, E.W.: Physiological yardsticks for bowel function and the rehabilitation of the constipated bowel, Pharmacol. **20**:88, 1980.

Gordon, J.: Nursing diagnosis: process and application, New York, 1982, McGraw-Hill Book Co.

Gordon, M., and Sweeney, M.A.: Methodological problems and issues in identifying and standardizing nursing diagnoses, Adv. Nurs. Sci. **2**(1):1, 1979.

Hahn, K.J.: Nursing diagnosis and the health belief model, Madison, Wis., 1981, Fourth Midwest Nursing Research Society Conference.

Kim, M.J., and Moritz, D.A.: Classification of nursing diagnoses: proceedings of the third and fourth national conferences, New York, 1982, McGraw-Hill Book Co.

McLane, A.M., and McShane, R.E.: Bowel elimination health practices of healthy adults, Study funded in part by a grant from the Nurses Foundation of Wisconsin, 1983a.

McLane, A.M., McShane, R.E., and Sliefert, M.: The nursing diagnosis of constipation: instrument development, Manuscript in preparation, 1983b.

Nunnally, J.C.: Psychometric theory, New York, 1978, McGraw-Hill Book Co.

Validation of a nursing diagnosis: role disturbance

TONI M. BALISTRIERI, R.N., M.S.N.
MARY K. JIRICKA, R.N., M.S.N.

The purpose of this paper was to validate the nursing diagnosis of *role disturbance* and to identify its defining characteristics. The methodology used was the retrospective identification model and the nurse-validation model described by Gordon and Sweeney (1979).

THEORETIC FRAMEWORK

Role can be conceptualized as a set of behaviors characteristic of or expected of an individual who is interacting with or reacting to another individual within the context of a particular social stratum or setting. Meleis (1975, p. 265) developed a conceptual framework to assess patients' roles. He defined role theory as "the notion that human behavior is not a simple matter of stimulus-response reaction, but rather the result of a complex interaction between ego and society. It synthesizes the culture and social structure from the individual's level."

Meleis (1975) discussed role transition and listed various categories of events that often predispose individuals to difficulties during a normal role transition. The first category is a developmental transition, which occurs naturally in an individual's life just by the fact of aging. The second category is a situational transition, which requires an individual to add or delete a role from a preexisting set of roles. The third category is the health-illness transition, which occurs anytime an individual moves from illness to wellness or from wellness to illness. Usually a transition period is easier if it occurs gradually. Each role transition encompasses simultaneous loss and gain. Often a nurse's first encounter with clients is in an altered role capacity—a sick role.

Meleis (1975, p. 266) defined role insuffiency as "any difficulty in the cognizance and/or performance of a role or of the sentiments and goals associated with role behavior as perceived by self or by significant others." It also includes behavorial and emotional components. Many patients admitted to a hospital experience role insuffiency, which is defined as role disturbance.

DESIGN AND METHODOLOGY

Gordon's PES (problem, etiology, and signs and symptoms) format (1976) for a nursing diagnosis was used. Role distrubance was identified as the diagnostic label to be examined. The etiology of the nursing diagnosis was based on Meleis' three categories of role transition (1975), specifically, transition on the health-illness continuum. The nursing diagnosis of role disturbance caused by transition on the health-illness continuum can be applied to any patient population. The investigators decided to apply it to a limited population of cardiovascular patients.

Retrospective identification model

The first method used was the retrospective identification model. Using a Delphi study, the retrospective identification model draws on the accumulated experiences of nurses. Nurses describe health problems they have treated in the past based on their memory of clinical encounters with patients and on their accrued nursing knowledge.

Gordon and Sweeney (1979, p. 6) stated that "the reliability and validity attained in a retrospective model depend to a great extent on the investigator's sample selection and training methodology." Twelve clinical specialists in the area of critical care who specialized in cardiovascular nursing were chosen for the study. Nursing experience for the group ranged from 5 to 12 years. The nurses practiced in various hospital settings in a large midwestern city. An introductory letter, with guidelines for constructing a diagnostic category, was given to each subject to increase reliability and validity. A verbal explanation and instructions were given by the investigators.

Six clinical nurse specialists from the list of 12 subjects were randomly chosen for the first part of the study. They identified signs and symptoms for the nursing diagnosis of role disturbance according to the retrospective identification model. The results are described later in Box 1, p. 183.

Next, consensual validity was sought for the nursing diagnosis of role disturbance. The set of signs and symptoms gathered by the investigators from signs and symptoms identified by the first group of clinical nurse specialists was used for phase two of the study. The remaining six clinical nurse specialists from the original 12 were asked to identify a problem label based on the signs and symptoms. An introductory letter and the same guidelines for constructing a diagnostic category were provided by the investigators along with a verbal explanation and instructions. The problem labels identified by the second group are discussed later in Box 2, p. 183.

Nurse-validation model

The second model used in the study was the nurse-validation model. With this method, validation of the diagnosis involves determining if the preidentified set of signs and symptoms actually occur in the clinical setting. Gordon and Sweeney (1979) stated that clinical validation is especially important when labels and defining characteristics are identified using the retrospective identification model, which is based on recall of clinical practice experience.

As with the previous model, reliability and validity depend on sample selection and training. Fifteen critical care nurses, identified as reliable diagnosticians by their head nurses, were selected to collect data for the study. Verbal and written instructions were provided. The nurses identified 36 cardiovascular patients displaying behaviors suggesting a role disturbance. The last four digits of their hospital numbers were used to prevent duplication. The nurses recorded which of the signs and symptoms of role disturbance, previously identified using the retrospective identification validation model, were actually present in the patients studied. Additional signs and symptoms could be recorded. The frequency of occurrence of each sign and symptom was tabulated, and percentages of occurrence were computed. A cluster of defining characteristics for the nursing diagnosis of role disturbance was identified from the findings. The results are discussed later in Table 1.

FINDINGS
Retrospective identification model

The first group of six clinical nurse specialists identified signs and symptoms of role disturbance, which were summarized by the investigators (Box 1). Problem-labels for the signs and symptoms were then developed by the second group of clinical nurse specialists (Box 2). One questionnaire was not returned. Role disturbance was identified by only one clinical nurse specialist. Consensual validity for the problem label role disturbance based on the set of signs and symptoms identified by the first sample was not established.

Nurse-validation model

Nine of the 15 critical care nurses completed and returned the work sheets. Most of the signs and symptoms were found to exist in the patient studied (Table 1). Six of the signs and symptoms were found to be present in 50% or more of the cases. The six signs and symptoms could be considered the cluster of defining characteristics for the nursing diagnosis of role disturbance.

DISCUSSION AND SUMMARY

Different results were obtained using the two methods to validate a nursing diagnosis. For the retrospective identification model, several reasons for the investigators' inability to establish consensual validity may be examined. The set of signs and symptoms identified from the first group may have been too encompassing, even though all the signs and symptoms listed were frequently identified by the first group. Another possibility for failure to establish consensual validity may be individual differences in ability and proficiency in constructing diagnostic labels. A review of the problem labels listed in Box 2 demonstrates that not all the items were constructed according to accepted guidelines (Gordon, 1982).

BOX 1 **Signs and symptoms identified by group 1 of the retrospective identification model**

1. Verbalization by patient/or family of doubts to fulfill role expectations
2. Physical inability to fulfill roles
3. Changes in client's health-care behavior
4. Manifestations of a grieving process
5. Manifestations of a stress response
6. Noncompliance with health regimen
7. Fear regarding ability to perform new role expectations
8. Conflict with significant other regarding role performance

BOX 2 **Retrospective identification model**

1. Altered self-concept caused by change in health status
2. Alteration in cardiac output—decreased
3. Alteration in body image
4. Role disturbance caused by change in health state
5. Coping patterns—maladaptive
6. Anxiety
7. Self-care deficit
8. Poor activity tolerance
9. Alteration in comfort
10. Normal grieving
11. Mild functional fear
12. Impaired self-esteem/self-actualization

TABLE 1 **Frequency of occurrence of signs and symptoms in the nurse-validation model**

Nurse-subject	Signs and symptoms*							
	1	**2**	**3**	**4**	**5**	**6**	**7**	**8**
1	4/5†	2/5	4/5	5/5	3/5	2/5	4/5	1/5
2	1/2	2/2	2/2	2/2	2/2	2/2	1/2	1/2
3	2/3	2/3	3/3	3/3	2/3	3/3	2/3	1/3
4	1/5	3/5	5/5	5/5	2/5	5/5	3/5	0/5
5	2/5	2/5	2/5	2/5	3/5	3/5	3/5	2/5
6	2/5	0/5	5/5	5/5	3/5	4/5	1/5	1/5
7	1/4	1/4	2/4	1/4	3/4	2/4	1/4	1/4
8	3/4	4/4	4/4	4/4	4/4	4/4	3/4	2/4
9	2/3	0/3	3/3	1/3	2/3	1/3	1/3	0/3
Percentage of occurrence	.50	.44	.83	.77	.66	.72	.52	.25

*Signs and symptoms 1 through 8 refer to those given in Box 1.
†Signifies the number of occurrences/the number of patients assessed.

One limitation in this study was the small number of nurse-subjects participating. Further study with a larger sample is recommended. Another limitation is generalizability, since only cardiovascular patients in the acute phase of their illness were studied. Nursing diagnoses frequently identified in critical care may preclude that of role disturbance. The infrequent use of role disturbance as a nursing diagnosis in critical care may have affected the results of the study. Further study of role disturbance in patients who are not critically ill is recommended.

Clinical nurse specialists in the sample selected for the retrospective identification model identified related problem labels, such as alteration of self-concept or alteration in body image. Role performance and body image are components of self-concept, and all are interrelated (Gebbie and Lavin, 1974).

Validating a nursing diagnosis is an important part of building a clinical science in nursing. As clients move from a state of health to a state of illness, role transition occurs and the potential for role disturbance exists. Nurses can play a role in assisting these clients in the transition.

REFERENCES

Gebbie, K.M., and Lavin, M.A.: Classifying nursing diagnoses, Am. J. Nurs. 74(2):250, 1974.
Gordon, M.: Nursing diagnoses and the diagnostic process, Am. J. Nurs. 76(8):1298, 1976.
Gordon, M.: Guidelines for reviewing and preparing diagnostic labels. In Kim, M.J., and Moritz, D.A., eds: Classification of nursing diagnoses: proceedings of the third and fourth national conferences, New York, 1982, McGraw-Hill Book Co.
Gordon, M., and Sweeney, M.A.: Methodological problems and issues in identifying and standardizing nursing diagnoses, Adv. Nurs. Sci. 2(1):1, 1979.
Meleis, A.I: Role insufficiency and role supplementation: a conceptual framework, Nurs. Res. 24(4):264, 1975.

A study to evaluate the validity of the rating system for self-care deficit

CAROL A. BAER, R.N., M.S.N.
MARCIA DELOREY, R.N., M.S.N.
JOAN B. FITZMAURICE, R.N., M.S.

An ongoing concern of nursing providers is quality care. Assisting patients with activities of daily living is recognized as one of its major components. To provide quality assistance requires a holistic approach and a systematic evaluation of patients' functional abilities. Most of the indices to evaluate these abilities, however, are "inadequate and clinically naive" (Feinstein, 1982). In fact, rating scales depicting patient requirements for nursing assistance in these areas did not even exist until recently (McCourt, 1981).

Recognizing this need, McCourt (1981) reviewed available classification methods, adapted a rating scale, and identified criteria of gradation to demarcate functional impairments. Thus evolved the nursing diagnosis of *self-care deficit* (SCD) in feeding, bathing, dressing, and toileting (Kim and Moritz, 1982, p. 379). Patients are rated in each area on a scale of 0 to 4 as their level of dependency increases (Table 1).

The purpose of this paper is to report the application of the SCD classification system to patients with spinal cord injury whose initial dependence on nurses for basic human needs progresses to varying levels of self-care. Promoting rehabilitation requires ongoing, accurate assessment of patients' deficits and identification of nursing interventions that will assist them in achieving optimal levels of independence.

Orem describes self-care as a human requirement necessary to sustain life and health (Foster and Janssens, 1980). Her theory defines self-care activities in the context of individuals' values/beliefs, roles/relationships, methods of coping, and so forth. Thus, despite similar physiologic indices, patients have different patterns of responding to stimuli (Orem, 1971). This study was conducted in this holistic framework.

The need for valid and reliable measures is considered one of the foremost problems of nursing research. Testing whether measures are "good" or "bad" along several dimensions is sorely needed. Diers (1979, p. 243) identifies several dimensions as measurement criteria, that is, the standards against which any measure is tested. The criteria are validity, reliability, meaningfulness, sensitivity, precision, and appropriateness. They are defined in Table 2 and will be used to evaluate the SCD rating system.

The researchers, a clinical coordinator and a head nurse on a spinal cord injury service, proposed McCourt's system in January 1981 to two other head

TABLE 1   SCD rating scale*

Numeric index	Definition
0	Independent, able to perform activity with no one present
1	Requires use of equipment or device
2	Requires help from another person for assistance, supervision, or teaching
2.2	Supervision—may include verbal reinforcement or stand-by assistance
2.4	Minimal assistance, patient does approximately 75% of the work
2.6	Moderate assistance, patient does approximately 50% of the work
2.8	Maximal assistance, patient does approximately 25% of the work
3	Requires help from another person and equipment or device
4	Dependent, does not participate in activity

*Modified from McCourt, A.E.: ANA Qual. Assur. Update **5**(1):1-3, 1981. Reprinted with permission of the American Nurses' Association.

TABLE 2   Measurement criteria

Criterion	Definition
Validity	The extent to which the measurement measures what it is suppose to measure
Reliability	The extent to which two measures can agree on the reading
Meaningfulness	The extent to which (1) the phenomena being measured are important to nursing and (2) the measurement can be used or abstracted from in practice
Sensitivity	The extent to which the measurement captures the "true" range of the possible variation in the phenomenon being measured
Precision	The extent to which the measurement can discriminate between individuals
Appropriateness	The extent to which the measurement "fits" the sample

nurses on the service. Following a 1-month trial evaluation, it was decided that the system lacked sufficiently precise criteria to rate patients accurately. Specific behavioral criteria were then identified to correspond with the numeric code. Evidence for the validity of the revised tool was obtained by its use from March through June, 1981 with patients with spinal cord injuries. Patients were individually assessed by head nurses, and the scores were recorded on a standardized sheet. Weekly meetings were held to discuss the scale and rater reaction. Interrater reliability was tested by the two researchers separately rating a preselected "blind" sample within 8 hours of each other and comparing the results.

The convenience sample included 110 male paraplegic and quadriplegic patients, 21 through 65 years of age, hospitalized on three units of a New England medical center. Injuries ranged from the first lumbar vertebra through the third cervical vertebra and had occurred anywhere from 2 months to 20 years before the study. Reasons for hospitalization included initial treatment and rehabilitation, annual physical examination, treatment for medical complications, and chronic care.

RESULTS AND DISCUSSION

Face validity requires that on inspection by experts the measure looks like it is a good indicator of the concept. It was tested by the researchers and head nurses. After a 1-month evaluation, disparities in scoring were apparent. In the area of feeding, for example, a quadriplegic patient eating with an adapted fork would receive a rating of 3 from one head nurse and a rating of 1 from the other. Criteria were too broad to achieve agreement among raters. Thus specific patient behaviors were identified to correspond with the numeric index in each of the four SCD areas. Toileting was expanded to toileting/bladder and toileting/bowel. There were some numeric ratings for which discriminating behaviors could not be identified (Table 3). There was unanimous agreement that explicit behavioral criteria were more specific indicators of numeric ratings, thus reducing individual interpretation

Construct validity requires application of the measure to groups that are *known* to differ on the construct involved to determine if the measure picks up the difference. Patients with spinal cord injuries have a wide range of mobility problems determined largely by their level of injury. Ratings of 104 patients with the revised SCD scale showed scores in all five categories reflecting a range of deficits (Figure 1). Before its use, patients were designated simply as "dependent" or "independent" on their nursing care plans, leaving much to interpretation.

The raters noted that as their familiarity with the scoring systems in each of the SCD areas increased so did their awareness of individual patient needs for nursing assistance. In the area of feeding, for example, a score of 2.6 indicates that the patient can feed himself if the food is prepared for him and appropriately "set up," for example, coffee poured, food cut. This information is far more helpful to nurses because they can focus their interventions and promote patient participation.

Future study should compare a patient's SCD score with other established ratings such as muscle testing. Concurrent validity could be established if a correlation between the measures was demonstrated.

Equivalence is demonstrated when two or more raters use the measure on the same sample to establish the amount of interrater agreement. Five patients, unknown to the researchers, were evaluated separately by them within 8 hours. The average percentage of agreement per SCD and per patient was 60% and considered unsatisfactory (Table 4). In the area of dressing, for example, when patients were on bed rest and not dressing routinely, the first rater determined a rating based on ability and the second rater did not rate

TABLE 3   Revised SCD rating scale

Numeric value	Definition
Self-feeding	
0	Independent
1	Requires use of equipment or device but can put it on by himself
2	
2.2	
2.4	Minimal assistance—needs only to have food cut
2.6	Moderate assistance—needs to have tray set up and food arranged, but can feed self
2.8	
3	Requires help from another person *and* equipment or device
4	Dependent
Self-dressing	
0	Independent
1	Requires use of equipment or device such as dressing stick
2	
2.2	
2.4	Minimal assistance—patient does 75% of the work; needs assistance with buttons, zippers
2.6	Moderate assistance—patient does 50% of the work; needs help with shoes or pants
2.8	
3	Requires help from another person *and* equipment or device
4	Dependent
Self-bathing	
0	Independent
1	Requires use of equipment or device such as mitt, adapted razor, toothbrush
2	
2.2	
2.4	Minimal assistance—patient does 75% of the work; needs back care
2.6	Moderate assistance—patient does 50% of the work; needs back and leg care
2.8	
3	Requires help from another person *and* equipment or device; needs to be washed but does light hygiene with adaptive devices
4	Dependent

TABLE 3 **Revised SCD rating scale—cont'd**

Numeric value	Definition
Self-toileting—bladder*	
0	Independent
1	Requires use of equipment or device
2	
2.2	
2.4	Minimal assistance—patient does 75% of the work; can put condom on, but needs to have bag attached
2.6	Moderate assistance—patient does 50% of the work; needs to have condom put on, but can percuss self
2.8	
3	Requires help from another person *and* equipment or device
4	Dependent
Self-toileting—bowel†	
0	Independent
1	Requires use of equipment or device such as suppository inserter
2	
2.2	
2.4	Minimal assistance—patient does 75% of the work; needs to be checked
2.6	Moderate assistance—patient does 50% of the work; needs to have suppository inserted and needs to be checked
2.8	
3	Requires help from another person *and* equipment or device
4	Dependent

*In this area, patient is considered independent if he can manage all areas of his bladder care such as putting condom on (condom drainage is not considered equipment).
†In this area, shower and bowel chairs are not considered equipment.

him, marking N/A (nonapplicable) because the patient was not actually dressing daily. Thus agreement could have been higher had the raters decided ahead of time to evaluate only by demonstrated performance of current activities.

Meaningfulness is evaluated by assessing the usefulness of the tool and seeing whether it tells anything about practice. Using the SCD rating system on spinal cord injury service demonstrated its administrative ease and value in identifying patient abilities. This information was used by the head nurses in making out assignments and advising staff on progressive interventions. A cumulative score calculated by adding all patients' SCD scores was "invented" by head nurses to discuss unit "heaviness" with peers, physicians,

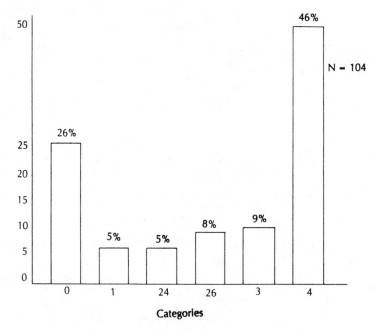

FIGURE 1   Distribution of self-care scores in 104 patients.

TABLE 4   **Interrater reliability on self-care scores**

Patient	Feeding A*	Feeding B*	Dressing A	Dressing B	Bathing A	Bathing B	Bladder A	Bladder B	Bowel A	Bowel B	Percentage of agreement per patient A
1	0	0	0	0	0	0	1	1	0	0	100
2	2.4	1	N/A	3	2.6	3	4	4	4	4	40
3	0	0	N/A	1	2.4	1	1	1	4	2.6	40
4	0	0	4	2.6	2.6	2.6	0	1	4	2.6	40
5	2.4	2.6	4	4	3	3	4	4	4	4	80
Percentage of agreement per SCD	60		40		60		80		60		

*A, Rater A; B, rater B.

and management staff. A census increase from 25 to 26 patients with spinal cord injuries, for example, does not demonstrate a significant change in nursing care requirements. But if that single patient escalates the cumulative SCD score by 46 points, others take notice. The raters agreed the cumulative score was a sensitive indicator for functional abilities and used it to help determine distribution of staff and placement of patients.

Sensitivity and precision are defined as the extent to which the measure can pick up the extremes as well as the small differences of the phenomena. It was evident in the rating of 104 patients that the majority of scores fell at the extremes of the scale (see Fig. 1). The remaining scores were fairly evenly distributed across the other three categories. Thus the scale provided a more accurate objective rating of an individual deficit. Serial ratings were also sensitive to changes in an individual's abilities over time.

Appropriateness is concerned with the relationship between the thing being measured and the characteristics of the sample. The SCD rating scale's appropriateness was determined by its usefulness to hospitalized patients with spinal cord injuries, a high proportion of whom had a deficit in one or more of the functional areas. Since all the patients were in wheelchairs and the philosophy of rehabilitation was that complete independence can be achieved, a 0 rating was assigned to those who could perform independently, despite the wheelchair.

It must also be emphasized that the rating scale behaviors were identified for patients in an institutional environment that was totally accessible and properly equipped. The rating would change if the patient were discharged to unfamiliar or inaccessible surroundings.

The SCD rating system is relevant to both the recipient of care and the nurse provider. It provides a system for easily and objectively rating individual self-care activities and monitoring progress. It provides a focus for identifying expected outcomes and nursing interventions. It provides an index that could be used to determine number and types of personnel required to assist patients with their self-care deficits. Certainly, it is another step toward achieving quality care through the measured expression of clinical observations that are nursing's unique clinical responsibility.

REFERENCES

Diers, D.: Research in nursing practice, New York, 1979, J.B. Lippincott Co.

Feinstein, A.R.: The Jones criteria and the challenges of clinimetrics, Circulation, **66**(1):1, 1982.

Foster, P.C., and Janssens, N.P.: Dorothea E. Orem. In George, J.B., ed.: Nursing theories, Englewood Cliffs, N.J., 1980, Prentice-Hall Inc.

Kim, M.J., and Moritz, D.A., eds.: Classification of nursing diagnoses: proceedings of the third and fourth national conferences, New York, 1982, McGraw-Hill Book Co.

McCourt, A.E.: The measurement of functional deficit in quality assurance, ANA Qual. Assur. Update 5(1):1-3, 1981.

Orem, D.: Nursing: concepts of practice, New York, 1971, McGraw-Hill Book Co.

Section III   **Poster presentation**

Nursing functions related to the nursing diagnosis *decreased cardiac output*

SUSAN L. WESSEL, R.N., M.S.
MI JA KIM, R.N., Ph.D., F.A.A.N.

The continuing effort to study both the empirical and theoretic components of nursing science is being conceptualized increasingly in terms of nursing diagnosis. Many educators and researchers such as Gordon (1979) and Soares (1978) have suggested that nursing diagnoses describe the patient problems that nurses diagnose and treat independently of physicians. However, some nursing diagnoses do not fit this criterion because they extend into areas in which physicians and nurses maintain mutual responsibility, which has produced confusion and controversy. For example, the appropriateness of the nursing diagnosis *decreased cardiac output* has been challenged because it does not describe a problem that is treated exclusively by nurses (Gordon, 1979). At the same time, studies of practicing nurses by Castles (1982), Halloran (1980), and Kim and others (1982) have shown this diagnosis to be one of the most frequently identified nursing diagnoses by both staff nurses and clinical specialists. This study addressed the appropriateness of decreased cardiac output as a nursing diagnosis by examining its nursing interventions.

PURPOSE OF THE STUDY

The purposes of this study were to (1) determine the nature and extent of independent nursing functions associated with decreased cardiac output, (2) describe the areas of collaborative practice in medicine and nursing for patients with decreased cardiac output, and (3) determine whether the use of a model that focuses on nursing problems (nursing diagnosis model) produces different nursing interventions than a medical model that focuses on disease.

REVIEW OF THE LITERATURE

A review of the literature on medical and nursing treatment of decreased cardiac output supported the complementary roles of both professions. Nursing textbooks did not describe decreased cardiac output, but both medical and nursing texts defined heart failure as a condition in which the heart pumped an inadequate amount of blood to meet the metabolic demands of the body

(Beeson, McDermott, and Wyngaarden, 1979; Beland and Passos, 1975; Harrison, 1977; Luckmann and Sorensen, 1980; Weber and Janicki, 1979).

Although the definitions for heart failure were similar, the interventions distinguished the nursing literature from the medical literature. The primary goal of medical treatment tended to be the improvement of ventricular function through pharmacologic and/or surgical means. The primary goal of nursing was to manipulate activity and availability of oxygen and nutrients to cells, provide comfort, adjust the level of physiologic and emotional stress to a level commensurate with heart function, and restore the patient's optimal level of functioning (Beland and Passos, 1975). Medical and nursing interventions overlapped for the prevention of heart disease and the preservation of life in cases of life-threatening heart dysfunction. The exact relationship between medicine and nursing in treating heart failure has not been studied in the clinical area.

METHOD
Definitions

Terms used in this study are defined as follows:

Nursing diagnosis—A statement of a patient problem derived from a nursing assessment that points to a specific intervention and outcome (Gebbie and Lavin, 1973). It is composed of a statement of the problem, the etiology, and the signs and symptoms (defining characteristics) (Gordon, 1976).

Nursing intervention—A specific behavior of a nurse based on a known scientific rationale that is expected to benefit the patient in a predicted way related to the diagnosed problem and accepted goal (Little and Carnevali, 1976).

Independent nursing intervention—Intervention that is within the scope of nursing practice as stated in the Nurse Practice Act (ANA, 1980) and that does not require a physician's order.

Dependent nursing intervention—Areas of patient treatment that require physicians' orders, including nurses making judgments on physicians' orders.

Decreased cardiac output—A cardiac output that is inadequate to meet the metabolic needs of the body's tissues (Luckmann and Sorensen, 1980). Defining characteristics include hypotension, bradyarrhythmias or tachyarrhythmias, angina, fatigue/weakness, jugular vein distention, increased pulmonary artery and/or wedge pressures, color changes of skin and mucous membranes, oliguria, decreased peripheral pulses, cold and clammy skin, abnormal breath sounds (rales), dyspnea/orthopnea, restlessness or anxiety, vertigo/syncope, decreased activity tolerance, and weight gain associated with edema (modified from Kim and others, 1982).

Samples

All registered nurses from one medical intensive care unit and two medical floors of a large medical center participated in the study. The hospital was not using nursing diagnosis but did practice primary nursing. The nurses were from 22 to 30 years of age. All the nurses had a baccalaureate degree, though this was merely coincidental. The patient sample included 21 patients with congestive heart failure (CHF) who were sequentially selected as they were admitted to the study units. Results of a chi-square test for differences in patient characteristics (age, sex, and medical diagnosis) between the two phases of the study were not significant.

Procedure

The medical diagnosis CHF was selected as a criterion based on results of a study by Kim and others (1982) in which this medical diagnosis was frequently associated with the nursing diagnosis *decreased cardiac output.* After the patients' consents were obtained, the investigator performed a cardiovascular assessment using a standardized assessment tool that included all the defining characteristics of decreased cardiac output. Patients diagnosed as having decreased cardiac output based on this assessment comprised the patient sample. Five CHF patients were judged by the investigator not to have decreased cardiac output. The cardiovascular assessment and nursing diagnosis were validated in a second independent assessment by a cardiovascular clinical specialist in half of the study patients. The agreement rate was 100%.

The staff nurses caring for the study patients recorded their nursing interventions during an 8-hour shift on an open-ended questionnaire. During Phase I of the study, each nurse used the framework of the medical diagnosis CHF to give nursing care to one patient. In Phase II the investigator presented a class about the concept of nursing diagnosis and asked the nurses to use *decreased cardiac output* as a framework for nursing care. All interventions in both phases were designated by the nurse as having been done either without a physician's order (independent) or with a physician's order (dependent). In each phase the nurse ranked five interventions as highest in priority.

RESULTS

From an examination of the data collected, the following 26 categories of nursing interventions were developed:

1. Vital signs
2. Swan-Ganz readings
3. Cardiovascular or peripheral vascular assessment
4. Pulmonary assessment (includes blood gases and lung sounds)
5. Physical assessment, nonspecific (includes neurologic)
6. Evaluating laboratory values
7. ECG monitoring

8. Fluid regulation (includes weights, I & O, and fluid restriction)
9. Nourishment (encourage eating, decision whether to feed patient)
10. Activities of daily living (bath, hygiene, comfort)
11. Therapeutic activity
12. Skin care
13. Therapeutic positioning
14. Deep breathing/coughing
15. Oxygen therapy
16. Asepsis (dressing change, Foley catheter care)
17. Intravenous therapy (starting and maintaining I.V. patency)
18. Patient teaching
19. Patient psychologic support
20. Family teaching and psychologic support
21. Therapeutic environment (sleep, quiet, safety)
22. Medication administration
23. Regulate/evaluate medications (I.V. drips, side effects)
24. Collaboration (M.D., dietition, psychiatrist)
25. Written communication (charting, care plan)
26. Overall evaluation/interpretation

The frequency of nursing interventions mentioned in Phase I using medical diagnosis and in Phase II using nursing diagnosis were compared by converting the frequency of use of each category to the proportion of the 12 nurses who completed the study. A test of difference of proportions was done for each of the categories. Only one category, patient teaching, showed a significant difference between Phase I, in which it was recorded by 75% of the nurses, and Phase II, in which it was recorded by 33% of the nurses ($Z = 2.10$, $p < .05$).

There was no significant difference in the proportion of independent nursing interventions performed for Phase I and Phase II. The scores of independence for both phases were therefore combined. Interventions were classified as independent if they were identified by the nurses as such over 80% of the time. Interventions between 80% and 20% independent were designated collaborative. Interventions less than 20% independent were classified as dependent. The independence scores for all interventions are presented in Table 1. Of the nursing intervention categories, 17 were independent nursing functions. Seven interventions were collaborative, and two were dependent.

Each nurse was instructed to rank the five most important nursing activities performed for the study patients. Importance scores were then derived for each category of intervention. To determine if the mean importance scores for each intervention differed between Phase I and II, a Spearman's Rank Correlation Coefficient was computed. The average importance of each nursing intervention was similar in both phases ($r_s = .64$, $p < .01$). The five most important interventions for Phase I were Swan-Ganz readings, physical

TABLE 1   Summary of independence of 26 categories of nursing intervention

Independent intervention*	Score (%)	Collaborative intervention†	Score (%)	Dependent intervention‡	Score (%)
Cardiovascular assessment	100	Vital signs	35	Medication administration	6.5
Pulmonary assessment	83	Swan-Ganz readings	53	Regulate/evaluate medications	19.0
Physical assessment	100	ECG monitoring	75		
Interpretation of laboratory data	100	Fluid management	31		
Nutrition	100	Therapeutic activity	64		
Activities of daily living	100	Oxygen therapy	59		
Skin care	100	Collaboration with other professionals	75		
Therapeutic positioning	100				
Deep breathing/coughing	100				
Aseptic environment	100				
Intravenous therapy	100				
Patient teaching	100				
Patient psychologic support	100				
Family teaching and psychologic support	100				
Therapeutic environment	100				
Written communication	100				
Overall evaluation/ interpretation	100				

*Mean independence scores 80% or more.
†Mean independence scores from 20% to 80%.
‡Mean independence scores less than 80%.

assessment, vital signs, medication administration, and cardiovascular assessment. The top five interventions in Phase II were physical assessment, Swan-Ganz readings, fluid regulation, family teaching and psychologic support, and patient teaching.

DISCUSSION

The high proportion of independent nursing functions associated with decreased cardiac output (65% of total) suggests that nurses need this diagnosis to describe their practice and to get proper credit for these activities, particularly in acute care settings, which should be considered in view of the questions surrounding the adequacy of medical diagnosis in describing nursing practice. The finding that several CHF patients did not have an actual decreased cardiac output (although it may have been a potential problem) further supports the need for a separate diagnostic category for nurses.

This diagnosis is not exclusively independent; that is, nurses are not licensed to treat it independently. Medication administration and regulation depend on a physician's order, and several other areas are collaborative. The roles of medicine and nursing are cooperative and complementary for this diagnosis.

It can be argued that some of the independent nursing interventions mentioned could be subsumed under other nursing diagnoses. In retrospect, it would have been more meaningful if the nurses had been instructed to identify as many nursing diagnoses as they could for each patient with CHF, which would have made the nursing interventions more sensitive and specific to each diagnosis.

The types of nursing interventions done for CHF and for decreased cardiac output were very similar. One possible explanation is that nurses respond to patients' needs as they perceive them, regardless of the diagnostic label. Another possibility is that the brief introduction to nursing diagnosis given by the investigator did not allow the nurses enough experience in using the concept to integrate it into practice.

The frequency of patient teaching done using medical diagnosis was significantly higher than that done using nursing diagnosis. The explanation for this result is unclear. It may be that under the nursing framework the nurses incorporated patient teaching as an integral part of their interactions with patients, whereas teaching was regarded as an extra task under the framework of medical diagnosis and therefore mentioned specifically as an intervention.

SUMMARY AND SUGGESTIONS FOR FURTHER STUDY

This beginning effort at establishing nursing interventions specific to decreased cardiac output will help to clarify and standardize the nurses' role for this diagnosis. The categories of nursing interventions developed here must be validated. In addition, nursing interventions must be studied in patients with heart disease other than CHF. Nursing interventions appropriate for outpatient settings should also be described.

REFERENCES

American Nurses' Association: Nursing: a social policy statement, Kansas City, Mo., 1980, The Association.

Beeson, P., McDermott, W., and Wyngaarden, J., eds.: Cecil's textbook of medicine, Philadelphia, 1979, W.B. Saunders Co.

Beland, I., and Passos, J.: Clinical nursing, New York, 1975, MacMillian Publishing Co., Inc.

Castles, M.R.: Interrater agreement in the use of nursing diagnosis. In Kim, M.J., and Mortiz, D.A., eds.: Classification of nursing diagnoses: proceedings of the third and fourth national conferences, New York, 1982, McGraw-Hill Book Co.

Gebbie, K.M., and Lavin, M.A.: Classifying nursing diagnoses, Mo. Nurs. **42**:10, 1973.

Gordon, M.: Nursing diagnosis and the diagnostic process, Am. J. Nurs. **76**:1298, 1976.

Gordon, M.: The concept of nursing diagnosis, Nurs. Clin. North Am. **14**:487, 1979.

Halloran, E.: Patterns of nursing diagnoses and drugs in 1167 hospitalized patients, Paper presented at the meeting of the Fourth National Conference on the Classification of Nursing Diagnoses, St. Louis, April 1980.

Harrison, T.: Principles of internal medicine, New York, 1977, McGraw-Hill Book Co.

Kim, M.J., and others: Clinical use of nursing diagnoses related to cardiovascular disease. In Kim, M.J., and Moritz, D.A., eds.: Classification of nursing diagnoses: proceedings of the third and fourth national conferences, New York, 1982, McGraw-Hill Book Co.

Little, D.E., and Carnevali, D.L.: Nursing care planning, Philadelphia, 1976, J.B. Lippincott Co.

Luckmann, J., and Sorensen, K.C.: Medical-surgical nursing, Philadelphia, 1980, W.B. Saunders Co.

Soares, C.A.: Nursing and medical diagnoses: a comparison of variant and essential features. In Chaska, N., ed.: The nursing profession: views through the mist, New York, 1978, McGraw-Hill Book Co.

Weber, K.T., and Janicki, J.S.: The heart as a muscle-pump system and concept of heart failure, Am. Heart J. **98:**371, 1979.

Nursing diagnosis—the state of the art as reflected in graduate students' work

SHIRLEY M. ZIEGLER, R.N., Ph.D.

The nursing process is the methodology of professional nursing. Legitimacy for this statement is provided in part by the 1973 Standards of Nursing Practice of the American Nurses' Association, by the focus of the new State Board Nurse Examinations on nursing process, and by the growing body of literature concerned with nursing process.

In reviewing historically the conceptualization of the nursingprocess, Stelzer and Becker (1982) traced the gradual evolution of nursing process into five steps. The five-step process has been identified by Mundinger and Jauron (1975) and by Aspinall (1976) as assessment, nursing diagnosis, planning, implementation, and evaluation.

Developing the nursing diagnosis statement is a crucial step and a major problematic area in using the nursing process in nursing practice. Mundinger and Jauron's definition of nursing diagnosis (1975, p. 97), "A nursing diagnosis is the statement of a patient response which is actually or potentially unhealthful and which nursing intervention can help to change in the direction of health," has been widely accepted.

Although no consensus exists on the components of the nursing diagnosis statement, the approach advocated by Gordon (1976), Henderson (1978), Mundinger (1980), Mundinger and Jauron (1975), and Ressler (1982) has been widely accepted. The components of the nursing diagnosis statement are perceived as consisting of two components joined with a "related to" phrase. The first component is the client's potential or actual unhealthful response. The second component is the reasons or etiology for the client's unhealthful response.

Mundinger (1980) provided the rationale for including these two components in the nursing diagnosis statement. The first component, the potential or actual unhealthful response, gives direction to the goals, objectives, or desired outcomes of nursing intervention and is the component on which the last step of the nursing process, evaluation, is based. The second component, the clause identifying the etiology, gives direction to nursing action. The planned interventions are specific regarding etiology; thus the second com-

☐The author would like to express appreciation to Karen Gartland, R.N., the research assistant on this project. This research was funded in part by a grant from the Institutional Research Fund, Texas Woman's University.

ponent individualizes nursing care. Nursing diagnosis statements that do not include both components do not give clear direction to the planning, implementation, and evaluation steps of the nursing process and have little value for professional nursing.

Although the nursing diagnosis statement is a crucial phase of the nursing process, little evidence exists indicating the state of the art, that is, how well practicing nurses can formulate nursing diagnosis. Indeed, some available evidence indicates that problems in formulating the nursing diagnosis are common.

Hefferin and Hunter (1975) studied the scope, specificity, and interrelatedness of patient problems and nursing intervention statements as reflected in nursing care plans. They found vagueness in the nursing interventions planned for identified patient problems and a large number of nursing interventions planned that were not related to identified problems. They concluded that nurses are having difficulty in stating problems and interventions in specific terms.

DeBack (1981) found a serious deficiency in the ability of baccalaureate senior nursing students to formulate nursing diagnoses. She speculated that nursing faculty may not understand and, therefore, not teach the skills of nursing diagnosis. Since the activities of the nursing process are based on the nursing diagnostic statement, DeBack's findings support a serious concern about the ability of professional nurses to carry out the nursing process.

The study reported here is part of a larger study concerned with validating a taxonomy for nursing diagnoses. Specifically, the purpose of this study was to determine the extent to which nursing diagnosis statements generated by graduate nursing students meet the criteria for nursing diagnosis statements considered necessary if the remaining steps of the nursing process are to be based on the statement. The common problems experienced in writing the statements were also to be determined.

METHOD
Design

The design of this study was retroactive, descriptive, exploratory, and evaluative.

Sample

The 168 nursing diagnosis statements that constituted the data of this study were generated by 90 master's level graduate nursing students attending a large master's program of nursing located in the southwestern part of the United States. The graduate nursing students were enrolled in their first clinical nursing course, and the nursing diagnoses were generated as part of course assignments. The assignments included case studies, client records, nursing care plans, and term papers. The students came from many geo-

BOX 1   **Instrument for evaluating the nursing diagnosis statement**

General criteria
1. Both components are present vs.
   a. Only one component present.
   b. No real response component; actually two etiologies identified.
   c. No real etiology component; actually two responses identified.
2. The clauses are joined with a "related to" phrase.
3. The response is written first and the etiology written second.
4. Asymmetric statement (the statement is not circular).

Response component
5. The response component is clearly unhealthy or written as a potentially unhealthy response.
6. Only one response for each diagnosis statement vs. multiple responses.
7. The response component must be potentially modifiable.
8. The identified unhealthy response is concrete enough to generate observable, measurable, and desired outcomes.

Etiology component
9. Only one etiology component for each diagnosis statement vs. multiple etiologies.
10. All the etiologies identified must be potentially changeable by someone.
11. The etiology addresses nursing's independent function.
12. The etiology is concrete enough to suggest a specific nursing activity vs. a variety of possible interventions, the choice of which requires more concise information.

---

graphic locations and had attended a variety of undergraduate curriculums. Students were enrolled in clinical nursing courses in one of the traditional nursing specialties: medical-surgical, pediatric, maternity, psychiatric-mental health, and community health.

Instrument

The *Instrument for Evaluating the Nursing Diagnosis Statement* (Box 1) was used in this study. Criteria were generated by the investigator from the desirable characteristics identified from the literature on nursing diagnosis and were believed to be necessary if the last three steps of the nursing process were to be based on the nursing diagnosis statement. The first four criteria address the nursing diagnosis statement in general; criteria five through eight address the response component; and the last four criteria address the etiology component of the diagnosis statement.

Procedure

No attempt was made to give the students special knowledge of nursing diagnosis for this project. The students, however, as part of regular course content attended a 3-hour class held in a core course and received varying input from the faculty teaching the different clinical nursing courses.

All the completed class assignments for each of the clinical nursing courses were made available to the investigator. The nursing diagnosis statements were extrapolated from the assignments by the investigator and a research assistant and recorded on separate 3 × 5 index cards.

The 168 nursing diagnosis statements recorded were evaluated against each of the 12 criteria by both the investigator and the research assistant working independently. Each criterion was judged as being met or not being met for each diagnosis statement. The ratings of the investigator and the research assistant were compared. If there was a disagreement, consensus was reached by discussion. In this way, a composite rating for each of the diagnostic statements for each of the criteria was recorded.

RESULTS

Of the 168 nursing diagnosis statements collected, all 12 criteria could be coded for only 94 (55%) of the statements; thus, 74 (45%) statements could not be used in tabulating the final results. The statements were lost in the following manner.

If the first criterion that both components for the statement be present was not met, the statements were classified into one of three categories: (A) only one component present, (B) two components present but both are response components, or (C) two components present but both are etiology components. If the statement was coded A, no further coding took place. If the statement was coded B or C, coding was continued for the second criterion and then discontinued.

Eighteen statements were lost because they failed to meet the first criterion and were coded A (consisted of only one component). Those coded B or C (43 statements) were lost after coding criterion 2. Consequently, 107 statements were coded beyond the second criterion.

If the fourth criterion was coded circular, coding was discontinued. Four statements were coded circular; therefore, 103 statements were available for coding the fifth criterion. This criterion required that the response component indicate a clearly unhealthy state. Nine statements failed to meet this criterion and further coding was discontinued. Thus 94 nursing diagnosis statements remained to be evaluated against the remaining 7 criteria.

Of the 168 statements collected, only 10 (6%) met all the criteria (Box 2). The results of the evaluation of the remaining statements are organized into three categories: general criteria, response criteria, and etiology criteria.

General criteria

Four criteria addressed the nursing diagnosis statement in general: both components are present, the components are joined with a "related to" phrase,

---

BOX 2   **Nursing diagnosis statements that met all the criteria**

1. Dental caries related to poor dental hygiene.
2. Potential teenage suicides related to parents demanding high achievement.
3. Anxiety related to lack of knowledge of relaxation methods.
4. Potential respiratory infection related to airway blockage with secretions.
5. Potential for physical injury related to lack of knowledge of medication and treatments.
7. Potential noncompliance to medical regimen related to lack of knowledge of pharmacologic aspects of medications.
8. Obesity related to lack of knowledge of normal nutrition.
9. Abdominal soreness related to lack of bowel movement.
10. Potential muscle degeneration related to immobility associated with fractured femur.

---

the response component is written first and the etiology component is written second, and the statement is asymmetric.

The first criterion was that both components of the nursing diagnosis statement are present. Of the 168 statements evaluated, 61 statements (36%) failed to meet this criterion. In 30% of the 61 statements, only one component was identified. In approximately 57% of the 61 statements, two components had been identified, but both components addressed etiology and no response component was identified. In 13% of the 61 statements, two components were identified, but they consisted of two response components and no real etiology was identified. Examples of diagnosis statements that consisted of only one component included inability to trust and feel confident regarding the reliability of others, lack of knowledge concerning fracture, and lack of independence. Examples of diagnosis statements that consisted of two response components included anxiety related to powerlessness, impaired physical mobility related to gross motor uncoordination, and dysfunctional family related to lower self-esteem among family members. Examples of diagnosis statements that consisted of two etiology components included psychologic trauma related to illness, joint motion discomfort related to arthritic changes, and inadequate knowledge of respiratory function related to seasonal hay fever and bronchial asthma.

The second general criterion was that the two components of the nursing diagnosis statement be joined by a "related to" phrase. Of the 150 statements in which at least two components were present (correctly or not), 32 (21%) failed to meet this criterion. Phrases used instead of the desired "related to" phrase included "associated with," "due to," and "resulting from."

The third criterion was that the response component was to be written first and the etiology component was to be written second. Only four of the 99 statements coded on this criterion failed to meet it. An example of a statement that failed to meet this criterion was: painful joint motion related to inability to move freely.

The last general criterion was that the components of the nursing diagnosis statement be asymmetric or noncircular. Only seven of the 99 statements coded on this criterion failed to meet it. An example of a statement that failed to meet this criterion was dysfunctional communication related to inability to receive and send clear messages.

Response criteria

Four criteria were related to the response component of the nursing diagnosis statement: the response component identifies a clearly unhealthy state or is written as a potentially unhealthy response, only one response is to be identified for each statement, the response component must be potentially modifiable, and the unhealthy response identified is concrete enough to generate observable, measurable, and desired outcomes.

The first response criterion stated that the response must be clearly unhealthy. Of the 102 statements evaluated on this criterion, 9% failed to meet it. Examples of diagnosis statements that failed to meet this criterion included grieving related to death of wife, grief related to loss, anxiety related to delay in preparation for kidney transplant, and anxiety related to change of residence.

The second response criterion stated that the statement must identify only one response. Approximately 11% of the statements consisted of multiple responses. Examples of multiple responses identified in single-diagnosis statements included shortness of breath and chest pain related to decreased cardiac output and inadequate tissue profusion; feelings of being alone, unloved, and isolated related to recent separation from husband, lack of finances, and failure to form new friendships; and susceptible to oral stomatitis and dental complications related to radiation to the neck.

The third response criterion stated that the response must be potentially modifiable. All of the 94 statements evaluated against this criterion met it.

The fourth response criterion stated that the identified response must be concrete enough to generate observable, measurable, and desired outcomes. Approximately 13% of the 94 statements failed to meet this criterion. Examples of statements in which the response component was vague included psychologic trauma related to adjustment to acute illness, and distress related to family disorganization.

Etiology criteria

Four criteria were related to the etiology component of the nursing diagnosis statement: only one etiology component for each statement, all the etiologies must be potentially modifiable by someone, etiology addresses nursing's independent function, and the etiology identified is concrete enough to suggest a specific nursing activity.

The first etiology criterion stated that only one etiology must be identified in each statement. Of the 94 statements evaluated on this criterion, 28% failed to meet it. Examples of multiple etiologies in single-diagnosis statements included feelings of being alone, unloved, and isolated related to recent separation from husband and lack of finances; profound disorientation associated with loss of spouse and arteriosclerotic heart disease; and predisposition to accidental injury because of immobility, obesity, and emotional status.

The second etiology criterion stated that the etiology identified must be potentially changeable by someone. This criterion was not met by 29% of the diagnosis statements. Examples of unchangeable etiologies included alteration in comfort related to menstruation, profound disorientation related to loss of spouse, inability to develop close relationships related to being raped, and decreased activity related to musculoskeletal changes.

The third etiology criterion stated that the etiology must address nursing's independent function. Almost 49% of the etiologies identified failed to meet this criterion. Examples of etiologies included in the statements that failed to meet this criterion were high blood pressure related to increased cardiac output and greater peripheral resistance, anxiety related to financial alterations, alterations in adaptation related to insertion of pacemaker, and elevated blood sugar level related to insulin deficiency.

The fourth etiology criterion stated that the etiology must be concrete enough to suggest a specific nursing activity. This was not met by 79% of the 94 statements. Examples of vague etiologies included painful joint pain related to inability to move freely, alteration in sleep patterns related to fear of living alone, and decreased muscle strength related to prolonged bed rest.

Problems in developing a nursing diagnosis

The problems with generating the nursing diagnosis statement are presented in Table 1. The first four problems concerned the etiology component of the nursing diagnosis statement. The most common problem (79%) was in writing an etiology concrete enough to generate a specific nursing action. The next most common problem (48%) was the identification of etiologies that not address nursing's independent function. The third most common problem (29%) involved the identification of an etiology not changeable by anyone. The fourth most common problem (28%) was the identification of multiple etiologies. The sample experienced fewer problems in identifying the response component. However, over one fourth of the diagnosis statements contained a response component that failed to meet one or more of the response criteria.

TABLE 1   **Rank order of problems in writing the nursing diagnosis statement by component**

		Frequency	
Rank	Problem	Number	Percentage
	Etiology component		
1	Etiology component not concrete enough to generate a specific nursing action	74	79
2	Etiology does not address nursing's independent function	46	48
3	Etiology identified not potentially changeable by anyone	27	29
4	Multiple etiologies identified	26	28
	Response component		
5	Response identified too vague to generate measurable goals	12	13
6	Multiple responses identified	10	11
7	Identified response not obviously unhealthy	8	9
8	Response identified not concrete enough to generate observable, measurable, and desired outcomes	0	0

DISCUSSION

Orlando (1961) introduced the concept of deliberate nursing action over 20 years ago. Deliberate nursing action is based on the etiology component of the nursing diagnosis statement. Little evidence is provided by this study that deliberate nursing action based on etiologic-specific nursing action is practiced by this sample. Of the 94 statements coded for the four criteria of the etiology component, over 75% were not concrete enough to generate a specific nursing action. Individualized nursing care depends on the etiology of the diagnosis being specific for nursing action. If nurses do not plan nursing action based on a specific etiology, individualized nursing care may be more of a slogan than a reality.

One of the benefits to nursing of writing nursing diagnosis statements identified in the literature (Viamontes, 1982) is autonomy. The nursing diagnosis statement is meant to reflect independent nursing action. Yet almost half the etiologies identified in this study did not address the area of nursing's independent function. Almost one third of the etiologies identified were not even potentially changeable; thus no known intervention on the part of any health care provider could be indicated.

Accountability is a client benefit identified by Viamontes (1982) for nurses writing nursing diagnoses. But evaluation of the outcomes of nursing care is based on the ability to generate observable, measurable, and desired outcomes that depend on the quality of the response component of the nursing diagnosis statement. No evidence is presented in the findings of this study that the nurses in the sample possess the skill to generate observable, measurable, and desired outcomes. Without an identified potential of actual unhealthful client response, no desired outcome or client goal can be identified. Without a client goal, no evaluation of the outcome of nursing care can be made. This finding suggests that quality assurance may be more a figment of nursing's imagination than a reality.

CONCLUSIONS

Assuming that the nursing process depends on the quality of the nursing diagnosis statement, the following conclusions are made. The state of the art of nursing diagnosis, if defined by findings of this sample of 90 graduate nursing students, is not well developed. The skills needed to generate a nursing diagnosis statement on which measurable goals, individualized nursing care, and evaluation of patient care can be based are lacking in this sample. The nursing diagnosis statements generated by this sample would not lead to the goals of accountability, autonomy, or individualized nursing care.

IMPLICATIONS

No claim can be made that the 90 subjects who generated the data for this investigation are representative of professional nurses in general. The nurses received their education from a variety of colleges, have had varied professional experiences, and came from many geographic areas. They have received some additional instruction beyond the undergraduate level in writing nursing diagnosis statements. One might speculate that the nurses in this study were better prepared educationally than the average nurse. If, however, they are representative in any way, the study supports DeBack (1981) in her questioning of whether faculty members are prepared to teach the skills of nursing diagnosis or whether practicing nurses have the skills needed to generate workable nursing diagnosis statements on which to base the last three steps of the nursing process.

If the findings of this study can be replicated or if one generalizes the findings to practicing nurses in general, a massive education program in the generation of nursing diagnoses is indicated for practicing nurses, nurse faculty, and nurse administrators. The need for writing the nursing diagnosis is evident. For without a usable nursing diagnosis statement, the nursing process cannot be implemented.

REFERENCES

Aspinall, M.J.: Nursing diagnosis—the weak link, Nurs. Outlook **24:**433, 1976.
DeBack, V.: The relationship between nursing students' ability to formulate nursing diagnosis and the curriculum model, Adv. Nurs. Sci. **3:**51, 1981.

Gordon, M.: Nursing diagnosis and the diagnostic process, Am. J. Nurs. **76:**1298, 1976.

Hefferin, E.A., and Hunter, R.E.: Nursing assessment and care plan statements, Nurs. Res. **24:**360, 1975.

Henderson, B.: Nursing diagnosis: theory and practice, Adv. Nurs. Sci. **1:**75, 1978.

Mundinger, M.O.: Autonomy in nursing, Rockville, Md., 1980, Aspen Systems Corp.

Mundinger, M.O., and Jauron, G.D.: Developing a nursing diagnosis, Nurs. Outlook **23:**94, 1975.

Orlando, I.: The dynamic nurse-patient relationship, New York, 1961, G.P. Putnam's Sons.

Ressler, M.M.: Formulation of a nursing diagnosis. In Carlson, J.H., Craft, C.A., and McGuire, A.D., eds.: Nursing diagnosis, Philadelphia, 1982, W.B. Saunders Co.

Stelzer, F.K., and Becker, A.M.: Historical development of nursing diagnosis. In Carlson, J.H., Craft, C.A., and McGuire, A.D., eds.: Nursing diagnosis, Philadelphia, 1982, W.B. Saunders Co.

Viamontes, C.M.: Nursing diagnosis: the client, the nurse, the nursing profession. In Carlson, J.H., Craft, C.A., and McGuire, A.D., eds.: Nursing diagnosis, Philadelphia, 1982, W.B. Saunders Co.

Nursing diagnoses in the chronically ill

LOIS M. HOSKINS, R.N., Ph.D.
CAROLINE S. BAGLEY, R.N., M.S.N.
ELIZABETH A. McFARLANE, R.N., D.N.Sc.
M. GAIE RUBENFELD, R.N., M.S.
ANN M. SCHREIER, R.N., Ph.D.
MARY B. WALSH, R.N., M.S.N.

Improved standards of living, health care, and technologies have lengthened the life span of persons with chronic illness. This lengthened life span increases the obligation of the health care system to respond to the health needs and problems of these patients and to improve the quality of their lives. Nurses, as the largest group of health care providers, have the responsibility to provide care to these patients based on sound decision-making practices. As defined by the ANA (1980, p. 9), "Nursing is the diagnosis and treatment of human responses to actual or potential health problems." It becomes increasingly evident that an organized system of terminology is necessary for nursing personnel so that the care of patients can proceed smoothly through the total process of nursing. The development and testing of nursing diagnoses in inherent in this process.

The questions this study addresses were: What are the nursing diagnoses of chronically ill patients? Do they have a common set of nursing diagnoses? Using direct assessment of the patient based on the human needs model, the specific aims of this study were to (1) derive the nursing diagnoses of two groups of chronically ill patients and (2) compare the frequency of occurrence of each nursing diagnosis in the two groups to determine commonalities.

THEORETIC FRAMEWORK

Human need and motivation theories provide an orderly framework within which client care can be examined, studied, analyzed, implemented, and evaluated. These theories are based on the belief that the human person is an integrated, organized entity who experiences motivations in various activities of living, which direct that person to seek and to use resources that aid in meeting human needs (Lederer, 1980; Maslow, 1970; McHale and McHale, 1978; Montagu, 1979; Yura and Walsh, 1978b).

☐This research was funded by an NRE/DP Grant from the Division of Nursing, Department of Health and Human Services.

Human beings are integrated holistic beings who are complex and multifaceted. They also possess a multitude of human needs that can be identified and studied as sets of similar needs or drives. Maslow identified the sets of needs as physiologic, safety and security, love and belonging, self-esteem, and self-actualization. Other scholars classify needs differently. For example, McHale and McHale (1978) classify needs according to biophysical and psychosocial needs with further subclassification according to sufficiency needs, deficiency needs, and growth needs.

Although there is evidence of an increased interest to study human needs, there is a gap in the means available to quantitatively measure these needs (Lederer, 1980). Human needs vary from person to person and from culture to culture, which poses problems in the quantitative measurement of needs, including the identification of what is the need as well as specific ways that the need can be satisfied (Lederer, 1980).

It is becoming increasingly evident that an organized system of terminology is necessary for nursing personnel to carry out the total process of nursing, assessment through evaluation. The professional nursing literature is experiencing an upsurge in writing, inquiry, curiosity, and study about the use of the nursing process and specifically about the need to establish nursing diagnoses in practice. Several authors reported positive results from their efforts to base nursing actions on nursing diagnoses (Aspinall, 1976; Gordon, 1982; Mundinger and Jauron, 1975). To provide a framework for the orderly analysis of the efforts to identify and label nursing diagnoses, there are also efforts to clarify the framework within which nursing diagnoses are determined. Kritek (1978) suggests a pragmatic approach to theory development. She contends that the efforts of nursing should be directed toward level one of theory development, that is, the development of factor-isolating theories. The next step is to define the nomenclature for nursing diagnoses. The final step is to classify these diagnoses to identify patterns and relationships (Gebbie and Lavin, 1975).

The implementation of nursing diagnoses in the care of the chronically ill adult person is considered a valuable and worthwhile endeavor for nurses and for the ultimate benefit of an increasing number of chronically ill persons. Recognition of patients' problems, actual and potential, and coordination of patient care planning by nurses can be enhanced by a tested and validated system of assessing and diagnosing the needs of patients.

METHODOLOGY
Research approach

The research is descriptive and comparative and uses a cross-sectional survey. No hypotheses are made.

Operational definitions

Definitions of terms used in this study are as follows:

Chronically ill patients—Patients 25 years of age and older who are diagnosed medically as having chronic disease. The National Conference on Chronic Disease (1952, p. 14) defines chronic disease as comprising "all impairments or deviations from the normal which have one or more of the following: are permanent, leave residual disability, are caused by non-reversible pathological alteration, require special training of the patient for rehabilitation, may be expected to require a long period of supervision, observation or care."

Nursing diagnosis—Label given to a cluster or group of signs or symptoms that indicate the absence of fulfillment or alteration of fullfillment of a human need. To be included as a specific nursing diagnosis, the signs and symptoms must be agreed on by 80% of the panel of judges (research associates).

Subjects

Data were collected from a sample of 200 subjects from the population of patients attending the medical outpatient clinic of a 900-bed health care facility serving a large metropolitan area. For comparison purposes, subjects were randomly assigned to two groups. Group membership was unknown to the data collectors and the judges, who analyzed the data and formed the diagnoses. Although a limitation exists in obtaining the subjects from one agency, the size of the sample and the randomization to comparison groups should improve the validity and reliability of the diagnoses.

Tool development

The development of the tool used to assess need alterations and assist in derivation of nursing diagnoses of chronically ill persons began in September 1980. The process was a collaborative effort of members of the research team and graduate students on the project staff.

With guidance from two research associates, two master's-level students reviewed the literature relevant to assessment tools and the 10 need categories in the study. The 10 need categories were air, nutrition, elimination, sleep and rest, activity, safety and security, love and belonging, sexual integrity, self-esteem, and self-actualization. The 10 need categories were operationally defined, and a 32-page tool eliciting data relating to need fulfillment and/or deprivation was developed.

Subsequent examination of the tool by the research team, a statistician, and consultants resulted in revisions in content and format, providing a more concise and clear tool without sacrificing the intent of gathering a broad base of data. To establish content validity, the revised 24-page tool was sent to 11 judges, nine of whom responded. The input from the judges was analyzed, and when appropriate, further revisions were made.

A pilot study for the purpose of determining reliability of the tool was begun in February 1981. The pilot study provided direction for further revisions. Some questions were reworded to improve clarity or to force choices; some redundant questions were eliminated. A consultant, who had been one of the validators of the first draft of the tool, reviewed the tool at this time and made suggestions for improvement in areas that could cause problems in establishing interrater reliability. These suggestions were incorporated. Interrater reliability was established in October 1981, and data collection was begun.

Data collection procedures

After the data collector obtained informed consent, the subject was interviewed using the previously described tool. Some information was obtained from the subjects' hospital records (data from physician's history, physical examination, and laboratory and x-ray reports). After collection of these data on all patients, a panel of judges analyzed them for content. Objective signs, such as pulse rate, weight, and blood pressure, were compared with standard parameters to determine normalcy. Subjective comments were analyzed for content. The panel of judges then independently clustered the signs and symptoms and labeled them with a nursing diagnosis. The clusters derived from the data collected should be agreed on by 80% of the panel of judges.

Data collectors

Five nurses, all with master's degrees and enrolled in doctoral study (four in a D.N.Sc. program and one in a Ph.D. program in education), performed the interviews and collected specified data from the clients' medical records. No physical examination skills were required.

Training

A combination of activities was used to train the data collectors. They were given a bibliography dealing with techniques of interviewing. Orientation to the interview guide consisted of reading and discussing each item in the tool during a group session with data collectors and tool developers and then practicing use of the tool in pairs. A videotaped interview of a client was conducted by one of the instrument developers for training purposes. The interview was observed and rated for agreement by the five data collectors and the five research associates as a group. Clarification and revisions of questions were made to improve agreement. Two of the research associates, one partic-

TABLE 1   Average percentage agreement of five interviewers over all subjects

Interviewers	1	2	3	4	5
1	1.00	.92	.92	.92	.90
2		1.00	.92	.91	.89
3			1.00	.91	.89
4				1.00	.90
5					1.00

ipant and one observer, conducted taped interviews of two clients in the actual research setting. The two audiotapes were rated independently by each of the five data collectors. A 95% agreement was reached by the seven raters, two research associates and five data collectors.

Reliability study

During a 1-month period in the medical outpatient setting, the five data collectors interviewed 11 subjects. Two data collectors were present at each visit, one as the participant interviewer and the other as an observer; each made an independent rating of the interview. The interview was also tape-recorded. Working in pairs, and alternating partners, each of the five data collectors (six pairings were necessary) interviewed one subject and observed the interview of another subject. Agreement of each of the five pairs was calculated, with a mean percent of agreement being .92. This gave an interrater reliability for direct observation of the subject. Using the audiotapes, the other three data collectors listened to the interview and made independent ratings. The interrater reliability from the taped recordings was .91. This sample included five raters each assessing 11 interviews for a total of 55 comparisons. Table 1 shows the average percentage of agreement of the five interviewers for all subjects.

This method made it possible to estimate interrater reliability without conducting extensive paired direct observations. It also provided the means for checking the stability of ratings over time. The data collector could listen to the audiotape of her direct interview, rate it, and compare it to her previous rating. Similar options were available for interrater stability.

Panel of judges

Five of the research associates of this project, who are all nurse educators adept in nursing diagnosis, are serving as the panel of judges. They will analyze the data and develop the nursing diagnoses. Interrater reliability among the panel determining the clusters of signs and symptoms to establish a nursing diagnosis is to be established as follows:

1. For the first 20 to 25 subjects, each of the five judges will determine the clusters independently.
2. A 5 × 5 correlation matrix will be formed, and the mean proportion of agreement among the judges will be determined.
3. If agreement is high, the remainder of the subjects' data could be broken into groups and pairs of judges would make the decisions.

This format eliminates the necessity of each judge analyzing the data on 200 subjects. With data from the pilot study, the judges are establishing agreements concerning analysis and coding of the content, which should lead to establishment of a high level of agreement for the final analysis.

This research is presently in progress. Currently, the judges are identifying the process they use in making the diagnoses and are establishing the percentage of agreement. Significant responses from each questionnaire are written on separate cards for each of the 10 needs, demographic data, medication data, and physical examination and laboratory data. Data from the latter three categories are indicators or sources of support from problems identified in the need areas. Responses are significant if they indicate abnormal behavior in comparison with an accepted standard or norm, a change in the subject's usual behavior, or a risk factor (potential for a problem). After extracting the data, which at this point are categorized according to a need, the individual items or responses are clustered. There is no limit on the number of clusters, but each cluster must have two or more indicators (significant responses). Information from one need may support a problem in another need. Cross-referencing and interrelationships are expected. Rules are being established for the process as the judges progress. The next step is to determine the percentage of agreement among the judges on the cluster formation.

Data analysis

A total list of nursing diagnoses will be derived for each group of 100 subjects. Then the frequency of each nursing diagnosis in each group of 100 subjects will be determined. A comparison of the two groups will be made, and tests for significance of the commonalities will be conducted.

In addition to the approach described, data will be subjected to descriptive analysis by means of a computer. The frequency of occurrence for each sign and symptom in each group of 100 will be determined and compared. Clusters of signs and symptoms may be formed, with weighting assigned to the signs and symptoms in the cluster based on the frequency of occurrence. Data obtained and conclusions formed in this manner will be compared with the judges' analysis.

REFERENCES

American Nurses' Association. Nursing: a social policy statement, Kansas City, Mo., 1980, The Association.

Aspinall, M.J.: Nursing diagnosis—the weak link, Nurs. Outlook **24**:433, 1976.

Gebbie, K.M., and Lavin, M.A., eds.: Classification of nursing diagnoses, St. Louis, 1975, The C.V. Mosby Co.

Gordon, M.: Nursing diagnosis—process and application, New York, 1982, McGraw-Hill Book Co.

Kritek, P.E.: The generation and classification of nursing diagnoses: toward a theory of nursing, Image **10**:33, 1978.

Lederer, K., ed.: Human needs, Cambridge, Mass., 1980, Oelgeschlager, Gunn, & Hain, Publishers, Inc.

Maslow, A.H.: Motivation and personality, ed. 2, New York, 1970, Harper & Row, Publishers.

McHale, J., and McHale, M.: Basic human needs—a framework for action, New Brunswick, N.J., 1978, Transaction Books.

Montagu, A.: The direction of human development, New York, 1970, Hawthorn Books, Inc.

Mundinger, M.O., and Jauron, G.D.: Developing a nursing diagnosis, Nurs. Outlook **23**:94, 1975.

National Conference on Chronic Disease: Conference proceedings, preventive aspects of chronic disease, Baltimore, 1952, Commission on Chronic Illness.

Yura, H., and Walsh, M.B.: Human needs and the nursing process, New York, 1978a, Appleton-Century-Crofts.

Yura, H., and Walsh, M.B.: The nursing process, ed. 3, New York, 1978b, Appleton-Century-Crofts.

ADDITIONAL READINGS

American Nurses' Association: ANA standards of nursing practice, Kansas City, Mo., 1973, The Association.

Avant, K.: Nursing diagnosis: maternal attachment, Adv. Nurs. Sci. **2**:45, 1979.

Carlson, J.H., Craft, C.A., and McGuire, A.D., eds.: Nursing diagnosis, Philadelphia, 1982, W.B. Saunders Co.

Chambers, W.: Nursing diagnosis, Am. J. Nurs. **62**:102, 1962.

Departmental Task Force on Prevention: Disease prevention and health promotion: federal programs and prospects. U.S. Department of Health, Education and Welfare, P.H.S. Pub. No. 79-55071 B, Washington, D.C. September 1978.

Dickoff, J., James, P., and Wiedenbach, E.: Theory in a practice discipline. Part I. Practice-oriented theory, Nurs. Res. **17**:415, 1968.

Durand, M., and Prince, R.: Nursing diagnosis: process and decision, Nurs. Forum **5**:50, 1966.

Gordon, M.: Nursing diagnosis and the diagnostic process, Am. J. Nurs. **76**:1298, 1976.

Gordon, M., and Sweeney, M.A.: Methodological problems and issues in identifying and standardizing nursing diagnosis, Adv. Nurs. Sci. **2**:1, 1979.

Kim, M.J., and Moritz, D.A., eds.: Classification of nursing diagnoses: proceedings of the third and fourth national conferences, New York, 1982, McGraw-Hill Book Co.

Levine, M.E.: Trophicognosis: an alternative to nursing diagnosis, Unpublished paper, February 1964.

The Surgeon General's Report on Health Promotion and Disease Prevention: Healthy people, U.S. Department of Health, Education and Welfare, DHEW (PHS) Pub. No. 79-55071, Washington, D.C., 1979.

Nurses' perceptions of rheumatic disease patient problems as evidenced in nursing diagnoses, etiologies, defining characteristics, expected outcomes, and interventions

TERESE M. HALFMANN, R.N., M.S.N.
JANICE S. PIGG, R.N., B.S.N.

Nurses base their actions on their perceptions of patient problems. These perceptions are evidenced in the nursing process that "encompasses all significant steps taken in the care of patients" (ANA, 1980, p. 12). In an attempt to advance the nursing care provided to rheumatic disease patients, this study examined rheumatology nurses' perceptions of patient problems by investigating the following questions:

1. What are the nursing diagnoses that rheumatology nurses identify clinically?
2. What are the etiologies identified for each nursing diagnosis?
3. What are the defining characteristics that substantiate each nursing diagnosis?
4. What are the expected outcomes listed for each nursing diagnosis?
5. What are the nursing interventions listed for each nursing diagnosis?

Specific terms used in this study were defined as follows:

Rheumatic disease patient—A person diagnosed as having a disease identified in the American Rheumatism Association Nomenclature and Classification of Arthritis and Rheumatism with the primary problem being medical (McCarty, 1979).

Nursing diagnosis—A title of an actual or potential health problem that had been accepted at the Fourth National Conference on the Classification of Nursing Diagnoses.

Positive indicator—A feature that describes a desirable patient behavior.

Subetiology—A term describing a contributing cause of the patient problem defined in the nursing diagnosis.

METHOD
Sample

The study was conducted at a large, private, urban hospital. Data were collected by retrospective audit of the nursing care plans of all rheumatic disease patients (N = 51) discharged from the hospital's 24-bed rheumatic disease unit (RDU) over a 30-day period. Although the RDU did not have primary nursing, nurses were assigned to patients with continuity of care as a major focus. Only those nursing care plans totally written by the RDU nurses were audited.

Nursing diagnoses, etiologies, defining characteristics, expected outcomes, and nursing interventions were documented by nurses in specific sections of the nursing care plan, which was considered a permanent part of the patient's hospital record. All the nurses on the RDU had received formal instruction about each component of the nursing care plan and the correct method for documenting information on the care plan. A copy of the Fourth National Conference List (NCL) of accepted nursing diagnoses was in each patient's nursing care plan folder.

Procedure

All the data recorded by the nurses in the nursing care plan sections designated for nursing diagnoses, etiologies, defining characteristics, expected outcomes, and nursing interventions were transcribed by the investigators. The labels for patient problems in the nursing diagnosis section of the nursing care plan were analyzed using a nursing diagnosis classification system developed by Halfmann and others (1981), which defines 16 categories for patient problem labels, for example, NCL nursing diagnosis, sign or symptom, and nursing problem. All the patient problem labels were further analyzed for frequency. The etiologies, defining characteristics, expected outcomes, and nursing interventions for the five most frequently occurring nursing diagnoses were analyzed. The etiologies and defining characteristics were compared with those accepted at the Fourth National Conference on the Classification of Nursing Diagnoses. The expected outcomes and nursing interventions were analyzed to determine natural groupings and frequency.

RESULTS
Nursing diagnoses

The investigators collected 161 labels for patient problems from the 51 nursing care plans. Analysis of these labels using the 16-category system of Halfmann and others (1981) revealed that 85% (137) of the 161 labels could be categorized as NCL nursing diagnoses; 6% (9) as sign and/or symptom, for example, *fatigue*; 4% (7) as non-NCL nursing diagnosis, for example, *alteration in comfort: stiffness*; 2% (4) as body system dysfunction, for example, *disturbance in GI system*; 2% (3) as medical diagnoses and/or surgical procedure, for example, *postoperative left hand tendon repair*; and 1% (1) as incomplete NCL nursing diagnosis, for example, *alteration in elimination*.

Examination of the 137 labels categorized as NCL nursing diagnoses revealed that 17 nursing diagnoses of the 42 accepted at the Fourth National Conference on the Classification of Nursing Diagnoses were represented (Table 1). Of the NCL nursing diagnoses, 39% (53) were *alteration in comfort:*

TABLE 1   **Percentage of 137 labels categorized as nursing diagnoses accepted at the fourth national conference on the classification of nursing diagnoses**

National conference list nursing diagnosis	Percentage
Alteration in comfort: pain	39
Knowledge deficit	19
Sleep pattern disturbance	9
Self-care deficit	9
Impairment of skin integrity: actual	8
Mobility, impaired physical	3
Noncompliance	3
Bowel elimination, alteration in: constipation	1
Coping, ineffective individual	1
Nutrition, alteration in: less than body requirements	1
Nutrition, alteration in: more than body requirements	1
Breathing pattern, ineffective	1
Gas exchange, impaired	1
Home maintenance management, impaired	1
Injury, potential for	1
Skin integrity, impairment of: potential	1
Thought processes, alteration in	1
TOTAL	100

pain. The other four most frequently occurring NCL nursing diagnoses were *knowledge deficit* (19%), *sleep pattern disturbance* (9%), *self-care deficit* (9%), and *impairment of skin integrity: actual* (8%).

The etiologies, defining characteristics, expected outcomes, and nursing interventions for the five most frequently occurring NCL nursing diagnoses were analyzed. For purposes of this presentation, the analysis of the nursing process components for only the nursing diagnosis *alteration in comfort: pain* will be discussed (Table 2).

Etiologies

There were no etiologies or "unknown" listed for the nursing diagnosis *alteration in comfort: pain* 24% (13) of the 53 times the diagnosis was documented by the nurses. All the 40 etiologies were injuring agents, with 38 relating to rheumatic diseases, for example, *inflammatory process*. Injuring agent is a defining characteristic identified by the Fourth National Conference Group.

TABLE 2   **Frequency of the nursing process components for *alteration in comfort: pain***

Component	Number	Component	Number	Component	Number
Etiology		*Subjective defining characteristics*		*Objective defining characteristics*	
Injuring agents*	40	Communication (verbal or coded) of pain des-criptors†	88	Physical assessment parameters	20
Unkown (5)				Treatment of pain (ef-fect not documented)	15
None listed (8)	—	Communication of ac-companying signs/ symptoms	40		
TOTAL	40			Effects of pain on ADL	7
Positive indicators		Factors positively af-fecting pain	14	Guarding behavior, pro-tective†	5
Subjective, e.g., denies radiation of pain	1	Factors negatively af-fecting pain	13	Distraction behavior†	1
Objective, e.g., no in-creased radiation of pain	5	Factors ineffective in relieving pain	6	TOTAL	48
				Interventions	
TOTAL	6	Factors positively af-fecting stiffness	2	Use of medications	56
Subetiologies		Factors negatively af-fecting stiffness	1	Assessment instruc-tions	34
Physical injuring* agents, e.g., arthralgia	17	TOTAL	164	Use of heat/cold	30
TOTAL	17	*Expected outcomes*		Requests for medical orders	16
		States decreased pain	35	Unrelated to problem	3
		Decreased stiffness	13	TOTAL	139
		Increased ROM	3		
		Increased mobility	2		
		Minimal joint pain	1		
		Verbalizes pain control and increased tolerance level	1		
		Increased ADL	1		
		Decreased fatigue	1		
		Decreased swelling	1		
		None listed (5)	—		
		TOTAL	58		

*An etiology identified at the Fourth National Conference on the Classification of Nursing Diagnoses.
†A defining characteristic identified at the Fourth National Conference on the Classification of Nursing Diagnoses.

Defining characteristics

The data documented by the nurses in the defining characteristic section of the nursing care plan were categorized by the investigators as subjective and objective characteristics, positive indicators, and subetiologies. The categorization was necessary because nurses documented data other than defining characteristics in the section of the nursing care plan designed for such data.

Subjective defining characteristics were 77% (164) of the 212 defining characteristics documented for the diagnosis *alteration in comfort: pain*. Of these subjective defining characteristics, 54% (88) were the patients' communication of pain descriptors, for example, location of pain and degree of pain. Of these subjective defining characteristics, 24% (40) were the communication of accompanying signs/symptoms with the most frequent sign/symptom being stiffness (26). The remaining 22% (36) of the subjective defining characteristics were factors that affected pain or stiffness.

The most frequent of the 48 objective defining characteristics were physical assessment parameters (20) related to the signs and symptoms of inflammation (for example, *joint swelling, reddened*) and treatment for pain (15). Only six of the objective defining characteristics, which included *guarding behavior* and *distraction behavior*, were identified at the Fourth National Conference.

Six positive indicators, which were subjective and objective, were listed, for example, *not hot* and *tests negative*. All the 17 subetiologies were injuring agents, with 82% (14) of these being related to medical diagnoses.

Expected outcomes

The most frequent expected outcome, *verbalization of decreased pain*, accounted for 60% (35) of the 58 outcomes listed. Of the outcomes, 22% (13) included stiffness as a measurement of the degree of comfort.

Nursing interventions

Interventions were grouped into five categories (Table 3). Of the 56 nursing interventions in the category *use of medications*, 73% (41) duplicated physicians' medication orders and 14% (8) were individualized to meet patient needs, for example, *medicate before x-ray*. Of the 34 assessment instructions, 85% (29) referred to parameters of pain such as type, duration, and location. Of the 30 interventions for use of heat/cold, 69% (25) included specific nursing instructions. The remaining interventions were requests for medical orders or were unrelated to the problem.

DISCUSSION
Nursing diagnoses

The high percentage of NCL nursing diagnoses documented by nurses may have been caused by their having the Fourth NCL of Nursing Diagnoses

TABLE 3   **Frequency of nursing interventions for *alteration in comfort: pain***

Percentage	Nursing interventions	Number
40	Use of medications	
	Duplication of medical orders	41
	Specific nursing interventions	8
	Unrelated to the identified problem	5
	Nonspecific	2
	TOTAL	56
24	Assessment instructions	
	Assess pain parameters	29
	Evaluate effectiveness of heat/cold	4
	Assess change in nature	1
	TOTAL	34
22	Use of heat/cold	
	Specific nursing interventions	25
	Nonspecific	5
	TOTAL	30
12	Requests for medical orders	
	Requests for OT and/or PT evaluation	10
	Requests for specific heat/cold treatment	6
	TOTAL	16
2	Unrelated to problem	3

available in each patient's nursing care plan folder. The use of the other types of patient problem labels may have resulted from the nurses' need to document a patient problem without having adequate assessment data to choose an NCL nursing diagnosis or from the lack of an acceptable NCL nursing diagnosis.

The five most frequent NCL nursing diagnoses documented could be expected because they are common health problems experienced by rheumatic disease patients. The high incidence of *alteration in comfort: pain* was anticipated because of the chronic nature of pain in rheumatic diseases. Also, the degree of pain a patient experiences is perceived by the patient as a measurement of control of the disease. Patient education is one of the primary focuses of RDU nurses that may explain the frequent documentation of *knowledge deficit* as an NCL nursing diagnosis. The low frequency of documentation of the patient problem labels *impaired physical mobility* and *noncompliance* was significant because they are considered common problems in rheumatic diseases.

Etiologies

Etiologies were not included in 25% of the *alteration in comfort: pain* nursing diagnostic labels. The data suggest that more emphasis is needed on the importance of including etiologies as a part of the complete nursing diagnostic label. The latter could be accomplished by making a copy of the NCL nursing diagnoses with their respective etiologies readily available to the RDU nurses. Gordon points out that "a different diagnosis exists and different treatment is required when the etiology is different" (Gordon, 1982, p. 9).

Defining characteristics

The high incidence of subjective defining characteristics, especially the patient's communication of pain descriptors, would be anticipated because of the importance placed on patient's perceptions of pain in determining nursing interventions (McCaffery, 1972). In addition, the investigators found it notable that 33 defining characteristics were factors affecting pain. Rheumatic disease, as well as many other chronic illnesses, requires pain management; therefore identifying factors that affect pain is vital. The investigators suggest that the National Conference Group consider the effects of pain management techniques as defining characteristics.

The investigators found it important that five patient problem labels were *stiffness* and that 26 of the signs/symptoms communicated by the patients when being assessed for pain were complaints of stiffness. With the findings of the study and since stiffness is a common rheumatic disease patient complaint (Polley and Hunder, 1978), the investigators recommended that an alternate nursing diagnosis, *alteration in comfort: stiffness*, be considered. The nurses' documentations of physical assessment parameters related to inflammation are not relevant to the nursing diagnosis because the degree of inflammation does not always correlate with the degree of pain.

Expected outcomes

The patients' statements of decreased or minimal pain are appropriate as expected outcomes because they reflect the subjective nature of pain; however, they should be expressed in more measurable terms. The inclusion of decreased stiffness as the second most frequent expected outcome may have occurred because of the lack of a separate nursing diagnosis for this problem or the nurses' correlation of pain with stiffness. The expected outcomes reflecting functional levels of the patient (ROM, mobility, ADL) and symptoms of disease (fatigue and swelling) are not always related to pain. The outcome *verbalizes pain control and increased tolerance level* relates to the investigators' suggested defining characteristic, *effects of pain management techniques.*

Nursing interventions

It is not surprising to find the use of medications as the most frequent intervention for pain. The high incidence of medication-related interventions that were duplicative of medical orders was of concern to the investigators. The nursing interventions relating to assessment of pain were those expected of acute pain evaluation. Chronic pain assessment might more properly be evaluation of change in nature (for example, location, degree, type) of the pain or the effectiveness of the pain management technique.

IMPLICATIONS

The 16-category system for classification of nursing diagnoses was useful in analyzing the sample patient problem labels. To further validate the tool, the investigators recommend its use in similar studies. Specific patient populations, such as patients with rheumatic diseases, can be used to validate and expand the NCL of nursing diagnoses. An example would be the investigators' suggestion to include *alteration in comfort: stiffness,* since this is a common rheumatic disease patient problem addressed by nurses but not recognized by the National Conference Group.

Now that the National Conference Group has developed a beginning list of nursing diagnoses and defining characteristics, it should proceed with identifying expected outcomes and nursing interventions. The investigators recommend that the process be facilitated through research of expected outcomes and interventions documented by nurses actually caring for patients. An NCL of accepted outcomes and nursing interventions may prevent nurses from documenting mainly nonmeasureable and nonspecific outcomes and inappropriate interventions such as was found in this study.

Investigation of the most frequently occurring nursing diagnoses for specific patient populations will aid in the development of standardized nursing care plans. The frequently occurring nursing diagnoses can be used as the basis for writing practice standards for a specialized nursing group. The findings of this study have been used in defining the standards of practice for rheumatic disease nursing (to be published by American Nurses' Association).

REFERENCES

American Nurses' Association: Nursing: a social policy statement, Kansas City, Mo., 1980, The Association.

Gordon, M.: Nursing diagnosis: process and application, New York, 1982, McGraw-Hill Book Co.

Halfmann, T., and others: The identification of clinically recorded nursing diagnoses and indicators, Manuscript submitted for publication, 1981.

McCaffery, M.: Nursing management of the patient with pain, Philadelphia, 1972, J.B. Lippincott Co.

McCarty, D.J.: Arthritis and allied conditions: a textbook of rheumatology, Philadelphia, 1979, Lea & Febiger.

Polley, H.P., and Hunder, G.G.: Rheumatologic interviewing and physical examination of the joints, Philadelphia, 1978, W.B. Saunders Co.

Incidence of nursing diagnoses

PATRICIA A. MARTIN, R.N., M.S.
KAREN A. YORK, R.N., M.S.N.

Primary nursing was instituted at Miami Valley Hospital in 1977. Historic perspective places this event between the Second and Third National Conferences on the Classification of Nursing Diagnoses. Although reference to nursing diagnosis is found in Fry's article (1953), the term *nursing diagnosis* did not begin appearing with regularity until around 1975 (Dodge, 1975; Gebbie and Lavin, 1975; LaMontagne and McKeehan, 1975; Lewis, 1975; Little and Carnevali, 1975; Mahomet, 1975; Marriner, 1975; Proder, 1975; Roy, 1975). Mundinger and Jauron (1975) and Yura and Walsh (1973) were the original primary references used at Miami Valley Hospital to define nursing diagnosis within the context of the nursing process. To implement the primary nursing concept, the nursing care plan documentation format was revised; *patient needs/problems* became *nursing diagnosis*. Since then Gordon's definition (1976) has been used.

Standardized mandatory in-service programs prepared the R.N. staff for the transition from team to primary nursing. Nursing diagnosis within the framework of the nursing process was a major part of the presentation, and pocket-sized reference cards containing the Second National Conference's list of nursing diagnoses were distributed. These programs continue as a part of the orientation program for all R.N.s, and the reference cards have been updated to reflect the most recent list from the National Conference on the Classification of Nursing Diagnoses. The standard form for a nursing diagnosis is a two-part statement: *patient problem related to etiology.*

In the fall of 1981, a survey that evaluated the documentation of the nursing process was conducted to establish appropriate indexes of growth (Field, 1979). The survey revealed a 67% incidence of care plans containing at least one statement in the nursing diagnosis portion of the care plan form. The range was from 0% to 100% on any given nursing unit. Informal discussions indicated that this incidence related to a wide variance of feelings among the R.N.s regarding their competency in making nursing diagnoses. Aspinall, Jambruno, and Phoenix (1977) discuss nurses' confidence in their assessment

□Thanks are expressed to the ten nurse experts who spent many longs hours evaluating these data: Kathy Eckerle, R.N., M.S.; Norma Keefer, R.N., M.S.; Barbara Kellerstraus, R.N., M.S.; Shirley McNamee, R.N., M.S.; Gail Moddeman, R.N., B.S.N.; Mary Murphy, R.N., A.D.; Kathy Percival, R.N., B.S.N.; Gwen Garber, R.N., B.S.N.; Louise Walther, R.N., M.S.; and Celeste Warner, R.N., B.S.N.

and intervention skills versus their lack of confidence in diagnostic skills. More than one nurse author (Aspinall, 1976; Shoemaker, 1979) has despaired at diagnosis being the "weakest link" in the nursing process.

STUDY FOCUS

The first purpose of the study was to provide a needs assessment of nursing diagnostic skills (Dalton, 1979; Gordon, 1979). This assessment included validation of the conclusion from the informal discussions that there was a skill deficit in identifying nursing diagnoses. In this study the criteria for nursing diagnoses were as follows: (1) being a patient problem, (2) being clear and consise, and (3) being treatable by independent nursing measures (Mundinger and Jauron, 1975; Gordon, 1976).

The second purpose was to determine the incidence of nursing diagnoses used in this clinical setting to obtain epidemiologic information (Brown, 1974; Friedman, 1974; Gebbie and Lavin, 1974, 1975; Gordon and Sweeney, 1979; Jones, 1979; and McKeehan and Gordon, 1982) that would be helpful to the Fifth National Conference on the Classification of Nursing Diagnoses. The findings will be used to prioritize nursing diagnoses to be addressed by staff development programs, quality assurance activities, and research studies.

In addition, the researchers were interested in measuring the concept of "valuing" (Steele and Harmon, 1979) based on the assumption that valuing the documented care plan would be expressed by using the care plan. The researchers considered the strong behavioral and motivational components of valuing important to planned change (Kritek, 1979). Therefore valuing is defined as "how useful the nurse perceives the documented care plan." Manthey (1981) emphasized the point that has been stressed since at least 1949: care plans must be useful to the care giver or they fail to meet their primary purpose.

RESEARCH QUESTIONS

The questions addressed by this study were as follows:
1. What diagnosis statements (in the Fourth National Conference terminology or as a similar concept) are being used most frequently by the staff nurses?
2. What is the representation of nursing diagnoses from the accepted Fourth National Conference list?
3. Which variations (if any) clarify the patient problem better than the Fourth National Conference wording?
4. How useful do the nurses think the documented care plans are in giving care, communicating, and charting?

STUDY SETTING

The study was conducted in an 800-bed, midwestern, metropolitan, voluntary hospital primarily featuring acute care medical-surgical units (16), with three high-risk maternity units and one physical rehabilitation unit. The nursing units have from 27 to 44 beds. The critical care and psychiatric units were not included in the study because of different record-keeping formats. The educational background of the more than 700 registered nurses at this hospital is diverse: 21% baccalaureate; 62% diploma; 15% associate; and 2% master.

STUDY METHODOLOGY

A stratified random sampling technique was used to identify four documented nursing care plans per nursing unit on which at least one nursing diagnosis was recorded. All the nursing diagnoses on each of these four care plans were recorded, as found, including problem and etiology clauses. Then the data gatherer interviewed the nurse caring for the patient that day. The nurse interviewed was not necessarily the same one who wrote the care plan. The interview consisted of five sample yes/no questions to determine the value the nurse placed on the care plan. The questions concerned the nurse's perception of the care plan as (1) helpful, (2) appropriate, and (3) useful. Data collection was conducted by a group of baccalaureate student nurses and by one staff nurse. These nurses, rather than an authority figure, were selected because the nurses interviewed would feel less threatened and would be more candid in relating their true feelings.

Data were collected on two separate occasions 2 months apart, sampling a total of eight care plans on 20 nursing units or 160 care plans and 156 nurse interviews. Other information collected included the date of sampling, the patient's admission date, the unit location, the patient's room number, and the date(s) of the nursing diagnoses. Goals or objectives were also recorded verbatim, but this portion of the data has not yet been examined.

ANALYSES

A panel of 10 nurse experts who had worked extensively with nursing diagnoses within the context of the nursing process was identified (Gordon and Sweeney, 1979). Of these experts, five have master's degrees in nursing, four are baccalaureate graduates (two of these are master's candidates), and one has an associate degree and is a B.S.N. student. Two of the experts are directors of nursing, two are clinical specialists, two are instructors in a diploma nursing program, two are primary level II nurses, and two were primary level I nurses at the time of their selection. One of the primary I nurses has since assumed the position of clinical nursing coordinator (CNC). Primary level I is the staff nurse, or first level bedside nurse. Level II is also a clinical position that requires demonstrated expertise in the nursing process as determined by peer review. The clinical nursing coordinator is a nursing unit manager/administrator with 24-hour responsibility. The nursing director is the next level of administration and supervises several CNCs in related patient care areas.

The nursing diagnoses collected were grouped verbatim under the heading of a diagnosis from the accepted listing of the Fourth National Conference as determined appropriate by the researchers. The 10 nurse experts evaluated the placement of the verbatim diagnoses in the categories as a fit or no fit. Frequency counts were used to determine which groupings of diagnoses were most commonly used by the nurses. In the first questionnaire, experts evaluated the problem clauses of the diagnoses collected as compared with the Fourth National Conference accepted diagnoses by indicating whether the in-house problem clauses of the nursing diagnoses were "better than," "equal to," or "less good than" the Fourth National Conference accepted nursing diagnoses. They also evaluated the diagnoses from the standpoint of their stating a clear, concise patient problem that could be treated by independent nursing actions. The experts found this task fatiguing and difficult to do in isolation of the assessment data. Their usual experience had been to fit words to a patient situation, not consider the verbiage in isolation. Their difficulties were not unlike those reported by Castles (1982). The frequency of these responses was tabulated. A questionnaire was developed based on these results to further evaluate the Fourth National Conference diagnoses list.

This second questionnaire to be used by the 10 experts asked the following questions regarding each of the Fourth National Conference diagnoses:

1. Is this a nursing diagnosis problem clause?
2. Is this a nursing diagnosis etiology clause?
3. Is this an inappropriate nursing diagnosis clause?
4. Is this clause too broad (encompasses too many concepts)?
5. Would you recommend keeping this clause as it is?

On some diagnoses, additional questions asked for ratings of various qualifiers, that is, ineffective vs. impaired, and different wordings of root statements, that is, respiratory status vs. breathing patterns.

The perceived usefulness of the care plans was addressed by the data from the 156 nurses interviewed. The frequency of yes/no responses from the nurse interviews was simply tabulated, and the percentages of the frequency totals were computed for the two nominal categories of yes and no.

FINDINGS

The number of diagnoses per care plan varied from 1 to 10. The mean number of diagnostic statements per care plan was 3 (2.56). Of the diagnoses, 65 (13%) did not fit into any of the Fourth National Conference diagnosis categories.

The most prevalent nursing diagnoses corresponded to the following diagnoses accepted by the Fourth National Conference: (1) alteration in comfort: pain (N = 46 or 11%), (2) ineffective breathing patterns (N = 33 or 8%), (3) knowledge deficit (N = 23 or 6%), (4) impaired mobility (N = 21 or 5%), (5) potential for injury (N = 21 or 5%), (6) potential impairment of skin integrity (N = 18 or 4%), and (7) actual impairment of skin integrity (N = 15 or 3%). These seven nursing diagnoses represented 176 or 43% of the 411 diagnoses collected in the study. Of these 411 in-house diagnoses, only 24% (N = 97) conformed to the Fourth National Conference terminology. The Fourth National Conference diagnosis *disturbances in self-concept* had the following three similar concepts preferred by five of the experts: (1) unrealistic role expectations, (2) changes in body image, and (3) alteration in body image.

The responses of the experts to the second questionnaire were tabulated by frequency of yes or no responses. Only totals of six or more were considered conclusive. Of the 49 diagnoses, 73% were evaluated by six experts as appropriate problem clauses, 71% were evaluated by six experts as inappropriate etiology clauses, and 75% were evaluated by six experts as appropriate diagnosis clauses. The experts judged 10% of the 49 as too broad. The experts believed 14% could be kept "as is." Gross examination did not show interrater consistency between various word choices for qualifiers, which supports the position for standardized wording linked to standardized defining characteristics for mutual comprehension among nurses.

The valuing of care plans by the nurses interviewed revealed the following:

1. Is this care plan helpful to you in caring for the patient? . . .82% yes
2. Is this care plan appropriate for the patient? . . . . .80% yes
3. Do you use this care plan:
   a. To give nursing care? . . . . .82% yes
   b. To chart? . . . . 68% yes
   c. To communicate with other nurses? . . . . .85% yes

CONCLUSIONS AND DISCUSSION

In this descriptive study of nursing diagnoses, the most prevalent nursing diagnoses were *alterations in comfort, ineffective breathing patterns, knowledge deficit, impaired mobility, potential for injury,* and *impairment of skin integrity.* These findings suggest that these diagnoses are a high priority in this setting (medical-surgical, obstetric, and rehabilitation patients) and serve as a guideline for development of educational programs, for quality assurance activities, and for research problems (Brown, 1974; Bruce, 1979). Their frequency may also indicate that the diagostic nomenclature of these particular problems is clear and useful to many nurses.

Of the 65 diagnoses that did not fit with the Fourth National Conference list, *anxiety* was a grouping frequently used (N = 25 or 6%) by these nurses. This diagnosis was deleted by the Fourth National Conference listing of diagnoses and was listed as a symptom of fear or ineffective coping (Kim and Moritz, 1982). The use of this diagnosis by these nurses may indicate that they perceive *anxiety* as a useful and clear concept, do not have the necessary assessment skills to differentiate the origins of the anxiety, or were using an earlier listing of diagnoses. After this data collection, pocket-sized reference cards of the Fourth National Conference diagnoses were distributed to all the nurses. Several standardized workshops on nursing diagnosis skills within the framework of the nursing process are now being conducted for the R.N. staff.

Although many guides to assessment are found in the nursing literature and articles on diagnosis dealing primarily with assessment skills (Avant, 1979; Mahomet, 1975), little is found regarding diagnostic skills. The diagnostic process is a complex cognitive process, but the end product must be concrete. A few nursing authors do lead the reader through the diagnostic process concretely (Guzzetta and Forsyth, 1979; Price, 1979). Myers (1973) shows an excellent diagram of the difficulties in developing objective diagnostic capabilities. Models of application of this skill need to appear in the nursing literature just as the assessment tools currently do.

Clear definitions of the concept of nursing diagnosis are found in the literature (Bircher, 1975; Gebbie and Lavin, 1974; Gordon, 1976; Mundinger and Jauron, 1975; Roy, 1975). These definitions identify the following common parameters for the concept of nursing diagnosis: (1) the problem must be that of the patient/client, not that of the nurse, (2) the problem must be a problem that can be successfully addressed by independent nursing approaches, and (3) the wording must clearly convey the same message to all nurses involved in the care of the patient. Researchers have found a documented two-part statement (Gordon, 1976; Lunney, 1982; Mundinger and Jauron, 1975) of the problem related to etiology (with signs and symptoms identified in the documented assessment) to be a workable method. This method is useful to the care giver, to the educator in evaluation research, to those performing quality assurance activities, and to nurse researchers. Bircher (1975) and Steckle, Fiennell, and Pragovan (1979) warn of the danger of stereotyping with the diagnosis. It must be individualized by the qualifiers and by the etiology segment.

Some of the nursing diagnosis categories that were very seldom found in this sample may represent complex problems that currently exceed many staff nurses' assessment and identification skills (Aspinall, Jambruno, and Phoenix, 1977; Fredette and O'Connor, 1979; Gordon, 1980; Matthews and Gaul, 1979; Roy, 1975). The exclusion of the psychiatric units of this hospital may have accounted for this lack in some categories. Another contributing factor may be the lack of understanding of the meaning of the diagnostic category, for example, *thought processes.* Further development of diagnosis skills among the nursing staff will be done by sharing not just the diagnosis but the defining characteristics and the etiology based on the end product of the Fifth National Conference.

At least 80% of the nurses interviewed positively valued the care planning process as helpful, appropriate to patient state, useful in giving care, and useful in communicating with other nurses. Only 68% of the nurses interviewed perceived the care plan as useful in charting, which is an important area of the care planning process and indeed is one often unspoken aim of the nursing process. Stevens (1974) addresses this issue in her critique of the ANA *Standards of Nursing Practice,* which clearly identify only the documentation of the assessment portion of the nursing process. Documentation is central to legal validation of our professional activities (Fortin and Rabinow, 1979) and necessary for reimbursement by third-party payers (Griffith, 1982; Mundinger and Jauron, 1975; Weber, 1979).

REFERENCES

Aspinall, M.J.: Nursing diagnosis—the weak link, Nurs. Outlook **24**(7):433, 1976.

Aspinall, M.J., Jambruno, N., and Phoenix, B.S.: The why and how of nursing diagnosis, Am. J. Matern. Child Nurs. **2**(6):354, 1977.

Avant, K.: Nursing diagnosis: maternal attachment, Adv. Nurs. Sci. **2**(1):45, 1979.

Bircher, A.U.: On the development and classification of diagnosis, Nurs. Forum **14**(1):10, 1975.

Brown, M.M.: The epidemiologic approach to the study of clinical nursing diagnosis, Nurs. Forum **13**(4):346, 1974.

Bruce, J.: Implementation of nursing diagnosis: a nursing administrator's perspective, Nurs. Clin. North Am. **14**(3):509, 1979.

Castles, M.R.: Interrater agreement in the use of nursing diagnosis. In Kim, M.J., and Mortiz, D.A., eds.: Classification of Nursing Diagnoses: proceedings of the third and fourth national conferences, New York, 1982, McGraw-Hill Book Co.

Dalton, J.: Nursing diagnosis in a community health setting, Nurs. Clin. North Am. **14**(3):525, 1979.

Dodge, G.H.: Forces influence move toward nursing diagnosis, AORN J. **22**(8):157, 1975.

Field, L.: The implementation of nursing diagnosis in clinical practice, Nurs. Clin. North Am. **14**(3):497, 1979.

Fortin, J., and Rabinow, J.: Legal implications of nursing diagnosis, Nurs. Clin. North Am. **14**(3):553, 1979.

Fredette, S., and O'Connor, K.: Nursing diagnosis in teaching and curriculum planning, Nurs. Clin. North Am. **14**(3):541, 1979.

Friedman, G.D.: Primer of epidemiology, New York, 1974, McGraw-Hill Book Co.

Fry, V.S.: The creative approach to nursing, Am. J. Nurs. **53**(1):301, 1953.

Gebbie, K.M., and Lavin, M.A., eds.: Classification of nursing diagnoses, St. Louis, 1975, The C.V. Mosby Co.

Gebbie, K.M., and Lavin, M.A.: Classifying nursing diagnoses, Am. J. Nurs. **74**(2):250, 1974.

Gordon, M.: Nursing diagnosis and the diagnostic process, Am. J. Nurs. **76**(8):1297, 1976.

Gordon, M.: The concept of nursing diagnosis, Nurs. Clin. North Am. **11**(3):487, 1979.

Gordon, M.: Predictive strategics in diagnostic tasks, Nurs. Res. **29**(1):39, 1980.

Gordon, M., and Sweeney, M.A.: Methodological problems and issues in identifying and standardizing nursing diagnosis, Adv. Nurs. Sci. **2**(1):1, 1979.

Griffith, H.M.: Strategies for direct third-party reimbursement for nurses, Am. J. Nurs. **82**(3):408, 1982.

Guzzetta, C.E., and Forsyth, G.L.: Nursing diagnosis pilot study: Psychophysiologic stress, Adv. Nurs. Sci. **2**(1):27, 1979.

Jones, P.: A terminology for nursing diagnosis, Adv. Nurs. Sci. **2**(1):65, 1979.

Kim, M.J., and Moritz, D.A., eds.: Classification of nursing diagnoses: proceedings of the third and fourth national conferences, New York, 1982, McGraw-Hill Book Co.

Kritek, P.: Commentary: the development of nursing diagnosis and theory, Adv. Nurs. Sci. **2**(1):73, 1979.

LaMontagne, M., and McKeehan, K.: Profile of a continuing care program emphasizing discharge planning, J. Nurs. Admin. **5**(8):22, 1975.

Lewis, E.P.: The stuff of which nursing is made, Nurs. Outlook **23**(2):89, 1975.

Little, D., and Carnevali, D.: The diagnostic statement: the problem defined. In Walter, J., Pardee, G., and Mallo, D., eds.: Dynamics of problem-oriented approaches: patient care and documentation, Philadelphia, 1975, J.B. Lippincott Co.

Lunney, M.: Nursing diagnosis: refining the system, Am. J. Nurs. **82**(3):456, 1982.

Mahomet, A.D.: Nursing diagnosis for the OR nurse, AORN J. **22**(5):709, 1975.

Manthey, M.: Nursing care plans, Nurs. Manag. **12**(9):28, 1981.

Marriner, A.: The nursing process: a scientific approach to nursing care, ed. 3, St. Louis, 1982, The C.V. Mosby Co.

Matthews, C.A., and Gaul, A.L.: Nursing diagnosis from the perspective of concept attainment and critical thinking, Adv. Nurs. Sci. **2**(1):17, 1979.

McKeehan, K.N., and Gordon, M.: Utilization of accepted nursing diagnoses. In Kim, M.J., and Moritz, D.A., eds.: Classification of nursing diagnoses: proceedings of the third and fourth national conferences, New York, 1982, McGraw-Hill Book Co.

Mundinger, M.D., and Jauron, G.D.: Developing a nursing diagnosis, Nurs. Outlook **23**(2):95, 1975.

Myers, N.: Nursing diagnosis, Nurs. Times **69**(38):1229, 1973.

Price, M.: The patient is starving—but why? RN **42**(11):45, 1979.

Proder, B.: What you should know about nursing diagnosis, Med. Rec. News **46**(4):87, 1975.

Roy, Sister C.: A diagnostic classification system for nursing, Nurs. Outlook **23**(2):90, 1975.

Shoemaker, J.: How nursing diagnosis helps focus your care, RN **42**(8):56, 1979.

Steckle, S.B., Fiennell, M.M., and Pragovan, A.: How nursing care can increase patient adherence rather than patient compliance, clinical and scientific session: 1979 ANA division of practice, Kansas City, Mo., 1979, American Nurses' Association.

Steele, S.M., and Harmon, V.M.: Values clarification in nursing, New York, 1979, Appleton-Century-Crofts.

Stevens, B.J.: ANA's standards of nursing practice: what they tell us about the state of the art, J. Nurs. Admin. **4**(5):16, 1974.

Weber, S.: Nursing diagnosis in private practice, Nurs. Clin. North Am. **14**(3):533, 1979.

Yura, H., and Walsh, M.B.: The nursing process, ed. 2, New York, 1973, Appleton-Century-Crofts.

An evaluation study of the implementation of nursing diagnosis

CHRISTINE MIASKOWSKI, R.N., M.S.N.
SANDRA SPANGENBERG, R.N., M.A.
GRAMATICE GAROFALLOU, R.N., M.S.

This study was an attempt to quantify and qualify preliminary data on the implementation of a nursing diagnosis project. The goal was to gather baseline data about the state of the art of nursing diagnosis. The study was conducted at a 431-bed tertiary care facility located in the New York metropolitan area.

The data presented are an initial attempt at evaluating a project that took 1½ years to complete. The Department of Nursing chose to implement nursing diagnosis–oriented care planning and charting after an evaluation of the present documentation system revealed numerous deficiencies and inconsistencies.

The change was accomplished in stages. Initially, a new nursing diagnosis assessment tool was introduced. The format and guidelines for nursing diagnosis–oriented care planning and documentation were then established. A hospital-wide 3-hour staff development program was mandated for the entire professional nursing staff. The didactic classes were followed up with on-unit clinical conferences during which concurrent reviews of charts were performed.

The authors conducted a quantitative study 3 months after initiating the nursing diagnosis project. This investigation supported compliance with the methodology of nursing diagnosis–oriented documentation. From the data obtained, the authors began to formulate the study questions for a qualitative analysis, which was completed 6 months after the project was started.

PURPOSE

This study was designed to evaluate the quality of nursing diagnoses being written 6 months after the implementation of the nursing diagnosis project. It was an initial attempt to define the state of the art and any parameters needing further clarification and revision.

SAMPLE

The sample consisted of a retrospective group of 155 medical-surgical charts. The sample included a cross section of nursing units within the hospital, including the intensive care unit and the coronary care unit. The pediatric and obstetric services were not included.

STUDY QUESTIONS

To define the quality of nursing diagnoses being written, the authors asked the following questions:

1. What are the most common nursing diagnoses being written?
2. Are new nursing diagnoses being created?
3. What are the correlations between the medical-surgical diagnoses and the nursing diagnoses?
4. Do specialty areas write unique diagnoses or the same nursing diagnoses as the general services?
5. How many nursing diagnoses address potential, actual, or health maintenance issues?
6. What is the average number of nursing diagnoses per patient?
7. When are the nursing diagnoses most frequently written?
8. Are signs and symptoms supporting the nursing diagnosis documented and valid?

RESULTS OF DATA COLLECTION

Based on the preliminary qualitative study and data reported in the literature, the authors formulated the following hypotheses in relation to the study questions.

Question 1. What are the most common nursing diagnoses being written?

Hypothesis 1. The most common nursing diagnoses written at this institution will be the same as those identified in the Halloran study (1980).

Results. The Halloran study was a research project presented at the Fourth National Conference on the Classification of Nursing Diagnoses. The data Halloran presented resulted in a list of the most frequently used nursing diagnoses (Halloran, 1980). These diagnoses were used as a point of comparison (Table 1). An analysis of the data in Table 1 reveals that the most common nursing diagnoses written at the authors' institution differ from the 10 most common diagnoses identified in the Halloran study by three diagnoses and by their rank order.

Question 2. Are new nursing diagnoses being created?

Hypothesis 2. There will be at least one new nursing diagnosis developed.

Results. For the purpose of this study, a new diagnosis was any diagnosis that differed in language or concept from those established in the institution's list of acceptable nursing diagnoses or those accepted by the Fourth National Conference on the Classification of Nursing Diagnoses. A total of 22 nursing diagnoses were identified. Examples of original nursing diagnoses are listed in Box 1.

Question 3. What are the correlations between the medical-surgical diagnoses and the nursing diagnoses?

Hypothesis 3. There will be an increase in the number and complexity of

TABLE 1   Halloran–study institution nursing diagnoses

Halloran	Study institution	Number of diagnoses
Discomfort	Anxiety*	77
Mild anxiety	Pain*	46
Impairment of mobility	Alteration in food, fluid, and electrolyte balance*	34
Altered ability to perform self-care	Alteration in circulatory integrity*	32
Pain	Alteration in respiratory integrity	28
	Postoperative complications*	28
Potential impairment skin integrity	Alteration in mobility*	26
Actual impairment skin integrity	Alteration in skin integrity*	20
Respiratory dysfunction	Alteration in intestinal integrity	18
Less nutrition than required	Alteration in urinary integrity	17
Decreased cardiac output	Alteration in sensory/perceptual/neurologic integrity	16
	Knowledge deficit	15
	Alteration in metabolism	14
	Alteration in personal integrity	13
	Alteration in protective mechanisms—infection	13
	Alteration in hemodynamics	9
	Miscellaneous	8
	Alteration in protective mechanisms—bodily injury	7
	Noncompliance	1

*Similar to Halloran (1980).

BOX 1   **Original nursing diagnoses**

Alteration in independence
Overweight related to sedentary life-style and restriction to wheelchair
Potential for mismanagement of diabetes related to insufficient knowledge of all aspects of diabetic self-care or to lack of motivation to comply with self-care regimen
Potential for contractures related to decreased mobility
Potential for falling related to increased weakness

TABLE 2   Correlation between medical-surgical diagnosis and number of nursing diagnoses

Medical-surgical diagnosis	Number of charts	Total number of nursing diagnoses	Number of nursing diagnoses per chart
Blood dyscrasias	7	10	1.4
Cancer—solid tumors	13	31	2.38
Cardiac	6	21	3.5
Eye	4	7	1.75
General surgery	22	60	2.7
Genitourinary	16	31	1.9
Gynecologic	3	6	2.0
Multiple medical problems	28	86	3.0
Neurologic	13	32	2.46
Open heart surgery	3	14	4.6
Orthopedic	4	10	2.5
Peripheral vascular disease	2	4	2.0
Plastic/ENT	4	7	1.75
Rehabilitation	13	35	2.69
Renal	9	18	2.0
Respiratory	5	7	1.4

nursing diagnoses based on the increased number of medical problems or surgical interventions, longer length of stay, and increased age of the patient.

Results. For the purpose of this study, the patient's medical-surgical diagnoses were grouped into 16 categories (Table 2). The data listed in Table 2 support the first part of the hypothesis. The more complex the medical-surgical problem, the more nursing diagnoses written. The data in Table 3 show the number of nursing diagnoses per length of patient stay. As can be seen, the second part of the hypothesis is supported: as the length of stay increases, the number of nursing diagnoses also increases. Table 4 represents the data obtained when patient age is correlated with number of nursing diagnoses. The highest number of nursing diagnoses was made for those patients 61 to 70 years of age.

Question 4. Do specialty areas write unique diagnoses or the same diagnoses as the general services?

Hypothesis 4. There will be common nursing diagnoses that cut across specialty areas.

Results. Table 5 shows the most common nursing diagnoses written in each medical surgical specialty listed previously. An analysis of the results

TABLE 3   Correlation between length of stay and number of nursing diagnoses

Length of stay (days)	Number of nursing diagnoses per patient									
	1	2	3	4	5	6	7	8	9	10
0-5	17	6	3							
6-10	8	17	13							
11-15	4	10	8							
16-20	3	1	10	8						
21-25		1	6	4	4					
26-30	1		3		1	1				
31-35			1		1	2				
36-40		1	1	1	2	1				
41-45					1					1
46-50										
51-55										
56-60										
61-65				1			1			

TABLE 4   Correlation between patient age and number of nursing diagnoses

Age group	Number of patients per group	Total numbers of nursing diagnoses per age group	Number of nursing diagnoses per patient									
			1	2	3	4	5	6	7	8	9	10
0-10	1	2		1								
11-20	7	16	3	1	1	2						
21-30	6	10	3	2	1							
31-40	9	19	2	4	3							
41-50	12	38	1	2	5	3	1					
51-60	29	69	10	8	6	2	1	2				
61-70	34	87	9	11	8	1	4		1			
71-80	29	80	4	10	8	3	4					
81-80	21	69	1	7	8	2	1	1				1
90-100	6	17		1	5							

TABLE 5   Nursing diagnoses related to medical-surgical specialty

Medical-surgical specialty	Number of charts	Number of nursing diagnoses per specialty
Blood dyscrasias	7	Pain—4 Anxiety—3 Alteration in hemodynamics—blood loss—3
Cancer—solid tumors	13	Pain—6 Anxiety—6 Alteration in fluid and electrolytes—3 Alteration in intestinal integrity—3
Cardiac	6	Pain—6 Alteration in circulatory integrity—6
Eye	4	Alteration in sensory-perceptual integrity—2 Potential for postop complications—2
General surgery	22	Pain—8 Anxiety—15 Potential for postoperative complications—1 Alteration in protective mechanisms—4
Genitourinary	16	Pain—6 Anxiety—7 Potential for postoperative complications—6 Alteration in urinary integrity—10
Gynecologic	3	Anxiety—3 Potential for postoperative complications—3
Multiple medical problems	28	Pain—9 Anxiety—7 Alteration in metabolism—6 Alteration in respiratory integrity—5 Alteration in circulatory integrity—10 Alteration in intestinal integrity—5
Neurologic	13	Pain—3 Anxiety—5 Mobility—3 Alteration in neurologic integrity—5
Open-heart surgery	3	Alteration in circulatory integrity—3 Alteration in respiratory integrity—2
Orthopedic	4	Pain—2 Anxiety—2
Peripheral vascular disease	2	Alteration in circulatory integrity—2
Plastics/ENT	4	Anxiety—2 Alteration in respiratory integrity—2
Rehabilitation	13	Anxiety—3 Alteration in intestinal integrity—4 Knowledge deficit—3 Alteration in skin integrity—3
Renal	9	Anxiety—4 Alteration in fluid and electrolytes—3 Alteration in circulatory integrity—3
Respiratory	5	Alteration in respiratory integrity—4

shows that the nursing diagnoses of pain and anxiety cut across all specialty areas and that each individual specialty generates diagnoses specific to its specialty.

Question 5. How many nursing diagnoses address potential, actual, or health maintenance issues?

Hypothesis 5. There will be more potential nursing diagnoses developed.

Results. This hypothesis was not supported by the study. Analysis of the data revealed 267 actual nursing diagnoses, 132 potential nursing diagnoses, and no health maintenance nursing diagnoses.

Question 6. What are the average number of nursing diagnoses per patient?

Hypothesis 6. The average number of nursing diagnoses per patient will be three.

Results. The investigators analyzed 155 charts. The total number of nursing diagnoses was 411. The average number of nursing diagnoses per patient was 2.65.

Question 7. When are the nursing diagnoses most frequently written?

Hypothesis 7. Nursing diagnosis are most frequently written on admission.

Results. The results of the study supported by hypothesis: 301 nursing diagnoses were written on admission, 97 were written during hospitalization, and 10 were written at discharge.

Question 8. Are the signs and symptoms supporting the nursing diagnosis documented and valid?

Hypothesis 8. There will be signs and symptoms supporting the nursing diagnosis 60% of the time.

Results. In reviewing the signs and symptoms that led the nurse to make a nursing diagnosis, the investigators found the data difficult to evaluate.

In many instances, descriptors were not documented in the progress notes or on the nursing assessment sheet that would lead the nurse to make a particular nursing diagnosis. Since anxiety was the nursing diagnosis that occurred most frequently in our study, the descriptors of this diagnosis were analyzed in detail. Of the 75 nursing diagnoses relating to anxiety, 37 did not have signs and symptoms documented. In fact, the investigator would find statements such as "friendly and cooperative," "appears calm," "does not seem overly anxious," and "depressed" in the nursing assessment sheet, and a diagnosis of anxiety would appear on the nursing care plan.

Another group of diagnoses that proved problematic was that dealing with potential problems. One example was a patient admitted with "intact skin, good turgor, and good nutritional status," but was confined to bed because of traction. Based on clinical experience, the nurse documented a nursing diagnosis of potential for alteration in skin integrity and developed a preventive plan of care.

Each nursing diagnosis or groups of diagnoses made in the study was analyzed in relation to the supporting signs and symptoms. In general, the study showed that the descriptors were not complete nor specific enough to be definitively diagnostic.

DISCUSSION

This study was undertaken with the purpose of defining a quality nursing diagnosis. The investigators' initial expectation was that each patient would have one diagnosis made on admission. As can be seen from the results of the study, the majority of the cases had more than one nursing diagnosis. Some of the charts had diagnoses that spanned admission, interim, and the discharge phases of the patient's stay. The number of diagnoses increased with the complexity of the patient's medical-surgical problems and length of stay.

Almost all the diagnostic statements written at this institution followed the format of the state of the patient related to a specific etiology. The best charts in the study were those on which:

1. The nursing diagnoses were written on admission and updated during the patient's stay with interim and discharge diagnoses
2. The nursing diagnoses were stated in precise state of the patient terms with specific etiologies
3. Signs and symptoms were documented supporting the nursing diagnosis
4. Progress notes were written in a SOAP format, identifying the nursing diagnoses by name in the patient progress record and "SOAPing" to the specific diagnosis (Weed, 1969)

Therefore the quality nursing diagnosis became one that was precisely written, updated, validated with signs and symptoms, and identified in the progress notes illustrating movement toward resolution or reevaluation.

Based on this initial study of the original documentation system, the investigators concluded that nursing diagnosis–oriented charting is a very effective way of implementing and documenting the nursing process. The formulation of nursing diagnoses requires the nurse to actualize the nursing process. Data obtained on admission and during ongoing assessment are synthesized into a diagnostic statement. The remainder of the documentation system requires that the practitioner complete the nursing process by formalizing goals, interventions, and evaluation criteria.

The study pointed out that certain nursing diagnoses cut across all specialty areas, yet specialty areas initiate unique nursing diagnoses. Further evaluation needs to be done on both the general nursing diagnoses and those unique to specialty areas. Defining characteristics must be specified and tested in the clinical laboratory. The data on the documentation of supporting signs and symptoms show that nurses need assistance in synthesizing assessment data to formulate a specific diagnosis and that practitioners need guidance in therapeutic interviewing, physical assessment skills, and correlation of laboratory data to determine a patient's problem. The results of the data indicate that nursing diagnoses are most frequently written on admission. Nursing diagnosis–oriented charting may facilitate the process of updating and revising the patient's plan of care.

IMPLICATIONS FOR FURTHER RESEARCH

Findings from this initial evaluation study have numerous implications for further research. The first question requiring investigation is: What are the defining characteristics that lead the nurse to make a specific nursing diagnosis? At the authors' institution, task force groups were initiated to analyze our most frequently occurring nursing diagnoses. The second area requiring further research is whether nurses have the interviewing and physical assessment skills needed to collect sufficient data, synthesize these data, and formulate a precise nursing diagnosis.

The third area for clinical investigation is how to achieve updating and revision of the patient's nursing diagnoses and the remaining components of the plan of care. At the authors' agency, the attempt to ensure revision was made by incorporating this standard into the evaluation tools. Further evaluation of this problem will be considered. A fourth problem for further research is whether educational preparation, that is, diploma, A.D., B.S., or M.S., makes a difference in the nurse's ability to formulate nursing diagnoses.

Finally, the ultimate questions are, What is the impact of nursing diagnosis on the quality of care the patient receives? Does the entire nursing process, with nursing diagnosis being one component, make a difference in the care the patient receives? Systems must be developed to evaluate the long-term impact on the delivery of patient care.

REFERENCES

Halloran, E.J.: Patterns of nursing diagnosis and diagnostic-related groups in a sample of 2560 hospitalized patients, Paper presented at the Fourth National Conference on the Classification of Nursing Diagnoses, St. Louis, Mo., April 11, 1980.

Weed, L.L.: Medical records: medical education and patient care, Cleveland, 1969, Case Western Reserve University Press.

The effect of teaching on documentation of nursing diagnoses

CATHY D. MEADE, R.N., M.S.
MI JA KIM, R.N., Ph.D., F.A.A.N.

Documenting nursing acts in a scientific manner has been a major problem in nursing practice. Lack of a scientific body of knowledge that is unique to nursing has been cited as one cause of the problem. The nursing profession needs research data to provide evidence of the extent of documentation of nursing acts by a scientific problem-solving process. Nurses must critically examine reasons why nursing documentation is composed primarily of technical procedures. Although frequent reference is made to the need for documentation of nursing diagnoses, research in the area is limited. However, the value of nursing diagnoses in providing quality patient care is supported in the nursing literature (Fry, 1953; Gerber, 1979; Gordon, 1976; Rothberg, 1967; Shoemaker, 1979).

Mundinger and Jauron (1975) collected data about the time involved in documentation of nursing diagnoses and found that accurate recording of one's activities requires time, thought, and synthesis of information and involves some risk taking. Mitchell and Atwood (1975) compared clinical recordings and case study data between two groups of beginning nursing students; one group was taught problem-oriented charting and the other was taught traditional charting. Their findings suggested that a problem-oriented format was superior in allowing students to identify, solve, and document patient problems. Findings from the study of Bertucci, Huston, and Perloff (1974) showed that nurses who applied the problem-oriented approach recorded more pertinent information than the nurses who used the traditional approach.

PURPOSE

The first purpose of this study was to examine the effect of teaching on staff nurses' documentation of nursing diagnoses in classroom and clinical settings. The second purpose was to identify problems associated with documentation of nursing diagnoses in patients' records. The third purpose was to explore the relationship of educational background and clinical experience to documentation of nursing diagnoses.

METHOD

The effect of teaching on documentation of nursing diagnoses was studied by two methods: case studies and patient records. The design was chosen to examine the effect of teaching in a simulated situation (case study) as well as in an actual setting (patient records). Each nurse served as his or her own control.

Two groups of subjects were selected for this study: nurses responsible for providing patient care and patients who received the nursing care. The nurse group consisted of 16 staff nurses who volunteered to participate in the study. They were employed at the institution for at least 6 months, had at least 6 months' clinical experience, and cared for patients with respiratory problems and/or diabetes. Written consent was obtained from the nurses for inclusion in this study. The patient group consisted of patients with respiratory and/or diabetic disorders who were not in the acute phase of illness and who were cared for by the participating nurses. A signed consent form was obtained from the patients for access to their charts.

The study was conducted on eight medical-surgical units of a 1265-bed Veterans Administration hospital. Data collection occurred during two phases, the control phase and the experimental phase. The control phase constituted the period in which no teaching session was offered.

Initially, nurses were given a case study from which they were instructed to identify nursing diagnoses with supporting data. They were given 20 minutes to complete the task. The case study was based on an actual clinical situation, one different from the area of proposed study. Content validity was established by a panel of clinical specialists. Following the case study exercise, the investigator reviewed the documentation of the same nurses from randomly chosen patient records during two 8-hour day shifts.

The experimental phase consisted of the period after a teaching session was offered. Approximately 1½ hours of instructions were given on the concept of nursing diagnoses, the diagnostic process, and the documentation of nursing diagnoses. The content of the session was developed by the investigator and was approved by content specialists in the area. At the completion of the teaching session, the nurses were given the same case study as in the control phase and were instructed to identify nursing diagnoses with supporting data. They were again given 20 minutes to complete the task.

At the completion of the teaching session, the nurses were given three research packets to complete in the clinical area. Each packet was for use with one patient. Research data sheets* for documenting nursing diagnoses and supporting data, an instruction sheet, and a list of nursing diagnoses from the Second National Conference on the Classification of Nursing Diagnoses were included in the packet. The research data sheets included such information as duration, severity, and etiology of the nursing diagnosis. Nurses

---

*The research data sheets were developed based on the PES system described by Gordon (1976) and Kim and others (1982).

were instructed to choose three patients to care for who met the patient selection criteria and to whom they would be assigned again in the same week.
They were asked to complete the research data sheets based on their assessment of the patients. They were encouraged to document their identified
nursing diagnoses in the patients' permanent record during the day shift. The
completed research packets were sealed and submitted to the investigator.

One of the three research packets was randomly selected to compare the
nursing diagnoses listed on the research data sheets with the actual nursing
documentation in the patient's chart. Again, nursing documentation during
two 8-hour day shifts was audited to determine the quantity and type of nursing diagnoses. The nurses were not aware of which charts were being reviewed in either the control phase or the experimental phase. They only
knew review of charts would take place during the study period, which
spanned 2 months.

On completion of the experimental phase, a questionnaire eliciting problems associated with documentation of nursing diagnoses was completed by
each nurse. The content validity of the questionnaire was based on an extensive review of the literature and on evaluation by a panel of clinical nurse
specialists. The content validity of the responses to questions one and two
was established based on the study by Kim and others (1982), in which five
content experts independently evaluated and agreed on the content.

RESULTS

Scoring of nurses' documentation of nursing diagnoses was measured by a
standard coding scale that was modified from the one used by Mitchell and
Atwood (1975). The standard scoring system ranged from 0 points to 3 points:
0 points when no documentation was made by the nurse, 1 point when only
isolated data were recorded, 2 points when a problem area was recorded without supporting data, and 3 points when a problem area plus supporting data
were recorded. To provide objective scoring, two independent raters were
used. There was 84% and 97% agreement between the two raters on their
scoring of simulated case study documentation and actual clinical documentation, respectively. Results showed that there was a significant difference
between the preteaching and postteaching in documentation of nursing diagnoses in the case studies (t [15] $= -4.683$, $p < .05$). No significant difference
was found in the actual clinical documentation (t [15] $= .0919$, $p < .05$).

A comparison between the nursing diagnoses recorded on the research
data sheet and the patients' clinical records was made. All nurses recorded a
total of 42 nursing diagnoses on the 16 patient assessments as evidenced by
the research data sheets. The range of identified nursing diagnoses per patient
was one to five, with a mean of three nursing diagnoses per patient. Of the
42 nursing diagnoses listed in the research data sheets, only six were actually

documented in the patient's clinical record, which is only 14% of the total nursing diagnoses identified. Twelve nurses (75%) did not record any nursing diagnoses on the patients records, although identification of the nursing diagnoses had occurred as shown on the research data sheets.

Responses of the 16 nurses to the questionnaire indicated that the majority of nurses did not find difficulty in determining acuity or severity of the diagnoses nor in identifying subjective or objective data. However, eight nurses (50%) stated that identifying and documenting etiology and selecting proper diagnosis nomenclature was somewhat difficult. Of particular interest is the finding that documentation of nursing diagnoses was more difficult than the actual use of nursing diagnoses. This finding agrees with the data that showed that all nurses were able to identify and document nursing diagnoses in the research data sheets, but only four nurses actually documented any of the diagnoses in patients' clinical records. The staff nurses identified factors that hindered documentation of nursing documentation. The three most frequently identified factors were not enough time, (all nurses—100%), short of staff, (14 nurses—88%), and care takes precedence over documentation, (10 nurses—63%) (Table 1).

The nurses' educational background and years of clinical experience were also examined to determine if these factors influenced increased documentation. Of the 16 nurses who participated in the study, one had a master's degree in nursing, four had baccalaureate degrees in nursing, four had diploma preparation, and seven had associate degrees. Nine nurses had less than 1 year of clinical experience, two had 1 to 5 years, three had 5 to 10 years, and two

TABLE 1   Factors that hinder documentation of nursing diagnoses

Factor	Number of nurses	Rank
Not enough time	16	1
Short of staff	14	2
Care takes precedence	10	3
Busy with clerical duties	3	4
Too much writing	1	5
Unclear on how to chart	1	5
Do not like to chart	1	5
Busy with doctors' orders	1	5
Lack of nursing support	0	—
Lack of administrative support	0	—
Lack of understanding of concept of nursing diagnoses	1	5
Other	1	5

had more than 10 years. Chi-square analysis of the data showed that there was no significant association between educational background and years of clinical experience in either classroom or clinical setting, respectively (χ^2 [15] = 0.1524 and χ^2 [15] = 0.1745 at $p > .05$ each).

DISCUSSION

The results of the study showed that the positive effect of teaching was significant only in simulated situations, as noted in documentation from the case study and the research data sheets but not in the actual clinical documentation. This indicates that the concept of nursing diagnosis and the diagnostic process were learned but application of the knowledge in a clinical setting was not apparent. One possible explanation for this finding is that there were intervening factors that prevented the nurses from actually recording the nursing diagnoses.

Documentation of nursing diagnoses can be viewed as a change from the nurses' traditional practice. Theoretically, change could occur as a result of learning, but it also depends on the individual's motivation or desire to alter past practices. While change in nurses' behavior in the clinical setting was not apparent in this study, change may have occurred subsequent to the study period.

If the nurses had been unable to identify nursing diagnoses for their patients, it would have been easier to explain why clinical documentation did not occur. However, this was not the case in the study as evidenced in the research data sheets. Another possible explanation as to why documentation did not occur could be that the nurses fear accountability for their judgments. To a degree, some risk taking is a part of documentation of judgments. Perhaps it must be stressed to professional nurses that accountability for judgments and documentation of judgments are part of being a professional.

Results of this study indicated that nurses' educational background and years of clinical experience were not factors in nurses improving documentation following teaching in either classroom or clinical situations. Theoretically, increased educational background or increased years of clinical experience should make some difference in the ability to make inferences or nursing judgments, such as nursing diagnoses. However, the small number of subjects in this study precludes any general conclusions from the results. However, the similarity of the one result to that of Kim and others (1982) may potentially indicate that educational background indeed makes no appreciable difference in the identification and use of nursing diagnoses in the clinical setting.

The three areas identified by nurses that most hinder documentation of nursing diagnoses were: not enough time, short of staff, and the feeling that care takes precedence over documentation. It is interesting to note that even though the nurses could not find time to document nursing diagnoses in patient's clinical records, all nurses found time to identify and document nursing diagnoses in the research data sheets. To a certain degree an increase in staff members might increase the time available for nurses to chart, yet if the nurse's beliefs in accountability and risk taking are not altered, more time would not alleviate nondocumentation of nursing acts.

One last point to mention was that there was no consistent use of the problem-oriented format by the nurses in clinical charting as was originally anticipated. Mitchell and Atwood (1975) showed that more patient problems were identified in a clinical setting in which nurses used problem-oriented format for recording than when traditional notes were used. When the findings of this study are compared with those of Mitchell and Atwood (1975), one is tempted to suggest that consistent use of a problem-oriented format would have yielded more documentation of patient problems in the clinical setting.

IMPLICATIONS

The results of this study indicate a need for an increased emphasis on staff nurse education about documentation. It is essential to stress to nurses that documentation is a part of nursing that cannot be overlooked. Every patient deserves an organized individual plan of care that is documented for future reference.

Nursing educators must continue to emphasize the importance of documentation of nursing diagnoses in the undergraduate curriculum. Staff development educators, clinicians, and clinical nurse specialists need to not only work closely with staff nurses to assess documentation difficulties but also must have clinical contact with nurses in the clinical setting to assist in solving documentation problems.

Nursing administrators must review their staffing patterns or develop new ones to ensure that quality care can be planned, delivered, and documented. Administrators must adopt a philosophy of patient care that places documentation of care at the same level of importance as the delivery of care. Increased emphasis must be placed on strengthening nursing service policies that hold individual nurses accountable for their documentation of nursing judgments and nursing acts.

CONCLUSIONS

The effect of teaching on documentation of nursing diagnoses was found to be significant in a classroom setting but not in a clinical setting. Educational background and years of clinical experience were not significant factors in increased documentation of nursing diagnoses in either classroom or clinical settings. Nurses identified not enough time, short of staff, and care takes precedence over documentation as the three factors that most hinder documentation of nursing diagnoses.

REFERENCES

Bertucci, M., Huston, M., and Perloff, E.: Comparative study of progress notes using problem-oriented and traditional methods of charting, Nurs. Res. **23:**351, 1974.

Fry, V.S.: The creative approach to nursing, Am. J. Nurs. **53:**302, 1953.

Gerber, F.G.: Diabetes out of control, RN **42:**65, 1979.

Gordon, M.: Nursing diagnoses and the nursing process, Am. J. Nurs. **76:**1298, 1976.

Kim, M.J., and others: Clinical use of nursing diagnoses related to cardiovascular nursing. In Kim, M.J., and Moritz, D.A., eds.: Classification of nursing diagnoses: proceedings of the third and fourth national conferences, New York, 1982, McGraw-Hill Book Co.

Mitchell, P.H., and Atwood, J.: Problem-oriented recording as a teaching learning tool, Nurs. Res. **24:**99, 1975.

Mundinger, M.O., and Jauron, G.D.: Developing a nursing diagnosis, Nurs. Outlook **23:**94, 1975.

Rothberg, J.S.: Why nursing diagnosis? Am. J. Nurs. **67:**1040, 1967.

Shoemaker, J.: How nursing diagnoses help focus your care, RN **48:**56, 1979.

The effects of an in-service program on nurses' ability to identify valid nursing diagnoses

JANET R. CARSTENS, R.N., M.S.N.

REVIEW OF LITERATURE

The literature review for this study focused on three major areas of influence on the diagnostic ability of nurses: (1) inferential ability of the nurse, (2) nursing in-service programs on nursing diagnosis, and (3) educational level of the nurse. Throughout the history of nursing, nursing observations and the use of inferences resulting from them have been deemed essential in planning nursing care. Florence Nightingale (1969) discussed the importance of nursing observations. Marsh (1909) noted the importance of the nurse's ability to observe and to use her imagination.

Two authors (K. Kelly, 1966; Hammond, 1966) identified the need to understand the process by which nurses make observations, collect data, and make inferences from these data. This inferential process involves the assessment of multiple patient cues, which may be fallible. If too much reliance is placed on invalid cues or if a highly significant cue is omitted, inferential accuracy declines (K. Kelly, 1964). Because of the complexity of this inferential task, nurses must have a theoretic background and be able to apply knowledge to a cognitive process to diagnose (Hammond, 1966).

Although it is essential for nurses to know how to make clinical judgments, a study by Aspinall (1976) indicated that most nurses are unable to use theoretic knowledge in the process of making a differential diagnosis. In a later study, Aspinall (1979) found that a decision tree can assist nurses in using theoretic knowledge and increase diagnostic accuracy. This study supports the need for a standard classification of nursing diagnoses to assist nurses to improve their diagnostic accuracy.

Matthews and Gaul (1979) conducted two studies to determine what variables relate to the nurses' cognitive ability to process thoughts. The variables were determined to be concept attainment, cue perception, and critical thinking. It was concluded that diagnostic ability depends on the ability to identify and discriminate cues and to make inferences based on these cues.

The second area of influence on diagnostic ability reviewed in the literature was that of nursing in-service programs. The implementation of nursing diagnoses in the clinical area requires an initiator who has expertise in the area and can be a model diagnostician for staff members (Feild, 1979). In a study by Gordon, Sweeney, and McKeehan (1980), staff nurses at the Boston Hospital for Women evaluated themselves on the use of nursing diagnoses.

Analysis of these evaluations indicated that 43% of the discharge diagnoses made by the staff were identical to those identified by the National Conference Group on the Classification of Nursing Diagnoses, which was believed to be the result of a hospital in-service program on diagnostic nomenclature.

Surveys conducted by O'Connor (1979) and by Curran (1977) explored the reasons nurses participate in continuing education. Maintenance of professional currency and improvement of nursing services were found to be significant motivating factors for participation in continuing education (O'Connor, 1979). Curran (1977) surveyed nurses in 11 different specialty areas to determine their perceptions concerning areas of priority in seeking continuing education. These nurses identified the need for information on nursing trends and on legal aspects of nursing to be of high importance. Therefore the fact that nursing diagnosis does have legal implications tends to give it priority in the continuing educational needs of nurses.

The third area reviewed was the effects of educational level on diagnostic ability. A recent study was conducted by Zuehls (1979) to determine the relationship between the types of nursing education and the ability to identify and rank cues in making a nursing diagnosis. Conclusions of the study were as follows: (1) the relationship between years of experience and identification of cues is not known, (2) associate degree programs and baccalaureate degree programs teach similar content for applying and analyzing knowledge regarding the patient, and (3) diploma programs tend to differ in their teaching of identification of nursing diagnoses. However, all three types of programs tend to teach the same content that applies to patient status.

Yura (1974) gives criteria essential to the promotion of utilization of the nursing process. One criterion is acceptance of the differences in the usage of the process by persons with varying academic backgrounds and years of experience. Separate competencies for the baccalaureate degree, associate degree, and diploma degree nurses in utilization of the nursing process are delineated. Johnson (1966) asserts that associate degree nurses have the ability to apply certain data to specific, concrete patient problems, whereas baccalaureate degree nurses have a larger framework of knowledge from which they can identify unique, complex problems.

Davis (1974) conducted a study to determine the effects of nursing educational levels and years of experience on the quality and quantity of patient care. Results indicated that the clinical nurse specialist made more patient observations than the baccalaureate degree nurse, and the baccalaureate degree nurse made more observations than the diploma nurse. Years of experience did not influence the number of patient observations made by the nurse.

Verhonick and others (1968) analyzed the responses of 1576 graduate nurses to identify relevant patient observations made from filmed patient situations. The number of relevant observations increased progressively with higher academic degrees held.

STATEMENT OF THE PROBLEM

The ability of nurses to master the task of making nursing diagnoses is essential to the development of the nursing profession. Yet nurses vary in their ability to master the complex inferential task of diagnosing. The literature suggests that nurses need assistance in developing their diagnostic skills, but few research studies indicate methods to assist the nurse in improving these skills. Recent studies indicated that nurses lack the theoretic knowledge needed to achieve the complex task of diagnosing. Gordon (1980, p. 45) suggests that "at present, in many health professions, including nursing, diagnoses is 'caught' more than taught." Knowledge about a subject can be taught but whether judgment and intuition can also be taught has been questioned (King, 1967). Matthews and Gaul (1979) identified the need for research studies to improve nurses' accuracy in the diagnostic task. Therefore the purpose of this experimental study was to determine if an in-service program focusing on nursing diagnoses can improve the nurse's ability to identify valid nursing diagnoses.

The two research hypotheses were as follows: (1) primary nurses who have attended a 5-hour in-service program on nursing process (experimental group) will be able to identify more accurate nursing diagnoses from a case study than primary nurses who have not had the in-service program (control group) and (2) primary nurses who have attended a 5-hour in-service program on nursing process (experimental group) will be able to identify more accurate supportive data for each nursing diagnosis identified than primary nurses who have not had the in-service program (control group). The research objective was to determine if baccalaureate, associate, and diploma nurses who have not attended the in-service program differ in the diagnostic abilities of (1) identification of nursing diagnoses and (2) identification of supportive subjective and objective data.

THEORY APPLICATION

The three theories on which this investigation was based were decision making, concept attainment, and Maslow's hierarchy of basic human needs. During assessment, many decisions are made by the nurse. The phases of the decision-making process are applicable to the processes required in making a nursing diagnosis (Griffiths, 1958). After collecting data, the nurse must use concept attainment to categorize this information. Categorization decreases the complexity of one's perceptions and enables one to focus on accurately identifying patients' problems (Bruner, Goodnow, and Austin, 1956). Maslow's hierarchy of basic human needs (1954) can be used to identify patient need deficits to formulate nursing diagnoses and set priorities.

SAMPLING PLAN AND DATA COLLECTION PROCEDURE

Subjects for the study consisted of 24 primary care nurses who met specific criteria for subject selection and gave informed consent to participate in the study. These nurses were of three educational levels (baccalaureate degree, associate degree, and diploma) with various years of experience. Eight nurses from each educational level were assigned to either the experimental or the control group. The 12 nurses in the experimental group were given a 5-hour in-service program on nursing process by hospital personnel from the education department. A 2-hour lecture was followed by a 3-hour practice session using case studies to identify nursing diagnoses. A test was given to both the control and the experimental groups 1 week after the in-service program was given. The test consisted of a patient case study followed by two diagnostic tasks: (1) identification of valid nursing diagnoses and (2) identification of supportive data.

DATA ANALYSIS FINDINGS AND FUTURE IMPLICATIONS

A percentage was calculated for these two tasks, and scores from both groups of nurses were compared. A 2×3 factorial analysis of variance was carried out for each of the dependent measures, which were the in-service program and the educational level. Results indicated that the in-service program did not have any statistical significant (.05 level) effect on ability to identify valid nursing diagnoses. However, the experimental group did score slightly higher than the control group on this task. The diploma subjects benefited more than the other subjects from the in-service program with regard to both diagnostic tasks.

From these findings, there are implications for both nurse educators and administrators. Faculty in schools of nursing must focus on teaching the diagnostic process to students. In addition, continuing in-service programs in hospitals may be a major focus to assist practicing nurses to develop their diagnostic skills. Future recommendations for research include a larger sample population, a more complete and updated course on nursing diagnosis, and use of a more reliable testing tool, which would all increase determination of the effects of an in-service program on one's diagnostic abilities.

REFERENCES

Aspinall, M.J.: Nursing diagnoses—the weak link, Nurs. Res. **24**(3):182, 1976.

Aspinall, M.J.: Use of a decision tree to increase accuracy of diagnoses, Nurs. Res. **28**(3):182, 1979.

Bruner, J.S., Goodnow, J.J., and Austin, G.A.: A study of learning, New York, 1956, Appleton-Century-Crofts.

Curran, C.L.: What kind of continuing education? Superv. Nurs. **8**(7):72, 1977.

Davis, B.J.: Effects of levels of nursing education on patient care: a replication, Nurs. Res. **23**(2):150, 1974.

Feild, L.: The implementation of nursing diagnosis in clinical practice, Nurs. Clin. North Am. **14**(3):497, 1979.

Gordon, M.: Predictive strategies in diagnostic tests, Nurs. Res. **29**(1):83, 1980.

Gordon, M., Sweeney, M.A., and McKeehan, K.: Nursing diagnosis: look at its use in the clinical area, Am. J. Nurs. **80**:672, 1980.

Griffiths, D.: Administration as decision-making. In Halpin, A., ed.: Administrative theory in education, New York, 1958, MacMillan Publishing Co., Inc.

Hammond, K.R.: Part II. Clinical inference in nursing: a Psychologist's viewpoint, Nurs. Res. **15**(1):27, 1966.

Johnson, D.E.: Competence in practice: technical and professional, Nurs. Outlook **14**:30, 1966.

Kelly, K.: An approach to the study of clinical inference in nursing. Part I. Introduction to the study of clinical inferences in nursing, Nurs. Res. **13**(4):314, 1964.

Kelly, K.: Clinical inference in nursing. Part I. A nurse's viewpoint, Nurs. Res. **15**(1):23, 1966.

King, L.S.: What is a diagnosis? Am. Med. Assoc. J. **202**(8):154, 1967.

Marsh, L.: Present methods used in medical nursing, Am. J. Nurs. **10**:155, 1909.

Maslow, A.: Motivation and personality, New York, 1954, Harper & Row, Publishers.

Matthews, C.A., and Gaul, A.L.: Nursing diagnoses: veiwed from the perspective of concept attainment and critical thinking, Adv. Nurs. Sci. **2**(1):17, 1979.

Nightingale, F.: Notes on nursing: what it is and what it is not, New York, 1969, Dover Publications, Inc.

O'Connor, A.B.: Reasons nurses participate in continuing education, Nurs. Res. **28**(6):354, 1979.

Verbonick, P.J., and others: I came, I saw, I responded: nursing observation and action survey, Nurs. Res. **17**(7):38, 1968.

Yura, H.: Climate to foster utilization of the nursing process, National League of Nursing Publication (20-1566), New York, 1974.

Zuehls, K.S.C.: Nursing diagnosis and clinical cues, Unpublished manuscript, 1979.

ADDITIONAL READINGS

Abdellah, R.G.: The nature of nursing science, Nurs. Res. **18**(5):391, 1969.

American Nurses' Association: Standards of nursing practice, Kansas City, Mo., 1973. The Association.

Aspinall, M.J., Jambruno, N., and Phoenix, B.S.: The why and how of nursing diagnosis, Am. J. Matern. Child Nurs. **2**(6):354, 1977.

Bailey, J.T., and Claus, K.E.: Decision making in nursing: tools for change, St. Louis, 1975, The C.V. Mosby Co.

Boyle, B.A.J.: Effects of an instructional program on use of nursing process in practice (abstract), Nurs. Res. **26**(4):309, 1977.

Brown, S.J.: Proposition: continuing education must impact on practice, J. Contin. Educ. Nurs. **11**(1):8, 1980.

Bruce, J.: Implementation of nursing diagnoses: a nursing administrator prospective, Nurs. Clin. North Am. **14**(3):509, 1979.

Bullough, B.: The law and the expanding nursing role, New York, 1975, Appleton-Century-Crofts.

Campbell, C.: Nursing diagnosis and intervention in nursing practice, New York, 1978, John Wiley & Sons, Inc.

Chatham, M.A.: Discrepancies in learning needs assessments—whose needs are being met? J. Contin. Educ. Nurs. **10**(5):18, 1979.

del Bueno, D.J.: Continuing education: spinach and other good things, J. Nurs. Admin. **4**:33, 1977.

Dincher, J.R., and Stidger, S.L.: Evaluation of a written simulation format for clinical nursing judgment, Nurs. Res. **25**(4):280, 1976.

Durand, M., and Prince, R.: Nursing diagnosis: process and decision, Nurs. Forum **5**(4):50, 1966.

Fatzer, C.: The relationship between logical reasoning and nursing diagnosis, Monograph of nursing diagnosis, Texas Woman's University, Fall 1979.

Fortin, J.V., and Rainbow, J.: Legal implications of nursing diagnosis, Nurs. Clin. North Am. **14**(3):553, 1979.

Fox, D.J.: Fundamentals of research in nursing, ed. 3, New York, 1976, Appleton-Century-Crofts.

Gebbie, K.M., and Lavin, M.A.: Classifying nursing diagnoses, Am. J. Nurs. **74**:250, 1974.

Gordon, M.: Nursing diagnosis and the diagnostic process, Am. J. Nurs. **76**:1298, 1976.

Gordon, M.: The concept of nursing diagnoses, Nurs. Clin. North Am. **14**(3):487, 1979.

Gray, J.E., and others: Do graduates of technical and professional nursing differ in practice? Nurs. Res. **26**(5):368, 1977.

Grier, M.: Decision making about patient care, Nurs. Res. **25**(2):105, 1976.

Hamdi, M.E., and Hutelmeyer, C.M.: A study of the effectiveness of an assessment tool in the identification of patient problems, Nurs. Res. **19**:354, 1970.

Hammond, K.R.: Part II. Clinical inference in nursing: a methodological approach, Nurs. Res. **13**(4):315, 1964.

Hefferin, E., and Hunter, R.: Nursing assessment and care plan statements, Nurs. Res. **24**(5):360, 1975.

Hertzka, A.A., and Guilford, J.P.: Logical reasoning test, Los Angeles, 1955, Sheridan Supply Co.

Jackson, C.: Promoting written care plans, Superv. Nurs. **9**(8):43, 1978.

Kelly, N.C.: Nursing care plans, Nurs. Outlook **14**(5):61, 1966.

Kepner, C.H., and Tregoe, B.B.: The rationale manager, New York, 1965, McGraw-Hill Book Co.

Lee, L.A.: An investigation of effects of clinical experience on cognitive gains, J. Nurs. Educ. **18**(7):27, 1979.

Marriner, A.: The nursing process: a scientific approach to nursing care, ed. 3, St. Louis, 1982, The C.V. Mosby Co.

Mauksch, I.G., and David, M.L.: Prescription for survival, Am. J. Nurs. **72**:2189, 1972.

Mundinger, M., and Jauron, G.: Developing a nursing diagnosis, Nurs. Outlook **23**(2):94, 1975.

Price, M.R.: Nursing diagnoses: making a concept come alive, Am. J. Nurs. **80**:668, 1980.

Raiffa, H.: Decision analysis: introductory lecture on choices under certainty, Reading, Mass., 1970, Addison-Wesley Publishing Co., Inc.

Rothberg, J.S.: Why nursing diagnosis? Am. J. Nurs. **76**:1040, 1976.

Roy, Sister C.: A diagnostic classification system for nursing, Nurs. Outlook **23**(2):90, 1975.

Shoemaker, J.: How nursing diagnosis helps focus your care, RN **42**(8):56, 1979.

Waters, V.H., and others: Technical and professional nursing: an experimental study, Nurs. Res. **21**(2):125, 1972.

Yura, H., and Walsh, M.B.: The nursing process: assessing, planning, implementing, and evaluation, ed. 3, New York, 1972, Appleton-Century-Crofts.

Nutrition, alterations in: more than body requirements: the pattern of yo-yo dieting

SUE POPKESS-VAWTER, R.N., Ph.D.

Obesity is a leading cause of morbidity in the United States. Each year thousands of Americans lose and regain millions of pounds. This pattern of weight gain, loss, and regain exists in a large percent of overweight and obese people. Mahoney (1976) has labeled this pattern the "yo-yo" dieter. (Popkess-Vawter, 1982).

The nursing diagnosis *nutrition, alterations in: more than body requirements*, the pattern of yo-yo dieting, is a specific subcategory that stems from the general health problem of obesity and overweight (Kim and Moritz, 1982). The investigator has observed a predominant pattern emerging among persons who attempt numerous weight loss programs but never permanently maintain a healthy weight. Defining characteristics for the pattern of yo-yo dieting may vary from those listed for the general nursing diagnosis. The research study described in this paper provided a means to explore defining characteristics of the yo-yo dieter. Although the purpose of the study was to test a specific nursing approach, subject characteristics and progress during the 1-year exploratory study provided data that clarified the nursing diagnosis.

Since the 1-year exploratory study will not be concluded until after the presentation of this paper, the posttest data are not available; however, pretest results will be discussed. Trends that have been observed in the subjects after 10 months of self-care counseling will be noted as potential defining characteristics for the yo-yo dieting pattern.

PURPOSE OF THE STUDY

This research is a 1-year exploratory study to investigate the feasibility of a 5-year longitudinal study. The specific purpose was to determine the long-term (1 year) effects of holistic, self-care counseling on the yo-yo dieter's physical and psychologic progress toward permanent weight control.

HYPOTHESES

Hypothesis 1. There will be no significant difference between subjects' pretest and posttest physical measurements of body weight, percent age of body fat, body proportions, resting pulse, and blood pressure after 1 year of holistic self-care counseling for permanent weight control.

Hypothesis 2. There will be no significant difference between subjects' pretest and posttest psychosocial scores as measured by the Self-Image Scale, the Tennessee Self-Concept Scale (TSCS), and the State-Trait Anxiety Inventory (STAI) after 1 year of holistic self-care counseling for permanent weight control.

BACKGROUND AND SIGNIFICANCE

Stuart (1972) stated that the average obese person went on 1½ diets per year and made over 15 major attempts to lose weight between 21 and 50 years of age. Many dieting attempts failed, resulting not only in regained weight but added pounds beyond the original weight. This never-ending cycle of feast and famine, yo-yo or see-saw pattern, is potentially hazardous to health (Mahoney and Mahoney, 1976). Nutritionist Mayer (1964) of Harvard called the pattern the "rhythm method of girth control." In general, only 5% to 20% of obese people can lose weight and keep it off after dieting, and no one diet has been found to be any better in terms of long-range results than others (Kolata, 1977).

Not only does the yo-yo dieter have physical health risks but also emotional and psychosocial well-being risks. As the body weight peaks and valleys, emotional highs and lows will occur, placing risks on the individual's self-concept, beliefs, attitudes, and interpersonal relationships (Popkess, 1978).

Both past and present therapeutic interventions for obesity have failed to assist most obese clients to achieve permanent weight control (Stunkard, 1973; Chlouverakis, 1975). Traditional weight reduction methods that specify a well-balanced, calorie-restricted diet complemented by a good exercise program can provide sound weight reduction (Lindner, 1976; Mayer, 1964; Stunkard, 1973). Fad weight reduction methods, including fad diets, reducing devices, and medications, can indeed augment rapid weight loss (Chlouverakis, 1975); however, the problem of weight regain, as well as added health hazards, haunt each method (Stunkard, 1973). Unfortunately, current statistical data indicate that the incidence of obesity is on the rise (Bruch, 1973; Mackenzie, 1976), and obesity itself, in spite of traditional and fad diets and treatments, has increased health-related hazards and risks. The obesity problem in the United States appears to be unsolved at present.

Leon, Roth, and Hewitt (1977) and Morelli (1977) document the efficacy of behavior modification techniques in the treatment of obesity. However, Mahoney and Mahoney (1976), Morelli (1977), and Stunkard (1973) report difficulty getting a client to implement behavioral procedures. Jeffrey (1974), Mahoney (1974), and Stunkard (1973) agree that the central theme underlying most behavioral approaches to obesity is the encouragement of the clients to assume greater responsibility for their treatment. Tobias and MacDonald

(1977) concluded that an individual's perceived responsibility in and of itself was not sufficient to instigate weight loss. Morelli (1977) stated the reason most often given for clients' unwillingness to implement behavioral procedures was an inappropriate attitude or cognitive expectancies about some aspect of either the diet or themselves. Some discrepancies exist among researchers concerning effective means of weight reduction. Traditional methods and behavior modification have proven successful; however, neither seems to be an all-encompassing means for permanent weight control.

I believe that a weight reduction program combining traditional and behavioral methods with counseling in self-care offers a balance of effective weight reduction practices. The nurse is educated and competent to assist the yo-yo dieter with such a long-term endeavor. Counseling in holistic, self-care provides clients with means to learn how to assume greater responsibility for their own well-being. Beck (1976), Ellis (1973), and Orem (1971) support self-care strategies and techniques to discover motivating, exploring, experiential learning, placing responsibility, facilitating, negotiating, and rewarding activities for the individual. This study could offer a new approach for nurses and other health professionals to assist the obese and/or overweight client with permanent weight control and a life-style compatible with health. The counseling techniques may also apply to other self-abusive habits such as smoking tobacco and drinking alcohol. A detailed account of the holistic, self-care approach is described by Popkess-Vawter (1982).

METHODS AND PROCEDURES

The subjects in the study were 11 females between 22 and 43 years of age. They volunteered to participate in the study in response to a verbal advertisement and called the investigator for more information. An appointment was made to discuss the study and to sign appropriate consent forms. Physical examination was performed by the investigator for each subject to identify any physical risk. Skinfold thickness (percentage of body fat measured by Lange calipers), actual body height and weight, pulse rate (resting), and blood pressure were measured, and biographic and dieting history data were obtained for each subject. Each subject completed the Self-Image Scale (Jackson, 1975), the Tennessee Self-Concept Scale (Fitts, 1964), and the State-Trait Anxiety Inventory (Spielberger, Richard, and Lushere, 1970) to obtain baseline data to measure the psychologic parameters. The investigator worked with each subject to develop an individual weight reduction program consisting of a well-balanced, calorie-reduced diet, aerobic exercise program, and self-care techniques. Subjects received weekly, 2-hour counseling sessions for the first month with the nurse investigator. Then the subjects met with the investigator every week for 1 hour the second month and then for 1 hour every 2 weeks the third month. After approximately 5 to 6 months, the nurse and client agreed to decrease the 1-hour sessions from once every 2 weeks to once every 3 weeks and finally to once every month. At the conclusion of the study, the subjects will be given the opportunity to continue with the investigator for additional counseling sessions.

The counseling sessions include study and discussions concerning anatomy and physiology of weight reduction, foods, and metabolism, aerobic exercise, life style analysis, body image and self-image, interpersonal relationships, sexuality, and stress management (Tables 1 and 2).

At the conclusion of the study, both physical and psychologic parameters will be measured. Thus a pretest and a posttest design will be used to analyze the data. I expect a reduction in subjects' physical parameters at the end of 1 year. The subjects are expected to demonstrate more positive self-image and self-concept scores and reduced anxiety reflected in the anxiety scale scores. Wilcoxin Matched Pairs Signed Ranks (Siegel, 1956) will be used to analyze the data.

TABLE 1   **Holistic self-care physical prescription**

Week	Assessment/plan	Intervention/evaluation/revision

1	1. Complete history and physical assessment
	  a. Cardiac risk factors
		1. Increase physical health state
		  a. Identify alterable risk factors
		  b. Review diet history and binges

2	2. Initial measurements
	  a. Height/weight
	  b. Skinfold iliac and arm
	  c. Body measurements
	  d. Resting pulse/BP
	  e. Diet history
		2. Measurement baseline vs. standards
		  a. Insurance tables
		  b. Percentage of body fat
		  c. Proportions
		  d. Monthly checks
		  e. 1-week diet log: foods like, dislike, cannot live without, daily requirements

3
4
	3. Verbalizes knowledge of
	  a. Calories, pounds, percentage of body fat
	  b. Metabolism, aerobics
	  c. Foods, body requirements
	  d. Binge eating behavior
		3. Self-reading/discussions
		  a. Negotiate healthy diet; use 1 week, then decrease discussions of foods
		  b. Negotiate aerobic plan
		  c. Renegotiate healthy diet
		  d. Identify and discuss binge eating behavior, allow for cravings in negotiated diet

5	4. Wardrobe and beauty
	  a. Colors best for self
	  b. Styles
	  c. Hair
	  d. Makeup
		4. Self-reading/experimentation with alternative rewards

TABLE 2   **Holistic self-care psychosocial prescription**

Assessment/plan	Intervention/evaluation/revision
1. Aerobics in life-style	1. Self-reading; renegotiate aerobic plan
2. Assertiveness	2. Self-reading and discussions; assignments
3. Self-concept, body image	3. Self-reading and discussions; assignments
4. Stress behaviors	4. Identify cues in everyday life (log); discussions; assignments
5. Coping mechanisms	5. Negotiate plan to increase healthy coping mechanisms
6. Life stresses	6. Plan to decrease stresses in life-style
7. Sexuality	7. Self-reading and discussions; assignments
8. Time management	8. Self-reading and discussions; assignments

TABLE 3   **Physical measurement means for 11 female subjects**

Physical measurement	Mean	Standard deviation
Height (cm)	166 (5 ft. 5½ in.)	5.11
Weight (pounds)	182.08	38.34
Percent body fat	34.32	6.32
Resting pulse (beats/minute)	73.55	11.66
Systolic blood pressure	110.83	11.27
Diastolic blood pressure	70.92	9.67

TRENDS OBSERVED AFTER 10 MONTHS OF SELF-CARE COUNSELING

The 11 female subjects completed both the physical and the psychologic pretests in June 1981. Means were calculated for physical measurements (Table 3). The psychologic scale means were then tested against the means of the normative values for each scale using a t-test (Table 4).

Two physical parameters were within the normal, health range for blood pressure (x = 111/71) and resting pulse (x = 74/min). Some subjects had healthy body weight. At first meeting, five of the 11 subjects did not outwardly appear to have a weight problem. However, they identified themselves as yo-yo dieters and did not feel in control of their weight. Thus the body weight means for the nonobese subjects lowered the means for the truly obese subjects. Mean height was 5 feet 5½ inches, and mean weight was 182 pounds. Only one subject met the criterion for healthy percentage of body fat (22% for women). The mean percentage for body fat was 34.32%.

Psychologic measurements consisted of three scales, Self-Image, Tennessee Self-Concept, and State-Trait Anxiety Inventory. Since posttest scores

TABLE 4   **Psychologic scale score means tested against normative values using *t*-test**

Scale	Group	Number	Mean	Standard deviation	*t*-value
Self-image	Norm	100	36	12	
	Sample	11	40.83	7.89	1.813*
Tennessee Self-Concept Scale					
Physical self	Norm	626	71.78	7.67	
	Sample	11	59.91	7.54	−4.787†
Moral ethical self	Norm	626	70.33	8.70	
	Sample	11	77.09	9.04	+2.293*
Personal self	Norm	626	64.55	7.41	
	Sample	11	61.18	6.66	−1.515
Family self	Norm	626	70.83	8.43	
	Sample	11	68.36	5.12	−1.308
Social self	Norm	626	68.14	7.86	
	Sample	11	69.36	7.65	.484
Self-criticism	Norm	626	35.54	6.70	
	Sample	11	39.64	4.90	2.395‡
State-Trait Anxiety Inventory					
State	Norm	231	35.12	9.25	
	Sample	11	38.27	9.04	1.128
Trait	Norm	231	38.25	9.14	
	Sample	11	46.78	11.01	2.528‡

*.05 level of significance.
†.001 level of significance.
‡.01 level of significance.

will not be available until after presentation of this paper, normative values for each scale were used to compare subject mean scores. Subject scores were significantly (*p* < .05) higher than normal on the Self-Image Scale, showing a poor or negative self-image.

The Tennessee Self-Concept Scale consists of six subscales that were pertinent for the study (Table 4). Most significant was the physical self subscale (*p* = .001). Subjects' self-criticism scores were also significantly higher than the norm (*p* < .01). Thus subjects held a poor self-concept regarding their physical self and were highly critical of themselves. An interesting finding occurred regarding the moral-ethical subscale scores. Subjects held a significantly higher self-concept of their moral-ethical self than the norm (*p* < .05). Six of the subjects identified their religious belief as one of their greatest strengths.

The State-Trait Anxiety Inventory scores showed that subjects had significantly higher than normal trait scores (*p* = .01) but normal state scores. Trait anxiety is the inherent anxiety that an individual has developed from childhood through life experiences. State anxiety expresses the anxiety felt as the result of an anxiety-producing situation. Therefore subjects inherently felt more anxiety than they would have if they had completed the scale in their own homes.

SUMMARY

Ten female subjects have each received approximately 30 hours of self-care counseling for permanent weight control over a 10-month period. One subject discontinued counseling after 1 month without giving an explanation. Another subject became pregnant after 9 months of counseling and therefore terminated for medical reasons.

Until posttesting for physical and psychologic progress is completed, after 1 year only general subject characteristics and trends can be summarized. Several physical and psychologic characteristics were determined by comparing subject data with normative data. The following list summarizes the preliminary results that may complement the current nursing diagnosis *nutrition, alteration in: more than body requirements.*

NUTRITION, ALTERATIONS IN: MORE THAN BODY REQUIREMENTS: THE PATTERN OF YO-YO DIETING

Etiology

Excessive intake in relationship to metabolic need

Defining characteristics: physical

Body weight greater than 10% of ideal for height and frame

*Percent of body fat greater than 26% for women and 19% for men (using 3 to 4 skinfold sites)

*Sustained participation in aerobic exercise less than once per week

*Binge eating behaviors

Eating used as a coping mechanism (stress/anxiety, anger, fear, depression, etc.) or as reward

Defining characteristics: psychologic

*External rather than internal locus of control

Rigid, "black and white" thinking

*Aggressive or nonassertive communication style

*Poor/negative, unrealistic body image and self-concept

Dissatisfaction with being single, married, divorced, or widowed

Poor organizational and time management skills

---

*Critical defining characteristic.

REFERENCES

Beck, A.: Cognitive therapy and the emotional disorders, New York, 1976, International Universities Press.

Bruch, H.: Eating disorders: obesity, anorexia nervosa, and the person within, New York, 1973, Basic Books, Inc., Publishers.

Chlouverakis, C.: Facts and fancies in weight control IV. National perspectives. Obes. Bariat. Med. **75**(4):208, 1975.

Ellis, A.: Humanistic psychotherapy, New York, 1973, McGraw-Hill Book Co.

Fitts, W.: Tennessee self-concept scale, Nashville, 1964, Counselor Recordings and Tests.

Jackson, J.: Standford University heart disease prevention program self-image scale, Unpublished instrument, 1975.

Jeffrey, E.: A comparison of the effects of external control and self-control on modification and maintenance of weight, J. Abnorm. Psychol. **74**(83):404, 1974.

Kim, M.J., and Mortiz, D.A., eds.: Classification of nursing diagnoses: proceedings of the third and fourth national conferences, New York, 1982, McGraw-Hill Book Co.

Kolata, G.: Obesity: a growing problem, Science **198**(4320):905, 1977.

Leon, G., Roth, L., and Hewitt, M.: Eating patterns, satiety, and self-control behavior of obese persons during weight reduction, Obes. Bariat. Med. **6**(5):172, 1977.

Lindner, P., and Blackburn, G.: Multidisciplinary approach to obesity utilizing fasting modified by protein-sparing therapy, Obes. Bariat. Med. **5**(6):198, 1976.

Mackenzie, M.: Obesity as failure in the American culture, Obes. Bariat. Med. **5**(4):132, 1976.

Mahoney, M.: Cognition and behavior modification, Cambridge, Mass., 1974, Ballinger Publishing Co.

Mahoney, M., and Mahoney, K.: Permanent weight control, New York, 1976, W.W. Norton & Co., Inc.

Mayer, J.: Reducing by total fasting, Postgrad. Med. **64**(35):279, 1964.

Morelli, G.: Behavior modification and obesity: a cognitive extension, Obes. Bariat. Med. **6**(2):44, 1977.

Orem, D.: Nursing: concepts of practice, New York, 1971, McGraw-Hill Book Co.

Popkess, S.: Assessment scales for determining the cognitive-behavioral repertoire of the obese client, Doctoral dissertation, The University of Texas at Austin, 1978.

Popkess, S.: Diagnosing your patient's strengths, Nursing **81**(11):34, 1981.

Popkess-Vawter, S.: The holistic self-care approach toward permanent weight control, Nurse Pract., Part I, 7(3), 45-50, and Part II, 7(4), 26-29, 1982.

Siegel, S.: Nonparametric statistics for the behavioral sciences, New York, 1956, McGraw-Hill Book Co.

Spielberger, C., Richard, L., and Lushere, R.: Stai manual for the State-Trait Anxiety Inventory. Palo Alto, Calif. 1970, Consulting Psychologists.

Stuart, R., and Davis, B.: Slim chance in a fat world, Champaign, Ill., 1972, Research Press.

Stunkard, A.: The obese: background and programs, U.S. nutrition policies in the seventies, San Francisco, 1973, W.H. Freeman & Co. Publishers

Tobias, L., and MacDonald, M.: Internal locus of control and weight loss: an insufficient condition, J. Consult. Clin. Psychol. **45**(4):647, 1977.

Problems in using nursing diagnoses: a descriptive study of graduate nursing students

JUDITH WARREN, R.N., M.S.

Nursing diagnosis is the end result of the assessment phase of the nursing process. It is the statement that defines and communicates to others the specific problems a patient is experiencing that require nursing care. Therefore the diagnosis can be used in several ways. Two major ways are documentation of ability and accountability in nursing practice and clear articulation of the domain of nursing practice (Dossey and Guzzetta, 1981; Gordon, 1976).

The use of a nursing conceptual model (Price, 1980) provides a framework that supports the use of nursing process—assessment, diagnosis, planning, implementation, and evaluation—and defines the domain of nursing practice. Without the ongoing use of a nursing model and evaluation of each nursing diagnosis, the nurse reverts back to using the medical model, a result too often seen in patient records. The use of a medical model for nursing practice makes identifying nursing diagnoses difficult because the model reflects only injury or disease (Dossey and Guzzetta, 1981). Nursing models, however, describe the whole patient, both in health and disease.

Although our graduate students based their practice on nursing models, we found that many were still using the medical model in the clinical area. The students expressed confusion about the roles of physicians and clinical nurse specialists. At the same time, faculty were looking for ways to improve the clinical component of the curriculum. The use of nursing diagnosis was introduced 2 years ago as a part of the solution to both problems.

Since the development and use of a nursing diagnosis outlines requisite clinical and theoretic knowledge for caring for patients with that particular problem, student knowledge and nursing model use can be evaluated. The student's ability to manage a case load of patients can be documented through review of the patient record and student interview. Accountability may also be evaluated by combining the use of the diagnostic framework and the POMR framework. The students must clearly communicate each nursing diagnosis, the plan of care, and an ongoing patient assessment and are therefore held accountable for their practices.

The process of making the nursing diagnosis requires an understanding of the nature of the diagnosis, the identification of a cluster of signs and symptoms, and the determination of appropriate patient outcomes (Mundinger and Jauron 1975). Based on the faculty's commitment and the curriculum plan of using nursing diagnoses, it was determined to present content of the diagnostic process as part of reviewing the student's plans of care and during seminar presentations. A list of readings and a list of the diagnoses accepted at the Fourth National Conference were provided.

At first students were enthusiastic and began to develop skills in using nursing diagnoses. Then a pattern of sporadic usage began to emerge. Students used nursing diagnoses while interacting with faculty and in their own private case records but did not use them consistently in the clinical agencies. A descriptive study was conducted to identify some possible causes of the pattern.

METHOD
Subjects

The study sample consisted of seven second-year graduate students enrolled in the third of four clinical courses of the medical-surgical nursing program at a state university. The students work at four different acute care hospitals. Generally the hospitals did not use the PES format of nursing diagnosis and the use of any nursing diagnosis was rare.

Instrument and procedure

Students were required to keep personal case records of all patients on their case load. The record was to include a list of all applicable nursing diagnoses and any information that the students thought was valuable to have in their own records. The record was to be developed in such a way as to reflect the student's nursing model of practice. The last component of the record had space for problem identification, for example, problems with staff, problems implementing role, and problems in care planning. One faculty member collected data at regularly scheduled student interviews throughout the semester. Patient records and personal records were reviewed with each student at the clinical agency. Specific questions were asked concerning the use or nonuse of nursing diagnoses. The data from the interviews were then analyzed and grouped into broad problem areas.

RESULTS

Five major problem areas were defined using the process just described. First, the students expressed a lack of experience in identifying nursing diagnoses—only one student had previously used nursing diagnoses. The other six had various experiences with formal nursing care planning. One had taught in an L.P.N. program and one was an in-service instructor, but all said that the development of nursing care plans on Kardexes or charts had been sporadic in their nursing careers. Actual problems in identifying nursing diagnoses were as follows: symptoms were used 45%, medical diagnoses were used 15%, expected outcomes were used 5%, and other types of statements were used 5%. Accurate and correctly stated nursing diagnoses, using the PES format, were identified approximately 30% of the time. The percentages are averages of the semester experience. Only a slight improvement was noted at the end of the semester.

Second, the nurses cited medical resistance to adding the nursing diagnosis to the problem list. Two students at different hospitals were told not to add anything to the problem list. Hospital A considered the list to be a medical list. Nurses were told to identify their problems on the Kardex. Hospital B, on one particular unit, required that all medical residents chart on every problem on the problem list. The residents expressed difficulty in charting on nursing diagnoses, so the chief of that division directed that nursing problems not be added. (The nursing service does not agree with this practice and actively supports nursing contribution but has not identified the nursing diagnosis format as that contribution.) The other five students, including one at Hospital A and one at Hospital B, experienced no problems with physicians' objecting to the addition of problems to the problem list. The second student at Hospital A worked closely with the physicians and explained her focus and practice. She was able to add nursing diagnoses to the list but only entered the problem and etiology portion. The other steps in the nursing process were documented in her charting. The second student at Hospital B received many comments from the medical residents that her additions to the problem list and charting had clarified the domain of nursing practice for them. The other three students received no specific comments from physicians regarding their entries on the problem list.

Third, all seven students complained of medical resistance to the use of the term *diagnosis*. Depending on the physician, the students changed the title to *problem*, which resulted in their questioning the validity of using the term *nursing diagnosis*. They stated that the term interfered with their working relationships with physicians, and therefore they quit using them. A few students, when meeting resistance, explained the concept and received varying degrees of understanding and support from physicians.

Fourth, staff nurses in all four hospitals resisted the use of nursing diagnoses. Examples of this resistance were (1) not enough room on the Kardex, (2) "that's used in POMR charting and we don't use that here," (3) diagnoses take too much time and too much room, (4) "you're using technical terms to show us how smart you are and how dumb we are," (5) "you're jealous of doctors," and (6) "I know your instructor makes you do that, but that's not what we do here." Since all the students were initially excited about nursing diagnoses and believed they had great potential to improve nursing practice, their reactions included (1) "what's the use," (2) "is it worth the effort," (3) "why don't they see how great diagnoses are," (4) "are we really jealous of doctors," and (5) "I'm committed to diagnoses; now how do I help them to see it."

Fifth, the students lacked experience and knowledge of how to conduct change. The four previous problems all had comments related to the fact that the students were doing something new and were meeting strong resistance. When asked if they had assessed promoting and restraining factors or explained what they were doing, comments varied from no to sometimes to always. One student was unfamiliar with change theory. Three had not systematically used the theory. Two used change theory constructively but believed the changes would occur only while they worked at the hospital. The seventh student expressed confidence that although the formal diagnosis statement usage may fade when she left, the way of viewing patient problems would remain.

DISCUSSION AND RECOMMENDATIONS

Although students were instructed in the proper use and development of nursing diagnoses during clinical experiences, they all expressed a lack of experience as a problem. On further inquiry, the students believed that a specific time in class needed to be set aside to discuss the nursing diagnostic process. They wanted the opportunity to work through case studies with the assistance of faculty. In response to this request and as a result of this study, a two-credit course will be offered to provide the experience. Faculty believed a course would be valuable, since evaluation of clinical and theoretic knowledge in nursing practice was facilitated when students identified nursing diagnoses. Students would also be better able to provide clear articulation of the domain of practice and implement a model-based nursing practice—goals of the graduate program. A question to be answered after the course is, Does increased knowledge and experience with nursing diagnoses lead to decreased problems with implementation by the student?

The problem of medical resistance to the listing of nursing diagnoses on the problem list leads to several interesting questions. Is there a relationship between the student's ability to use nursing diagnoses and the amount of medical resistance? In two hospitals, one student had difficulty; the other did not. What was different in the four approaches or the situation? The same question could be asked in reference to staff nurse resistance. Also, would the commitment of nursing administration to the use of the nursing diagnosis format decrease physician and staff nurse resistance to the term and its use in nursing care planning? The issues of resistance to terminology and student role confusion lead to the question, Would the consistent use of nursing diagnosis in practice lead to or be correlated with decreased role confusion?

Finally, all the identified problems related to lack of experience with and knowledge of the change process. If the students learned this skill early in their graduate program, would their use of nursing diagnoses meet with less resistance? Faculty have decided to present change theory in the first semester and to develop it as a curricular thread in the remaining semesters. Evaluation of the approach is being planned.

A major limitation of the study is the small sample size. The study needs to be replicated in other graduate programs to validate the findings. The three major benefits of the study are (1) identification of variables and possible relationships to be tested, (2) evaluation of a curriculum strategy with recommendations for improvement, and (3) validation of the idea that the use of nursing diagnoses provided documentation of clinical competence and articulation of nursing practice.

REFERENCES

Dossey, B., and Guzzetta, C.E.: Nursing diagnosis, Nurs. 81 **11**(6):34, 1981.

Gordon, M.: Nursing diagnoses and the diagnostic process, Am. J. Nurs. **76**(8):1298, 1976.

Mundinger, M.O., and Jauron, G.D.: Developing a nursing diagnosis, Nurs. Outlook **23**(2):94, 1975.

Price, M.R.: Nursing diagnosis: making a concept come alive, Am. J. Nurs. **80**(4):668, 1980.

Differences in documentation of nursing services according to recording format

SUZANNE K. GUZELAYDIN, R.N., M.S.
SUSAN K. PFOUTZ, R.N., M.S.

Documentation of service in nursing has undergone many format changes in the last 2 decades. This process has occurred to assist practitioners in the delivery of service, to facilitate the retrieval of information, and for reimbursement purposes. Presently little research compares various recording formats in practice settings. Bertucci, Huston, and Perloff (1974) compared narrative recording with problem-oriented recording (POR) in simulated client situations. They found that POR facilitated the recording of an increased amount of subjective data when compared with narrative methods. However, interpretation of data and planning for care was often lacking with both methods. Rieder and Wood (1978) documented an increase in problem identification with a POR system as compared with traditional recording. A descriptive study of the implementation of nursing diagnosis was conducted at Boston Hospital for Women. The results showed a wide range of nursing diagnoses. Another finding was that 57% of the listed diagnoses differed from those developed by the National Conference on the Classification of Nursing Diagnoses. The need for further expansion of accepted diagnoses was suggested (Gordon, Sweeney, and McKeehan, 1980).

PURPOSE

The purpose of this study was to evaluate the effectiveness of three recording formats on community health nursing service documentation. The definitions for the three formats follows:

> **Descriptive, narrative recording (narrative)**—A format in which observations relevant to nursing service are organized in paragraph form. This recording usually follows a chronologic sequence.
>
> **Problem-oriented recording (POR)**—A format that structures data into categories consisting of baseline data, problem list, plan of service, flow sheets, progress notes, and discharge summary. The progress notes include subjective data, objective data, analysis of that data, and plan for action.
>
> **POR with nursing diagnosis (PORND)**—A recording format that includes all the elements of POR with nursing problems labeled according to the diagnoses of the Third National Conference on the Classification of Nursing Diagnoses.

The study was designed to (1) examine documentation of community health nursing service by three recording formats, (2) describe the range and focus of nursing diagnoses used in a practice setting, and (3) describe the sample.

METHODS AND SAMPLING

A retrospective record audit was performed on a random sample of inactive records in a metropolitan community health nursing agency located in a large midwestern city. The audited records were randomly sampled from one inner city and one suburban district office that were considered to be representative of the agency. Eleven narrative, 11 POR, and 11 PORND records were selected from each office for a total sample of 66 records. A minimum of three home visits was required for inclusion in the study.

The Phaneuf Nursing Audit (Phaneuf, 1976) was used to evaluate records. This instrument consists of 50 items that result in a total score and subscores for each of the seven nursing functions developed by Lesnick and Anderson (1950). These nursing functions are as follows:

1. Application and execution of physician's legal orders
2. Observation of symptoms and reactions
3. Supervision of the patient
4. Supervision of those participating in care
5. Reporting and recording
6. Application and execution of nursing procedures and techniques
7. Promotion of physical and emotional health by direction and teaching

Each item is scored as being present, absent, or uncertain in the record being audited. The various functions have scores that are weighted differently. The bases of these weightings have not been described (National League for Nursing, 1978; Phaneuf, 1968, 1976).

The content validity of this instrument has been supported by its wide acceptance in practice. Stanhope (1981) has reported this instrument to be reliable with respect to time for a single auditor and to be internally consistent. In this study the interrater reliability of the instrument was evaluated by auditing a subsample of five simulated records. The percentage of item disagreements for the two raters was 42%. However, the instrument is developed around function and total scores. Comparisons showed more agreement in function and total scores than in individual item scores. Because of questionable interrater reliability, the differences in recording formats were analyzed both as a total sample and as individual rater samples.

RESULTS

Descriptive data were collected on the clients whose records constituted the sample. Clients were from 9 to 89 years of age with a mean age of 67.3 years for the total sample. The clients consisted of 23 males and 43 females. Length of service ranged from 1 to 10 months. The number of home visits ranged from 3 to 49. These data suggest a largely female elderly group who received home visits for a short period. As might be expected, the largest single source of payment for this elderly population was Medicare. (See Tables 1 and 2 for a description of clients by district office.)

The effect of recording format on documentation of service was analyzed through a one-way analysis of variance. Narrative, POR, and PORND formats were analyzed by total score and individual function scores. Only one function, reporting and recording, showed a significant difference in function score according to recording format (F [2, 63] = 5.78, p = .005) for the total sample. Post hoc analysis showed the difference in the mean scores of the narrative and PORND records to be significant, at the level of p = .0012. No other pairs of formats showed a significant difference in mean scores for this function. (Analyses of variance results are reported in Table 3.)

A feature of the Phaneuf (1976) audit is the classification of the recording quality into the following categories: excellent, good, incomplete, poor, or unsafe. Because of the sample size and distribution, only a 2 × 3 table could be constructed to test the distribution of record quality by record format (see Table 4). The obtained chi-square statistic was not significant (p > .20). Al-

TABLE 1   **Client description by district office**

Descriptor	Suburban	Inner city
Number	33	33
Male	39%	30%
Female	61%	70%
Mean age	72.2	62.6
Mean length of service (mo)	2.0	1.6
Mean number of home visits	11.7	9.4

TABLE 2   **Frequency distribution of clients' payment sources by district office***

Source	Suburban	Inner city
Medicare	26	17
Medicaid	0	4
Blue Cross or other insurance	6	10
Self or free	1	2

*The cell sizes were too small to test differences in proportions.

TABLE 3   **One-way analysis of variance of nursing audit scores according to recording format**

Type of score	Mean square between formats	Mean square within formats	F*	P
Total score	2372.8	1039.6	2.28	.110
Application of orders	91.2	77.4	1.18	.314
Observation of symptoms	75.9	70.8	1.07	.348
Supervision of client	146.9	36.3	4.04	.022†
Supervision of care givers	26.7	13.5	1.98	.147
Reporting and recording	147.7	25.6	5.78	.005‡
Procedures	22.1	22.0	1.00	.372
Direction and teaching	0.4	14.2	0.30	.971

*$df_1 = 2$, $df_2 = 63$.
†p values for two raters: .336 and .071.
‡p values for two raters: .061 and .066.

TABLE 4   **Frequency distribution of records by quality and recording format***

Recording format	Record quality	
	Excellent/good	Incomplete/poor
Narrative	8	14
POR	11	11
PORND	14	8

*$df = 3$; chi-square = 3.27; $p > .20$.

though this approach did not show a significant difference in the record quality by the recording format, a trend showing more high-quality records with PORND deserves further investigation with a larger sample.

Table 5 describes the range and frequency of nursing diagnoses for the PORND subsample. The number of nursing diagnoses per client ranged from 2 to 10, with a mean of 4.18 and a standard deviation of 1.82. Most of the diagnoses represented physiologic problems. Eighteen of the diagnoses from the Third National Conference on the Classification of Nursing Diagnoses were represented, and 9 additional diagnoses were generated by the nurses.

DISCUSSION

This study did not demonstrate consistent differences among the recording formats. The level of interrater reliability and moderate sample size could be

TABLE 5   **Frequency distribution of nursing diagnoses**

Standardized nursing diagnoses*	Frequency	Additional diagnoses†	Frequency
Mobility, impairment in	10	Difficulty starting stream	1
Bowel elimination, alteration in	9	Hypertension and/or unstable status	1
Functional performance, variations in	7	Lives alone and/or unsafe	1
Lack of knowledge	7	Terminal care caused by discontinuing treatment	1
Skin integrity, impairment of	7		
Cardiac output, alteration in	7	Malnourished regarding cancer of lung	1
Urinary elimination, alteration in	6	Undernourished regarding decreased appetite	1
Blood flow, alterations in	4		
Respiratory function, alterations in	5	Dietary restriction caused by fluid balance	1
Nutritional requirements, alterations in	3	Alteration in metabolism caused by diabetes mellitus	1
Self-concept, alterations in	3	Depression caused by alteration in life-style	1
Comfort, alteration in—pain	3		
Anxiety	1		
Sensory perception, alteration in	1		
Environment, impairment in	1		
Family coping, alteration in	1		
Grieving	1		
Nonadherence	1		

*Those accepted by the agency and generated by the Third National Conference on the Classification of Nursing Diagnoses.
†Not included on the standardized agency list.

contributing factors. Ventura, and others (1980) discuss methods for increasing interrater reliability that could be used in future research. Yet the outcome of this study was not differing results but the lack of differences among the three recording formats. The reporting and recording function that did show differences included items related to the facts on which future care depends: reporting to the physician, evaluation of facts, client information needs, and continuity of intramural and extramural care. The structure of POR recording and standardization of terminology with nursing diagnosis should facilitate organization and retrieval of information to enable continuity of care. The qualitative evaluation of records did show a trend toward better recording with PORND, a fact that should be pursued.

Examination of the descriptive characteristics provided insight into the use of nursing diagnoses in this setting. As previously described, this population was elderly and predominately female and received reimbursement through third-party payers. The distribution of nursing diagnoses focused on problems that reflect physical impairment or dysfunction. Perhaps the nature of physical problems lends them more easily to identification and intervention than does the nature of psychosocial problems. Another interpretation is that physical problems and subsequent care more easily fit into the framework of skilled nursing care for which reimbursement is available. Thoma and Pittman (1972) describe documentation of service for reimbursement purposes as one important function of recording. The nurse-generated diagnoses represent an attempt to adapt nursing diagnoses to this practice setting. Additional diagnoses are being developed to encompass the practice of nursing. Experience with nursing diagnoses in practice settings will also result in more standardized use.

REFERENCES

Bertucci, M., Huston, M., and Perloff, E.: Comparative study of progress notes using problem-oriented and traditional methods of charting, Nurs. Res. **23:**351, 1974.

Gordon, M., Sweeney, M.A., and McKeehan, K.M.: Nursing diagnosis: looking at its use in the clinical area, Am. J. Nurs. **80:**672, 1980.

Lesnick, M.J., and Anderson, B.V.: Nursing practice and the law, Philadelphia, 1950, J.B. Lippincott Co.

National League for Nursing: Instruments for measuring nursing practice and other health variables (DHEW #78-53, Vol. 1), Hyattsville, Md., 1978, The League.

Phaneuf, M.C.: Analysis of a nursing audit, Nurs. Outlook **16:**57, 1968.

Phaneuf, M.C.: The nursing audit, New York, 1976, Appleton-Century-Crofts.

Rieder, K.A., and Wood, M.J.: Problem-orientation: an experimental study to test its heuristic value, Nurs. Res. **27:**25, 1978.

Stanhope, M.K.: The Phaneuf nursing audit: a psychometric evaluation, Presentation at American Public Health Association, Los Angeles, 1981.

Thoma, K., and Pittman, K.: Evaluation of problem-oriented nursing notes, J. Nurs. Admin. **2:**50, 1972.

Ventura, M.R., and others: Interrater reliabilities for two measures of nursing care quality, Res. Nurs. Health **3:**25, 1980.

ADDITIONAL READINGS

Bloom, J.T., and others: Problem-oriented charting, Am. J. Nurs. **71:**2144, 1971.

Dickoff, J., James, P., and Wiedenbach, E.: Theory in a practice discipline, Nurs. Res. **17:**415, 1968.

Donaldson, S.K., and Crowley, D.M.: The discipline of nursing, Nurs. Outlook **26:**113, 1978.

Feinstein, A.R.: The problems of the problem-oriented medical record, Ann. Intern. Med. **78:**751, 1973.

Fessel, W.J., and Van Brunt, E.E.: Assessing quality care from the medical record, New Engl. J. Med. **286:**134, 1972.

Gebbie, K.M., and Lavin, M.A.: Classifying nursing diagnosis, Am. J. Nurs. **74:**250, 1974.

Gebbie, K.M., ed.: Summary of the Second National Conference: classification of nursing diagnoses. St. Louis, 1976, Clearinghouse National Group for the Classification of Nursing Diagnoses.

Gordon, M.: The concept of nursing diagnosis, Nurs. Clin. North Am. **14:**487, 1979.

Linn, B.S., and Linn, M.W.: Validity impairment ratings made from medical records and from personal knowledge, Med. Care **12:**363, 1974.

Lyons, T.F., and Payne, B.C.: The relationship of physician's medical recording performance to their medical care performance, Med. Care **12:**463, 1974.

Morgan, M.K., and Irby, D.M.: Evaluating clinical competence in the health professions, St. Louis, 1978, The C.V. Mosby Co.

Price, M.R.: Nursing diagnosis: making a concept come alive, Am. J. Nurs. **80:**668, 1980.

Recording the home visit, Nurs. Outlook **15:**38, 1967.

Schell, P.L., and Campbell, A.T.: Problem-oriented medical records: POMR—not just another way to chart, Nurs. Outlook **20:**515, 1972.

Weed, L.L.: Medical records that guide and teach, New Engl. J. Med. **278:**593, 1968.

Weed, L.L.: Medical records, medical education, and patient care, Chicago, 1969, Year Book Medical Publishers, Inc.

Woody, M., and Mallison, M.: The problem-oriented system, Am. J. Nurs. **73:**1168, 1973.

CHAPTER 5

Practice and education

Papers primarily related to practice and education areas are included in this chapter. Admittedly, some papers do include research data, but they were judged to be more pertinent to the concerns of this chapter. All abstracts submitted were reviewed by a blind review process in the same manner as the research papers. Presentations ranged from development of nursing diagnoses and implementation strategies used in the clinical setting to scholarly expositions of the theories underpinning nursing diagnoses. It is noteworthy that some of the presentations stem from doctoral dissertation work.

Various frameworks for generating and categorizing nursing diagnoses have been proposed, and specific examples of how nursing diagnoses interface with medical practice are offered in several papers. All of these papers should benefit nursing practice and therefore our patients/clients. Teaching methods and strategies are also presented that will enhance the integration of nursing diagnoses into the formal academic settings. In particular, the process of developing a baccalaureate curriculum incorporating nursing diagnoses may give impetus for other schools that are struggling with similar concerns. Such diverse topics, creative approaches, critical thinking about nursing diagnoses, and definitive experiences of using nursing diagnoses indeed have constituted the health of the conference.

Section I   **Formal presentation**

The implementation of nursing diagnoses using a computerized information system

SUSAN SIMMONS, R.N., M.S.N.
LAURA RYAN, R.N., M.S.N.

In this presentation we will describe the process by which nursing diagnoses were introduced into a nursing department using a computerized information system. We hope that our experience may be helpful to others launching a similar program.

We are truly in an era of technology when the word *apple* for many may suggest a machine. Just 7 years ago, when the Technicon Medical Information System (MIS) was installed at the Clinical Center, National Institutes of Health, the impact of this innovation on nursing practice was not predicted. The Clinical Center is a 541-bed research hospital of the National Institutes of Health in Bethesda, Maryland. A variety of research programs are carried out by the nine NIH facilities, which are located in Bethesda, using inpatient beds on 26 nursing units and a large ambulatory care department. The nursing department of the Clinical Center supports the biomedical research programs through the provision of nursing care for patients and support for their families or significant others. The 351 members of the nursing staff reflect a fairly high nurse to patient ratio, based on a complex mix of acute care needs and research-related activities.

Nursing and medicine are the critical dyad in care delivery at the Clinical Center. Nursing also supplies enormous support for the data-collecting efforts of the medical research component. Increasingly a more collaborative relationship between nursing and medicine has emerged in which care planning is a joint process and a variety of professional support systems are called in to assist in the coordination of patient care.

External forces, such as the consumer movement, the Joint Commission on Accreditation of Hospitals, American Nurses' Association, and Nurse Practice Acts, have influenced changes in nursing practice. As nurses advocate for expanded practice, they must in turn demonstrate their accountability through documentation. At the Clinical Center, nursing personnel demonstrated a readiness to establish a data base to handle the documentation of its practice.

The MIS is a "computer system whereby all services for all patients are ordered by physicians or their agents and in which most of the clinical findings and observations based on these findings are recorded" (Romano, McCormick, and McNeely, 1982, p. 44). Nurses record vital signs, medications, intravenous administrations, all care planning data, and activities in the terminal located at each nursing unit. Printers are available in the nursing units to provide printed copies of the information for the patients' clinical records.

Before the implementation of the MIS, nurses charted manually on the nursing notes using the SOAP format. Kardexes were used to record pertinent care plan data and activities, medications, diet, and treatments. The arrival of the computer served as a catalyst for change in nursing practice. A task force chose a nursing framework and developed a paradigm for documentation in the MIS. The content on the nursing screens was developed by various committees, task forces, and cadres in the Clinical Center Nursing Department.

A holistic, human needs framework was selected with strong emphasis on the nursing process (Maslow, 1970; Yura and Walsh, 1978). In this framework, identified patient needs are organized into categories to provide a systematic method of assessment (Romano, McCormick, and McNeely, 1982) allowing the patient to be seen as a biopsychosocial unit. Figure 1 shows the cluster of 13 need categories that initiate the assessment process. The need categories are air, circulation, food/fluid, elimination, neuro/sensory, sleep/rest, physical safety, mobility, comfort/pain, hygiene/skin, sexuality, sociopsychologic, and teaching/learning. The sociopsychologic pathways are growth and development, psychologic state, stress, safety/security/trust, communication, self-concept, strengths, psychosexuality, family/social relationships, sociocultural, perception, and suicide risk potential. Following completion of the assessment, the planning phase of the nursing process begins. This documentation begins the nursing care planning sequence. The MIS subdivides again into the same 13 patient need categories to contain one or more subcategories of nursing diagnoses. These nursing diagnoses replaced the problems that could be typed in and selected approximately 1½ years ago.

While this may be state of the art nursing assessment today, in 1975 it was a radical change in the way most nurses at the Clinical Center approached patient problems. At that time, many of the staff were not using the nursing process and relied heavily on the medical model to direct practice. The introduction of primary nursing provided a new model for accountability. Clinical nurse specialists began working closely with primary nurses to strengthen their competencies in relation to the nursing process. We realized early that the process of clinical inference leading to an accurate diagnosis for the client was not a simple cognitive bridge to cross.

Before the adoption of nursing diagnosis, the nurses would type in their identified patient problems from the assessment data. Initially, there were

NURSING ADMISSION ASSESSMENT

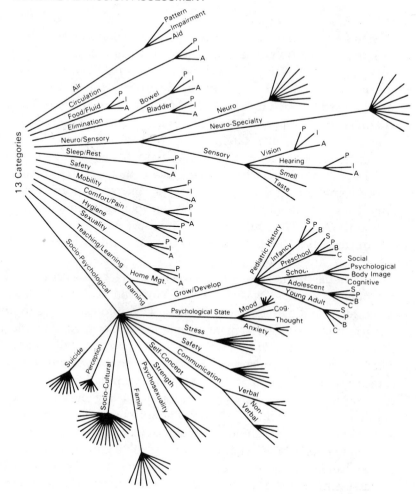

FIGURE 1   Nursing assessment categories.

From Romano, C., McCormick, K.A., and McNeely, L.D.: Adv. Nurs. Sci. **4**:43, 1982.

BOX 1   **Sample nursing problems from which to select before implementation of nursing diagnosis**

Decubitus ulcer	Altered sleep pattern
Anemia	Dyspnea
Somatic complaints	Depression
Dehydration	Nausea and vomiting
Grief over loss of limb	Edema
Anxiety	Immobility
Altered body image	Pain
Short stature/cystinosis	Fever

177 items from which to select, and these diagnoses reflected the mixed level of nursing practice. Many were the same as the disease entity being researched, for example, diabetes, orthostatic hypotension, and cystic fibrosis. Other diagnoses were procedure titles, signs, symptoms, or expressed patient concerns. Box 1 illustrates the diversity of diagnostic nomenclature that nurses were choosing. This initial period of "floundering" may have been needed as nurses began to master the conceptual steps necessary to organize data more systematically. The computer served as an excellent evaluative tool as we tracked the process of change.

Current nursing diagnoses that may be selected from the assessment categories were accepted at the Fourth National Conference (Box 2) To implement nursing diagnoses, the nursing Administrative Council agreed with the suggestion of the Clinical Center Nursing Diagnosis Task Force to provide gradual exposure to the concept and not mandate an in-service program as a major initiative. This quiet conversion to programming the computer and supplying resource persons to assist in the change was met favorably by the clinical nurses.

Actual use of the nursing diagnoses varies with the state of the art of practice for each clinical nurse. Those who are competent with the nursing process are most skilled in using the nursing diagnoses. In planning for the transition, the assessment tool was carefully evaluated to ensure that all the defining characteristics of the accepted diagnoses were included. To achieve a valid data base to arrive at a diagnosis requires a relationship with the client that will elicit the unique variability affecting the person. Nurses must possess interviewing and communication skills to achieve this sophisticated practice. The computer provides a logical structure to guide the nurse's thinking about the patient's problems.

In retrospect, the stages of development followed very closely the socialization model of Parsons as a model for "managing behavioral change in conjunction with technological change in organizations" (Farlee, 1978, p. 24).

The first, or permissive, stage provided critical information opportunities for learning expectations of new behavior. In stage two, stage one behaviors were continued and external rewards were given for new behavior. For example, as nurses identified accurate nursing diagnoses for patients in their specialty areas, they were encouraged to develop standard care plans and submit them to the Care Plan Review Committee. Final approval and acknowledgment came from the Nursing Practice Committee, and the care plan was entered into the MIS system. In stage three, external rewards were reduced and new patterns were internalized. This stage corresponded to the situation 2 years ago when the Clinical Center Nursing Diagnosis Task Force was formed, through the initiation of the Clinical Nurse Specialist Group, to assess progress, solidify gains, and move the process forward. Renewed educa-

BOX 2   Nursing diagnoses related to assessment categories

Air
  Altered respiratory function
  Aspiration
  Potential altered respiratory
    function
Circulation
  Alteration in tissue perfusion
  Alteration in cardiac output
  Potential fluid imbalance
  Potential disruptions in wound
    healing
Food/fluid needs
  Dysphagia
  Nausea
  Nutrition alteration
    (more than body
    requests)
  Nutrition alteration
    (less than body
    requests)
  Potential fluid imbalance
Elimination
  Altered pattern of elimination
    related to ostomy
  Altered pattern of urine
    eliminated
  Constipation
  Fecal incontinence
Neuro/sensory
  Alteration in thought processes
  Difficulty with communication
  Difficulty with mobility
  Dysphagia
Sleep/rest
  Altered sleep pattern
  Inability to sleep
  Insomnia
Physical safety
  (Safety) physical injury potential

Mobility
  ADL—inability/limited ability to
    perform
  Difficulty with mobility
Comfort/pain
  Pain
Hygiene/skin
  ADL—inability/limited ability to
    perform
  Impaired skin integrity (actual)
  Impaired skin integrity (potential)
  Mouth integrity, alterations in
    (actual, potential)
  Potential disruptions in wound
    healing
Sexuality
  Sexual difficulties
Sociopsychologic
  Adolescence and prolonged illness
  Alteration in thought processes
  Altered body image
  Boredom related to physical
    restriction
  Coping, ineffective individual
    (anger, anxiety, mood alteration)
  Difficulty with communication
  Difficulty with interaction with
    others
  Disturbance in child's self-concept
    related to altered development
  Low self-esteem
Teaching/learning (lack of
    knowledge of)
  Diagnostic tests
  Diet management
  Follow-up care
  Medications
  Physical and/or psychosocial
    limitation

tional efforts were launched, a consultant was hired, and a decision was made to include in our MIS system only those nursing diagnoses approved by the Fourth National Conference. The Task Force used Feild's assessment factors (1979) to assist staff members in identifying special needs, resources, and resistances.

The nursing staff is now moving toward the fourth and final stage, in which self-reward and satisfaction for performance of the new task are increased and old behaviors are given up. Stage four has not yet been totally achieved. As Bircher, (1982, p. 35) pointed out, "Nursing diagnosis is a complex concept and a central formulating notion for nursing." She also cautioned that it should not be used as a magic wand.

In an attempt to evaluate the current status of nursing diagnosis at the Clinical Center, two commonly used diagnoses were selected for a comparison. Assessment data were selected at random from 50 patient records in which these diagnoses had been recorded. The two diagnoses were (1) *alteration in comfort: pain*, and (2) *ineffective individual coping related to anxiety*. These two diagnoses were chosen because pain and anxiety had been the most frequently chosen diagnoses before the adoption of the standard nomenclature. It was hypothesized that if nurses were making accurate nursing diagnoses, evidence should be found of the defining characteristics in the assessment data. Of the two diagnoses, more complete data were documented for *alteration in comfort: pain*, which may be summarized as follows:

1. In every case in which a diagnosis of pain was entered, a nursing assessment had been done.
2. At least one defining characteristic was documented in the assessment data.
3. Most often, the defining characteristic was a subjective report of the patient with few objective descriptors.
4. The diagnosis was not an end in itself but served as the cornerstone for the care plan.
5. Documentation throughout the record consistently referred to the problem of pain. But it was sometimes charted under multiple categories, for example, mobility, respiratory, or sociopsychologic.

In an effort to respond to the identified need of nurses at the Clinical Center, a standardized care plan for the diagnosis *ineffective individual coping related to anxiety*, was submitted by the Clinical Specialists in Mental Health. This need was based on the data that anxiety was the most frequently selected problem, with a frequency of 1685 in the year before conversion to the standard nursing diagnoses.

The deletion of anxiety by the Fourth National Conference was recognized. But the need existed to respond to the widespread use of this problem. This retrieval indicated that nursing care was directed toward the intervention of the cause of the anxiety rather than the symptom itself as discussed by the Fourth National Conference. Documentation of the defining characteristics—for example, verbalization of inability to cope or to ask for help; inability to meet role expectations and basic needs or solve problems; destructive behavior to self or others; inappropriate use of defense mechanisms; change in communication patterns; verbal manipulation; high illness or accident rate—was not always in agreement with the assessment. The critical characteristic, verbalization of inability to cope, was generally placed under a sociopsychologic assessment category as a subjective verbalization. Some assessments revealed no documentation to support the diagnosis. As with *alteration in comfort: pain,* the sociopsychologic observations revealed ongoing notations, especially if the behavior was more disruptive to routines or the unit as a whole. As one might expect in the mental health area, there were more supporting data in the assessment subcategories. An explanation for the latter may be that mental health nurses are more skilled in the interpersonal process.

Analyzing the results gives rise to several questions:

1. Is there inadequate conceptual knowledge related to diagnostic categories?
2. Are the clinical reasoning skills of nurses in this agency lacking, underdeveloped, or nonrewarded?
3. Is there an inherent intuitive conclusion nurses make that relates to certain populations?
4. Is there a diagnostic formulation that is not documented?

Looking at Gordon's schema (1982), is the absent link in the diagnosis process the ability to acquire, evaluate, interpret, and cluster the clinical information? Following this investigation, we concurred with Gebbie (1982): "The computer-based records system provides an excellent resource for data collection and storage, retrieval of clinical data around diagnostic categories, and could put the Clinical Center in a clear position to provide leadership to nurses in other settings." In contrast to that strength, an identified weakness in the system, as Gebbie (1982) points out, is the present MIS programming that "does not follow a natural diagnostic process." This is currently being evaluated by nursing practice and data base committees.

Future directions will include clinical nursing rounds focused on nursing diagnosis. The use of role modeling by the Clinical Specialist Group to strengthen competencies of the clinical nurses will enhance a diagnosis-based practice. Additionally, a performance-based evaluation will assist head nurses in focusing on this area of practice.

The Clinical Center experience with a computerized system to implement nursing diagnoses revealed that it assisted the nursing staff to shift from a medical focus to a nursing perspective. It served as a form of programmed learning and made the nursing process more visible. Retrospectively, it is believed that the gradual approach to implementation was a useful strategy. However, education related to the defining characteristics should occur simultaneously in the implementation process. Of all the changes in practice in our setting, conversion to the concept of nursing diagnoses met with the least resistance and has led to a new language for nursing.

REFERENCES

Bircher, A.U.: The concept of nursing diagnosis. In Kim, M.J., and Moritz, D.A., eds.: Classification of nursing diagnoses: proceedings of the third and fourth national conferences, New York, 1982, McGraw-Hill Book Co.

Farlee, C.: The computer as a focus of organizational change in the hospital, J. Nurs. Admin. **8**:20, 1978.

Feild, L.: The implementation of nursing diagnosis in clinical practice, Nurs. Clin. North Am. **14**(3):497, 1979.

Gebbie, L.: Personal communication, February 8, 1982.

Gordon, M.: The diagnostic process. In Kim, M.J., and Moritz, D.A., eds.: Classification of nursing diagnoses: proceedings of the third and fourth national conferences, New York, 1982, McGraw-Hill Book Co.

Maslow, A.H.: Motivation and personality, New York, 1970, Harper & Row, Publishers.

Romano, C., McCormick, K.A., and McNeely, L.D.: Nursing documentation: a model for a computerized data base, Adv. Nurs. Sci. **4**:43, 1982.

Yura, H., and Walsh, M.: The nursing process, ed. 3, New York, 1978, Appleton-Century-Crofts.

Discussion

Mi Ja Kim: You mentioned many complex branches in your model. If you count all those complex subcategories of the 13 categories, how many are there in total?

Susan Simmons: I refer you to the article by Romano, McCormick, and McNeely.*

Mi Ja Kim: That must be an awfully comprehensive assessment guide. My next question is a very pragmatic one. How long does it take for any nurse to use this complex, comprehensive assessment guide?

Susan Simmons: I think it really varies. I would say probably a nurse who is new to our system and who has to learn to use the mechanics of the computer might take around 2 hours. We have some staff nurses here today who I think can probably go through the assessment in ½ hour.

Laura Ryan: It just depends on how much in-depth the patient's problems are. It can go anywhere from ½ hour to 2 hours.

Susan Simmons: Our standards say that a holistic assessment is to be done during the first 8 hours. I think that probably some nurses can get data and document them in ½ hour to 1½ hours.

Laura Ryan: I think the other thing is that nurses set priorities around an acute problem. The assessment is an ongoing process and so is continued if we do not get it finished during the first patient interview.

Mi Ja Kim: What were the most frequently used nursing diagnoses?

Susan Simmons: The best that we can assess, it is still those two diagnoses *(coping, ineffective, individual* and *comfort, alteration, pain)*. That is why we selected them. They continue to be the most frequently selected diagnoses.

---

*Romano, C., McCormick, K.A., and McNeely, L.D.: Nursing documentation: a model for computerized data base, Adv. Nurs. Sci. **4**:43, 1982.

Comment: I am wondering, do your nurses document things on a manual report first and then go to a CRT? I see the answer is yes, and I am wondering how they see that total process. Do they see it as a waste of their time?

Laura Ryan: Well, we developed a worksheet sometime after we had programmed the computer, and the staff see it as a useful tool rather than as a duplication. It does help them to direct their observations and their whole assessment. So I think that they see this as something beneficial to their practice rather than as a waste of their time.

Susan Simmons: It is interesting, too, because the clients are very interested in knowing what the nurses are asking about and whether they are looking at them as a whole person, because in a biomedical research institution, you are classified under a disease entity on entering the door. Therefore it is nice to have that rapport with someone who is interested in meeting you as a whole person.

Laura Ryan: In fact, we have found that clients are beginning to use nursing diagnoses, and they are questioning their ability to cope. They are sort of telling us what their diagnosis might be. I think it is this language that is catching on, both with the client and with other disciplines.

Anxiety revisited—from a practice perspective

PHYLLIS E. JONES, R.N., M.S.
DOROTHEA F. JAKOB, R.N., M.A.

At the Fourth National Conference on the Classification of Nursing Diagnoses, the diagnostic label *anxiety* was deleted from the list of accepted nursing diagnoses on the recommendation of the work group discussing anxiety. The rationale for this recommendation rested on two considerations: (1) anxiety "is a symptom rather than a problem," and (2) anxiety "in and of itself is not a problem which is amenable to nursing" (Kim and Moritz, 1982, p. 280). At the same time the work group anticipated that in view of its present widespread use in clinical practice the deletion of anxiety may create difficulties.

The purpose of this paper is to present and discuss some findings from recent research on nursing diagnostic terms used by nurses. It is hoped that these findings may stimulate further discussion and reconsideration of the recommendation to delete anxiety as a nursing diagnosis. Included are a brief overview of the research, selected findings regarding anxiety and fear, and implications and suggestions.

OVERVIEW OF THE PROJECT

The project from which this paper emerges is the final phase of research underway since 1974,[*] aspects of which have been reported at previous National Conferences on the Classification of Nursing Diagnoses (Kim and Moritz, 1982). Previous conferences have also approved nursing diagnostic categories developed in association with this project: *impaired home maintenance management; potential for injury; ineffective family coping, compromised and disabling* (Kim and Moritz, 1982).

The purpose of this three-phase investigation was to determine and document the terms used by nurses to describe the human conditions for which they provide care (nursing diagnoses). The design and procedures have been described fully elsewhere (Jones and Jakob, 1980) and will be summarized here only briefly. In each of the three phases, nurses who volunteered to report data from a predetermined number of nurse-client encounters were provided with a list of nursing diagnoses, developed or refined in a previous

☐The authors wish to acknowledge the joint development of this paper and the effort and interest of more than 214 nurses who contributed to this project in its various phases.

[*]An Investigation of the Definition of Nursing Diagnoses, supported by National Health Research and Development Projects Nos. 606-1399-49, 6606-1610-46, and 6606-1830-46, Canada.

phase. Participants were asked to select terms from this list (or to suggest others) that labeled the conditions for which they were providing care and to report these together with related contributing factors, that is, those historic or situational factors related to the existence, intensity, or duration of the reported client response. Also requested was information about the clients, the nurse-participants, and the nurses' opinions about the list of nursing diagnoses concerning its usefulness and completeness and the clarity of the terms. Review of the returns by two nurses associated with the project was designed to ensure that the data met the investigation's criteria for a nursing diagnosis. For purposes of this investigation, a *nursing diagnosis* was defined as the statement of a person's response to a situation or illness that is actually or potentially unhealthful and that nursing intervention can help to change in the direction of health, a modification of the definition by Mundinger and Jauron (1975). Data that did not meet the criteria were deleted. The nursing diagnoses resulting from these procedures made up the sample that was analyzed. It is from this sample that the following findings are selected.

The third phase of the investigation generated a total of 2772 nursing diagnoses submitted by 147 nurses from 427 nurse-client encounters in a wide variety of clinical settings. All 64 of the listed nursing diagnoses were reported, with frequencies ranging from 2 (for *maladaptive parenting*) to 179 (for *impaired hygienic self-care*).

FINDINGS

In terms of frequency of occurrence, *anxiety* ranked third (148 incidents, 5.3% of the total) and *fear* ranked fourth (140 incidents, 5.0% of the total), outranked only by *impaired hygienic self-care* and *mobility deficit* (Figure 1). In terms of clients affected, *anxiety* was reported for 35% and *fear* for 33% of the total of the 427 clients. *Anxiety* and *fear* were diagnosed in persons of all ages with health status at all levels and were associated with all categories of medical diagnoses. Furthermore, these client/patients were reported from a wide range of health care settings.

Contributing factors were reported at an average rate of 1.9 per diagnosis. The range was 1.2 contributing factors associated with *motor incoordination* to 2.7 associated with *difficult grieving* and *difficult role adaptation*. The patterns of these contributing factors have been of interest to the investigators, and Table 1 shows categories of these factors associated with *anxiety* and *fear* as well as mean rates associated with all reported nursing diagnoses. As in the total sample, other nursing diagnoses were most frequently reported as factors contributing to *anxiety* and to *fear*. For example, *impaired communication*, a listed nursing diagnosis, was frequently reported as contributing to *anxiety* identified in clients and *knowledge deficit* was reported as contributing to *fear*.

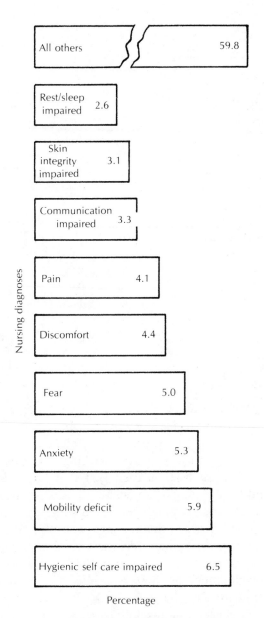

FIGURE 1 Most frequently reported nursing diagnoses, phase 3, by percentage: N = 2772.

TABLE 1   **Percentage distribution of all nursing diagnoses, *anxiety*, and *fear* by type of contributing factor (Phase 3)**

Type of contributing factor	Nursing diagnoses		
	All (2772) (%)	Anxiety (148) (%)	Fear (140) (%)
Other nursing diagnosis	48.9	42.5	41.4
Disease entities (medical diagnosis)	18.0	13.1	13.6
Medical test or treatment	10.1	15.3	19.1
Unknown, undetermined	7.3	5.7	3.1
Family-related	2.0	6.8	3.1
Nursing care or treatment	1.6	1.9	2.8
Life-style or choice	1.3	0.3	—
Death-related	1.1	3.8	9.0
Life-style change	1.1	2.2	0.6
Institutionalization	0.8	0.8	0.9
Occupational situation	0.7	0.8	0.6
Community home environment	0.6	0.8	0.6
Financial inadequacy	0.5	1.1	0.3
Other, not classified	6.0	4.9	4.9
TOTAL	100.0	100.0	100.0

IMPLICATIONS AND SUGGESTIONS

These data from the recently completed third phase are similar to those from the second phase. They suggest that *anxiety* and *fear* are phenomena, each of which is found with relatively high frequencies in clinical settings or, at the least, are terms that are useful to nurses in describing client responses for which they provide care. The findings also suggest that many factors that contribute to *anxiety* and to *fear* may be amenable to nursing intervention.

Analysis of data from the second phase suggested some confusion among the nurses about *anxiety* and *fear* as nursing diagnoses, since there was evidence of difficulty in differentiating between the two terms. This analysis has been reported (Jakob and Jones, 1981) together with a review of selected literature tracing the development of these concepts. The review itself reflected a similar confusion. As Bowlby (1973, p. 101) has pointed out in reviewing literature from a variety of disciplines, "'anxiety' and 'fear' are closely related. In just what way they are related is the puzzle." "Terminology problems abound, not least in the numerous and varied attempts to distinguish anxiety from fear" (Bowlby, 1973, p. 112). On the other hand, nurses seem generally in agreement that appropriate care for anxious and fearful

BOX 1   **Definitions of nursing diagnoses:** *anxiety* **and** *fear*

> *Anxiety*   A vague, uneasy sense of worry, nervousness, anguish, or marked
> ambivalence. The client appears not to have yet expresses the underlying
> feelings involved, such as fear, grief, conflict, insecurity. The client may or
> may not be aware of the particular display pattern of the anxiety or the
> factors contributing to it. Once the underlying feelings and sources are
> identified, a new diagnosis can be formulated.
> Contributing factors may be impaired communication, knowledge deficit,
> separation from a significant other especially a caretaker, ineffective coping,
> interpersonal transmission, as well as the underlying fear, grief, conflict, or
> insecurity.
> *Fear*   A client-expressed or client-confirmed response of apprehension or
> dread of the presence of a recognized, usually external, threat or danger to
> one's limb, autonomy, self-image, or community with others.
> Contributing factors may be the presence of external threat or danger,
> knowledge deficit, separation from significant other, especially a caretaker,
> interpersonal transmission, impaired communication, past experience of
> threat, danger, pain, discomfort, or confusion.

clients differs. Nursing literature suggests that effective intervention for anxiety aims to help the client recognize the presence of clues to anxiety, to gain insight into the contributing factors, and to enhance the use of constructive coping strategies to deal with and perhaps master the threat. On the other hand, effective care for fear involves scrutiny of the types of learning involved and the use of stimulus exposure to extinguish fear, positive inoculation to forestall potential fear, and active participation in strategies to lower the risk of threat and maximize one's resiliency (Jakob and Jones, 1981).

This evident difficulty in differentiating anxiety and fear, together with the seeming agreement regarding nursing intervention, led to the development of definitions for these terms rather than their deletion as nursing diagnoses. The definitions were based on the view that anxiety and fear are differentiated by the presence or absence of a known or recognized stimulus or focus. Fear and anxiety, together with definitions, were listed among the 64 nursing diagnoses developed in the second phase of this investigation (Jones and Jakob, 1980). These diagnoses and their definitions have been field tested by a sample of nurses, as reported earlier, and reviewed by a group of expert clinicians who have been involved in at least two phases of this research. The definitions shown in Box 1 have resulted from this work.

Consideration of these findings points to the inclusion of both *anxiety* and *fear* as nursing diagnoses. Although this proposed acceptance of *anxiety* as a nursing diagnosis is contrary to the decision of the Fourth National Conference to delete it, its inclusion is consistent with other current compilations of nursing diagnoses (Campbell, 1978; Castles, 1982; New Jersey State Department of Health, 1979; Simmons, 1980). Current nursing research on aspects of stress and coping (Guzetta and Forsyth, 1979; Llewellyn-Thomas, 1982) suggests that it is premature to exclude *anxiety* as a possible nursing diagnosis.

SUMMARY

Anxiety may well be usefully viewed as "a symptom rather than a problem" (Kim and Moritz, 1982, p. 280) amenable to nursing intervention as recommended at the Fourth National Conference. However, the findings just discussed suggest that the human response, anxiety, is prevalent and widely distributed in nursing practice settings. Furthermore, examination of the reported contributing factors suggests that they are amenable to nursing intervention. Ruling out *anxiety* as a nursing diagnosis therefore seems premature at this time. The seeming ambiguity in the terms *anxiety* and *fear* point to the need for definitions. Continued inclusion of *anxiety* stimulates further clinical nursing investigation leading to clarification of the concept and therefore to improved nursing care.

REFERENCES

Bowlby, J.: Attachment and loss, volume II—separation: anxiety and anger, Baltimore, Md., 1973, Penguin Books, Inc.

Campbell, C.: Nursing diagnosis and intervention in nursing practice, New York, 1978, John Wiley & Sons, Inc.

Castles, M.R.: Interrater agreement in the use of nursing diagnosis. In Kim, M.J., and Moritz, D.A., eds.: Classification of nursing diagnoses: proceedings of the third and fourth national conferences, New York, 1982, McGraw-Hill Book Co.

Guzetta, C.E., and Forsyth, C.A.: Nursing diagnostic pilot study: psychophysiologic stress, Adv. Nurs. Sci. **2**(1):27, 1979.

Jakob, D.F., and Jones, P.: Nursing diagnosis: differentiating fear and anxiety, Nurs. Papers **13**:20, 1981.

Jones, P.E., and Jakob, D.F.: The definition of nursing diagnoses: report of phase 2, Toronto, 1980, University of Toronto.

Kim, M.J., and Moritz, D.A., eds.: Classification of nursing diagnoses: proceedings of the third and fourth national conferences, New York, 1982, McGraw-Hill Book Co.

Llewellyn-Thomas, H.: Patient and spouse perceptions in malignant lymphoma: a research proposal. In Cahoon, M.C., ed.: Cancer nursing, Edinburgh, 1982. Churchill Livingstone.

Mundinger, M.O., and Jauron, G.D.: Developing a nursing diagnosis, Nurs. Outlook **23**:(2):94, 1975.

New Jersey State Department of Health: Case-mix nursing performance study: nursing diagnoses key for scaling (App. A), Trenton, N.J., 1979, The Department.

Simmons, D.A.: A classification scheme for client problems in community health nursing, Hyattsville, Md., 1980, U.S. Department of Health and Human Services, Public Health Service, Division of Nursing.

Implementation of nursing diagnosis in the trauma setting

LYNN TOTH, R.N., B.S.N.
DENISE COST, R.N., C.C.R.N.
BARBARA KEYES, R.N., B.S.
SANDRA DELI, R.N.
BARBARA BERKOWICH, R.N.

The nursing diagnosis model developed by Mundinger and Jauron (1975) has been adopted and implemented successfully as an integral part of primary nursing at the Shock Trauma Center of the Maryland Institute of Emergency Medical Services Systems (MIEMSS). The Mundinger and Jauron model was chosen because (1) it is a fairly straightforward model that is easily understood and followed by nursing personnel, (2) it actualizes the nursing process, (3) it has inherent flexibility that permits easy alteration of diagnoses as a patient's condition changes, and (4) by having two distinct parts, it enables the nurse to differentiate specific behaviors that define a patient's problems. For example, a specific behavior in several patients may be caused by several different etiologies; conversely, many different behaviors of several patients can result from the same underlying etiology or unhealthful response. This diagnostic flexibility and updating promotes continuity of care during hospitalization.

MODEL

Mundinger and Jauron (1975, p. 96) defined nursing diagnosis as "a statement of a patient problem which is arrived at by making inferences from collected data." A nursing diagnosis is a two-part statement—a definition of the patient's unhealthful response related to the causes of that response or the contributing factors maintaining that response (Box 1). The criteria for an unhealthful response are as follows: (1) the response must be clearly unhealthful, (2) the response must be validated with data (supported by both objective and subjective data), (3) the response must be stated in terms of patient behavior, and (4) the response must be able to be changed or altered by independent nursing interventions. The criteria for the causative factors are as follows: (1) they must be amenable to or influenced by independent nursing measures or therapy (nursing interventions that can be initiated without a physician's order), (2) they must be changeable, and (3) they must be validated with data.

Mundinger and Jauron (1975) have defined three types of nursing diagnosis: actual, potential, and possible. An *actual* nursing diagnosis occurs in the

---

BOX 1   **Nursing diagnosis**

Unhealthful patient response related to   Causative factors
        ↓   ↓
    Goal   Plan
     ↓   ↓
  Evaluation   Implementation

Patient behavior   Nursing activity

1. Clearly unhealthful   1. Influenced by nursing
2. Validated with data   therapy
3. Stated in patient behaviors   2. Changeable
4. Altered by nursing interventions 3. Validated with data

---

present and is easily validated with data (for example, retained secretions related to immobility). A *potential* nursing diagnosis calls for preventive measures to maintain or protect a healthful state (for example, potential for infection related to interrupted skin integrity). A *possible* nursing diagnosis indicates diagnostic uncertainty based on unclear data concerning the response or the related factors (for example, possible depression related to alterations in body image).

IMPLEMENTATION
Background

Nursing diagnosis implementation was facilitated by the existing system of nursing care delivery, primary nursing, in which one nurse (a primary nurse) assumes 24-hour responsibility and accountability for the nursing management of a patient and the patient's family (Mallison, 1980). The primary nurse is responsible for developing a written patient care plan that includes the patient's problems (identified as a medical diagnosis before nursing diagnosis implementation) and the nursing interventions.

Education

The first step of implementation was the education of the primary and staff nurses. In 1979 clinical specialists at the Shock Trauma Center, aware that nursing diagnosis could improve the quality of care delivered, enhance nursing accountability and responsibility, and more clearly define the role of the nurse, conducted a search for published theories on nursing diagnosis. They chose the Mundinger and Jauron format as best fitting the complex and frequently changing needs of the trauma patient. This model was presented in a 2-day nursing workshop. The first day Mundinger presented and explained the model for nursing diagnosis. Small-group work followed to allow hands-

TABLE 2   Nursing diagnosis evolution

Original diagnosis	Problem/error	Revised diagnosis
Potential for infection related to *facial laceration*	Medical diagnosis	Potential for infection related to loss of skin integrity secondary to multiple facial lacerations
Family in crisis related to *sudden hospitalization of son*	Too vague Unchangeable	Crying, withdrawal, and fear related to need for information and uncertainty of hospital routines secondary to hospitalization of son
Potential for pneumonia related to *mechanical ventilator*	Can be more specific Unchangeable	Retained secretions related to immobility secondary to mechanical ventilator and multiple fractures

on practice with the new idea. The second day Mundinger helped primary nurses to identify existing patient problems and to translate them into nursing diagnoses while the clinical specialists conducted educational group meetings for the staff nurses.

Initial effort and revision

The primary nurses, backed by clinical specialists serving as resource people, reviewed all available written material on the Mundinger and Jauron format, began using nursing diagnoses for patient care plans, and maintained a continual reassessment of this nursing diagnosis implementation. Over the next year, the first efforts at nursing diagnosis evolved into more sophisticated and efficient tools for patient problem identification. The diagnoses were kept in a manual as a reference resource. Table 1 shows some examples of nursing diagnosis evolution.

Evaluation

Mundinger returned in 1980 to review the progress of nursing diagnosis at the Shock Trauma Center and found that nursing diagnoses were well-defined and appropriate for the trauma patient. She also believed that the frustration primary nurses experienced in "wanting to get it right all the time" would ease as the process of implementing nursing diagnosis continued to evolve.

Introduction to medical staff

The medical staff was introduced to nursing diagnosis in a patient-oriented conference. The nurses gave a brief summary of each patient's injuries and status. Then several medical diagnoses were compared with the corresponding nursing diagnoses, and recommended nursing interventions were derived.

Standardized plans with individuality

Since many patients at the Shock Trauma Center exhibit the same unhealthful responses in relation to specific injuries, the same nursing diagnoses and nursing interventions have had to be repeated on the majority of written care plans (Table 2). To conserve valuable nursing time, primary nurses have developed a standardized care plan incorporating the most common nursing diagnoses and interventions, for example, potential for retained secretions, skin breakdown, contractures, vascular stasis, and constipation related to decreased mobility. There is flexibility, and patient care is individualized. A standardized care plan outlines one of four major areas of concern: (1) head injuries, (2) immobility, (3) infection, or (4) orthopedic injuries.

CLINICAL EXAMPLE

The implementation of nursing diagnosis in the trauma patient can be understood more clearly when it is applied to a clinical situation. The following case study illustrates the development and utilization of nursing diagnosis.

Case study

M.D., a 24-year-old white man, was injured in a motor vehicle accident and transported to the Shock Trauma Center by helicopter. Initial assessment showed that he sustained the following injuries: closed head injury, LeForte II facial fractures with facial lacerations, lung contusion, fractured ribs on left (3-6) with flail, ruptured spleen, and left acetabular fracture. Hemopneumothorax ruled out myocardial contusion, exploratory laparotomy led to splenectomy, and the acetabular fracture was stabilized with a tibial pin and 20 pounds traction.

While the patient was in surgery, the primary nurse met his mother and girlfriend in the waiting room, compiled a patient history (Box 2), and assessed the family's needs. After surgery, the patient was taken to the Critical Care Unit where a physical assessment was performed, which included a review of all systems, vital signs, laboratory data, intake and output, and dressings. The assessment presented a typical picture of a trauma patient.

After the data collection phase was completed, the primary nurse began to formulate nursing diagnoses, set goals, and outline a plan of care to achieve the goals. Many nursing diagnoses were generated by the patient's needs: (1) altered level of consciousness related to changes in cerebral edema, (2) potential for impaired wound healing and/or infection related to facial swelling and loss of skin integrity, (3) potential for hypoxia and/or atelectasis related to retained secretions, (4) potential for infection related to loss of skin integrity, and (5) potential for skin breakdown, contractures, and constipation related to immobility. Two of the diagnoses and the process used to derive them are shown in Tables 3 and 4.

TABLE 2   Common identified nursing diagnoses in the trauma setting

Unhealthful response	Cause/contributing factors
Altered level of consciousness	Changes in cerebral edema
Potential for impaired wound healing and/or infection	Facial swelling and loss of skin integrity
Potential for hypoxia and/or atelectasis	Retained secretions
Potential for infection	Loss of skin integrity secondary to _____
Potential for skin breakdown, contractures, constipation	Decreased mobility
Potential for prolonged anxiety, anger	Change in body image
Fear of being left alone	Impaired ability to communicate
Potential for life-threatening cardiac dysrythmias	Wide fluctuations in body electrolytes secondary to _____
Alterations in vital organ perfusion	Fluid volume imbalances
Impaired motor and sensory function of an extremity	Disrupted musculoskeletal integrity and swelling

BOX 2   Patient history summary

Mike is a 24-year-old single student who presently lives at home with his mother and younger brother Joe. His parents have been divorced for 5 years, and Dad just remarried 1 month prior. Mike has been concerned about this remarriage because it means his father will be moving out of state. His normal stress reaction is to become very verbal when angry, and his mother describes him as not liking authority figures. Mike is athletic and likes skiing and jogging; he also enjoys working on cars. He has a significantly close relationship with his girlfriend Laurie who was also present at the time of the interview. Mike enjoys good health with no significant previous illnesses or hospitalizations; no eating or sleeping problems, no bowel or bladder dysfunction, and no drug intake. He does smoke one pack of cigarettes per day and drinks alcohol moderately. He is employed part time as a busboy in a restaurant in addition to attending college as a second-year pharmacy student.

TABLE 3   Nursing diagnosis from patient assessment immediately after surgery

Step 1	Step 2	Step 3
A. Medical diagnosis: lung contusion	A. Nursing diagnosis: potential for hypoxia and/or atelectasis related to retained secretions	A. Nursing diagnosis: potential for hypoxia and/or atelectasis related to retained secretions; short-term goals: chest x-ray film will be clear within 1 week, PA_{O_2} will remain >90 while intubated
B. Unhealthful patient response: hypoxia, hypercapnea, retained secretions, possible airway obstruction, pneumonia, atelectasis	B. Validating criteria: chest x-ray film showing infiltrates and rib fractures, arterial blood gases, bloody secretions, mechanism of injury, medical diagnosis of lung contusion, coarse breath sounds	B. Interventions: 1. Chest physiotherapy (CPT) 94° 2. Patient may not be turned onto left side 3. Trendelenburg for 15 minutes as long as intracranial pressure <25 4. No vibration over rib fractures 5. Patient becomes bradycardiac when off ventilator; bag before and after suctioning with Puritan Resuscitator using 100% O_2 6. May lavage with ½-strength normal saline and sodium bicarbonate every 2 hours as needed 7. Medicate before CPT 8. Monitor daily chest x-ray films and arterial blood gases (covered in nursing standards)
C. Nursing diagnosis: potential for hypoxia and/or atelectasis related to retained secretions secondary to left lung contusion		C. Evaluation

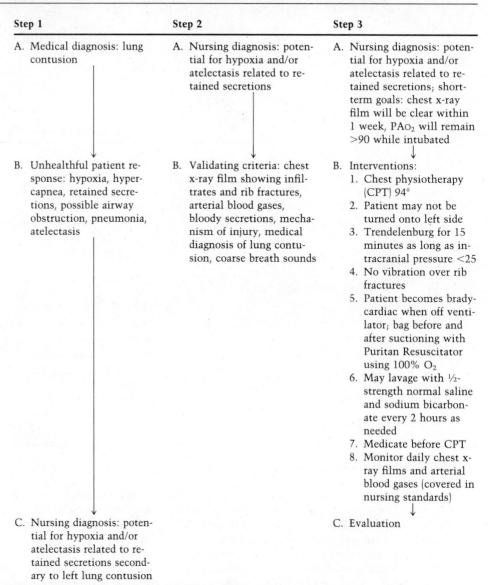

TABLE 4   Second nursing diagnosis*

Step 1	Step 2	Step 3
A. Medical diagnosis: psychologic needs	A. Nursing diagnosis: restlessness and disorientation related to sensory overload and unfamiliar surroundings	A. Nursing diagnosis: restlessness and disorientation related to sensory overload and unfamiliar surroundings; short-term goals: Mike will be consistently oriented to person and place by _____; Mike will show cooperation by participating in respiratory treatments and turning by _____; Mike will be able to sleep for at least 4 hours each night.
B. Unhealthful patient response: self-destructive behavior, restlessness, noncompliance, disorientation	B. Validating criteria: hypertension, tachycardia, patient needs restraints, diaphoresis, patient pulls at I.V.s and tubes, patient tries to get out of bed, patient writes notes that are undiscernable, facial expressions of fear, patient doesn't close eyes unless heavily sedated	B. Interventions: 1. Michael is waking up from closed head injury. He needs to be reoriented to person, time, and place. He is especially confused on awakening. 2. He calms down with gentle touch and soft voice. 3. Do not restrain when with him. 4. Remind him of family contact. Laurie, Mike's girlfriend, was in accident. Let him know she is okay and at home. 5. Mike is feeling overwhelmed by constant stimulation. He is more cooperative when allowed to get adequate rest. 6. Block care. 7. Allow sleep time after midnight assessment until AM. Give sleeping medication q.h.s. Even if Mike wakes up, DO NOT initiate treatments. He may fall back asleep.
C. Nursing diagnosis: restlessness and disorientation related to sensory overload and unfamiliar surroundings		C. Evaluation.

*This diagnosis was formulated 1 week postadmission. The patient was awake and following commands; he remained intubated.

SUMMARY

In summary, nursing diagnosis now provides nurses with an established mechanism for defining the domain of nursing practice more clearly and for attaining a higher level of professionalism. According to Feild (1979, p. 505), "it influences the quality of nursing practice positively by facilitating the nursing process, more clearly defining the scope of nursing accountability, and enhancing professional responsibility identity." The nurses at the Shock Trauma Center of MIEMSS believe that nursing diagnosis more clearly identifies the needs of a trauma patient who has complex injuries because it defines a patient's response to an illness and it delineates more specifically what a nurse can treat independently. Nursing diagnosis also provides documentation of the steps the nurse has taken to prevent complications, steps that before went unnoticed (Logsdon, 1973).

Nurse Practice Acts throughout the nation define and legislate this idea. The Maryland Nurse Practice Act (1981) defines *practice of registered nursing* as the performance of acts requiring substantial specialized knowledge, judgment, and skill based on biologic, physiologic, behavioral, or sociologic sciences for assessment, nursing diagnosis planning, implementation, and nursing practice evaluation.

Because nursing diagnosis is a relatively new concept, information and documentation about its impact on the nursing profession and health care field are scarce. The Shock Trauma Center nurses will continue to research, revise, and improve nursing diagnosis and document its changing impact on patient care.

REFERENCES

Feild, L.: The implementation of nursing diagnosis in clinical practice, Nurs. Clin. North Am. **14**(3):497, 1979.

Logsdon, A.: Why primary nursing? Nurs. Clin. North Am. **8**(2):283, 1973.

Mallison, M.: An editorial, Am. J. Nurs. **80**(12):2165, 1980.

Maryland Nurse Practice Act, Charlottsville, Va., 1981, Michie Co.

Mundinger, M.O., and Jauron, G.D.: Developing a nursing diagnosis, Nurs. Outlook **23**(2):94, 1975.

Discussion

Michelle Bockrath: I think one of the issues is whether an etiology can be a medical problem. I found that extremely interesting that you could use "secondary to a medical problem." Since you are in a critical care area, I am wondering if you had difficulty initially when you instituted that, and if you did, how you did you go about it?

Denise Cost: Yes, we did have a great problem. It is still an evolving process. The one concrete thing I can offer you in terms of that process is to ask yourself, "What is it about the medical diagnosis that you are concerned with? What do you see in the patient as a result of the medical diagnosis that you are responsible for and that you can treat?"

Carolyn Yocom: One of your nursing diagnoses was restlessness and disorientation related to sensory overload and unfamiliar surroundings. I consider restlessness and disorientation to be signs and symptoms. Why were the signs and symptoms not further grouped/clustered and then given a label, a nursing diagnosis?

Denise Cost: That is an excellent point, and it is something that we have been discovering; that is, we are learning, we need additional education, and we need to further delineate the diagnostic process.

Carolyn Yocom: Do you use a problem-oriented record? If so, where do you place validating criteria?

Denise Cost: We do not use a problem-oriented record, and we do not, at this time, record our validating criteria anywhere.

Carolyn Yocom: What about the time factor if you are primary nurses going through this whole process?

Denise Cost: Well, our administration has been extremely supportive of primary nursing and the work that we need to do. We work on a flex-time schedule, that is, 10-hour days with 8 hours of patient care and 2 hours for related activities such as developing care plans, interacting with patients and families, and consulting with other health care specialists.

Nursing diagnoses of abusive patients

VIRGINIA LUETJE, R.N., M.S.N.
MARYELLEN McSWEENEY, R.N., Ph.D.

INTRODUCTION

By the mid-1960s, psychiatric nursing text authors were beginning to arrange discussion on nursing care according to the predominating behavior patterns the nurse might see. Texts had chapters on socially aggressive patterns (Matheney and Topalis, 1965), behavior characterized by antisocial attitudes (Mereness and Karnosh, 1966), and patients with feelings of distrust (Brown and Fowler, 1966). These were early attempts at departing from the medical model chapters about schizophrenia, mania, and sociopathy. The early attempts may have helped nurses realize that patients can behave in a manner that places great stress on other people in the environment regardless of the psychiatric diagnosis. This study was particularly concerned with developing nursing diagnoses of abusive patients. The question it attempted to answer was: Is there a way to recognize a group of nursing diagnoses that classifies what nurses assess and do as intervention when they use their nursing skills with people who "dis-stress" others?

SELECTED LITERATURE REVIEW AND RATIONALE

A cursory review of literature was begun. Papers were not reviewed for what they were uniquely saying but rather for what words they were commonly using to describe behaviors that negatively affected other people. We cataloged 43 literature sources, many of which were entire books. Many other articles and books were scanned without cataloging because certain themes became so apparent that the sources were adding nothing new. Past reviews of client histories, medical notes, and nursing notes were also used.

It became apparent that the behaviors that were affrontive to others could be arranged in a few basic categories of outwardly directed behavior: anger, active aggression, impulsiveness, self-exhaltation (grandiosity), manipulation, subtle obstructivism (which is an indirect form of aggression), and overdependency. One assumption that appeared to be supported by experience was that the duration and persistence of affrontive behaviors were highly varied. The behavior might be temporary, lasting only minutes or hours or perhaps only during a particular crisis. For such temporary behaviors the classification

□Partial funding for this project was granted by the Office for Nursing Research, St. Louis University, School of Nursing.

scheme we developed used the modifying word *state*. A *state* is defined as the condition of a person or thing with respect to circumstances or qualities. Colloquially, people are sometimes described as being in "a nervous state" or "just in a terrible state." Abusive behavior can also be observed as a long-standing characteristic pattern of behavior of some individuals. The behaviors become a style or mode of acting that one comes to expect a given individual to manifest from time to time. For these patterned behaviors the classification scheme we developed used the modifying word *mode*.

By using mode and state as modifiers with the seven basic categories identified, nine categories were developed. One of the nine categories, the rational anger state, is viewed as a healthy response pattern. It is still a response, however, that must be addressed by quality nursing care so that anger does not degenerate into more unacceptable behavior. The other eight categories are viewed as unhealthy behaviors amenable at varying levels (depending to an extent on etiology) to independent nursing therapy. The nine categories and literature sources that specifically influenced their development are given in Box 1. Four of the categories have no references cited. Sources citing impulsiveness as a behavior are countless, but none were found that list phenomena for assessing impulsiveness. Self-exhaltation is described in references discussing mania, but it also occurs in the absence of other manic

---

BOX 1   **Diagnoses with references**

    I. Rational anger state
      (Cuthbert, 1969; Gruber and Schniewind, 1976: Kiening, 1970; Moritz, 1978; Rogers, 1962; Sundeen and others, 1976)

    II. Aggressive response state
      (APA, 1980; Coleman, 1972; Loomis, 1970; Moyer, 1971; Scherer, Abeles, and Fischer, 1975)

    III. Aggressive coping mode
      (Bandura, 1973, 1978; Carney, 1976; Karshner, 1978; Kiening, 1970; Sherer, Abeles, and Fischer, 1975; Wolfgang, 1978)

    IV. Impulse-dominated state
    V. Impulsive coping mode
    VI. Self-exhaltation state
    VII. Manipulative coping mode
      (Bursten, 1973)

    VIII. Subtle obstructive mode
    IX. Dependent coping mode
      (G.A.P., 1970; Gruber and Schniewind, 1976; Kyes and Hofling, 1974; Rouslin, 1975)

symptoms. Subtle obstructiveness has also been referred to as passive-aggressive behavior or oppositional disorder by diagnosticians.

INITIAL STUDY

A central question was raised: Would nurses who were giving direct care find that these nursing diagnoses we developed were useful and had content validity?

Design of tool

Using the definitions, assessment criteria, and interventions identified (Luetje, 1983), a nine-page checklist tool was developed (Box 2). Each tool included two pages of instructions and information about its use. Data on interventions were collected using this tool. (These data have yet to be fully analyzed.) All nine diagnoses were included on the tool. Each tool could be used for five client assessments. The assessor checked off diagnoses that seemed appropriate for the client on the final page of the tool (Box 3).

Use of Tool

The potential patients on whom the data could be collected were the entire population of a 105-bed acute care psychiatric setting that was part of a hospital affiliated with a large private university. All registered nurses who were providing primary care between the hours of 0700 and 2300 were invited to serve as data collectors. These 26 registered nurses were asked to do five assessments on five shifts of their choice during a 3-week data collection period. The instructions asked that they use the tool particularly for patients they believed had one or more of the listed assessment behaviors. They could assess the same patient on more than one shift, if they were assigned the same patient. An evening nurse might do an assessment of the same patient who had been assessed by the day primary care nurse.

All 26 nurses turned in the data collection tool at the end of the 3 weeks. One tool was unusable because the nurse had not completed the final page of the form. One other nurse had completed the form on only three patients rather than five. The total number of assessments that were usable was 123.

The nurses had an average of 6½ years of direct care nursing experience. The range was from 1 to 23 years. The mean was 3 years, with five nurses indicating this amount. At the time the assessments were done, 13 nurses worked the day shift, six worked the evening shift, and six rotated day and evening shifts.

Data analysis

The total number of nursing diagnoses made in 123 assessments was 256 for an average of two diagnoses per assessment. The range was from one to nine.

BOX 2   **Sample checklist page**

I. Rational anger state: A temporary condition in which the individual is
angry for understandable, valid reasons, and the expression of the anger is
direct but socially and morally acceptable. Others are not abused by this
behavior except in the sense that it is often anxiety provoking to be
confronted by another's anger.

Assessment criteria present

		Patient			
	A	B	C	D	E
01 Direct appropriate communication of anger					
02 Degree of anger appropriate to stimulus					
03 Goal-directed behavior					
04 Alert					
05 Oriented					
06 Organized thinking					
07 Angry facies					
08 Verbalizes frustration					
09 Valid basis for anger					
10 Socially condoned behavior					
Other (describe)					
Intervention used					
Active listening					
Clarification of issue creating the anger					
Validated appropriateness of angry feelings					
Apology from person who caused the anger					
Explained own viewpoint of situation					
Assisted patient in planning a way to resolve anger					
Validated whether anger was resolved					
Other or comments:					

However, only one assessment resulted in all nine diagnoses being used. No
assessment used eight of the diagnoses, only two used seven. There was a
marked skewing toward using three or fewer of the diagnoses. In 71 of the
123 assessments, only one diagnosis was used.

Frequencies were obtained for each global diagnosis, each assessment criterion, and each nursing intervention. The presence or absence of each global
diagnosis was cross-tabulated against the presence or absence of each assessment criterion. The associated percentages of consistent criteria and diag-

BOX 3   **Final data page**

In my global opinion, the following nursing diagnoses would have been appropriate on this shift for:

	Patient				
	A	**B**	**C**	**D**	**E**
I. Rational anger state					
II. Aggressive response state					
III. Aggressive coping mode					
IV. Impulse-dominated state					
V. Impulsive coping mode					
VI. Self-exhaltation state					
VII. Manipulative coping mode					
VIII. Subtle obstructive mode					
IX. Dependent coping mode					

Estimated time spent this shift with patient A _____

B _____

C _____

D _____

E _____

Estimated time required to complete this form: _____

Number of months'/years' experience in direct care nursing: _____

Date _____ Shift _____ Division _____

Do you wish your identity to remain confidential?   YES   NO

Name _____

Home phone number (if willing) _____

noses (that is, both present or both absent) and inconsistent criteria and diagnoses (that is, false positives, consisting of the criterion present but the diagnosis absent; false negatives, consisting of the criterion absent but the diagnosis present) were determined for each possible pairing of a diagnosis with an assessment criterion (9 diagnoses × 85 criteria = 765 pairings). In addition, Kendall's tau b was used to measure the association between the presence of an assessment criterion and the presence of the global diagnosis. Tau b has a theoretic range from -1, indicating perfect negative association, to $+1$, indicating perfect positive association. The values of tau b are given in Table 1.

Text continued on p. 310.

TABLE 1   Kendall's Tau B Correlations

Assessment criteria	Rational anger state D1(N=26)	Aggressive response state D2(N=34)	Regressive coping mode D3(N=31)	Impulse-dominated state D4(N=39)	Impulsive coping mode D5(N=30)	Self-exaltation state D6(N=20)	Manipulative coping mode D7(N=29)	Subtle obstructive mode D8(N=20)	Dependent coping mode D9(N=33)
1. Direct anger appropriately comm.[b] (0=40)	.58[f]	.07	.04	−.06	−.03	.02	−.14	−.21[d]	−.07
2. Degree of anger appropriate to stimulus (0=17)	.43[f]	−.03	.04	−.03	−.01	−.05	−.11	−.05	.02
3. Goal-directed behavior (0=21)	.35[f]	.00	−.06	−.08	−.01	.03	−.15[c]	−.08	−.13
4. Alert (0=65)	.49[f]	.07	.10	−.09	−.07	−.16[c]	−.17[c]	−.29[e]	−.13
5. Oriented (0=60)	.45[f]	.09	.03	−.08	−.02	−.12	−.12	−.21[d]	−.04
6. Organized thinking (0=18)	.18[c]	.00	−.03	−.09	−.13	.00	−.07	−.06	−.09
7. Angry facies (0=46)	.30[e]	.09	.09	.14	−.09	−.16[c]	−.11	−.25[d]	−.05
8. Verbalizes frustration (0=59)	.40[f]	.05	−.09	−.16[c]	−.22[d]	−.19[c]	−.25[d]	−.28[e]	−.05
9. Valid basis for anger (0=29)	.51[f]	.08	.03	−.08	−.05	.06	−.13	−.14	−.03
10. Socially condoned behavior (0=21)	.29[e]	.11	.04	−.13	−.01	.03	−.15	−.08	−.03
11. Agitated (0=60)	.09	.34[f]	.22[d]	.36[f]	.01	.19[c]	.07	−.21[d]	−.19[c]
12. Argumentative (0=54)	.06	.47[f]	.35[f]	.24[d]	−.01	.14	.05	−.21[d]	−.31[e]
13. Behavior not rational (0=50)	−.10	.30[e]	.28[e]	.25[d]	−.05	.04	.01	−.14	−.16[c]
14. Fearful of others/environs (0=31)	.02	−.02	−.07	.24[d]	−.02	−.05	−.15[c]	−.15[c]	−.06
15. Hostile (0=53)	.03	.35[f]	.36[f]	.36[f]	−.04	.06	−.06	−.12	−.23[d]
16. Impaired judgment (0=66)	.12	.36[f]	.20[d]	.31[e]	.07	.19[c]	.02	−.12	−.21[d]

[a]O = number of times that assessment criterion was reported in 123 assessments.
[b]N = number of times the diagnosis was a conclusion judgment in 123 assessments.
[c]Level of significance at or greater than 0.05.
[d]Level of significance at or greater than 0.01.
[e]Level of significance at or greater than 0.001.
[f]Level of significance at or greater than 0.0001.

Continued.

TABLE 1   Kendall's Tau B Correlations—cont'd

Assessment criteria	Rational anger state D1(N=26)	Aggressive response state D2(N=34)	Regressive coping mode D3(N=31)	Impulse-dominated state D4(N=39)	Impulsive coping mode D5(N=30)	Self-exaltation state D6(N=20)	Manipulative coping mode D7(N=29)	Subtle obstructive mode D8(N=20)	Dependent coping mode D9(N=33)
17. Impaired reality testing (0=48)	.12	.33[e]	.19[c]	.23[d]	.05	.05	−.01	−.13	−.25[d]
18. Limited self-insight (0=64)	.10	.41[f]	.29[e]	.29	.09	.07	.00	−.28[e]	−.12
19. Perceives goal conflict/blockage (0=40)	.19[c]	.15[c]	.12	.25[d]	.08	.12	.02	−.07	−.15[c]
20. Rejecting toward intervention (0=50)	.01	.30[e]	.32[e]	.28[e]	.03	.13	.09	−.05	−.16[c]
21. Tense (0=55)	.17[c]	.32[e]	.19[c]	.19[c]	.02	.05	.04	−.17[c]	−.18[c]
22. Verbal threats (0=39)	−.05	.28[e]	.21[d]	.18[c]	−.02	.08	−.01	−.16[c]	−.25[d]
23. Other: describe (0=7)	−.04	.16[c]	.02	.09	−.06	.08	−.05	−.11	−.07
24. Hx: repeated assaultiveness (0=31)	−.02	.06	.35[f]	.28[e]	.06	.15[c]	.12	.05	−.18[c]
25. Hx: property destruction (0=27)	.11	.07	.42[f]	.26[d]	.02	.19[c]	.03	.03	−.19[c]
26. Hx: using force to achieve wants/goals (0=25)	.03	.09	.31[e]	.15[c]	.00	.16[c]	.01	.11	−.21[d]
27. Tense (0=57)	.15[c]	.15[c]	.29[e]	.25[d]	.19	−.01	.02	−.14	−.19[c]
28. Sullen expression (0=46)	.18[c]	.17[c]	.38[f]	.23[d]	.04	.03	.02	−.06	−.16[c]
29. Resentful (0=43)	.13	.16[c]	.40[f]	.25[d]	.15[c]	.16[c]	.20[d]	.11	−.13
30. Perceptually distorted world view (0=43)	.12	.30[e]	.44[f]	.17[c]	.22[d]	.14	.11	.05	−.14
31. Rationalizes actions (0=44)	.07	.22[d]	.47[f]	.16[c]	.17[c]	.13	.22[d]	.08	.07
32. Projects responsibility (0=37)	.05	.19[c]	.40[f]	.16[c]	.12	.19[c]	.26[c]	.10	−.12
33. Impoverished resolving anger via discussion (0=45)	.10	.17[c]	.38[f]	.30[e]	.12	−.06	−.02	−.11	−.12
34. Other: describe (0=4)	−.09	.30[e]	.32[e]	.20[d]	.22[d]	.17	.11	.04	−.11

Continued.

35. Restless (0=57)	.15^c	.12	.17^c	.54^f	.27^d	.08	−.06	−.14	−.19^c
36. Excitable (0=45)	−.02	.02	.14	.50^f	.20^d	.17^c	−.06	−.11	−.27^d
37. Unpredictable (0=44)	.07	.18^c	.27^e	.54^f	.29^e	.08	.06	−.05	−.22^d
38. Exposed self or others to harm or danger (0=24)	−.05	−.03	.09	.35^f	.01	.12	−.03	−.05	−.16^c
39. Impaired concentration (0=52)	.04	.10	.18^c	.52^f	.24^d	.11	−.09	−.15	−.26^d
40. Disregard for realistic consequences (0=46)	−.07	.09	.21^d	.56^f	.19^c	.16^c	−.05	−.11	−.13
41. Limited insight (0=60)	.09	.12	.15^c	.47^f	.20^d	.05	.03	−.17^c	−.04
42. Bafflement post-action (0=16)	.03	.08	.00	.26^e	.12	.03	−.04	−.10	−.13
43. Dismay post-action (0=14)	−.06	−.16^c	.09	.13	.08	−.02	−.08	−.16^c	−.22^d
44. Anxiety post-action (0=26)	−.02	.04	.11	.32^e	.12	−.01	−.10	−.17^c	−.08
45. Guilt post-action (0=24)	.04	−.02	.04	.30^e	.05	.01	.02	−.11	−.07
46. Other: describe (0=5)	.10	.05	.07	.34^f	.07	.24^d	−.02	.02	−.03
47. Hx: hasty, heedless actions (0=44)	.11	.03	.31^e	.43^f	.56^f	.13	−.05	.00	−.11
48. Hx: nonviolent disciplinary problems (0=32)	.06	.05	.13	.23^d	.44^f	.14	−.02	−.11	−.15^c
49. High overall activity level (0=37)	.14	.03	.11	.36^f	.45^f	.14	.05	−.10	−.12
50. Affect labile and dependent on moment concern (0=52)	.02	.06	.26^d	.30^e	.47^f	.11	−.01	−.15^c	−.04
51. Low tolerance for frustration (0=58)	.11	.07	.20^d	.35^f	.37^f	.03	.05	−.15^c	−.06

[a] 0 = number of times that assessment criterion was reported in 123 assessments.
[b] N = number of times the diagnosis was a conclusion judgment in 123 assessments.
[c] Level of significance at or greater than 0.05.
[d] Level of significance at or greater than 0.01.
[e] Level of significance at or greater than 0.001.
[f] Level of significance at or greater than 0.0001.

TABLE 1   Kendall's Tau B Correlations—cont'd

Assessment criteria	Rational anger state D1(N=26)	Aggressive response state D2(N=34)	Regressive coping mode D3(N=31)	Impulse-dominated state D4(N=39)	Impulsive coping mode D5(N=30)	Self-exaltation state D6(N=20)	Manipulative coping mode D7(N=29)	Subtle obstructive mode D8(N=20)	Dependent coping mode D9(N=33)
52. Impaired social judgment (0=55)	.05	.07	.16[e]	.30[e]	.44[f]	-.04	+.12	-.04	-.10
53. Lack of meaningful friendships (0=52)	.08	.05	.15[e]	.22[d]	.40[f]	.02	.03	-.06	-.15[c]
54. Longstanding tumultuous family relationship (0=42)	.09	.13	.37[f]	.30[e]	.43[f]	.05	.13	-.08	-.09
55. Hx: sudden school/job changes (0=20)	.10	.02	.10	.23[d]	.37[f]	.16[c]	.01	-.07	-.12
56. Hx: sudden moves (0=20)	.04	.02	.05	.03	.26[d]	.04[c]	-.04	.04	-.07
57. Hx: many romantic liasons (0=10)	.00	.08	.10	.09	.32[d]	.11	.12	-.05	-.18[c]
58. Pervasive grandiose thinking (0=26)	.07	-.01	.20[d]	.18[c]	.08	.47[f]	-.10	-.07	-.22[d]
59. Impaired judgment (0=51)	.04	.07	.12	.20[c]	.02	.34[f]	.04	-.06	-.21[d]
60. Impaired insight (0=58)	.06	.00	.09	.16[c]	.03	.38[f]	.01	-.11	-.20[d]
61. Impaired reality testing (0=39)	.03	.01	.21[d]	.22[c]	.02	.41[f]	.03	-.16[c]	-.29[e]
62. Irritable if ideas challenged (0=41)	-.02	-.01	.19[c]	.19[c]	-.08	.34[f]	-.07	-.17[c]	-.19[c]
63. Other: describe (0=2)	-.07	.06	-.07	.07	-.07	.29[e]	-.07	-.06	-.08[c]
64. Client perceives goal conflict with others (0=53)	.11	-.10	.06	.10	.00	.02	.52[f]	.15[c]	.02
65. Conscious intent to influence other person (0=36)	.10	-.08	.08	.05	.01	.06	.44[f]	.10	.01
66. Conscious deception and insincerity (0=25)	-.01	-.09	.13	.06	.00	-.17[c]	.39[f]	.05	-.12
67. Feeling of "putting something over" on other (0=23)	-.09	-.11	.06	.06	-.07	-.10	.32[e]	.13	.04

68. Hx: above behaviors are a pattern (0=34)	.00	-.10	.06	.08	-.01	-.08	.51[f]	.27[d]	.12
69. Excess concern with inconsequential ideas (0=32)	.05	.28[e]	-.13	-.07	-.08	-.11	.15[c]	.14[f]	.06
70. Procrastinates (0=32)	.01	-.12	.04	.10	.05	-.06	.19[c]	.34	-.11
71. Neglects keeping promises or agreements (0=25)	-.01	-.22[d]	-.04	.01	-.05	.00	.10	.27[c]	-.12
72. "Intentional" failures (0=29)	-.05	-.17[c]	-.05	.01	.00	-.04	.28[e]	.38[f]	.18[c]
73. Indirect aggression (0=35)	.11	-.03	.17[c]	.19[c]	.06	-.03	.24[e]	.31[c]	.02
74. Passively resistent (0=44)	.07	-.12	.04	.20[d]	.09	-.01	.34[f]	.41[f]	.16[c]
75. Other: describe (0=3)	-.08	-.10	.09	.14	.16[c]	.07	.16[c]	.07	.14
76. Resistance to self-care (0=32)	-.08	-.16[c]	.00	.14	.06	-.11	-.06	-.06	.39[f]
77. Statements of helplessness (0=47)	.00	-.26[d]	-.18[f]	-.02	.04	-.12	.02	.02	.58[f]
78. Frequent demands on staff (0=52)	-.04	-.12	.00	.08	.22[d]	-.06	.11	.11	.44[f]
79. Overly sweet (0=25)	-.06	-.18[c]	-.10	-.12	.05	.00	.00	.00	.24[d]
80. Clinging (0=23)	-.04	-.20[d]	-.18[c]	-.05	.12	-.15	.07	.07	.36[f]
81. Overt anxiety (0=36)	.01	-.20[d]	-.17[c]	-.06	.15[c]	-.14	.00	.00	.42[f]
82. Unverifiable somatic complaints (0=40)	.06	-.24[d]	-.20[d]	-.10	.15[c]	-.16[c]	.02	.02	.40[f]
83. Attention seeking (0=55)	-.14	-.17[c]	-.07	.05	.12	-.17[c]	.14	.14	.34[f]
84. Extreme compliance (0=12)	-.04	-.14	-.19[c]	-.19[c]	.08	-.14	.15[c]	.15[c]	.30[e]
85. Other: describe (0=12)	-.02	-.05	.04	.05	.14	.00	.21[d]	.21[d]	.29[e]

[a] 0 = number of times that assessment criterion was reported in 123 assessments.
[b] N = number of times the diagnosis was a conclusion judgment in 123 assessments.
[c] Level of significance at or greater than 0.05.
[d] Level of significance at or greater than 0.01.
[e] Level of significance at or greater than 0.001.
[f] Level of significance at or greater than 0.0001.

Results

If a particular assessment criterion is relevant to a particular diagnosis, there should be a positive correlation between the two. Moreover, if the criterion is specific to that diagnosis, their correlation should be greater in value than those of the same criterion with other diagnoses. Table 1 shows that this pattern is true for all the assessment criteria placed with the following seven diagnoses on an a priori basis: rational anger state, aggressive coping mode, impulse-dominated state, impulsive coping mode, self-exhaltation state, manipulative coping mode, and dependent coping mode. In the two remaining cases of nursing diagnoses, aggressive response state and subtle obstructive mode, over two thirds of the criteria were more highly positively correlated with the a priori diagnosis than with any other diagnosis. The pattern of correlation of aggressive response state with its associated criteria is similar to that of both aggressive coping mode and impulse-dominated state with the same criteria, although as already noted, the values of the correlations are higher for aggressive response state than for aggressive coping mode or impulse-dominated state in over two thirds of the cases. Specificity of the assessment criteria seems to be somewhat less in the case of aggressive response state than for the remaining eight diagnoses. The data in Table 1 strongly suggest that the assessment criteria are both relevant to and specfic to the a priori nursing diagnoses.

Limitations

The criteria were presented with an a priori diagnostic heading and definition. However, the instructions requested global diagnoses regardless of the a priori headings (see Boxes 2 and 3). The placement of an a priori diagnosis on the same page as the assessment criteria may have encouraged the nurses to pair that diagnosis with the criteria to a greater extent than would be true if the criteria had not been so presented. In judging the incidence of false positives and false negatives, the global diagnoses were treated as correct decisions although they were not confirmed independently.

Suggestions for further research

A Q-sorting technique could be used to verify that nurses would classify the assessment criteria with the a priori diagnoses, given no prompting by the typography of the instrument. If the Q-sorted classifications of the criteria and diagnoses parallel those presented in the original instrument, there would be little reason to believe that the strong association of criteria and a priori diagnoses reflects the typographic structure of the instrument.

A study of nurses' ratings of criteria and diagnoses on the basis of videotapes of clinical simulations could be used to study the consistency of nurses in applying the assessment criteria and the nursing diagnoses under uniform conditions.

SUMMARY AND CONCLUSIONS

Gordon (1982) calls for the involvement of all professional nurses in identifying, developing, and testing diagnostic categories. This paper has presented one method of doing this. An approach using literature and clinical experience posited nine nursing diagnoses related to anger and aggression. These posited definitions and criteria were used by 26 nurses to conduct 123 client assessments in acute inpatient psychiatry.

Cross-tabulation of each diagnosis with each of the 85 assessment criteria indicated statistical support for each of the nine a priori diagnoses: rational anger state, aggressive response state, aggressive coping mode, impulse-dominated state, impulsive coping mode, self-exhaltation state, manipulative coping mode, subtle obstructive mode, and dependent coping mode. The project generated data to use in considering the new diagnoses and indicated that further research in this area would be useful.

REFERENCES

American Psychiatric Association: Diagnostic and statistical manual of mental disorders, ed. 3, Washington, D.C., 1980, The Association.

Bandura, A.: Aggression: a social learning analysis, Englewood Cliffs, N.J., 1973, Prentice-Hall, Inc.

Bandura, A.: Learning and behavioral series of aggression. In Kutash, I., and others, eds.: Violence: perspectives on murder and aggression, San Francisco, 1978, Jossey-Bass, Inc., Publishers.

Brown, M., and Fowler, G.: Psychodynamic nursing, ed. 3, Philadelphia, 1966, W.B. Saunders Co.

Bursten, B.: The manipulator: a psychoanalytic view, New Haven, Conn., 1973, Yale University Press.

Carney, F.: Treatment of the aggressive patient. In Madden, D., and Lion, J., eds.: Rage, hate, assault, and other forms of violence, New York, 1976, Spectrum Publications, Inc.

Coleman, J.: Abnormal psychology and modern life, ed. 4, Glenview, Ill. 1972, Scott, Foresman & Co.

Cuthbert, B.: Switch off, tune in, turn on, Am. J. Nurs. **69**(6):1206, 1969.

Gordon, M.: Historical perspective: the national conference group for classification of nursing diagnoses (1978, 1980). In Kim, M.J., and Moritz, D.A., eds.: Classification of nursing diagnoses: proceedings of the third and fourth national conferences, New York, 1982, McGraw-Hill Book Co.

Group for the Advancement of Psychiatry: Toward therapeutic care, ed. 2, New York, 1970, Group for the Advancement of Psychiatry.

Gruber, K., and Schniewind, H.: Letting anger work for you, Am. J. Nurs. **76**(9):1450, 1976.

Karshner, J.: The application of social learning theory of aggression, Perspect. Psychiatr. Care **16**(5-6):223, 1978.

Kiening, M.: Hostility. In Carlson, C., ed.: Behavioral concepts and nursing intervention, Philadelphia, 1970, J.B. Lippincott Co.

Kyes, J., and Hofling, C.: Basic psychiatric concepts in nursing, ed. 3, Philadelphia, 1974, J.B. Lippincott Co.

Loomis, M.: Nursing management of acting-out behavior, Perspect. Psychiatr. Care **8**(4):168, 1970.

Luetje, V.: The person whose behavior is abusive. In Murray, R., and Huelskoetter, M., eds.: Psychiatric-mental health nursing: giving emotional care, Englewood Cliffs, N.J., 1983, Prentice-Hall, Inc.

Matheney, R., and Topalis, M.: Psychiatric nursing, ed. 4, St. Louis, 1965, The C.V. Mosby Co.

Mereness, D.A., and Karnosh, L.J.: Essentials of psychiatric nursing, ed. 7, St. Louis, 1966, The C.V. Mosby Co.

Moritz, D.A., Understanding anger, Am. J. Nurs. **78**(1):81, 1978.

Moyer, K.E.: The physiology of aggression and the implication for aggression control. In Singer, J., ed.: The control of aggression and violence, New York, 1971, Academic Press, Inc.

Rogers, C.: Characteristics of a helping relationship, Can. Ment. Health **27**(suppl.):1, 1962.

Rouslin, S.: Developmental aggression and its consequences, Perspect. Psychiatr. Care. **8**(4):170, 1975.

Scherer, K., Abeles, R., and Fischer, C.: Human aggression and conflict, Englewood Cliffs, N.J., 1975, Prentice-Hall, Inc.

Sundeen, S., and others: Nurse-client interaction: implementing the nursing process, St. Louis, 1976, The C.V. Mosby Co.

Wolfgang, M.: Violence in the family. In Kutash, I., and others, eds.: Violence: perspectives on murder and aggression, San Francisco, 1978, Jossey-Bass, Inc., Publishers.

I am nursing diagnosis . . . color me DSM-III green: a comparative analysis of nursing diagnoses and diagnostic categories of the *Diagnostic and Statistical Manual III* of the American Psychiatric Association

MARGA S. COLER, R.N., Ed.D.

The prevailing problem of the application of nursing diagnoses in the clinical setting continues to be overcoming inertia. Often what seems ideal to academic nurses remains but a theoretical exercise to the service sector of nursing. To facilitate the introduction of nursing diagnoses into the clinical area, it seems logical to link them with an already existing protocol—the *Diagnostic and Statistical Manual III* (DSM-III) of the American Psychiatric Association (1980). As with nursing diagnoses, DSM-III has been in a developmental stage since the 1970s. Both are products of our computer culture. Because every consumer of traditional mental health services must receive a DSM-III–based diagnosis, a synergism between nursing diagnoses and DSM-III diagnoses might be feasible. Before such an implementation, however, an assessment of the interrelationship between the systems is indicated.

The DSM-III was prepared to compensate for some of the gross deficiencies of the second manual, which did not address a theoretic framework for the comprehension of nonorganic mental disorders. It was long believed that diagnostic categories required a greater reliability factor. The meaning of certain terms had become diffuse. Research data were inconsistent with the taxonomy of classification. Most importantly, diagnostic labels were being applied indiscriminately, arbitrarily, and inconsistently, which led not only to errors in diagnosing but also to errors in the prescription of medications and treatments.

Consequently, the DSM-III used the input of 14 advisory committees of different clinical expertise. This approach was then supplemented by comments from allied professional groups. Disease classifications were presented over 4 years to local, national, and international groups for critical review and consideration. A special conference was held in St. Louis in June 1976 to examine DSM-III in midstream. Following a series of field trials, the review process culminated in a 2-year project sponsored by the National Institutes

☐The author wishes to acknowledge with graditude the contribution of the Class of 1982, the first nursing majors to graduate from the College of Our Lady of the Elms.

of Mental Health in which thousands of patients were examined in over 200 facilities by clinicians using successive drafts of the DSM-III. Reliability was assessed by "having pairs of clinicians make independent diagnostic judgments of several hundred patients" (APA, 1980, p. 5).

As a result of this project, each DSM-III category was associated with a behavior or set of behaviors representing a disability in one or several areas of functioning. The manual does not classify individuals but only maladaptations that individuals may have at a given time.

DSM-III is descriptive only and leaves the analysis of etiology to others. It is also atheoretic with regard to pathophysiology except in cases in which both etiology and pathophysiology are "well established and therefore included in the definition of that disorder" (APA, 1980, p. 7). It does however have a mechanism for describing the statement of prognosis and severity, which appears in the fifth digit of the diagnostic classification number. Aside from this number, DSM-III diagnoses are defined along five axes (APA, 1980):

> Axis I is for the clinical diagnoses and other conditions on which treatment is focused except for categories specified for the second axis.
>
> Axis II is for personality and developmental disorders.
>
> Axis III is for medical and physical conditions that are not pertinent to the psychiatric state.
>
> Axis IV is for the severity of psychosocial stressors in the client's life.
>
> Axis V is an indicator of the highest level of functioning attained during the year preceding the dysfunction.

An individual, then, can have an Axis I diagnosis with or without a notation on Axis II or Axis III, or an Axis II disorder without the presence of pathology in either Axes I or III, or both. Although nursing is presently not defining axes nor thinking in that direction, such a protocol might be an interesting concept to pursue. Nursing diagnosis, on the other hand, consists of a problem statement, amplitude, and etiology. It began as a mere discussion by McManus in 1950 (Gordon, 1978), rapidly gaining momentum toward its present stage at the First National Conference on the classification of Nursing Diagnoses in the early 1970s. Its history was comprehensively cited by Gordon (1982) at the Fourth National Conference. Table 1 illustrates the similarity of the developmental process in both systems in spite of the difference in terminology.

As is common in professional diagnostic practice, all diagnoses evolve from what Soares (1978) called an "invariable component," in this case, problem solving, which is a requisite for the derivation of all diagnoses, be they nursing or medical. Problem solving begins with the collection of data and becomes the guide for the entire process. The variable aspects, one of which is the diagnostic statement, are specific to individual professions. It is at this

TABLE 1   **The derivation of diagnoses—nursing diagnoses compared with DSM-III diagnostic categories**

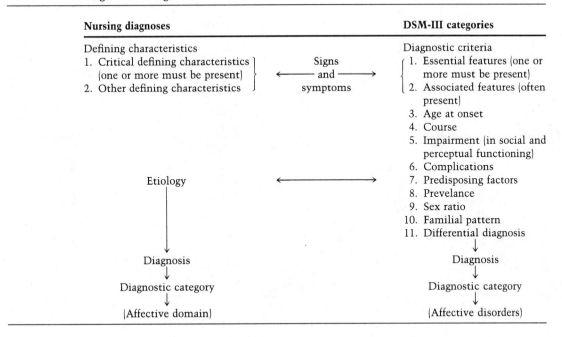

Nursing diagnoses	DSM-III categories
Defining characteristics 1. Critical defining characteristics (one or more must be present) 2. Other defining characteristics	Diagnostic criteria 1. Essential features (one or more must be present) 2. Associated features (often present) 3. Age at onset 4. Course 5. Impairment (in social and perceptual functioning) 6. Complications 7. Predisposing factors 8. Prevelance 9. Sex ratio 10. Familial pattern 11. Differential diagnosis
Etiology	
Diagnosis	Diagnosis
Diagnostic category	Diagnostic category
(Affective domain)	(Affective disorders)

juncture that the autonomous aspect of nursing (Soares, 1978) becomes self-actualizing.

Table 2 is profession-specific representation of the diagnostic process. The nursing diagnosis affective domain (Fredette and O'Connor, 1979), which is contained in most DSM-III categories was selected. The DSM-III order has been rearranged to conform with the format of nursing diagnoses proposed at the Fourth National Conference. The similarities are evident, and it is this intertwining of nursing diagnoses with DSM-III categories that prompted this study. The purpose of the study was to correlate identified nursing diagnoses specific to psychiatric–mental health nursing with the diagnostic categories of the DSM-III and to establish a measure of validity for the diagnoses in psychiatric–mental health nursing.

METHODOLOGY

The identification process consisted of three components. The first two consisted of student designations of nursing diagnoses in the classroom and in the clinical setting. The third component was similar to the first component

TABLE 2　Nursing diagnosis (affective domain) applied to selected DSM-III categories

Nursing diagnosis	DSM-III diagnoses			
	Affective disorders	Schizophrenia		Organic mental disorders
Affective domain	Bipolar disorder, manic depression	Schizophrenia, residual	Schizophrenia, paranoid	Dementia
Coping, ineffective, individual	**Diagnostic criteria**			
Etiology				
Situational crises (E1)	Frequently following psychosocial stressor →		Onset later in life than other schizophrenia	CNS infection CNS degeneration
Maturational crises (E2)				
Personal vulnerability (E3)	←—— Endogenous ——→ ?Genetic	←— Premorbid personality —→ ←— Endogenous —→ ?Genetic Continuing evidence of illness		Anxiety Depression
Defining characteristics	**Features**			
Verbalization of inability to cope or inability to ask for help*	Predominant mood ↑, >, irritable† Rapid shifts to anger or depression	←Poverty of content of speech†→		Disturbances of higher cortical† function
	Slowed thinking† ↓Concentration Suicidal ideation		Grandiosity† Persecution†	
Inability to meet role expectations	Inflated self-esteem† Delusions	Bizarre delusions† Inappropriate affect†		Impaired abstract thinking
Inability to meet basic needs	↓Need for sleep† Hyperactivity†	←— Illogical thinking† — Bizarre hallucinations†		Memory impairment†
	Feeling of worthlessness† ↓Appetite† Insomnia/hyper-somnia†			
Inability to solve problems*	Flight of ideas† Distractability† (CC4) Hallucinations	←—— Incoherence† —→		Impaired judgment
	Loss of energy†			
Alteration in social participation	High potential for unrecognized pain-ful consequences†	←— Disorganized behavior† — ←— Social isolation† —→		
	Psychomotor agitation or retardation† Loss of interest†			

*Critical defining characteristics for nursing diagnosis.
†Essential features for DSM-III diagnosis.

of the student project, but involved registered nurses employed by our affiliate agencies. The relationships between student-classroom, student–clinical–DSM-III, and the registered nurse designations were correlated by Spearman rho.

Specifically, this identification began in the classroom following the presentation and discussion of the terminal psychiatric module in an integrated baccalaureate nursing program. Thirty senior students were asked to check those nursing diagnoses on the Fourth National Conference list they believed were most applicable to the consumers of psychiatric–mental health services. The results were tabulated, and the diagnostic list was rearranged in rank order with the most prevalent diagnosis at the top. The list became the vertical column of a comparative grid. The horizontal row constituted the DSM-III categories of the client sample, which was derived from nursing process recordings initiated on two patients by each of 20 students in the psychiatric rotation. The task was to identify at least three nursing diagnoses per individual. These diagnoses were derived from subjective and objective assessment data clustered into functional categories. The nursing process recordings (including identification data and DSM-III diagnoses) were submitted weekly to the faculty clinician. The pertinent information for this study was noted on a data entry form before being transferred to the grid to identify the relationship between (1) the two diagnostic systems, (2) the diagnoses selected in the classroom, and (3) the diagnoses identified clinically. The reliability of the student rankings was assessed by comparing their ranked priorities with those identified by the registered nurses employed in the clinical settings. Eight psychiatric nurses participated in the study.

DATA ANALYSIS

Table 3 indicates that the clinical assessment priorities of the students correlated with the priorities of their classroom speculations ($r_s = 0.63$, $p <$ .001). It may be noted that the highly prioritized nursing diagnoses appear throughout the majority of the medical categories. For instance, the nursing diagnosis *ineffective individual coping* was identified 37 out of 56 times and in all of the DSM-III categories. The second most prevalent clinical nursing diagnosis, *injury, potential for,* was appropriately ranked by the registered nurses but appeared in eleventh rank in the student rankings. This diagnosis was chosen for 25 patients and appeared in all but two of the DSM-III categories. *Thought process, alteration in* was ranked second by the students in class, third by the nurses, and third clinically. This nusing diagnosis, involving 22 of the patients was identified in all but four of the DSM-III categories. The ranks of other identified nursing diagnoses are given in Table 4.

TABLE 3   **Nursing diagnoses as identified through DSM-III categories by senior student nurses**

Nursing diagnoses	Affective disorders					
	Bipolar disorders		Mixed	Major depression	Cyclothymic	Dysthymic
	Manic disorder	Depressed				
Coping, ineffective individual	8	1	1	8	1	3
Thought process, alterations in	8		2	1		1
Self-concept, disturbance in	1	1	3	2	1	2
Sensory perceptual alterations	2		3			1
Sleep pattern disturbance	5		1	4		1
Fear			1		1	3
Coping, ineffective family disabling						
Coping, ineffective family compromised	2			1		1
Violence, potential for	1		2			
Spiritual distress						
Injury, potential for	5		2	6	1	1
Coping, family potential for growth						
Grieving, dysfunctional				2		1
Noncompliance	3		1	2		
Rape-trauma syndrome						
Parenting, alterations in actual						
Parenting, alterations in potential	1			1		
Self-care deficit	2					
Sexual dysfunction						
Diversional activity deficit				1		
Grieving, anticipatory						
Communication, impaired verbal	1			1		1
Role disturbance (TBD)						
Social isolation (TBD)			1		1	
Nutrition, alterations in ↓	1			1		
Nutrition, alterations in ↑						
Nutrition, alterations in: pot. ↑			1			
Home maintenance mgt., impaired	1				1	

Schizophrenic disorders			Organic mental disorders (OMD)		Personality disorders	
Catatonic	Paranoid	Undifferentiated	Degenerative dementia	Substance-induced OMD	Borderline	Total through DSM-III categories
1	6	2	1	1	4	37
1	4	3		2		22
	1			1	1	13
		1	1			8
	1	3	1	1	2	19
1	2				1	9
1	3				1	5
						4
	1	2	1		3	10
	1					1
		3	1	2	4	25
	1			1		2
		1				4
1	1	1				9
						0
		1				1
						2
1	1	1	1	1		7
						0
	1			1		3
						0
1		1				5
						0
1	2	2				7
1	2	1	1			7
	1					1
						1
						2

Continued.

TABLE 3   **Nursing diagnoses as identified through DSM-III categories by senior student nurses—cont'd**

Nursing diagnoses	Affective disorders					
	Bipolar disorders					
	Manic disorder	Depressed	Mixed	Major depression	Cyclothymic	Dysthymic
Memory deficit (TBD)						
Rest activity pattern, ineffective (TBD)						
Knowledge deficit						
Cognitive dissonance (TBD)						
Family dynamics, alterations in (TBD)	1			1		1
Bowel elimination, alterations in						
Fluid volume deficit, actual						
Fluid volume deficit, potential						
Mobility, impaired physical	1			1		
Participation, alteration in ↓						
Growth, potential for, fam.	1					
Cardiac output, alteration in ↓					1	1
Comfort, alteration in			1		1	
Skin integrity, impairment of	1		1			
Urinary elimination						
Breathing pattern, ineffective			1			
Total number of individuals	12	1	3	8	1	5

It may be noted from the data presented in Tables 3 and 4 that there also exists a significant agreement between registered nurse and the student theoretic selections ($R_s = 0.50$, $p < .001$). A missing link at this time is the clinical input from the registered nurses, important because of the positive correlation between theoretic options of registered nurses and student clinical selections ($r_s = 0.48$, $p < .001$).

The signficance of the study is that it serves to demonstrate the overlap of the diagnostic labels of nursing and psychiatry. The importance of the collaborative component in the clinical specialty is documented in the literature of the professions, including the American Nurses' Association's *Statement on Psychiatric and Mental Health Nursing Practice* (ANA, 1976). The diffusion of boundaries, however, has left nursing the "weaker" collaborator with no secure base of reference for nursing input, which has often been confined

Schizophrenic disorders			Organic mental disorders (OMD)		Personality disorders	
Catatonic	Paranoid	Undifferentiated	Degenerative dementia	Substance-induced OMD	Borderline	Total through DSM-III categories
						0
						0
	2	1				3
						0
1						4
1						
						1
		1				1
						0
						2
						0
						1
		2				4
						2
						2
		1				1
						1
1	8	6	2	3	5	55

to ideas, feelings, and intuitive hunches (Soares, 1978). The strong interaction of specific nursing diagnoses with the already identified, published, and used medical nomenclature can provide such a reference base. For example, the majority of psychiatric–mental health settings, be they inpatient or crisis intervention, operate within a nurse-mediated and nurse-implemented therapeutic milieu (Devine, 1981). Integrated with the accountable and requisite DSM-III diagnoses, nursing diagnoses can become essential components contributing to patient growth and to the foundation for standardized interventions. These interventions, in turn, can become a reservoir from which individual adaptations might be tailored toward specific DSM-III categories. Finally, whereas the DSM-III diagnoses remain throughout a patient/client's contact with an agency, a nursing diagnosis could vary with changes in patient/client status (Purushotham, 1981).

TABLE 4   Comparative rankings of nursing diagnoses

Nursing diagnoses	Student rankings—classroom (prioritization)	RN rankings—classroom (prioritization)	Student rankings—clinical setting (patient/client assessment)
Coping, ineffective individual	1.5	11	1
Thought process, alterations in	1.5	11	3
Self-concept, disturbance in	4.5	5.5	5
Sensory perceptual alterations	4.5	5.5	10
Sleep pattern disturbance	4.5	5.5	4
Fear	4.5	15.5	8
Coping, ineffective family disabling	7	15.5	14
Coping, ineffective family compromised	8	11	18
Violence, potential for	9.5	1	8
Spiritual distress	9.5	15.5	31.5
Injury, potential for	11	11	2
Coping, family potential for growth	12	21	24
Grieving, dysfunctional	13.5	5.5	18
Noncompliance	13.5	34.5	8
Rape-trauma syndrome	15	21	40
Parenting, alterations in actual	17.5	21	31.5
Parenting, alterations in potential	17.5	26.5	24
Self-care deficit	17.5	15.5	11.5
Sexual dysfunction	17.5	5.5	40
Diversional activity deficit	20.5	21	14
Grieving, anticipatory	20.5	5.5	40
Communication, impaired verbal	23	5.5	14
Role disturbance (TBD)	23	26	40
Social isolation (TBD)	23	26	11.5
Nutrition, alterations in ↓	25	15.5	6
Nutrition, alterations in ↑	35	21	31.5
Nutrition, alterations in: pot. ↑	26.5	31.5	31.5
Home maintenance mgt., impaired	33	15.5	24
Memory deficit (TBD)	26.5	26.5	40
Rest activity pattern, ineffective (TBD)	34	26.5	40
Knowledge deficit	28.5	31.5	19.5
Cognitive dissonance (TBD)	28.5	31.5	40
Family dynamics, alterations in (TBD)	30	26.5	18

TABLE 4   Comparative rankings of nursing diagnoses—cont'd

Nursing diagnoses	Student rankings—classroom (prioritization)	RN rankings—classroom (prioritization)	Student rankings—clinical setting (patient/client assessment)
Bowel elimination, alterations in	31	39.5	24
Fluid volume deficit, actual	37	39.5	31.5
Fluid volume deficit, potential	39	39.5	40
Mobility, impaired physical	36	34.5	24
Participation, alteration in ↓	44	39.5	40
Growth, potential for, fam.	43	39.5	31.5
Cardiac output, alteration in ↓	38	39.5	19.5
Comfort, alteration in	31	31.5	24
Skin integrity, impairment of	41	39.5	24
Urinary elimination ↓	40	49.5	31.5
Breathing pattern, ineffective	42	39.5	31.5

Student/client r_s = 0.63 $p<0.001$

Student/RN r_s = 0.50, $p<0.001$

RECOMMENDATIONS

To facilitate acceptance of nursing diagnoses, it is proposed that psychiatric–mental health nursing incorporate the top 10 identified taxonomic labels into admission forms, kardexes, problem lists, and care plans. A printed checklist would facilitate their identification and circumvent the necessity of carrying a list of nursing diagnoses as prescribed by Dossey and Guzzetta (1981). Once printed, the diagnoses would become fixed and less subject to individual variation. A list containing a space designated for individualized patient/client diagnoses would provide the consistent nomenclature discussed by Gebbie (1976). This tactic would provide the substrate for the subsequent phase of standardized interventions collated from a stockpile of client-specific implementations.

These recommendations are currently being implemented in two Massachusetts agencies. In the inpatient unit the students are writing nursing diagnoses on the Kardex. It is encouraging that the diagnoses currently appear intermingled with other "problems." They are no longer erased by the nursing staff. In the crisis agency, it has become necessary to come to grips with who may make nursing diagnoses. In contrast to some of our leaders who contend that nursing diagnoses should remain the task of professional nurses only, I defer to the collaborative element in psychiatric nursing. There exists a viable potential in the use and training of other professional staff to implement these diagnoses. Many of our support and co-workers in mental health have adequate credentials. Other professional staff could be an asset in the establishment of a discrete nursing territory and in the establishment of nursing boundaries.

Nursing diagnoses provide the beginnings of territorialism in a clinical area that has long struggled for a strong professional role image (Coler, 1983). Not only do the data presented mark a step forward in the collaborative process of mental health professions, but they serve as a vehicle for the dissemination of information among nurses within the system. I speak for collaboration in the same breath that I speak for territorialism—I speak for nursing diagnoses colored a DSM-III green.

REFERENCES

American Nurses' Association: Statement on psychiatric and mental health nursing practice, Kansas City, Mo., 1976, The Association.

American Psychiatric Association: Diagnostic and statistical manual of mental disorders (DSM-III), Washington, D.C., 1980, The Association.

Coler, M.: A semiquantitative method to assess role image in nursing through the application of semantics, Manuscript submitted for publication, 1983.

Devine, B.: Therapeutic milieu/milieu therapy: an overview, J. Psychiatr. Nurs. **19**(3):20, 1981.

Dossey, B., and Guzzetta, C.: Nursing diagnosis, Nursing 81 **11**(6):34, 1981.

Fredette, S., and O'Connor, K.: Nursing diagnosis in teaching and curriculum planning, Nurs. Clin. North Am. **14**:541, 1979.

Gebbie, C.: Development of a taxonomy of nursing diagnosis, In Walter, J., and Pardee, G., eds.: Dynamics of problem-oriented approaches: patient care and documentation, Philadelphia, 1976, J.B. Lippincott Co.

Gordon, M.: Nursing diagnoses and diagnostic process. In Chaska, N., ed.: The nursing profession: views through the mist, New York, 1978, McGraw-Hill Book Co.

Gordon, M.: Historical perspective: the national conference group for classification of nursing diagnoses (1978, 1980). In Kim, M.J., and Moritz, D.A., eds.: Classification of nursing diagnoses: proceedings of the third and fourth national conferences, New York, 1982, McGraw-Hill Book Co.

Purushotham, D.: Nursing diagnosis: a vital component of nursing process, Can. Nurs. **77**:46, 1981.

Soares, C.: Nursing and medical diagnoses: a comparison of variant and essential features. In Chaska, N., ed.: The nursing profession: views through the mist, New York, 1978, McGraw-Hill Book Co.

ADDITIONAL READINGS

Feild, L.: The implementation of nursing diagnosis in clinical practice, Nurs. Clin. North Am. **14**:497, 1979.

Gane, D.: Systems/computer application. In Walter, J., and Pardee, G., eds.: Dynamics of problem-oriented approaches: patient care and documentation, Philadelphia, 1976, J.B. Lippincott Co.

A reformulation and methodologic approach to the diagnosis of chronic pain

JACQUELINE D. FORTIN R.N., M.S.

There is a current upsurge of interest in the study of the acute pain experience, stimulated by the work of Melzack and Wall (1965, 1970). The interest, however, does not seem to have a parallel in the chronic pain experience. Yet perusal of the pain literature suggests that the chronic pain experience is far broader in scope than the acute pain experience. As in most conditions of a chronic nature, pathologic mechanisms blend with complex psychosocial experiences to alter personal perceptions and response patterns. Therefore repatterning of the patient with chronic pain can only be understood in a multidimensional context. However, assessment and inquiry in the area of chronic pain have been impeded by ambiguity in terms, inadequate theory development, and methodologic shortcomings. An interim approach suggested here proposes (1) an operational definition, (2) an eclectic theoretic model, and (3) a sequential criterion analysis as a first methodologic step in instrument development.

This discussion deals with both a need and a reality. The need is to examine isomorphic concepts from related disciplines to determine their usefulness to the holistic practice and inquiry of nursing. The reality is that nurses must continue to develop conceptual models at a level of abstraction that will guide clinical practice, further elucidate the uniqueness of nursing, and contribute to theory building.

CONSIDERATIONS IN REFORMULATION

Schwab (1978) critiques the role of theory, particularly borrowed theories, in applied practice. The weakness of theory, he states, results from the "inevitable incompleteness . . . and the partiality of view . . . of its already incomplete subject" (Schwab, 1978, p. 296). He proposes that weaknesses can be brought to light and to some extent resolved by eclectic reformulation. Although the reformulation will itself be incomplete, it may help to resolve the practical problem at hand. However, such an undertaking must be based on (1) clear identification of the problem, (2) evaluation of the theories at hand, (3) reformulation, and (4) evaluation of the reformulation.

The first step requires that the problem and related variables be clearly identified and when possible operationally defined. The second step suggests that theories or models under consideration require evaluation and analysis (Ellis, 1968; Hardy, 1974) to determine what each has done to "disconnect it

from related (areas) and give it the appearance of an independent whole"
(Schwab, 1978, p. 298). The third step is to predetermine which concepts
central to nursing (that is, man coextensive or interacting with the environment), if juxtaposed with the theory or reformulated into the theory, lend the
most pragmatic utility or explanatory potential. The fourth step requires
identifying the purpose, the scope, and the limits of the reformulated model
as well as its biases to determine its usefulness across and within the subdis-
ciplines of nursing. In short, whatever phenomena we view we tend to do so
from our own conceptual reference. Thus as Hardy (1978) cautions, our biases
may permit us to attribute meaning where it does not exist. However,
through careful analysis of borrowed theories and models and cautious development of eclectic approaches, we may shed light on some of the problems
that confront clinical nursing practice. The chronic pain experience is one
such problem.

TOWARD A DEFINITION OF THE CHRONIC PAIN EXPERIENCE

Ambiguity in definitions of chronic pain arises from the failure to operationally and conceptually distinguish between the concepts of chronic pain as a
psychosensory stimulus condition and the chronic pain experience, a dynamic blending of the pain sensation in the context of person-environment
interaction. This idea is a departure from the traditional acute pain (sensory-
response) model and suggests instead that the chronic pain experience is a
sensory-transactive process. The current literature and theoretic and empirical evidence support the latter view.

Despite current recognition that acute and chronic pain experiences are
very different, there is a scarcity of theoretic definitions and empirical evidence to guide research in this area. Therefore to provide a rationale for the
use of an eclectic theoretic approach, I will briefly contrast the acute and
chronic pain experiences, review the gate control theory of pain, and examine
the psychologic dimensions from three theoretic frameworks: intrapsychic,
situational, and interactional.

THE EXPERIENCE OF CHRONIC PAIN

Compared with short-term pain episodes that lend themselves more readily
to a sensory reactive model, the chronic pain experience reflects a dynamic
composite of physiologic and psychosocial variability. The pattern of response seems to arise from the interaction of the two factors. Thus both sensory mechanisms and environmental influences mold the experience of
chronic pain.

Eland (1978, p. 430) describes chronic pain most poignantly: "The world
of chronic pain is truly a living hell where, little by little, people are de-

stroyed until they hardly recognize their former selves." Loss of sleep, disinterest in food, overmedication, and lack of activity lead to progressive physical deterioration (Bonica, 1980). Eventually the debilitating effects of the chronic pain experience and loss of coping reserves alter the individual's perceptions, personality, and social functioning. As the person changes, the environment to which he responds changes; that is, personal variability in pain sensation and psychophysiologic responses become intrinisically woven into the situational milieu. Problems of altered self-esteem, social identity, changes in roles and social interaction, and the responses that feed back into the problems, depression, anxiety, and irritability become integral to the chronic pain experience. Thus attempts to explain the chronic pain experience outside the environmental context in which it occurs distort empirical reality and lead to separate investigation of sensory experiences and behavioral responses. The approaches fragment person-environment interaction and thus obscure a knowledge of the whole.

In an effort to determine how the sensory mechanisms might interact with psychosocial variables, two theoretic constructs are reviewed here: pain sensation and self-concept. The first construct is exemplified in the psychophysiologic model proposed by Melzack and Wall (1970). The second construct, self-concept, provides a representative example of psychosocial interaction. A holistic approach to the inquiry of chronic pain experience might best be served by juxtaposing two theoretic approaches: the gate control theory (Melzack and Wall, 1970) and an interactionist model. Juxtaposing of two models allows each to maintain its own integrity. From a systems perspective this approach provides a mechanism from which each system, psychophysiologic and interactional, can be examined as well as the relationships and interactions at the boundaries.

THE PSYCHOPHYSIOLOGIC ASPECTS OF PAIN

Over a decade ago Melzack and Wall (1965, 1970) offered an explanation of the neurophysiologic events that may occur in the modulation of clinical pain. Unlike other sensory theorists, they recognize that psychologic determinants interact with sensory mechanisms to modulate the transmission of neural impulses before they are consciously perceived as pain. Their goal was simply to establish a relationship between pain perception and the underlying physiologic processes thought to initiate that perception. The purpose here, however, is not to explicate the neurologic mechanisms of the gate control theory but rather to clarify the postulate that higher nervous system functions modulate sensory input (Melzack and Casey, 1968).

The key assumption of the gate control theory of pain proposed by Melzack and Wall (1965) is that nociceptive information is repeatedly modulated, filtered, and abstracted by a neurologic "gating mechanism" as it ascends toward the brain. In part this modulation is the result of descending influences from neurologic activity in the brain that may open or close the gate. More specifically, neural information delivered at the time of sensory input is postulated to (1) "prime" selective brain processes (that is, memories, preset response strategies) so that they may more effectively interpret information arriving over slower conducting pathways and (2) influence, by means of efferent fibers, the gating mechanism. However, general arousal states such as anxiety or excitement may open or close the gate, respectively, to all input. It is important to recognize that these activities are proposed to take place below the level of awareness; thus they do not give rise to pain experience. In short, the cognitive, affective, and sensory dimensions of pain are believed to interact below the level of awareness to influence motor mechanisms responsible for the characteristic overt responses to pain. Put another way, nociceptive information traveling over neural pathways does not mark the beginning of the pain process. As Melzack and Dennis (1978, p.1) state: "Stimulation produces neural signals that enter an active nervous sytem that . . . is already the substrate of past experience, culture, anxiety, and so forth."

In addition, the theory suggests that a relative balance exists between presumably nonpainful impulses carried in large-diameter fibers, which act to close the gate, and potentially painful impulses in small-diameter fibers, which open the gate. In summary the modulating properties of cells that make up the "gate" are influenced by two modes: the activity in small- and large-diameter fibers and the descending influences from the brain (Crue and others, 1980; Melzack and Dennis, 1978).

The ability of this theory to lend a theoretic basis to a variety of psychologic (for example, anxiety reduction, distraction, placebo, suggestion) and sensory (for example, massage, acupuncture, and electrical stimulation) research and therapy attests to its pragmatic adequacy in the area of pain. However, of primary interest to this presentation is the scope of the gate control theory. Essentially the theory characterizes pain as a sensation arising from the dynamic interaction of neural mechanisms below the level of awareness. Although Melzack and Wall (1965, 1970) and Melzack and Dennis (1978) acknowledge the role of simultaneous psychosocial events, memories, and so on, the purpose of their theory is not to explicate this dimension but rather the physiologic processes underlying pain perception and response. Therefore development of a more comprehensive model requires an eclectic approach. Toward the development of an eclectic model, one dimension of the personality is reviewed here to suggest the potential viability of an interactionist approach.

A PSYCHOSOCIAL PERSPECTIVE

In the review of chronic pain, altered self-concept is representative of the intricate psychologic phenomena associated with the experience and an example of current theorizing and research. Three variations of the self-construct are pertinent here: (1) self-concept as an intrapsychic phenomena, (2) self-concept molded by environmental contingencies, and (3) self-identity arising from person-environment interaction (Cartwright, 1980).

The presupposition of intrapsychic theories is that the pain experience is organized around personal attributions, self-concept, and trait characteristics. Elton, Stanley, and Burrows (1978) delineate these as punishment, anger, guilt, fear, and doubts concerning one's ability to cope. Other authors suggest that pain response patterns evolve from a neurotic personality (Bond, 1971 Robinson and others, 1972). Based on a study of rheumatoid arthritis patients, Robinson and co-workers coined the phrase "R.A. personality" to describe the neurotic tendencies. Although a subsequent study failed to support their earlier findings, the term persists in the literature. In sharp contrast, social learning theorists contend that behavior is a function of social contingencies in the environment. From this perspective, Wooley, Blackwell, and Winget (1978) argue that the characteristic helplessness, hostility, manipulativeness, and reluctance to assume responsibility seen in chronic pain patients is shaped and reinforced by situational antecedents. Similarly, Craig (1978) maintains that pain behavior is in part influenced by social modeling.

In a direct criticism of situational behaviorism and social learning assumptions, Bowers (1973) presents a cogent argument for an interactionist perspective. He chides trait theorists for ignoring situational contingencies and criticizes the situationists for their preoccupation with metaphysical and methodologic issues that obscure reality. Quoting Wachtel, Bowers (1973, p. 330) notes that "situations [are] largely of one's own making and . . . characteristic of one's personality." Thus he proposes that understanding of the personality arises from the theoretic blending of inferential and empirical observations of the person and the situation. One way to examine this idea is to look at self-identity in the context of one's social identity.

Self-identity is defined by Pruss (1975) as a pattern that arises out of interactions with others in which each person potentially alters the perception of the others and himself in the process. In contrast, social identity can be viewed as a set of preconceived expectations that determne the nature of social interactions (Lorber, 1967). As such, it represents a classification system that provides the quick reference categories that allow us to anticipate social contingencies operating in the situation (Goffman, 1963).

The viability of an interactionist approach for the investigation of chronic pain has been suggested in a few studies, although many of these discuss the broader issue of chronic illness. For example, Armentrout (1979) reported that chronic pain patients had significantly lower self-concepts than general medical patients. He concluded that this finding reflected several interactive influences, namely, alterations in physical ability, family patterns, and occupation. Coulton (1979) found that chronically ill patients perceived a discrepancy between themselves and their environment on several dimensions. Subjects in this study described unmet needs for affiliation, social interaction, and support and difficulty in meeting expectations of self and others. Hopper (1981) cited loss of employment, limited mobility, dependence, impotence, and other negative life changes as factors affecting both self-identity and social identity. She contends that these changes may be most problematic in familial and intimate relationships, where they are most apparent.

Ablon (1981, p. 5) reports that when social identity is perceived as different and that "differentness is negatively valued [it may be] perceived as deviance" and lead to stereotyping. The notion of deviance may seem somewhat harsh, but examples appear in the literature and research on chronic pain. Although disfigurement is not prevalent, life changes that alter social and occupational roles may act collectively to discredit the chronic pain patient in social interaction. Armentrout (1979) paraphrased Frank's findings (1977, p. 520), which showed that "Physicians, nurses and the general public all have negative stereotypes of the chronic pain patient." Thus chronic pain is not an individual concern; "it affects and is affected by the attitudes of the family, society . . . and the health team" (Callahan and others, 1966, p. 895). Notably, however, there is a scarcity of attention given to the potential positive aspects for adaptation or rehabilitation (Adams and Lindeman, 1974; Turk and others, 1980).

In summary, the idea that self-perception is altered by the chronic pain experience is supported in this limited sampling from a variety of conceptual positions. Changes in pattern and organization of self are influenced by changes in both the internal and external environment through a transactive process. Therefore it might be argued that the difference between self-concept (personal) and self-identity (person-environment interaction) is the difference between conceptual invention and empirical reality. Although operationally justified, intrapsychic and situational approaches bring about premature closure, creating gaps in our knowledge of experiences.

TOWARD A REFORMULATION

The purpose here is to examine the model (dimensions of the pain experience) proposed by Melzack and Wall (1970) to determine its adequacy in guiding nursing practice and research in the chronic pain experience and to suggest an eclectic model that may facilitate nursing assessment, intervention, and inquiry. The following discussion is based on the premise of Rogers

(1970) that both man and environment are four-dimensional energy fields characterized by pattern and organization. The assumption is made that knowledge of the whole may be derived from examination of concepts and relations (the parts) taken collectively. All events and experiences are recognized as inseparable from and parts of larger wholes. Three assumptions of the work of Melzack and co-workers are accepted a priori: stimuli enter an active nervous system; in part, cognitive and higher central nervous system activities take place below the level of awareness; and these activities influence the pain experience.

The model, dimensions of the pain experience (Melzack and Wall, 1970), proposes that the system's action (response) stems mainly from internal psychophysiologic forces. The importance of the personal sensory experience is not denied. It is argued, however, that exclusion of the person-environment transactions prohibits adequate explanation of the behaviors associated with chronic pain. Therefore it is suggested that for this model to be maximally useful to nursing, its structure must lend itself to holistic considerations. One resolution is to take an eclectic approach to reformulation of the existing model—a reformulation that allows us to explain the interactional and transactional processes that influence the pain experience. Interaction is defined here as "process of perception and communication" (King, 1981, p. 145), whereas transaction refers to the ongoing relationship of person-environment in which each alters the other and itself in the process (repatterning).

For clarity in articulation, the environment of the person is arbitrarily defined as four simultaneously interacting fields: experiential, personal-social, social-cultural, and universal. The experiential field encompasses the internal environment of the person and the immediate external energy field. It is viewed from Lewin's field theory perspective as expanding and contracting and changing in permeability and density at the boundaries. Thus the boundaries act as a "gating" mechanism in the flow of psychic energy. It is postulated that the experiential field is in constant and simultaneous interaction with all other fields but varies in openness to them. The purpose of this distinction is to facilitate assessment of interaction at the boundaries, (that is, social-self-identity). This model, however, is not accurately depicted by the traditional, sensory-reactive (Beecher, 1965; Johnson, 1972; Melzack and Wall, 1965) model of acute pain.

Based on the assumption that the syntax of theory determines the way in which substantive knowledge is used (Schwab, 1964; Whall, 1980), the model might be more comprehensively defined as an integrated pattern of sensory, sentient, and interactive components. Sensory refers to the quality and intensity of the pain sensation. Sentience refers to the motivational and affective qualities of the experience. Interactive refers to the simultaneous interaction between the individual and the environment. It is suggested that in the experience of chronic pain, these forces act collectively to repattern the person and the environment in a transactional process.

In summary, the eclectic reformulation juxtaposes a transactional model and the pain dimensional model. Thus repatterning arises from the blending of psychosocial forces with those of the somatosensory system. However, the "cement" that brings the two models together has yet to be clearly formulated. Interactional approaches are rudimentary and lack adequate instrument development. Thus explication of experiences can best be served by moving along both routes: theory development and research. This discussion proposes one approach to instrument development: criterion analysis.

CRITERION ANALYSIS

Recently, Turk and others (1980) have suggested the use of a behavior analytic model (Goldfried and D'Zurilla, 1969) for the investigation of specific clinical problems. It is the premise of Turk and co-workers that each clinical entity poses a distinct array of problems that require different modes of response, adaptation, and management. The behavior analytic approach facilitates the examination of the individual's response to a clinical problem in the context of the environment to which they are responding. "The model consists of three stages: criterion analysis, instrument development, and assessment application" (Turk and others, 1980, p. 36). It is the first phase, criterion analysis, that is of interest to us in further exploring the experience of chronic pain. This phase is "comprised of three interrelated phases: problem identification, response enumeration, and response evaluation" (Turk and others, 1980, p. 36).

The first phase, problem identification, focuses on the collection of a wide range of data, gathered from several sources, across settings, and using a variety of techniques, for example, self-report, diary, and participant observation. The data gathered by this technique points up problems that are transient, short-term, or static and are sampled from a population that represents different periods in the sequence of the experience, for example, recently diagnosed. Furthermore, data collection is not limited to the individual but encompasses significant others, for example, family, health care providers, over time, and across settings. Commonly identified problems may then be clustered into categories and tested to determine their actual occurrence in the population.

The second phase, response enumeration, is designed to collect samples of coping strategies, feelings, and overt and covert behaviors used to modulate responses when problems, identified in the initial phase, are encountered. Whether the responses are adaptive or detrimental depends, in part, on the individual's "cognitive appraisal" (Cohen and Lazarus, 1979) of the situational demand and the resources they have to meet them. Thus a response that is adaptive for one person may not be for another (Turk and others, 1980).

The third phase, response evaluation, is conducted to determine the relative effectiveness of the responses elicited in Phase 2. Information concerning the efficacy of these responses in promoting a high level of adaptation is determined by sampling another group of patients and health care providers. According to Turk and others (1980), this three-stage approach facilitates the development of an assessment framework from which multiple treatment alternatives may be identified and applied to specific cases.

The importance of indivdual variability has been brought out in recent investigations. In a review of studies, Turk and others (1980) found that characteristically there is a wide range of variability in individual responses to the same clinical diagnosis. Similar attendant problems have been described from severe and incapacitating to mildly disrupting. Criterion analysis provides a mechanism for examining both the adjustive demands and coping strategies used by persons in specific clinical populations. Knowledge of why some people adapt well when others do not will help us to devise growth-producing interventions.

In addition to providing an assessment framework, the behavior analytic approach yields data that may be used to formulate instruments to test specific hypotheses. More importantly, it may help to reduce the incongruence between the assumptions of health care providers and researchers and issues the patients see as most relevant (see, for example, studies by Bond and Pilowsky, 1966; Jacox, 1980). However, the collection of voluminous data outside a theoretic framework will severely limit the explanatory value of the findings.

Establishing lists of common problems and response patterns may be more or less beneficial in devising select treatments. But failure to examine the interrelationships between personal problems and the contextual environment in which they occur impedes our understanding of the process and the experience as a whole. Current research findings in chronic pain management attest to the need for multivariate approaches (Shealy, 1980; Wooley, Blackwell, and Winget, 1978). However, as Leventhal, Meyer, and Nerenz (1980, p. 8) warn, if a discipline develops as a "collection of technologies . . . to be applied to specific practice problems and ignores the underlying explanatory mechanisms, it will fail both as a science and as a problem solving technology."

SUMMARY

This discussion reviews the gate control theory and research findings related to the experience of chronic pain from a variety of theoretic orientations. The purpose of the analysis was to examine the potential for juxtaposing the dimensional model of the pain experience, developed by Melzack and co-workers, and an interactionist approach. It is proposed that an eclectic reformulation provides, at least, an interim model by which the chronic pain experience can be viewed from a holistic perspective. A behavior analytic approach is suggested as one method of exploring complex clinical experiences.

CONCLUSION

Theories and conceptual frameworks are essentially relative. They are based on presuppositions and the conceptual schemes with which the authors set out and encompass their belief in the field in question. Therefore each discipline must examine the assumptions of isomorphic theories from their own unique perspective. The growth of scientific knowledge, however, may be enhanced by the judicious use of eclectic reformulations. Although such an approach does not result in the development of one coherent theory, it does provide guideposts that may be useful in directing research and practice. In addition, crude models can pave the way to more rigorous thinking and dialogue in the profession.

REFERENCES

Ablon, J.: Stigmatized health conditions, Soc. Sci. Med. **15:**5, 1981.

Adams, J.E., and Lindeman, E.: Coping with long-term disability. In Coelho, G.E., Hamburg, D.A., and Adams, J.E., eds.: Coping and adaptation, New York, 1974, Basic Books, Inc.

Armentrout, D.P.: The impact of chronic pain on the self-concept, J. Clin. Psychol. **35:**517, 1979.

Beecher, H.K.: Quantification of the subjective pain experience. In Hoch, P.H., and Zubin, J., eds.: Psychopathology of perception, New York, 1965, Grune & Stratton, Inc.

Bond, M.R., and Pilowsky, I.: Subjective assessment of pain and its relationship to the administration of analgesics in patients with advanced cancer, J. Psychosom. Res. **10:**203, 1966.

Bond, M.R.: The relation of pain to the Eysenck Personality Inventory, Cornell Medical Index, and Whiteley Index of Hypochondriosis, Br. J. Psychiatry **119:**671, 1971.

Bonica, J.J.: Cancer pain. In Bonica, J.J., ed.: Pain, New York, 1980, Raven Press.

Bowers, K.S.: Situationism in psychology: an analysis and a critique, Psychol. Rev. **80:**307, 1973.

Callahan, E.M., and others: The "sick role" in chronic illness: some reactions, J. Chron. Dis. **19:**883, 1966.

Cartwright, D.S.: Exploratory analyses of verbally stimulated imagery of the self, J. Ment. Imag. **4:**1, 1980.

Cohen, F., and Lazarus, R.S.: Coping with the stresses of illness. In Stone, G.C., and others, eds.: Health psychology—a handbook, San Francisco, 1979, Jossey-Bass, Inc., Publishers.

Coulton, C.: A study of person-environment fit among the chronically ill, Soc. Work Health Care **58:**5, 1979.

Craig, K.D.: Social modeling influences on pain. In Sternbach, R.A., ed.: The psychology of pain, New York, 1978, Raven Press.

Crue, B.L., and others: The continuing crisis in pain research. In Smith, W.L., Merskey, H., and Gross, S.C., eds.: Pain: meaning and management, New York, 1980, SP Medical and Scientific Books.

Eland, J.M.: Living wth pain, Nurs. Outlook **26:**430, 1978.

Ellis, R.: Characteristics of significant theories, Nurs. Res. **17:**217, 1968.

Elton, D., Stanley, G.V., and Burrows, G.E.: Self-esteem and chronic pain, J. Psychosom. Res. **22:**25, 1978.

Frank, R.: Pain patients: the observers perspective, unpublished doctoral dessertation, Columbia, Mo., 1977, University of Missouri.

Goffman, E.: Stigma, Englewood Cliffs, N.J., 1963, Prentice-Hall, Inc.

Goldfried, M.R., and D'Zurilla, T.J.: A behavioral analytic model for assessing competence. In Spielberger, C.D., ed.: Current topics in clinical and community psychology, New York, 1969, Academic Press, Inc.

Hardy, M.E.: The nature of theories, Nurs. Res. **23:**100, 1974.

Hardy, M.E.: Perspectives on nursing theory, Adv. Nurs. Sci. **1:**37, 1978.

Hopper, S.: Diabetes as a stigmatized condition: the case of low income clinic patients in the United States, Soc. Sci. Med. **15B:**11, 1981.

Jacox, A.K.: The assessment of pain. In Smith, W.L., Merskey, H., and Gross, S.C., eds.: Pain: meaning and management, New York, 1980, SP Medical and Scientific Books.

Johnson, J.E.: Effects of structuring patients' expectations on their reactions to threatening events, Nurs. Res. **21:**499, 1972.

King, I.M.: A theory for nursing: systems, concepts, process, New York, 1981, John Wiley & Sons, Inc.

Leventhal, H., Meyer, D., and Nerenz, D.: The common sense representation of illness danger. In Rachman, S., ed.: Contributions to medical psychology, vol 2, New York, 1980, Pergamon Press, Inc.

Lorber, J.: Deviance as performance: the case of illness, Soc. Problems **14:**302, 1967.

Melzack, R., and Casey, K.L.: Sensory, motivational, and central control determinants of pain. In Kenshalo, D., ed.: The skin senses, Springfield, Ill., 1968, Charles C. Thomas, Publisher.

Melzack, R., and Dennis, S.G.: Neurophysiological foundations of pain. In Sternbach, R.A., ed.: The psychology of pain, New York, 1978, Raven Press.

Melzack, R., and Wall, P.D.: Pain mechanisms: a new theory, Science **150:**971, 1965.

Melzack, R., and Wall, P.D.: Psychophysiology of pain, Int. Anesthesiol. Clin. **8:**3, 1970.

Pruss, R.C.: An extension of attribution theory, Sociol. Inquiry **45:**3, 1975.

Robinson, H., and others: A psychological study of patients with rheumatoid arthritis and other painful diseases, J. Psychosom. Res. **16:**53, 1972.

Rogers, M.: An introduction to the theoretical basis for nursing, Philadelphia, 1979, F.A. Davis Co.

Schwab, J.J.: Structure of the disciplines: meanings and significances. In Ford, G., ed.: The structure of knowledge and the curriculum, Skokie, Ill., 1964, Rand McNally & Co.

Schwab, J.J.: The practical: a language for curriculum. In Westbury, I., and Wilkof, N.J., eds.: Science, curriculum and liberal education: selected essays, Chicago, 1978, University of Chicago Press.

Shealy, N.C.: Holistic management of chronic pain, Top. Clin. Nurs. **2:**1, 1980.

Turk, D.C., and others: A sequential criterion analysis for assessing coping with chronic illness, J. Human Stress **6:**35, 1980.

Wachtel, P.: Psychodynamics, behavior therapy, and the implacable experimenter: an inquiry into the consistency of personality, J. Abnorm. Psychol. **82:**35, 1973.

Whall, A.L.: Congruence between existing theories of family functioning and nursing theories, Adv. Nurs. Sci. **3:**59, 1980.

Wooley, C., Blackwell, B., and Winget, C.: A learning theory model of chronic illness behavior: theory, treatment, and research, Psychosom. Med. **40:**379, 1978.

ADDITIONAL READING

Space, L.G., and Cromwell, R.L.: Personal constructs among depressed patients, J. Nerv. Ment. Dis. **168:**150, 1980.

Section II **Small group presentation**

Brothers/keepers: ethical implications of the self-care deficit nursing diagnosis

PRISCILLA A. LOGUE, R.N., M.A.

Am I my brother's keeper?
GENESIS 4:9

The idea that individuals have the responsibility to direct and control their own health has important ethical implications for nursing practice. The practice of this responsibility is called self-care and was originally defined in the nursing literature by Orem (1971, pp. 13, 19): "Self care is the practice of activities that individuals personally initiate and perform on their own behalf in maintaining life, health, and well-being. . . . Self care action is practical in orientation. . . . Performing a self care measure involves a decision, a choice."

Ethics involves the scrutiny of human choices based on the assumption of shared moral obligations. The ethical implications of the self-care concept will be examined from the three perspectives inherent in each clinical nursing encounter: the patient, the nurse, and the dominant political society. An individual nurse's value orientation toward the concept of self-care will influence the choices that must be made every day.

THE PATIENT

"Please your majesty," said the knave, "I didn't write it and they can't prove I did; there's no name signed at the end." "If you didn't sign it," said the King, "that only makes the matter worse. You must have meant some mischief, or else you'd have signed your name like an honest man."

Alice's Adventures in Wonderland

If health is regarded as a choice that individuals make, individuals who choose to ignore their self-care responsibilities can be readily identified. In 1980 a recognized nursing diagnosis was *self-care deficit* (Bennett, 1980). It is important to examine potential value judgments implicit in this diagnosis and their ethical implications for nursing intervention. The way in which nurses regard patients with a self-care deficit—as victims who are derelict in their duties or as free agents with infinite resources—will influence the ethical decisions they must make about such patients and will dictate their choice of nursing interventions.

The idea of individual responsibility for one's own health is not new. Butler (1927, p. 88) envisioned a system of justice for individuals who did not take care of themselves:

> Prisoner at the bar, you have been accused of the great crime of labouring under pulmonary tuberculosis and after an impartial trial before a jury of your countrymen, you have been found guilty. This is not your first offence: you were convicted of aggravated bronchitis last year. And I find that though you are only twenty three years old, you have been imprisoned on no less than fourteen occasions for illnesses of a more or less hateful character.

> It is all very well for you to say that you come of unhealthy parents and had a severe accident in your childhood which permanently undermined your constitution; excuses such as these are the ordinary refuse of the criminal; but they cannot for one moment be listened to by the ear of justice.

In 1979 Moore's sentiments (1979, p. 207) echoed Butler's remarks:

> Wards, clinics, and homes are full of debilitated bodies made wretched by irresponsibility and individual wantonness—ruined by wilful disregard for personal well-being. People who have choked the blood from their heart with cigarettes and torn the air from their lungs; who have squandered their body through lethargy; who have been digging their own graves with gluttonous gums; whose organs have been eroded with alcohol; whose bones have been splintered by delinquent driving; whose nerves have been snapped on the rack of ambition or anxiety; whose personality has become a plague through drugs; whose kidneys have been gnawed by aspirin; and whose mind has been sludged with sedatives.

With a more positive regard toward individual responsibility, Cousins (1976) was instrumental in raising the general public's awareness about the power of enlightened self-care. In his account of an illness in which he used laughter and positive emotions to facilitate his self-care, he speculated on the efficacy of self-administered placebos and related psychosomatic phenomenon:

> At this point, of course, we are opening a very wide door, perhaps even a Pandora's box. The vaunted "miracle cures" that abound in the literature of all the great religions, or the speculations of Charcot and Freud about conversion hysteria, or Lourdes phenomena—all say something about the ability of the patient, *properly motivated or stimulated*, to participate actively in extraordinary reversal of disease and disability" (Cousins, 1976, p. 1463, emphasis added).

Is it the role of the nurse to "properly motivate or stimulate"? According to Joseph (1980), it is. "The nursing system is generated by the nurse and patient to assist the patient in meeting his or her demands and *overcoming deficits* and is composed of the nursing actions necessary to accomplish certain *therapeutic self care demands*" (Joseph, 1980, p. 132, emphasis added).

An ethical implementation of a self-care deficit nursing plan would involve a careful personal analysis of the nurse's own value orientation toward individual responsibility.

Inherent in the ideologic concept of self-care is the idea of "victim blaming." This ideology, much like Butler's system, could impose economic sanctions on individuals who do not practice self-care:

> In the new system, the pariahs of the medical world and larger numbers of people in general could be diagnosed as having life-style problems, referred to a health counselor or social worker, and sent home. At the very least, the victim blaming ideology will help justify shifting the burden of costs back to users. If you are responsible for your illness, you should be responsible for your bill as well.

> The common themes apparent in all these and similar statements emphasize the need to reduce expectations and utilization of ineffective and costly medical services, the necessity instead for individual responsibility, and the requirement for either education or economic sanctions to enlighten and reinforce one's sense of responsibility (Crawford, 1977, p. 668).

Crawford finds this idea of self-care and individual responsibility representative of a class strategy as well as an attempt to divert attention from the social causation of disease in the commercial and industrial sectors. Such a behavioral model of illness directs attention toward individuals and their ability or inability to change external causative factors such as environment, occupational hazards, or even culture. UAW President Leonard Woodcock summed up industry's attitude toward self-care and individual responsibility succinctly when he stated "fix the worker, not the workplace" (Crawford, 1977, p. 665).

Implicit in the concept of self-care is the assumption that people make themselves sick, mentally and physically. Illness is a psychologic, if not moral, failure; cancer is a state of mind. LeShan (1977), an experimental psychologist, expands this idea. If this implication is followed to its logical conclusions, patients' abilities or inabilities to change or cope, emotionally or physically, have consequences that are critical to their health and their very survival. The role of the nurse as a self-care agent, then, assumes awesome and perhaps unwarranted proportions. Nurses must be aware of these and similar issues inherent in the self-care concept if they are to make ethical decisions in daily practice.

THE NURSE

> "Where do you come from?" said the Red Queen. "And where are you going? Look up, speak nicely, and don't twiddle your fingers all the time."
>
> *Through the Looking Glass*

An important "self" to consider in the clinical nursing encounter is, of course, the nurse. Historically, the role of the nurse has been that of self-abnegating service to mankind. Maslow's concept of the actualized self is perhaps antithetical to this historic precedent (Maslow, 1968). If nurses regard themselves as unique individuals capable of self-love, they will be most effective in meeting the therapeutic self-care demands of patients.

One of the first books on nursing ethics was published by Hampton in 1900. This early attempt to establish an ethical basis for nursing practice was essentially a code of etiquette.

> Like most etiquette books, it was designed to enable the reader to acquire the standards of a higher social class. The complex history of nursing, however, imparted to the code a distinctive emphasis on stringent discipline.

> Historically, this element was in part a legacy from the military, religious, and nursing orders going back to the Middle Ages with their traditions of obedience, subordinations, and self-abnegation (James, 1979, p. 220).

Assertiveness has replaced abnegation in nursing practice only within the last 10 years. As nurses collectively begin to experience the freedom of greater self-awareness, more attention will be focused on professional and ethical behavior.

Nurses have a right as well as an obligation to practice their own self-care. Such rights and obligations include the right to organize and engage in collective bargaining, the right to reasonable legal protection, and the right to refuse to participate in nursing actions that they personally consider morally wrong, such as assisting in abortions.

Transactional analysis teaches an awareness of self and one's own weaknesses. In unhealthy encounters the helping professional may play the untherapeutic role of "the rescuer" who offers unsolicited aid, "the persecutor" who enters with a preconceived idea of a moral imperative, or "the victim" who is apparently defenseless with no recognized resources (Berne, 1964). The belief has been expressed that some student nurses view themselves as "rescuers" (Glott-Maine, 1981). For nurses to practice their own self-care effectively, they must critically assess their own perceptions of their role. This is the first step toward one's own healing.

Self-awareness requires critical analysis and a receptive attitude toward learning and change, however painful it may be. The possibilities for creative nursing practice begin here.

> Healing is more than repairing, more than not destroying, it is creating. It is an article of faith with us and one without which we cannot work or live, to believe that things can be improved, that the patient can be helped, and that we ourselves can always be better than we are. We must improve ourselves to improve those who seek our help. This aspiration is in itself creative (Menninger, 1957, p. 106).

THE SOCIETY

"I'm glad they've come without waiting to be asked," she thought; "I should never have known who were the right people to invite!"

Through the Looking Glass

The influence of the larger group on individual behavior must be considered as well as the nurse's professional obligation, if any, to that group. The nurse's therapeutic relationship extends beyond the individual to the broader society. The Social Policy Statement of the ANA considers the relationship as mutually beneficial: "Nursing can be said to be owned by society, in the sense that nursing's professional interest must be and must be perceived as serving the interests of the larger whole of which it is a part" (ANA, 1980, p. 3). "For nursing, the public good must be the overriding concern" (ANA, 1980, p. 2).

Still there are many instances when the rights of the individual may seem contrary to the public good. The welfare recipient who continually abuses the use of the emergency room, the terminal cancer patient who requests death, or the patient who refuses a blood transfusion on religious grounds all have belief systems and values that may be contrary to prevailing norms and ideas about the public good. The ANA concedes the supremacy of the public good: "Section 1:1. The nurse must also recognize those situations in which individual rights to self determination in health care may temporarily be altered for the common good" (ANA, 1976, p. 4). Appropriate nursing action following such recognition is not discussed. Central to this idea of the common good is how nurses conceptualize the health of their patients: as a right or as a responsibility. Generalizations made about the public good will rest on this conceptualization.

According to the ANA, authority to practice is legislated: "This legal authority to practice stems from the social contract between society and the profession; the social contract does not derive from legislation" (ANA, 1980, p. 3). Where, then, does the nurse turn to clarify the nature of the social contract, and what are appropriate nursing actions regarding the public good? The study of ethics is perhaps the best area for purposeful investigation of the answers to these questions. The philosophy and ethics that guide nurses will directly impinge on their nursing actions and how they regard the public good. How nurses regard the public good depends on their value orientations toward the concept of self-care.

The economics of the society also directly affect the implementation of the concept of self-care.

Within a given society, however, the dominant type of treatment depends in part on the class position and group affiliation of the recipient. In America, religio-magical forms of healing are practiced by certain religious groups. Lower class patients, who view treatment as something the doctor does to one, are more likely to receive directive treatment, often accompanied by medication. Middle and upper class patients, who put a high value on self-knowledge and self-direction are more likely to receive permissive forms of treatment stressing insight" (Frank, 1961, p. 182).

It would seem that self-care is probably most highly valued by the middle and upper classes, whereas lower class patients would need more direction to increase self-care abilities. This is an important element for nurses to consider in the diagnosis of self-care deficit and in assessing their own value orientations toward which nursing actions would be appropriate. A compassionate and reasoned approach toward self-care must consider the holistic milieu of the patient's illness and what specific nursing actions will encourage the development of a patient's self-care abilities to meet therapeutic self-care demands.

The implementation of the self-care concept must never become a justification for victim blaming or a political or economic weapon to hinder access to medical services in the public sector. The diagnosis of self-care deficit must be sufficiently broad to include the social, economic, and cultural context in which an individual's health choices are being made.

SUMMARY

"Would you tell me, please, which way I ought to go from here?"

"That depends a good deal on where you want to get to," said the Cat.

"I don't much care where—so long as I get *somewhere*," Alice added as an explanation.

"Oh, you're sure to do that," said the Cat, "if you only walk enough."

Alice's Adventures in Wonderland

The ethical implementation of the self-care concept is a process, a creative and healing journey with as many destinations as there are travelers. The idea that individuals have responsibility for their own health is not new. The application of the self-care concept in nursing practice is quite recent, however. Careful attention must be given to the ethical implementation of this concept.

The nursing diagnosis of self-care deficit must be based on a positive regard for individual patients their existing strengths and weaknesses, and an awareness of the possibility for uniquely creative solutions to individual health care problems. An ethical implementation of the self-care concept in nursing practice will consider the social and economic environment in which an individual's choices are made. The beauty and the challenge of the self-care concept lies in the recognition of all "selves" involved: the patient, the nurse, and the collective self, or society.

REFERENCES

American Nurses' Association: Code for nurses with interpretive statements, Kansas City, Mo., 1976, The Association.

American Nurses' Association: Nursing: a social policy statement, Kansas City, Mo., 1980, The Association.

Bennett, J.: Symposium on the self-care concept of nursing, Nurs. Clin. North Am. **15:**123, 1980.

Berne, E.: Games people play, New York, 1964, Grove Press, Inc.

Butler, S.: Erehwon, ed. 2, New York, 1927, Random House, Inc.

Cousins, N.: Anatomy of an illness (as perceived by the patient), N. Engl. J. Med. **295:**1458, 1976.

Crawford, R.: You are dangerous to your health: the ideology and politics of victim blaming, Int. J. Health Serv. **7:**663, 1977.

Frank, J.: Persuasion and healing, New York, 1961, Schocken Books, Inc.

Glott-Maine, C.: Personal communication, Sept. 18, 1981.

James, J.W.: Isabel Hampton and the professionalization of nursing. In Chertok, L., and De-Sassure, R., eds.: The therapeutic revolution: from Mesmer to Freud, New York, 1979, Brunner/Mazel, Inc.

Joseph, L.S.: Self-care and the nursing process, Nurs. Clin. North Am. **15:**131, 1980.

LeShan, L.: You can fight for your life: emotional factors in the causation of cancer, New York, 1977, M. Evans & Co., Inc.

Maslow, A.H.: Toward a psychology of being, New York, 1968, Van Nostrand Reinhold Co.

Menninger, K.: Psychological factors in the choice of medicine as a profession, Bull. Menninger Clin. **21:**99, 1957.

Moore, A.R.: Letter from Australia, J. Med. Ethics **5:**207, 1979.

Orem, D.E.: Nursing: concepts of practice, New York, 1972, McGraw-Hill Book Co.

Alienation: a basic concept underlying social isolation

WINNIFRED C. MILLS, B.Sc.N., M.Ed.

This paper examines the concept of alienation, the existing diagnostic labels that incorporate forms of alienation, and that aspect of alienation known as social isolation together with its positive referents: solitude and social interaction. The possibility will be discussed of considering alienation as a syndrome for further development.

In reviewing the work of the past two conferences, two areas of intense intellectual activity are evident. The Nurse Theorist Group and their associates have proposed a framework for the classification of nursing diagnosis incorporating characteristics of unitary man/human) (Roy, 1982). Patterns such as communicating, relating, and valuing (Roy, 1982) offer structure for deductive reasoning to elicit diagnostic labels. Other groups using inductive approaches have refined existing diagnoses together with the related etiology and defining characteristics. Clusters of concepts such as body image, role performance, self-esteem, and personal identity have emerged in this way, and the possibility of syndromes is suggested (Kim and Moritz, 1982).

Baccalaureate nursing students with whom I work in the psychosocial domain of oncology nursing practice have generated diagnostic statements using the behavioral systems model. The concept of alienation was presented in a senior nursing course. The students have recognized aspects of alienation in the categories *ineffective individual coping, knowledge deficits,* and *disturbance in self-concept,* although they have suggested additional defining characteristics for these categories.

Isolation as an aspect of alienation seems not to be addressed in any of the existing diagnostic categories, and *social isolation* is a diagnosis to be developed. It is believed that isolation is a state of the individual closely related to the other forms of alienation. It is this thinking that leads to the consideration of alienation as a syndrome and the forms of alienation as possible subcomponents. In discussing alienation, present usage of the sociologic term includes two aspects: alienation as a social condition and alienation as the state of the individual (Bloch, 1978). For the purpose of this paper, alienation refers to the state of the individual.

THE FIVE FORMS OF ALIENATION

Seeman (1959) has described five forms of alienation: powerlessness, meaninglessness, normlessness, isolation, and self-estrangement. Feelings of *powerlessness* originate from a person's belief that he is subject to the influence of outside forces such as luck or chance and that he lacks any resources to control the situation or to determine the consequences of his behavior. *Meaninglessness* refers to the inability of the individual to determine who or what to believe. There is no way to choose alternatives with confidence because clear information to help in decision making is lacking. The disabled person often experiences this feeling when others, wishing to "help," attempt to make all the decisions without consulting the person. *Normlessness* results when social values are changing and the individual chooses alternatives that may be in conflict with previously held values. Gay clients are examples of this category. *Isolation* is a condition of "aloneness" when the individual experiences rejection and no longer expects to be included and accepted. From these situations, people sometimes come together in subcultures and ghettoization results. Substance abusers are examples of this category. *Self-estrangement* occurs when a person experiences a lack of congruence between what he is and what he wants to be. This condition can be especially true of the educationally and economically disadvantaged person. The urban housewife who discontinued her education to "see hubby through" is an example of this category. An individual may experience one or more of these forms of alienation simultaneously.

SOURCES OF ALIENATION

At least two sets of factors produce a state of alienation. Social conditions can produce feelings of alienation in which people feel powerless to influence conditions of their environment and experience hopelessness leading to despair. Psychologic factors underlying alienation are related to developmental tasks. Individuals are unable to build a strong ego identity and experience repeated failure in establishing satisfying relationships. A particularly interesting theory is that of *learned helplessness* proposed by Seligman (1975). He states that for some people the feeling of helplessness only follows repeated, unremitting hardships, whereas for others a minor mishap can trigger helpless feelings. How readily a person believes in his own helplessness, or mastery, is shaped by his experience (beginning in infancy) with controllable and uncontrollable events. At about 8 weeks of age, a new capacity emerges in the infant. It is the perceived response of the environment to self. The infant learns that responding works, and this perception of control leads the child to learn that he is an effective human being. Here begins the lifelong struggle to make the world respond—the struggle for control. In humans, opportunities to learn successful control of outcomes are necessary. Experience with uncontrollable events may predispose a person to lack of trust and hope, and eventually to depression; on the other hand, early experience with mastery may immunize him, by giving him hope that he can again succeed.

IDENTIFICATION OF CLIENTS SUSCEPTIBLE TO ALIENATION

Bloch (1978) identifies the following persons and groups as most likely to experience alienation in our society: women; elderly people; disadvantaged people; educationally or economically; handicapped people, or those suffering from chronic disease; members of an ethnic/racial minority; and sick people. In working with any of these individuals, the nurse must be aware of the potential for alienation. The condition can be identified by careful observation and through the use of questions that imply caring. Nursing assessment should include an estimation of the client's feelings about himself as a person, his ability to control the situation in which he finds himself, his hopes, and the coping mechanisms he uses to deal with his world. With this information, it is then possible to plan and implement appropriate interventions.

ALIENATION AS A SYNDROME

The proposed schema (Figure 1) suggests alienation as a state of negative energy in which deficits occur in the individual's ability to feel normal, recog-

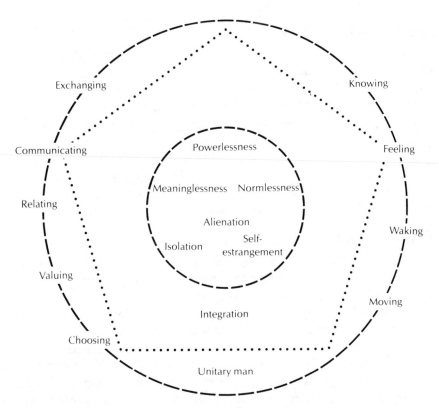

FIGURE 1 Alienation depicted as a state of negative energy.

nize meaning in life, feel in control, and feel as an intact human in touch with the environment. Aspects of alienation could impinge on all the patterns of unitary man/human. Although there seems to have been some reaction to the term *unitary man/human* at the 1980 conference, this discussion of the concept of alienation could apply equally to such terms as *human existence* (Chin, 1982) or *holism* in its many variations (Rogers, 1982a, p. 248). The negative energy field described as *alienation* occurs as a result of forces both inside and outside the individual, that is, personal and social. This idea is congruent with the concept of man as a dynamic, open-energy field involving "mutual simultaneous interaction" within self and between self and environment (Rogers, 1982b).

In the schema described (Figure 2), the five aspects of alienation are suggested as a syndrome, each subcomponent of which may produce negative energy or an energy deficit. The subcomponents are depicted as continua and are balanced by positive forces supporting integration. Behaviors of human beings may be generated to correct the energy deficit that occurs with alienation. If the energy deficit is not corrected, the individual's integrity is threatened and death may occur.

SOLITUDE AND SOCIAL INTERACTION

In identifying dimensions of self-care, Orem (1971, p. 24) describes solitude and social interaction as "conditions of existence which affect human development and health." Solitude exists when a reduced number of social stimuli are present and when the individual is required to make fewer social responses. Solitude allows for reflection and introspection and exists as a need in relation to the individual's usual pattern of activity. The individual whose family or occupational role involves high visibility and constant social interaction requires periods of solitude for recovery. Social interaction involves satisfying personal relationships, development of a realistic self-concept, and satisfaction in group membership.

SOCIAL ISOLATION AND LONELINESS

Rogers (1982b) reminds us that the behaviors of unitary man/human constitute an open system and that there are no dichotomies. Social isolation and loneliness can be considered as states in the negative energy field of alienation, with positive or negative energy being contributed to the individual's state of integration as the person experiences both internal and external forces (Figure 3). Corresponding states within the positive energy field would include solitude and social interaction. It is possible to consider solitude versus loneliness and social interaction versus isolation as continua in the context of the alienated individual versus the integrated individual.

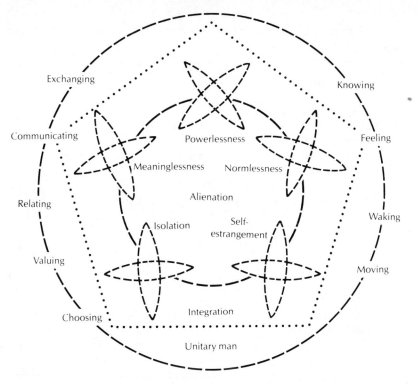

FIGURE 2   The five aspects of alienation depicted as a syndrome.

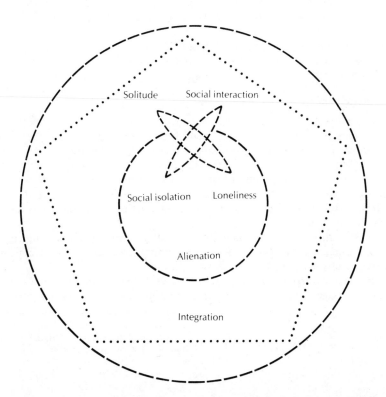

FIGURE 3   Social isolation and loneliness depicted as states in the negative energy field of alienation.

BOX 1   **Diagnostic concept format**

Title: Concept label (diagnosis).

Overall definition: General description of the category, problem, or phenomena.

Etiology: Antecedent or current events, factors in environment, changes or predicted changes in internal or external resources that predispose an individual or group to this problem.

High risk factors: Prediction of categories of persons who have a higher probability of having this diagnosis. Consider also presenting situations or time periods that increase risk of occurrence.

Dynamics: The variables involved and their relationships, leading to an understanding of the underlying mechanisms of the problem.

Differential diagnosis: Other diagnostic concepts that must be considered as a basis for making the most precise clinical decision.

Manifestations (signs and symptoms): Patterns of cues, subjective and objective, that together present the profile needed to assign the problem to this diagnostic category.

Complications: Additional undesired sequellae or side effects that can occur secondary to the primary problem.

Prognosis: Predicted direction, duration, and range of outcomes together with the factors that contribute and thus enable prediction.

Prevention and management: Guidelines for prescription of actions to most effectively prevent the phenomenon or manage living with its presence. (These are general guidelines and must be individualized based on the presenting data in a given situation.)

Evaluation: Guidelines for areas of data collection on client status and response to treatment together with criteria for interpreting the data in terms of improvement or lack of it.

Diagnostic concept—example

Title: Social isolation

Overall definition: Condition of aloneness experienced by the individual and perceived as imposed by others and as a negative or threatened state.

Etiology: Inability to engage in satisfying personal relationships; delay in accomplishing developmental tasks; immature interests; alterations in physical appearance; alterations in mental status; unaccepted social behavior; unaccepted social values; altered state of wellness; inadequate personal resources.

High-risk factors: Elderly; female; member of an ethnic or racial minority; disadvantaged status, educationally or economically; being handicapped; suffering physical, mental, or chronic illness.

Dynamics: Socal isolation is like pain: it is real if the sufferer says it exists. Objective signs of isolation may be present but are not necessary to the

BOX 1   **Diagnostic concept format—cont'd**

diagnosis, although one objective sign has been deemed critical and two subjective symptoms are similarly labeled.

Differential diagnosis: Must be differentiated from solitude, which has no negative connotations for the individual, and loneliness, which is not perceived as imposed by others.

Manifestations (defining characteristics)

Objective	Subjective
absence of supportive significant other/s: family, friends, group.*	verbalizes feelings of aloneness imposed by others*
sad, dull, affect.	verbalizes feelings of rejection.*
inappropriate or immature interests or activities for developmental age or stage.	experiences feelings of difference from others, inadequacy in or absence of significant purpose in life, inability to meet expectations of others, insecurity in public.
uncommunicative, withdrawn, no eye contact.	
preoccupation with own thoughts, repetitive, meaningless actions.	expresses values unacceptable to the dominant cultural group.
projects hostility in voice, behavior.	expresses values acceptable to the subculture.
seeks to be alone or exists in a subculture.	describes an altered state of wellness.
evidence of physical or mental handicap or altered state of wellness.	verbalizes interests inappropriate to developmental age or stage.
shows behavior unacceptable to dominant cultural group.	

Complications: Increased alienation; decreased will to live; increased depression, suicide; violence to others; noncompliance with health prescriptions.

Prognosis: Depends on the alleviation of other aspects of alienation. Factors to be considered include the degree of alienation (how many of the five forms are involved?); the duration of the alienated state (after a number of years, habits are formed that are hard to eradicate); the willingness of the individual to be involved with others; and the social situation contributing to the condition.

Prevention and management:
   Identify cause of the isolation.
   Identify willingness of individual to seek others.
   Expose individual to resources available and guide use of the resources.
   Teach needed skills, for example, problem solving, communication, personal care.
   Support risk-taking as individual moves toward other human beings.
   Reinforce positive behavior and successes in achieving developmental tasks, establishing identity.
   Suggest role models, mentors.
   Support social action programs for the disadvantaged.
   Foster development of peer groups and mobilize action among indigenous nonprofessionals.

*Critical defining characteristics

SOCIAL ISOLATION: A DIAGNOSTIC CATEGORY

Gordon (1982) has pointed out three problems underlying current work in establishing diagnostic categories: (1) lack of clarity in diagnosis, (2) inadequate theoretic knowledge of the health problem represented by the diagnosis, and (3) deficiencies in clincial reasoning skills that direct the search for information. The proposed diagnostic category may suffer any of these inadequacies but may, nevertheless, stimulate further productive thinking. The Diagnostic Concept Format (Box 1) was developed by Carnevali (1981) and is modified from that presented by Bircher (1982) at a previous conference.

CONCLUSION

This discussion has examined the concept of alienation and identified existing diagnostic labels that incorporate forms of alienation. Social isolation was discussed as an aspect of alienation together with its positive referents: solitude and social interaction. A schema was presented that suggested alienation as a syndrome. Social isolation as a diagnostic category was developed within that syndrome.

Kuhn (1970) refers to puzzles and paradigms in the world of science. We are reminded that it is possible to recognize a paradigm without a full interpretation or rationalization of it and that "Lack of a standard interpretation . . . will not prevent a paradigm from guiding research" (Kuhn, 1970, p. 44). This schema, developed around the concept of alienation, is a structure offered to stimulate thinking and effort toward the development of diagnostic categories.

REFERENCES

Bircher, A.: The concept of nursing diagnosis. In Kim, M.J., and Moritz, D.A., eds.: Classification of nursing diagnoses: proceedings of the third and fourth national conferences, New York, 1982, McGraw-Hill Book Co.

Bloch, D.W.: Alienation. In Carlson, C., and Blackwell, B., eds.: Behavioral concepts and nursing interventions, Philadelphia, 1978, J.B. Lippincott Co.

Carnevali, D.: Conceptualizing: storage of knowledge for diagnosis and management. In Mitchell, P., and Loustau, A., eds.: Concepts basic to nursing, ed. 3, New York, 1981, McGraw-Hill Book Co.

Chin, P.: Small group reactions to the theoretical framework "unitary man." In Kim, M.J., and Moritz, D.A., eds.: Classification of nursing diagnoses: proceedings of the third and fourth national conferences, New York, 1982, McGraw-Hill Book Co.

Gordon, M.: The diagnostic process. In Kim, M.J., and Moritz, D.A., eds.: Classification of nursing diagnoses: proceedings of the third and fourth national conferences, New York, 1982, McGraw-Hill Book Co.

Kim, M.J., and Moritz, D.A., eds.: Classification of nursing diagnoses: proceedings of the third and fourth national conferences, New York, 1982, McGraw-Hill Book Co.

Kuhn, T.: The structure of scientific revolutions, ed. 2, Chicago, 1970, University of Chicago Press.

Orem, D.: Nursing: concepts of practice, New York, 1971, McGraw-Hill Book Co.

Rogers, M.: Development of a new knowledge base for nursing, In Kim, M.J., and Moritz, D.A., eds.: Classification of nursing diagnoses: proceedings of the third and fourth national conferences, New York, 1982a, McGraw-Hill Book Co.

Rogers, M.: Theoretical frameworks for classification of nursing diagnosis. Panel discussion. In Kim, M.J., and Moritz, D.A., eds.: Classification of nursing diagnoses: proceedings of the third and fourth national conferences, New York, 1982b, McGraw-Hill Book Co.

Roy, Sister C.: Historical perspective of the theoretical framework for the classification of nursing diagnosis. In Kim, M.J., and Moritz, D.A., eds.: Classification of nursing diagnoses: proceedings of the third and fourth national conferences, New York, 1982, McGraw-Hill Book Co.

Seeman, M.: On the meaning of alienation, Am. Sociol. Rev. **24:**783, 1959.

Seligman, M.E.: Helplessness: on depression, development and death, San Francisco, 1975, W.H. Freeman & Co. Publishers.

The differentiation of fear and anxiety

CAROLYN J. YOCOM, R.N., M.S.N.

At the Fourth National Conference the nursing diagnosis of *fear* was accepted and the diagnosis of *anxiety* was subsumed under it. In addition, the diagnoses of *functional* and *nonfunctional fear* were deleted. The defining characteristic of *fear* was identified as the "ability to identify the object of fear"; the etiology for this diagnosis was to be developed (Kim and Moritz, 1982). It was also noted in the proceedings (Kim and Moritz, 1982) that some group members expressed concern that fear may be a symptom of *ineffective coping* and other diagnoses or that fear may be a symptom analogous to the symptom of anxiety.

The purpose of this paper is to examine the differences between anxiety and fear so that careful consideration can be given to reversing the 1980 decision to subsume the diagnosis of *anxiety* under the diagnosis of *fear*. It is also anticipated that sufficient information will be provided to lend support to the fact that *fear* and *anxiety* are, in fact, diagnoses in their own right and not symptoms of other diagnoses.

To differentiate between fear and anxiety, it is first necessary to identify the stimulus for such reactions. In the process of interacting with the environment, human beings are exposed to situations that may pose a danger to their physical and personal well-beings. Whether or not a particular individual interprets a situation as threatening depends on his or her subjective appraisal of the potential for harm or danger. This appraisal is determined by aptitudes, skills, personality traits and personal experiences with similar experiences (Spielberger, 1972).

The response to an actual or potential danger can be manifested as a startle reflex or the affective reactions of anxiety and fear. The emotions of fear and anxiety can be differentiated by the fact that they occur on different psychologic levels of the personality (May, 1950, 1977) as well as by neurophysiologic, behavioral, and subjective characteristics (Borkovec, Weerts, and Bernstein, 1977; Izard, 1972; May, 1950, 1977; Spielberger, 1972). To differentiate these two affects, the characteristics of fear will be addressed first, followed by those of anxiety.

CHARACTERISTICS OF FEAR

Imagine yourself standing on a small ladder changing the bulb in a ceiling light. All of a sudden the ladder begins to shake and sway because your cat has begun to climb up after you. Or imagine the feelings you would experience just before receiving an injection of Inferon when you first see the 2½-inch needle used for the deep intramuscular injection. In both of these situations you probably would experience feelings of apprehension and fright and a desire to withdaw from the situation. The stimulus of your fear has been a threat to your physical integrity; you have perceived a potential, which may be either real or imagined, for physical injury.

In fear the feelings of apprehension have a tangible quality to them because their source is identifiable (Sarason, 1975). Fear is a reaction to a specific danger, but once the threat is removed the associated feelings are often quickly forgotten (May, 1950, 1977). May (1977) has stated that fear is experienced as a result of a threat that can be located spatially and to which an adjustment can be made by removal of the object, reassurance, or flight. Once this adjustment is made, the feeling of apprehension disappears. Subjectively, the fearful individual can identify feelings of increased tension and impulsiveness and decreased self-assurance. A fearful individual will also experience feelings of being afraid, scared, terrified, panicked, frightened, and/or jittery (Izard, 1972).

The neurophysiologic manifestations of fear are caused by sympathetic nervous system stimulation. This stimulation results in the classic "fight or flight" response consisting of cardiovascular excitation, superficial vasoconstriction, decreased gastrointestinal activity, and pupil dilation. Dryness of the mouth and palmar sweating are also present (Izard, 1972; May, 1950, 1977). Behaviorally, increased alertness and concentration on the source of the threat are present. In addition, the individual is wide-eyed and may experience avoidance or attack behavior (Izard, 1972; May, 1977; Sarason, 1975). The severity of these manifestations varies greatly from individual to individual and from situation to situation. However, the major characteristic of fear is the individual's ability to identify the specific source and object of the threat. In addition, the manifestations of fear subside shortly after the source of the threat has been removed.

CHARACTERISTICS OF ANXIETY

Recall the first time in your professional career that you had to make a formal presentation (a classroom lecture or a continuing education presentation) or had to lead a clinical conference or seminar. You probably experienced what are commonly referred to as "butterflies" in your stomach and had vague feelings of uneasiness and apprehension. You knew you were afraid of something but were unable to specifically identify what you were afraid of and what was actually being threatened. A clinical correlate of this experience may be the feelings experienced by the patient about to undergo anesthesia and surgery. He knows that the procedure must be performed and what the benefits, risks, and outcomes should be. However, he still has a vague feeling of apprehension, helplessness, and uneasiness. In both of these situations, the affect being experienced is anxiety.

The threats responsible for these responses were to values that the individual considered essential to his existence as an individual distinct from everyone and everything about him. In the first situation, the threat was to values associated with feelings of self-worth or self-esteem. In the clinical situation, even though the patient knew basically what to expect, he could anticipate a lack of control over the findings and over his interaction with the environment while under the effects of the anesthesia. He could also have a fear of dying that goes beyond the fear of actual physical death. His fear of death could include an anticipated loss of the psychologic and religious meanings that are identified with one's existence. A threat of meaninglessness also exists in anxiety (May, 1977, 1980).

Anxiety is a subjective, objectless experience. The diffuse and undifferentiated quality of anxiety refers to the level in the personality at which the threat is experienced. One is afraid but is unable to specify the exact object of which one is afraid because the value system on which the core or essence of the personality is based has been threatened. In contrast to fear, which is experienced on the basis of a security pattern that has been developed, it is the security pattern itself that is threatened in anxiety (May, 1977).

The subjective manifestations of anxiety include feelings of tension, apprehension, and worry (Izard, 1972; Spielberger, 1972); having painful and persistent feelings of helplessness (Izard, 1972; May, 1977; Sarason, 1975); and uncertainty (Sarason, 1975). Additional subjective manifestations include complaints of feeling anxious, jittery, shaky, inadequate, fearful, scared, overexcited, rattled, regretful, and distressed (Izard, 1972). There is a fear of unspecified consequences of unspecified noxious stimuli (May, 1950, 1977, 1980; Sarason, 1975).

The neurophysiologic response to anxiety is characterized by both sympathetic and parasympathetic activity. Therefore a mixed reaction is manifested, as may be seen by the presence of both cardiovascular excitation, an example of sympathetic stimulation, and an increase in gastrointestinal activity, an example, of parasympathetic stimulation (Izard, 1972; May, 1977).

Behaviorally the anxious person is characterized by a general restlessness, insomnia, wariness, and glancing about even though no specific "enemy" exists (May, 1977). In addition, poor eye contact with others, foot shuffling, trembling, extraneous hand and arm movement, hand tremors, facial tension, quivering voice, and increased perspiration may be present (Paul, 1966). There is also a preoccupation with "me " as opposed to "it out there" as is seen in a fear response (Sarason, 1975).

The intensity and duration of the manifestations of anxiety are determined by the amount of the threat that is perceived and by the persistence of the individual's appraisal of a situation as being dangerous (Spielberger, 1972). Individuals cannot avoid anxiety. However, they are able to reduce its level by admitting that apprehensiveness exists and by moving ahead in spite of it. Anxiety reduction is facilitated when the individual is convinced that the values to be gained, by moving ahead are greater than those to be gained by escape (May, 1980).

CONCLUSION

In conclusion, it can be seen that distinct differences exist between fear and anxiety. Fear is experienced as a result of a threat that can be located spatially. It is characterized by a sympathetic response and behavioral signs of increased alertness and concentration on the source of the threat. Subjectively, individuals experience feelings of apprehension and fright and can identify the source of their feelings. Fear can be allayed by withdrawal from the situation, by removal of the offending object, or by reassurance. In contrast, anxiety is caused by a threat to the value systems that are essential to a person's existence as an individual. The person is afraid but is unable to distinguish either the specific source of the threat or the object that is threatened. Anxiety is characterized by both sympathetic and parasympathetic responses. Behaviorally, depending on the level of anxiety, general restlessness, purposeless movement, facial and voice distortion, and sleep disturbances are prominent. The subjective experiences are characterized by feelings of uncertainty, helplessness, and apprehension. Anxiety reduction is promoted by admitting its presence and by moving on with the task at hand. This movement is facilitated once the individual is convinced that the values to be gained by moving ahead are greater than those to be gained by escape.

REFERENCES

Borkovec, T., Weerts, T., and Bernstein, D.: Assessment of anxiety. In Ciminero, A., Calhoun, K., and Adams, H., eds.: Handbook of behavioral assessment, New York, 1977, John Wiley & Sons, Inc.

Izard, C.: Patterns of emotion, New York, 1972, Academic Press, Inc.

Kim, M.J., and Moritz, D.A., eds.: Classification of nursing diagnoses: proceedings of the third and fourth national conferences, New York, 1982, McGraw-Hill Book Co.

May, R.: The meaning of anxiety, New York, 1950, The Ronald Press Co.

May, R.: The meaning of anxiety, rev. ed., New York, 1977, W.W. Norton & Co., Inc.

May, R.: Value conflict and anxiety. In Kutash, I., and others, eds.: Handbook on stress and anxiety, San Francisco, 1980, Jossey-Bass, Inc., Publishers.

Paul, G.: Insight vs. desensitization in psychotherapy, Stanford, Calif., 1966, Stanford University Press.

Sarason, I.: Test anxiety, attention, and the general problem of anxiety. In Spielberger, C., and Sarason, I., eds.: Stress and anxiety, New York, 1975, John Wiley & Sons, Inc.

Spielberger, C.: Conceptual and methodological issues in anxiety research. In Spielberger, C., ed.: Anxiety: current trends in theory and research, vol. II, New York, 1972, Academic Press, Inc.

Proposal for a category of nursing diagnosis: alteration in level of consciousness caused by nervous system dysfunction

MARGARET C. LANNON, R.N., M.S.

CONCEPTS RELATED TO ALTERED CONSCIOUSNESS

Silverman (1975, p. 91) stated that "normal, waking consciousness—'rational consciousness' as William James called it—is but one state of consciousness. There are others." For any individual the normal state of consciousness is the one in which the majority of time is spent. An altered state of consciousness is one in which the qualities of the mental functions are different from the baseline state (Tart, 1969). Armstrong (1977) reminds us that environmental factors also play a part. What is considered a normal level of consciousness is influenced by one's culture.

In most medical literature any discussion of altered states (or level) of consciousness refers to reduced consciousness. Although not all changes in level of consciousness are considered pathologic (for example, sleep, daydreaming, and dreaming are recognized as normal deviations from the waking state), those usually discussed at length have as their etiology some dysfunction in the central nervous system (CNS). Certain fluctuating and transient levels of consciousness are also recognized. Delirium is a fluctuating alteration in consciousness often listed with confusion and disorientation as a "confusional state" (Luckman and Sorensen, 1974). These three conditions are seen as excitatory states, differing from the levels of depressed consciousness such as stupor and coma.* Epilepsy and syncope are listed by Walton (1975) as two other transient disorders of consciousness.

NEUROLOGIC CAUSES OF ALTERATION IN LEVEL OF CONSCIOUSNESS

Disturbances of consciousness may arise from altered function of the cerebral cortex, the diencephalon, and the brainstem. Any factor that impairs the supply of oxygen and essential nutrients to the brain causes an alteration in an individual's level of consciousness. Likewise, an interruption of neural pathways and/or cerebral structures affects level of consciousness. Excluding changes caused by anesthesia and psychiatric conditions, the neurologic

---

*In describing the states between alert wakefulness and coma, many different terms are used. Examples are apathy, automatism, brain death, clouded consciousness, confusion, deep coma, deep stupor, disorientation, drowsiness, excitatory unconsciousness, lassitude, lethargy, light coma, obtundation, semicoma, semiconscious, somnolence, and stupor.

causes of changes in level of consciousness can be divided into three categories: (1) occurrences in the CNS, (2) metabolic disorders, and (3) exogenous materials/influences that affect the CNS.

Intracranial pathology, such as vascular thrombus or embolus, hemorrhage, cerebral edema (causing increased intracranial pressure and possible herniation), neoplasm, epilepsy, or infection (meningitis, encephalitis, abscess), is a common cause of altered consciousness. External damage to the skull can also directly affect the brain and cause changes in level of consciousness. Metabolic disturbances may affect the CNS and thus cause alterations in consciousness. Examples are hypoglycemia, diabetic ketoacidosis, renal and liver failure, and severe fluid and electrolyte imbalances. Respiratory or circulatory disorders may compromise metabolic processes and thus be indirect causes of altered consciousness. Examples of exogenous materials that affect the CNS either directly or indirectly are toxic chemicals (poisons or drugs), snake venom, and antigens that cause anaphylactic shock.

SIGNIFICANCE OF LEVEL OF CONSCIOUSNESS

A survey of nursing and medical literature shows total agreement in one area—the level of consciousness is the most important single indicator of cerebral function. As Teasdale (1975, p. 914) states: "No single aspect of the patient's physiological state which we can measure mechanically contains information about the sum total of the activity of the brain which is implied in assessment of 'conscious level.' "

Although every brain disorder does not cause an alteration in level of consciousness, impaired consciousness is definitely an indication of "diffuse dysfunction of the brain as a whole" (Teasdale, 1975, p. 914). Level of consciousness is also the most sensitive, first indicator of a change in intracranial pressure. This sensitivity is a result of the highly specialized cortical cells being supplied by terminal arteries rather than by the large vessels that supply the brainstem (Jimm, 1974). The higher cognitive functions are therefore especially vulnerable to neurologic disease and will show impairment sooner than the more basic processes of attention, language, and memory (Strub and Black, 1977).

The level of consciousness must be accurately described and communicated to others if two major questions are to be answered: (1) Is the patient's condition improving or deteriorating? (2) What is causing the alteration in consciousness? To answer the first question, or assess the direction of change, it must be understood that as patients lose consciousness they go from alert and purposeful behavior to purposeless behavior. As the patient improves, the reverse is true. A patient who is generally deteriorating may show an orderly downward progression in motor function, which would be apparent if serial assessments were carried out and the results charted or communicated. Teasdale, Galbraith, and Clarke (1975) believe that the evidence of progressive changes in a patients condition is often more important than the findings at any one (however thorough) neurologic examination. The answer to the second question cannot be answered by assessment alone. Many important cues can be picked up. Patients with alterations in level of consciousness, especially those with head injuries, are particularly vulnerable to rapid intracranial changes that can lead to irreversible brain damage or death if undetected and untreated. For this reason, a complete assessment includes attention to focal signs such as pupillary reaction and limb movement, which can help to localize the cause of altered consciousness.

ASSESSMENT

In a patient with an alteration in level of consciousness caused by neuologic dysfunction, assessments are done to (1) determine the direction of change— is the patient's condition getting better or worse? and (2) pick up cues as to the possible cause of the altered state.

All neurologic assessments begin with a determination of a patient's level of consciousness. Although classifying labels alone are not sufficient to describe the various states or levels of consciousness, neither are behavioral descriptions alone a practical way to communicate observations. Rather than giving a number, label, or definition, it seems best to describe a patient's behavior with respect to content and arousal and refer to a common list of behaviorally defined terms for the communication of the information. Included in such behaviorally defined descriptions of level of consciousness would be reflections on how the patient appeared, what was done to stimulate the patient, and a description of the response.*

After determination of a patient's level of consciousness, an assessment continues, including measurement of vital signs, pupil and eye movement, motor response, and reflex activity.

DEFINING CHARACTERISTICS

A continuum of consciousness ranges from alert and oriented behavior to comatose and unresponsive behavior. Each of the intermediate levels has characteristic signs and symptoms, although no clear-cut boundaries are defined. In Box 1, these defining characteristics have been grouped under the headings of level of consciousness, speech, pupil and eye movement, vital signs, motor response (to tactile-painful stimuli), and reflex activity. Al-

---

*A good example of a behaviorally defined way of describing a patient's level of consciousness ia the Glasgow Coma Scale (Teasdale and Jennett, 1974). When paired with Teasdale's Observation Record Chart, the Coma Scale provides a comprehensive picture of the patient's condition.

BOX 1   **Defining characteristics of altered consciousness**

Level of consciousness
Opens eyes, responds to name
Obeys simple commands
Confused
Drowsy, easily arousable
Unarousable (unresponsive)
Speech
Moaning
Inappropriate speech (rambling, incomprehensible)
Dysphasia
Aphasia (no speech)
Pupil and eye movement
Visual field disturbances (homonymous hemianopia, diplopia)
Involuntary eye movements (doll's eyes, roving, nystagmus, disconjugate gaze)
Pupillary reaction to light (constriction dilation, uneven reactions, sluggishness, fixed)
Absence of blinking
Vital signs
Depressed respirations
Neurogenic hyperventilation
Arrhythmic breathing (apneustic, cluster, ataxic, Cheyne-Stokes)
Mechanically assisted breathing
Fluctuating hypothermia, hyperthermia
Elevated blood pressure
Widening pulse pressure
Tachycardia, bradycardia
Pathologic brain wave patterns
Increased ventricular pressure
Motor response (to tactile-painful stimulus)
Involuntary (inappropriate) response (decorticate posturing, decerebrate posturing)
No response to stimulation
Paralysis
Loss of sphincter control (incontinent)
Altered muscle tone (hypotonia [flaccid], Hypertonia [spastic], clonus)
Reflex activity
Normal reflexes absent
Presence of pathologic reflexes
No reflexes

---

though level of consciousness, the most important determinant of nervous system dysfunction, has been the major focus of this paper, a thorough neurologic assessment should also include assessment of the remaining parameters. Depending on the severity of the alteration in level of consciousness, many or few of the defining characteristics in each category would be present. In general the defining characteristics are listed from mild to severe. Changes in these body processes will correlate with nursing diagnoses of mild, moderate, or severe alteration in level of consciousness caused by nervous system dysfunction.

REFERENCES

Armstrong, M.E.: Use of altered states of awareness in nursing practice, AORN J. **1**:49, 1977.

Jimm, L.R.: Nursing assessment of patients for increased intracranial pressure, J. Neurosurg. Nurs. **6**(1):27, 1974.

Luckman, J., and Sorensen, K.: Medical-surgical nursing: a psychophysiologic approach, Philadelphia, 1974, W.B. Saunders Co.

Silverman, J.: On the sensory bases of transcendental states of consciousness. In Altered states of consciousness: current views and research problems, Washington, D.C., 1975, Drug Abuse Council.

Strub, R.L., and Black, F.W.: The mental status examination in neurology, Philadelphia, 1977, F.A. Davis Co.

Tart, C., ed.: Altered states of consciousness: a book of readings, New York, 1969, John Wiley & Sons, Inc.

Teasdale, G.: Acute impairment of brain function. 1. Assessing "conscious level," Nurs. Times **71**(24):914, 1975.

Teasdale, G., Galbraith, S., and Clarke, K.: Acute impairment of brain function. 2. Observation record chart, Nurs. Times **71**(25):972, 1975.

Teasdale, G., and Jennett, B.: Assessment of coma and impaired consciousness, Lancet **2**:82, 1974.

Walton, J.: Essentials of neurology, ed. 4, Philadelphia, 1975, J.B. Lippincott Co.

Nursing staff as victims: implications for a nursing diagnosis

MARILYN L. LANZA, R.N., M.S.

Violence is more and more a public concern as demonstrated by daily media attention. Violence ranges from acts of international war and terrorism to personal threats to safety in school, home, and community. According to F.B.I. Uniform Crime Reports, violent crimes of murder, forcible rape, robbery, and aggravated assault have been steadily increasing (Statistical Abstracts of the U.S., 1979). Whereas there has been much recent interest in assault as an example of violence, there has been relatively little acknowledgment that assault is a problem for nurses.

Although nursing staff are required to report when they are assaulted by a patient, little evidence of patient-nurse assault exists in the literature. An extensive literature review in 1980 and 1981 concluded that assaults on nurses were infrequent (Brooks, 1967; Kalogerakis, 1971; Lange, 1966). When patient violence was addressed, the nurse was often blamed. For example, patient violence may be attributed to the nurse's expectation of assault, thus representing a self-fulfilling prophecy (Levy and Hartocollis, 1976).

In an effort to bring recognition to the problem of patient assault on nursing staff and to document nursing staff's reactions as victims, a descriptive exploratory study entitled "Nursing Staff's Responses to Violence" was conducted at a federal hospital. Part of that study will be discussed as it relates to the formation of a tentative nursing diagnosis: *victim (abuse) reaction, related to intentional physical abuse.*

METHODOLOGY

All reports of assault were reviewed retrospectively over a 1-year period. From a potential sample of 67 nurses and nursing assistants who were assaulted 91 times, 40 nursing staff members (17 RN's and 23 nursing assistants), from both psychiatric and medical wards, volunteered to complete a self-administered questionnaire. The questionnaire included closed- and open-ended questions and a five-level response rating scale. The questionnaire focused on the victims' and patients' demographic data; descriptions of the last reported assault and prior assaults; short- and long-term emotional, social, biophysiologic, and cognitive responses to the assault; and prediction

□The opinions expressed in this article are those of the author and do not necessarily reflect those of the Veterans Administration Hospital.

of assault. Descriptive statistics, chi-square analysis, and analysis of variance were used in data analysis.

FINDINGS

The emotional, social, biophysiologic, and cognitive responses (Table 1) on defining characteristics were reported by at least 30% of the victims.

TABLE 1   **Emotional, social, biophysiologic, and cognitive responses from questionnaire**

Emotional	Social	Biophysiologic	Cognitive
Short-term			
Helplessness	Change in relationship with coworkers	Startle response	Denial of thoughts about assault
Irritability		Sleep pattern disturbance	
Fear of returning to scene of assault	Difficulty returning to work	Soreness	Preoccupation with thinking about assault
	Fear of other patients	Headaches	
Feelings of resignation	Feeling sorry for patient who hit them		Considering change in life-style
Depression	Should have done something to prevent assault		
Anger			
Anxiety			
Shock			
Apathy			
Disbelief			
Self-blame			
Dependency			
Long-term			
Fear of patient who hit them	Feeling sorry for patient who hit them	Body tension	Anger toward authority
Anger		Soreness	Wanting protection by authority and from authority's criticism
Anxiety			

RECOMMENDATIONS FOR FURTHER RESEARCH

Two avenues for further research are suggested. The first is a continuation of the research on victim reactions, which is currently in progress. Two purposes of this research are to (1) refine and expand the defining characteristics of victim abuse reaction and (2) determine what variables influence the presence or absence of the defining characteristics exhibited by victims (Lanza, 1982). The second suggestion is to compare the defining characteristics reported in this study with those reported by other populations of victims. Similarities of victim reactions resulting from different types of physical assault have already been reported (Frederick, 1980; Krupnick and Horowitz, 1980; Symonds, 1980).

REFERENCES

Brooks, B.: Aggression, Am. J. Nurs. **67:**2519, 1967.

Frederick, C.J.: Effects of natural vs. human induced violence upon victims, Evaluation and Change, special ed., 1980, 71-75.

Kalogerakis, M.: The assaultive psychiatric patient, Psychiatr. Q. **45:**372, 1971.

Krupnick, J.L., and Horowitz, M.J.: Victims of violence: psychological responses, treatment implications, Evaluation and Change, special ed., 1980, 42-47.

Lange, S.: Scientific bases for therapeutic nursing practice—approaches to coping with problem patients, the violent patient, ANA Clin. Sess. **54:**54, 1966.

Lanza, M.: Attributions to nurses and assault victims, Unpublished doctral dissertation, Boston, 1982, Boston University.

Levy, P.M., and Hartocollis, P.: Nursing aids and patient violence, Am. J. Psychiatry **133:**429, 1976.

Statistical Abstracts of the U.S., ed. 100, Washington, D.C., 1979, U.S. Department of Commerce.

Symonds, M.: The second injury to victims, Evaluation and Change, special ed., 1980, 36-38.

Alteration in health maintenance: conceptual base, etiology, and defining characteristics

KAREN K. PERET, R.N., M.S., C.N.A.A.
BARBARA STACHOWIAK, R.N., B.S.

Concepts of health are central to our efforts in defining parameters of our professional practice. One such concept particularly relevant to nursing practice is health maintenance. Current literature repeatedly refers to health maintenance as an appropriate nursing function. Most often this reference is general and abstract. This concept must be defined in more concrete and clinically useful terminology to advance nursing practice in the realm of health maintenance. An appropriate means for achieving this end is through the mechanism of nursing diagnosis. The diagnostic label *alteration in health maintenance* designates the client problem in this need area. *Alteration in health maintenance* is conceptualized along a continuum from complete dependence (dysfunctional) on a second party for all health needs, to a partial level of dependence, to relative independence. A link to formal nursing theory is provided by Orem's conceptual model of self-care (1980).

Alteration in health maintenance has been developed into a nursing diagnosis and has been used at the Monson Developmental Center in Palmer, Massachusetts for more than 1 year. This nursing diagnosis defines a need area evidenced in 98% of the client population. Because of our clinical experiences with the diagnosis, it is believed that it is applicable to a wide segment of clients, particularly in long-term care and community settings.

This paper will review a portion of the current literature and the nursing theory that provides the conceptual base for *alteration in health maintenance* and will discuss the definition of *alteration in health maintenance* and its etiology and defining characteristics. We will also present several examples of how *alteration in health maintenance* at the Monson Developmental Center.

REVIEW OF THE LITERATURE

Current literature generally looks at the function of health maintenance from two perspectives: as a role of the nursing profession and as a self-care role of the patient. An example of the first perspective is provided by the ANA (1980). Their Social Policy Statement has several references to the role of the nurse in assisting the client in maintaining and managing usual health practices "both during periods of wellness and when faced with a progressive or long-term health problem" (ANA, 1980, p. 6). Chang (1980) further specifies the nursing role in health maintenance as one of assessing the level of ability clients have in meeting their health maintenance needs. These two works support the concept of health maintenance as (1) a legitimate concern for the nursing profession and (2) applicable to the general client population. The proposed nursing diagnosis *alteration in health maintenance* is one mechanism for providing a clear, more concrete focus for this accepted nursing role.

Health maintenance as a nursing function occupies a central focus in developmental disabilities nursing. The ANA (1978) lists the following nursing goals:

1. "Promoting and teaching health maintenance and a high level of wellness throughout the life span" (p. 4)
2. "Determining the level of adaptive behavior" (to self-care) (p. 7)
3. "Observation of the client's level of knowledge and skills related to health maintenance and environmental safety" (p. 7)

McNelly (1978, p. 80) looks at the role of the nurse in developmental disabilities as one that incorporates a "concern with the ability of the individual to perform self-care activities necessary for daily living and for maintaining health." Other aspects of the nurse's role include assessment and interpretation of the individual's adaptive behavior, the ability to communicate "basic health care and health maintenance needs, including prevention, growth and development factors, strength and limitations in coping abilities, and social and environmental factors" (McNelly, p. 1978, p. 81).

As the literature indicates *alteration in health maintenance* is a primary problem for people with developmental disabilities. Nurses' concern with this problem is seen as both appropriate and prescriptive of a new, more professional nursing role. This new role is currently being called for by nursing leaders in the field of developmental disabilities (Curry and Peppe, 1978).

The second perspective of health maintenance, the self-care role of the client, is discussed by Chang (1980). She includes in her definition of client self-care "health maintenance, disease-prevention, self-diagnosis, self-medication, self-treatment, and patient participation in the use of professional services" (Chang, 1980, p. 43). Skills, knowledge, and the ability to adapt to changing conditions are prerequisites to self-care.

Given (1979) discusses the legislative and research concensus that consumers hold the key to disease prevention, health maintenance, and health promotion through their participation in self-care. She researched the relationship between client knowledge and beliefs and clients' contributions to their own care. She found that the "importance patients assign to the barriers they encounter in their daily activities in attempting to participate in their prescribed care" is quite high (Given, 1979, p. 27). She postulates that reducing barriers may be a very effective means of gaining client participation.

The review of the literature up to this point supports our contention that health maintenance is discussed in abstract and elusive terms from both the nurse and the client perspectives. The proposed diagnosis of *alteration in health maintenance* is an attempt to answer the need for a more clinically useful definition. The appropriateness of health maintenance as a nursing concern can further be established when it is linked to nursing theory. We believe the nursing theory that is most appropriate is Orem's (1980). According to Orem's self-care concepts (1980, p. 6), "nursing has as its special concern the individual's need for self-care action and the provision and management of it on a continuous basis in order to sustain life and health, recover from disease or injury, and cope with their effects." "Self-care is based on deliberate and thoughtful judgment that leads to appropriate action" (Joseph, 1980, p. 132). Orem calls the ability to meet basic health needs *self-care agency*. Self-care agency is more specifically defined in terms of behaviors essential to self-care, such as prerequisite knowledge, skill, resources, and motivation. Basic health needs for which self-care activities are directed are the following:

> The maintenance of a sufficient intake of air, water and food; the provision of care associated with elimination processes and excrements; the maintenance of a balance between activity and rest; the maintenance of a balance between solitude and social interaction; the prevention of hazards to human life, human functioning and human well-being; and the promotion of human functioning and development within social groups in accord with human potential, known human limitations and the human desire to be normal (Orem, 1980, p. 42).

In addition, there are developmental and health-deviation needs that arise as a result of life cycle events, illness, or injury or from the therapy or procedures used to treat an illness or injury or to assist in a life cycle event (Joseph, 1980). Nursing care is required when the clients's ability to perform self-care is absent or compromised or "whenever the maintenance of continuous self-care requires the use of special techniques and the application of scientific knowledge in providing care or in designing it" (Orem, 1980, p. 7).

Orem's conceptual model (1980) provides the framework on which to structure a definition of *health maintenance* and of *alteration in health maintenance*. She outlines the basic health-related need areas that people must meet on a continual basis to remain healthy. She also identifies the four components of an individual's self-care ability (self-care agency). When one or more of these components is missing, the individual is in jeopardy of lacking sufficient self-care abilities to meet health needs required in a particular situation. The client may be diagnosed as having a *potential alteration in health maintenance*. *Alteration in health maintenance*, therefore, describes the condition in which clients are unable to meet their fundamental health needs.

HEALTH MAINTENANCE: ALTERATION IN, POTENTIAL ALTERATION IN, DYSFUNCTIONAL

The formal definition of *alteration in health maintenance* that is proposed is an inability to identify, manage, and/or seek help to maintain a basic level of health (Box 1). The etiology parallels Orem's fundamental concept of self-care. "Self-care is based on deliberate and thoughtful judgment that leads to appropriate action" (Joseph, 1980, p. 132). The lack of the ability to make deliberate and thoughtful judgments is the underlying foundation of *alteration in health maintenance*. It can be measured by a demonstrated lack of adaptive behaviors to internal or external environmental changes. The other etiologies are deduced from Orem's four factors (1980) that people must have to be capable of self-care:

1. Knowledge
   a. Demonstrated lack of knowledge regarding basic health practices
2. Physical abilities
   a. Lack of significant communication skills (written, verbal, and/or gestural)
   b. Unachieved developmental tasks
   c. Complete/partial lack of gross motor skills
   d. Perceptual/cognitive impairment
3. Resources
   a. Disabling ineffective family coping
   b. Lack of material resources
4. Motivation
   a. Ineffective individual coping
   b. Spiritual distress
   c. Dysfunctional grieving

Alteration in health maintenance is therefore a condition that arises when several signs and symptoms are present. If only one of the etiologic factors is operational in a client condition, the nurse should use the specific nursing diagnosis that identifies the immediate problem. If, however, a large number of these etiologic factors are present to a varying degree, the client's condition warrants a more fundamental, perhaps even compensatory, focus in the nursing care provided. This fundamental focus is represented by *alteration in, potential alteration in,* or *dysfunctional health maintenance.*

The defining characteristics further clarify the nature of *alteration in health maintenance*. They include a demonstrated lack of adaptive behaviors to internal/external environmental changes; a reported or an observed inability to take responsibility for meeting basic health practices in any or all functional pattern areas; a history of a lack of health-seeking behavior; an expressed client interest in improving health behaviors; a reported or an observed lack of equipment and financial and/or other resources; and a reported or an observed impairment of the client's personal support system.

BOX 1   **Health maintenance: alteration in, potential alteration in, dysfunctional**

Definition
  Inability to identify, manage, and /or seek help to maintain health.
Etiology
  Lack of, or significant alteration in, communication skills (written, verbal,
    and/or gestural)
  Lack of ability to make deliberate and thoughtful judgments
  Perceptual/cognitive impairment
  Complete/partial lack of gross and/or fine motor skills
  Demonstrated lack of knowledge regarding basic health practices
  Ineffective individual coping
  Spiritual distress
  Dysfunctionl grieving
  Ineffective family coping: disabling
  Unachieved developmental tasks
  Lack of material resources
Defining characteristics
  Demonstrated lack of adaptive behaviors to internal/external
    environmental changes
  Reported or observed inability to take responsibility for meeting basic
    health practices in any or all functional pattern areas
  History of lack of health-seeking behavior
  Expressed client interest in improving health behaviors
  Reported or observed lack of equipment and financial and/or other
    resources
  Reported or observed impairment of personal support system

Example

In our facility, two objectives of care for a client with *dysfunctional health maintenance* have been identified. First, the client's baseline patterns of health must be monitored—vital signs, weights, and normal patterns in the eight universal need areas. Second, deviations from normal patterns, such as signs and symptoms of illness or injuries, or illness-producing behaviors, such as behavioral outbursts, are identified. A sample health care plan follows.

Objectives	Interventions
1. The client will have baseline patterns of health monitored.	1. Mental retardation assistant will weigh client during the first week of each month and document on the Health Care/Maintenance Checklist
	2. Blood pressure will be read quarterly/monthly during the first week of the month by the nurse.
	3. The nurse will perform a breast examination during the second week of each month.

Objectives	Interventions
	4. The nurse will schedule, coordinate, and monitor the results of routine and specially ordered lab tests and medical/other consults and confer with staff of ancillary services.
	5. The nurse will review the data on the Health Care/Maintenance Checklist on a weekly basis and will summarize and evaluate it monthly in the Progress Notes.
2. The client will have signs and symptoms of potential and/or actual changes in health status assessed.	1. The nurse will observe the client twice daily while administering medications.
	2. The nurse will investigate, evaluate, and document all reports of client injury or accident immediately and will provide care when necessary and appropriate.
	3. An RN will review the medication record for client response to medication therapy administered, potential adverse reactions, allergic interactions, contraindications, an lab test modifications and will document the review in the record.
	4. The nurse will confer with other health professionals to evaluate how their program interventions affect the health status of the client.

The level of *alteration in health maintenance* is a function of the severity of one or any combination of defining characteristics. If the client depends on the nurse for all basic health needs, the client has *dysfunctional health maintenance*. If the client can independently meet some portion of basic health needs, the client has *alteration in health maintenance*. If the client is at risk or in an at-risk population such as severe brain injury or a developmental disability, the client may have *potential alteration in health maintenance*. Nursing interventions range from wholly compensatory to supportive/educative.

Since implementing this nursing diagnosis in our facility, the nursing staff has decreased its dependence on the physician for direction in health care. *Alteration in health maintenance* has generated the identification of a number of other nursing needs. The types of interventions that nurses plan have become much more concrete and realistic. In short, *alteration in health maintenance* has actually helped to foster a higher caliber of professional nursing care in our facility.

Significance

Alteration in health maintenance is significant because it is one of the first nursing diagnoses that operationalizes a recognized nursing theory. Practicing nurses readily identify with the diagnosis because it is what they have known intuitively for years. *Alteration in health maintenance* provides the words with which nurses can articulate those intuitions.

Alteration in health maintenance, with its basis in the *self-care theory of nursing*, gives form and measurability to the current literature that speaks of health maintenance as a role of the nurse. With this form and measurability, client need areas can be specifically identified and treated. Health maintenance is less of an abstract idea and more of a concrete list of knowledge, skills, resources, and motivation.

The level of independent nursing judgment involved in treating *alteration in health maintenance* is high. The condition it describes is one that confronts nurses daily in nursing homes, convalescent homes, psychiatric facilities, and facilities for the mentally retarded. Nurses in community care see it as do school nurses and clinic nurses. Not only does *alteration in health maintenance* describe the client's underlying need for nursing care, but it also supplies the structure and the direction to respond to that need, to develop nursing objectives, and to plan interventions for client care.

SUMMARY AND CONCLUSION

In summary, the literature regarding the role of the nurse and the role of the client in health maintenance was reviewed. Theoretic constructs of Orem's concepts of self-care and *alteration in health maintenance* were outlined and compared. An example of the application of *alteration in health maintenance* was given. The significance of *alteration in health maintenance* was discussed. Feedback from colleagues with whom we have shared *alteration in health maintenance* has been positive. Colleagues are enthused about *alteration in health maintenance* and are eager to share it with their peers. We recommend that the diagnosis of *alteration in health maintenance* be included on the accepted list of nursing diagnoses.

REFERENCES

American Nurses' Association: Guidelines for continuing education in developmental disabilities, Kansas City, Mo., 1978, The Association.

American Nurses' Association: Nursing: a social policy statement, Kansas City, Mo., 1980, The Association.

Chang, B.L.: Evaluation of health care professionals in facilitating self-care: review of the literature and a conceptual model, Adv. Nurs. Serv. **3**(1):43, 1980.

Curry, J., and Peppe, K., eds.: Mental retardation: nursing approaches to care, St. Louis, 1978, The C.V. Mosby Co.

Given, B.: Patient participation. In American Nurses' Association, ed.: Nursing's influence on health policy for the eighties: 1978 scientific session of the American Academy of Nursing, Kansas City, Mo., 1979, The Association.

Joseph, L.S.: Self-care and the nursing process, Nurs. Clin. North Am. **15**(1):131, 1980.

McNelly, P.: Quality assurance in residential settings. In Curry, J., and Peppe, K., eds.: Mental retardation: nursing approaches to care, St. Louis, 1978, The C.V. Mosby Co.

Orem, D.: Nursing: concepts of practice, New York, 1980, McGraw-Hill Book Co.

ADDITIONAL READING

Maloney, M., and Ward, M.: Mental retardation and modern society, New York, 1979, Oxford University Press, Inc.

Family diagnoses that work

LEONA C. HAYES, R.N., M.S.N.

The purpose of this paper is to describe a systems approach to family diagnosis that makes it possible to obtain family participation in improving health-related behaviors, health status, and/or the environment in which the family lives. Authors such as Robischon and Smith (1977) provide helpful guidelines for the collection and classification of data from family assessment. Their kind of help is most valuable for the essential function of assessment of families. Community health nurses, educated to use information from various supporting disciplines, have a great receptivity to cues relating multiple factors to the health of the families. They do not wear blinders that screen out all information that does not apply to physiologic, economic, or psychologic problems. Once data are collected, how are they used? Is it ethical to collect all data and then proceed as if only one part of it was available? Can nurses resist the temptation to grab at a smaller, more easily defined diagnosis so that they can rush on with the planning and intervention?

Nurses are not unlike the six blind men in the Hindu fable who used different sensory data collection devices to assess the essence of an elephant. The blind man who grabbed the elephant's tail and exclaimed, "The elephant is very like a rope!" resembles a professional who concentrates only on improving medical or social conditions in a family. "No, " said the man at the other end of the elephant with his arms around the elephant's swaying trunk. "The elephant is very like a snake!" He could be likened to a professional who focuses on family interactions to do family therapy. "Aha!" shouts the third man who is hugging the big leg of the elephant. "You have seen only a small part of the elephant. He is very like a tree!" This man is similar to a professional who plans restorative care without allowing the family decision-making process to select a level of self-care to which they are willing to commit themselves. The essential wholeness of the elephant must be perceived before one can say one knows what an elephant is. Likewise, the wholeness of the family must be recognized and dealt with in any attempt to develop a workable family diagnosis. Long-range goals that are prerequisite to effective care cannot be formulated without a holistic view of the family.

A holistic view of the family can be made operational by using a systems approach to the family. This framework for family diagnosis is based on an underlying proposition identified by Bredemeier: "The family is a complex system, which requires adaptive, integrative, and decision-making processes for survival, continuity, and growth" (Horton, 1977, p. 102). Bredemeier has suggested that the process of family adaptation consists of four boundary maintenance functions of obtaining, containing, retaining, and disposing of matter, energy, information, and services (Horton, 1977). Therefore in this paper the adaptation process is called *boundary maintenance*. Boundary maintenance deals with such things as maintenance of privacy and safety of the home environment, use of economic resources, use of matter such as nutrients, and use of resources outside the family such as community services and support systems.

The term *family interaction* is used to describe internal patterns of interdependence that are unique to the family being studied. Family role relationships, coping methods, and communication patterns are considered, along with the influence culture.

Family decision making is the third process necessary to family survival, continuity, and growth. Omitting this essential area of decision making is a costly mistake. Optimum use of the energies of a nursing staff and a family dictates that full consideration be given to the desires of the family before writing care plans. Nurses might be surprised to learn that many of their clients were merely being polite when they acquiesced and said they would follow the staff's directions (as long as professionals are in sight, that is). Decision making relates to choices made by families regarding growth and health care. Alliances and the use of power in family decision making are assessed. Decision making in a family involves group consent and commitment to the course of action chosen (Horton, 1977).

METHODOLOGY

Senior students in a baccalaureate nursing curriculum gave nursing care to 120 families using a systems approach to the organization of nursing care. Families were assessed by the students and faculty separately, and the data were examined together in weekly conferences. Each family was analyzed for a diagnosis in each of the three general areas—adaptation, interaction, and decision making.

The three organizing diagnoses arose from the classification of cues perceived in the early part of the assessment. Gordon (1982) calls them spacer diagnoses or problem space areas. The broad organizing diagnoses served as skeleton hypotheses available for verification and double checking when there was conflict among cues. Diagnoses were tested by assuming optimal health until the data indicated family dissatisfaction or the nurse had data supporting a pattern of dysfunction. The descriptive terms *adequate, inadequate*, or *potentially inadequate* were used to qualify the diagnoses.

The thinking process thus completed involved both inductive and deductive reasoning. Inductive reasoning, using the sensory data collected from the

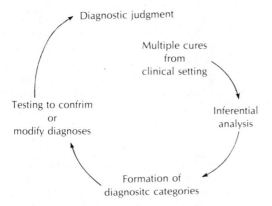

Diagnostic judgment

Multiple cures
from
clinical setting

Inferential
analysis

Testing to confrim
or
modify diagnoses

Formation of
diagnositc categories

FIGURE 1   Diagnostic judgment spiral.

clinical setting, gave rise through inferential analysis to the general diagnoses (Figure 1). The deductive reasoning process was used in the collection of confirming or contrasting data to support the original conclusions or to provide alternative explanations. Confirming or contrasting data were collected from consultants, cooperating agencies, and, most importantly, from the family. Such information as family perceptions of vulnerability, perceived seriousness of the problem, and confidence in the value of early action (Pender, 1975) was obtained. Based on the new data and interpretations, a diagnostic judgment was formulated (Figure 1).

After formulating diagnoses and validating them with a family, the nurse and family members collaborated in establishing goals for care. Long-term goals were designated for the family, that is, goals toward which the family would be moving after the relationship with the nurse was terminated. Intermediate goals were developed to be achieved by the end of the relationship. Immediate or short-term goals were established for weekly visits.

The following case study shows how family diagnoses were used to assist in organizing nursing care for one family.

Case study

The *A* family lived in a suburban, three-bedroom home that was 5 years old. The family had four children ranging from 14 to 28 years of age. Mr. and Mrs. *A* ran an insurance–tax service business in one part of their home. The oldest child was married and lived in Arizona with her husband and two children. Robert, the next eldest, was 22 years of age and a quadriplegic with an injury at the C-4 level. Robert had extensive rehabilitation assistance through the Department of Rehabilitation Service, including a home designed especially for him, training in operation of "slip-n-puff system" gadgets, and a specially adapted van. With his disability income, he paid for the house and utilities plus gas and insurance for the van. Although he could operate a wheelchair anywhere in the house, he spent most of the day in his room. Mrs. *A* fed Robert all his meals because it was easier than cleaning up food spills. Physical care was adequate and included visits by a physical therapist 6 days per week.

Mr. *A* was on medication to control high blood pressure. The family unit had communication difficulties. Robert intended to make a trip to Arizona to see his older sister, accompanied by his two younger sisters. If he liked the area, he would stay. The plan was acceptable to his parents. He intended to enter college at a local university or in Arizona.

A boundary maintenance diagnosis for this family related to several areas of family involvement in the care of Robert. An example was adequate boundary maintenance related to infection control and preventing urinary tract complications for Robert. A long-term goal was a normal life expectancy resulting from preventing interference with adequate urinary elimination by maintaining a barrier to bacterial growth in the urine and by maintaining adequate resistance to infection in Robert. Achievement of the goal required family-based care.

Another area of family care for Robert involved controlling the environmental temperature for the protection of Robert who had lost the physiologic mechanisms needed to maintain normal body temperature. A diagnosis was *potential inadequate boundary maintenance* related to environmental changes for Robert when he entered college. If he attended college in Arizona or in Illinois, he needed to anticipate the effects of temperature extremes in the climates found in either place. A long-range goal for care of the client and the family was stated as protection from temperature extremes so that he could pursue his educational goal in a severe climate. The care involved his parents, sisters, and other caretakers.

The diagnosis relating to family interaction for the *A* family was *inadequate family interaction* related to patterns of communication or *inadequate family interaction* related to level of responsibility Robert had assumed. Cues to this area of inadequacy were the presence of stress-related hypertension in the father, Robert's dependency for feeding, and his lack of participation in the family business, which was conducted in the home. This diagnosis had to be validated by determining the family desires regarding the level of independence Robert should have. Goal formation in this area depended on the family decision as to how much responsibility for the business was to be shared by Robert, whether or not Robert wanted to feed himself, and how much the younger sisters were willing to invest in the care of Robert at mealtime. A long-range goal was healthy family interaction that promoted the growth of all family members.

Decision making in the *A* family was considered potentially inadequate based on the patterns of family communication. The family mode of decision making appeared to be de facto; the mode had to be explained more clearly as the family decided whether Robert would attend college. The possibility of Robert leaving the family was the focus of future decision making. Family alliances of the siblings against the parents appeared possible, and the maturation of Robert seemed to be a possible outcome of the process. Goals were the development of open communication lines and improved decision making. Nursing functions were to help family members look at the consequences of the various alternate plans available and to support family members in implementing the chosen course of action that related to health. Organization of family diagnoses into the three functions necessary to system survival, continuity, and growth appeared to facilitate obtaining family participation in improving their own health.

SUMMARY

Was the experience in formulating nursing diagnoses for families related to an improved ability to make a diagnostic judgment? DeBack (1981) examined the relationship between the curriculum model and the ability of senior nursing students to formulate nursing diagnoses. Curriculum design did not appear to be significantly related to differences in students' ability to formulate nursing diagnoses.

In describing the experiential learning theory, Kolb (1981) emphasizes the important role that experience plays in the learning process. He describes how concrete experience serves as the basis for observation and reflection, leading to the formation of generalizations. The generalizations are tested for aptness, and the outcomes are used to design new experiences for learning. This experience in working with senior nursing students in formulating nursing diagnoses for 120 families suggests that laboratory experience may be more important than curriculum design or methods of classroom evaluation in determining how well students can formulate nursing diagnosis. Further study of a possible relationship is indicated.

REFERENCES

DeBack, V.: The relationship between senior nursing student's ability to formulate nursing diagnoses and the curriculum model, Adv. Nurs. Sci. 3(3):51, 1981.

Gordon, M.: Nursing diagnosis process and application, New York, 1982, McGraw-Hill Book Co.

Horton, T.: Conceptual basis for nursing intervention with human systems: families. In Hall, J.E., and Weaver, B.R., eds.: Distributive nursing practice: a systems approach to community health, Philadelphia, 1977, J.B. Lippincott, Co.

Kolb, D.A.: Today's students and their needs. In Chickering, A.W., and others, eds.: The modern American college, San Francisco, 1981, Jossey-Bass, Inc., Publishers.

Pender, N.J.: A conceptual model for preventive health behavior, Nurs. Outlook 23(6):385, 1975.

Robischon, P., and Smith, J.A.: Family assessment. In Reinhardt, A.M., and Quinn, M.D., eds.: Current practice in family-centered community nursing, vol. 1, St. Louis, 1977, The C.V. Mosby Co.

Nurses' assessment of a person's potential for violence: use of grounded theory in developing a nursing diagnosis

PATRICIA CLUNN, R.N., Ed.D.

The recognition of formulating nursing diagnoses as an independent, legal function of the nurse distinguishes clinical inference as a professional nurse behavior and underlies the premise that appropriate assessment and diagnostic formulation are critical to effective nursing practice (Fortin and Rabinow, 1979; Lesnick and Anderson, 1955). Definitions of assessment usually imply the existence of substantive theory, providing the nurse clinician with a framework for cue identification and utilization. Facts are derived from theoretic or conceptual frameworks providing criterion measures to evaluate outcomes of the diagnoses/hypotheses formulated from assessment variables.

The diagnostic process investigated in this study was the nurse's assessment of a person's potential for violence. Violence, defined as the intent to inflict injury on another person, is a transitory emotional state for which there is no substantive theoretic framework (Fromm, 1973; Gelles and Strauss, 1979). Nurses generally lack formal preparation for making potential for violence diagnoses; present practice represents the nurse's intuitive inferences drawn from "practice wisdom" and trial-and-error learning. The identification of cues nurses use in making inferences about a person's potential for violence was an initial effort toward replacing intuitive responses with a deliberate nursing inference process.

Previous relevant nursing research consisted of a cognitive-perceptual project (Hammond, and others, 1966; Hammond and Summers, 1965, 1972) and the cue utilization and prioritization of nurses from different role groups (Thomas and Hansen, 1966, 1970). These research projects drew on the diagnostic decision-making strategies of practicing nurses to identify cue utilization, configuration, and prioritization.

Clinical inference studies using Len's model computation formula to establish relationships between cue utilizations differ from this descriptive study. In most simulated situation studies, clinicians are provided a specific set of cues on the basis of which judgments are to be made. By controlling the cues in the stimuli, it is possible to rule out unidentified cues influencing the subject's decision. The problem in these studies is the utilization and configuration of cues that are known and controlled. The steps required to

□Portions of this writing were adapted from the author's doctoral dissertation (Clunn, 1975).

achieve the level of conceptualization appropriate to using Len's model necessitate (1) identification of information that constitutes a cue, (2) availability of the cue, and (3) cue utilization and configuration. This research represented a preliminary step in identifying some of the cues used in violence assessment, drawing on the statement by Dickoff, James, and Wiedenback (1968) that level one theory must evolve from practice and from Wald's and Leonard's earlier advocacy (1964) that nursing researchers build knowledge directly from a systematic study of nursing experiences derived from and tested in the actual nursing arena.

Assumptions underlying this study were:

1. Nurses assess and predict potentially violent behavior using specific cues.
2. Nurses judge degrees of potential for violence by using cues to which they attach weights of importance in different situational contexts.
3. Nurses are natural figures in settings in which violent behaviors occur, and the predictive cues they use are derived from naturalistic observations that are reliable and valid (LeCompte, Butts, and Busch, 1972).
4. Cues nurses use in clinical inferences of a person's potential for violence are not necessarily the same cues identified by behavioral scientists in contrived, artificial, experimental, and ex post facto studies of violence.

The research sought answers to two questions:

1. What cues do nurses rely on in formulating a diagnosis of potential for violence?
2. Do nurses discriminate degrees of potentially violent behaviors by using and weighting cues differently, that is, varying cue configurations or using different cue configurations?

A two-part questionnaire with structured and unstructured sections was developed, and two concurrent, though interrelated, methodologies were used. The structured section of the questionnaire was designed to answer the latter question of cue utilization and configuration. Subjects were requested to assess a person's potential for violence depicted in six simulated situations written by nurses describing work encounters with potentially violent people. The situations were revised for the purposes of the study. Two scales followed the presentation of each situation—a Likert scale, on which subjects rated the described client's potential for violence, and a cue scale on which, in order of priority, the five salient cues used to make the violence inferences were listed. Since it was not possible to know which data served as cues, all phrases in the six situations were underlined and consecutively numbered so respondents could select any of the information presented in the anecdote.

The Likert scale had five points ranging from nonviolent (0) to violent (4). Each point was operationally defined by specific nurse interventions. For example, moderate potential for violence (2) was: "A person potentially violent with the likelihood of injuring others if the state escalates; requires a controlled environment and supervision." Ratings of nonviolent (0) and low potential for violence (1) did not require removing the client from the environment. Ratings of high potential for violence (3) required restriction and supervision. Violent (4) referred to an acute emergency situation that required immediate protective security and active restraining actions.

The unstructured section of the questionnaire consisted of open-ended questions referring to demographic variables: age, ancestry, education, preparation for violence prediction, years of active nursing, years in present position, number of times per week violence diagnoses were formulated, and self-assessment of violence assessment competencies. Respondents listed five clues they relied on most in violence prediction, wrote an anecdote depicting a recent potentially violent client situation, and rated and ranked the encounter on the scales used in the structured section. The cues identified in personal encounters contributed to the ongoing generation of cues and conceptual categories, following grounded theory methodology (Glaser and Strauss, 1968). An analysis of variance (ANOVA) technique for assessment of configural cue utilization in clinical judgment (Hoffman, Slovic, and Rarer, 1968) was used to discern interactions of violence ratings and cue category saliency. The .05 level of significance was selected for the study, and .01 findings were specified when they were found.

METHODOLOGY

The focus of this descriptive research was that of generating information rather than the verification of an existing theory. Grounded theory is a sociologic-anthropologic method that involves systematic choices and the study of theoretically relevant groups that can be of any size. The role groups studied ranged from 15 to 25 subjects, representing nurses employed in six metropolitan New York health agencies, including private, public, acute, and long-term care settings. The subjects were limited to nurses whose work roles placed them strategically in direct client encounters requiring the independent formulation of diagnoses of potential violence:

Agency	Number of subjects	Percentage of total sample
State mental hospital	15	11.2
Private hospital emergency	25	18.5
Department of corrections	20	14.8
Municipal hospital, inpatient psychiatric unit	25	18.5
Municipal hospital emergency	25	18.5
Public health agency	25	18.5
TOTALS	135	100

Theoretic completeness for the generation of grounded theory occurred with the analysis of the 60th critical incident, at which point cue saturation was reached. However, the number of subjects in the sample was predetermined, since both qualitative and quantitative measures were used (Devons and Gluckman, 1964; Jick, 1979). The rationale for sampling nurses employed in various work role settings was from the etiologic perspective that viewed violence as a "component of emotional reactivity that occurs over a broad range of physical and psychopathological disorders that by and in of itself is not diagnostically differential" (Ackerman, 1959, p. 236).

QUESTIONNAIRE DEVELOPMENT AND PILOT STUDY

The initial empirical grounded theory data were situations collected as preliminary survey materials for formulating continuing education programs. Nurses working in metropolitan New York health agencies were asked to write patient encounters that depicted their greatest need for additional education (Siegel, 1971). A comparable survey in a southern community and a workshop published as a result of a similiar survey (Flynn, 1969) corroborated that potential violence was among the most problematic client behaviors encountered in practice. From these surveys, over 280 practitioner-generated situations were collected and thematically analyzed, using Flanagan's critical-incident technique. The concrete, real-life accounts were considered one step away from field observations, and the subjective nature of the incidents was not considered a limitation, since subjective data were sought.

An extensive search of the theoretic and research literature was conducted to draw on the existing knowledge of violence potential and research methodologies. The pervasive rationale given for the lack of adequate violence theory development found in the literature was methodologic limitations imposed by ethical/legal concerns for subjects participating in life-threatening experiments, lack of definitional clarity, and researchers' adversion to the topic. As to the latter, Bettelheim (1966, p. 51) cogently commented:

> Aggression is by now a respectable object of study among students of human behavior. But in this paper, I should like to refer to violence, which the same scholars tend to ignore or treat with contempt. By simply agreeing violence is bad resolves nothing. To study aggression in detail while we close our eyes to its source is like wishing to clean out all filth without soiling our hands. If we are serious about our understanding of aggression and its role in society, we have to start with a good look at the desire to do violence. . . . if we are the children of Cain, it behooves us to know Cain well, and examine his behavior and what causes it, and not look away in disgust.

The literature review did not produce additional cues other than those derived from thematic analysis of the nurse-generated situations.

Twelve situations were selected, three from each of the four areas of clinical nursing practice, presenting a sample of young, middle-aged, and older adult males in simulated client encounters. Situations (4%) depicting females, children, sexual acting-out, and instrumental aggression were excluded. The 12 selected situations were edited, refined, and further developed by two groups of pilot study participants. These groups included 22 nurses in work roles comparable to the projected research subjects and a 10-member expert panel whose expertise was determined through publications and recognition for violence assessment and intervention knowledge and skills.

The initial 22-member nurse pilot group found the 12 situations excessively time consuming, and the expert panel was formed to select six of the 12 situations most supportive to the study purposes. After the developmental study group and the expert panel completed the unstructured section of the questionnaire, data were collected from their input and used as a data base for the initial generation of a cue listing and the conceptualization of 11 broad cue categories for the specific cues. This data base provided a conceptual framework for categorizing the 176 cues in the simulations. Whereas the six simulated situations were discrete and unrelated, the 11 conceptual categories facilitated comparisons of cues that spanned the simulations and allowed for data analysis.

RELIABILITY AND VALIDITY

The limited knowledge of violence necessitated reliance on the developmental study group for validation. Although this was a weak test for content validity, it was superior to mere reliance on the face value of practitioner-submitted situations. Two tests-retests for reliability and validity were performed. The expert panel completed test-retesting in 3 months, and 16 members of the 22-member nurse pilot group completed test-retesting in 2 weeks.

Although reliability and validity were major concerns, pilot study results were also used to ascertain the nature of the diagnostic decision-making tasks and applicability of the Hoffman, Slovic, and Rarer (1968) model. Use of the model depended on verification that cue usage in violence assessment was both linear and configural. If judgment stimuli were regarded as continuous random variables and judgments made to cues considered dependent variables, the inferential and descriptive capabilities of the ANOVA technique could be applied to this study of judgment. Brunswick's probabilistic model provides for this discrimination when cues used in decision making are known. The pilot study group provided data to replicate Hoffman's research (1968) and to validate the research model's usefulness. Except for Gordon's research (1980) identifying strategies nurses use to select or eliminate hypothesis in the process of decision making, little attention has been given to defining how nurses use probabilistic information in the decision-making process.

Bruner, Goodnow, and Austin (1956) have set fourth two basic diagnostic strategies: simultaneous and successive. Simultaneous scanning strategies involve the simultaneous use of information to test multiple hypotheses. It is generally assumed that inductive inferences are primarily linear, and it is not yet understood how subjects cope with linear and nonlinear data simultaneously in the cognitive and perceptual domains (Hammond and Summers, 1965).

Review of reliability studies of clinical inferences showed low reliability and validity, with about one third of the variation attributed to inconsistencies among the diagnosticians (interrater) and other variations attributed to the rater's professional identity and theoretic orientation and the setting in which the rater functioned (Fleiss, Spitzer, and Burdock, 1965). Bias and unreliability are the two components of inaccuracy in clinical inference. Bias can be eliminated by deleting results that are widely divergent when compared with other qualified raters. To eliminate bias error, cumulative violence scores were computed and extreme scores were deleted from the pilot study. Thus two of the original 12 expert panelists and four of the original 26 nurse pilot subjects were excluded because of bias error.

The reliability of the expert panelists' violence ratings were computed by percentage comparisons, which averaged 70%; product-moment correlation coefficients were established at 0.91. Percentage rating agreements varied among the situations, ranging from 90% for situation 6 to 50% for situation 1. The percentage rating agreement was 68% for situations 2, 3, and 4 and 80% for situation 5. The nurse pilot group ratings showed a percentage comparison reliability average of 71% and a product-moment correlation of 0.88. As with the expert panel, there were situational variations; situations 1, 2, and 6 had 75% agreement, situations 3 and 4 had 78%, and situation 5 had 56%. The most marked divergence between nurse and expert groups was for situation 5 (56% for the nurse groups, 80% for the expert panel). These differences could be explained by regional orientation and setting diversity—the expert panel represented broad geographic areas and the nurse pilot group practiced regionally in New York.

Replication of cue usage and cue sequencing was analyzed for additive (linear) or configural indices of the diagnostic task. The nurse pilot group used 70% of the same cues on retesting. Of these cues 37% were replicated in the same order. The expert panel used 67% of the same cues on retesting, but only 26% of the cues were replicated in the same order. The low sequential and high replication of cue usage suggests that the nurse pilot group used configural and linear clinical inference processes in scaling replications, a complexity noted in earlier studies (Kelly, 1966). Use of the ANOVA model was deemed appropriate given these findings.

DATA COLLECTION

Agencies from which research participation was requested were located in metropolitan New York. The major concern in administering the questionnaire was the need for debriefing and providing feedback to participants. Supervisors arranged for the researcher to meet with potential participants to clarify the questionnaires, which were completed during work hours, and to provide follow-up review of the group responses.

DATA ANALYSIS

Data analysis is presented with supporting figures of results. The statistical procedures move in stepwise complexity, and descriptive data were progressively analyzed until cue configurations emerged. Several propositional statements emerged during data analysis, and although they were specific to the simulated situations, they provided answers to the questions posited by the study. The methodology is presented in detail with strong recommendation that techniques using grounded theory be considered in developing and validating nursing diagnoses. Data analysis consisted of four aspects:

    I. Violence ratings of the six simulated situations
        A. One-way ANOVA to discern between-group differences in violence ratings
        B. Two-way ANOVA with Scheffé's correction to discern interaction of demographic variables with role group affiliation and violence ratings
        C. Chi-square cross tabulations to discern within-group differences in violence ratings
    II. Cue category usage
        A. Frequency distributions of cue categories ranked on cue saliency scales
        B. Percentages of subjects in role groups using cue categories on the cue ranking scales.
    III. Violence ratings of the six simulated situations and cue category saliency scores
        A. One-way ANOVA to discern differences between cue category saliency scores and role groups
        B. One-way ANOVA to discern differences between cue category saliency scores and violence ratings
    IV. Formulation of conceptual categories with specifying properties of cues practitioners reported most reliable in practice

Two-way ANOVA tests (235) with Scheffé's correction were computed on demographic variables, role group affiliation, and violence ratings. Cue category saliency scores (36) were tested using one-way ANOVA tests. Some of the significant findings could have occurred by chance. The demographic characteristics of the 135 nurse subjects were as follows:

1. Age ranged from 20 to over 50, with over half (55%) 30 years of age or less.
2. Fifty-seven subjects (55%) were single; 76 (57%) were married.
3. Sixty-six subjects (49%) were white Americans; 43 (32%) were black Americans; and 25 (19%) were of Caribbean, Hispanic, or West Indian ancestry.
4. One-hundred-fourteen subjects (86%) were Protestants.
5. Forty-eight percent had basic educational preparation in hospital programs, and 52% had collegiate-based educational preparation (29% BSN, 16% ADN).
6. Thirty-six subjects (27%) held baccalaureate degrees.
7. Fifty-three percent of the public health group held baccalaureate degrees.
8. The majority (51%) had 6 or more years active nursing experience; thirteen (10%) had 20 years or more; and 6% had between 25 and 36 months' experience.
9. Although an older experienced group, 59% had been in their present work role for less than 23 months.
10. Fifty-two subjects (38%) reported six or more potentially violent encounters per week, and 18% reported 11 to 20 per week. Long-term subjects employed in acute psychiatric and emergency room settings (39 subjects) reported 10 to 15 violent or potentially violent encounters per week, twice the number of encounters reported by subjects employed in long-term psychiatric and correctional settings.
11. Forty-two percent (57) had no preparation for prediction of violence potential.
12. In self-assessment of competency for violence prediction, two subjects rated themselves inadequate, 53 above average, and seven excellent.
13. One hundred six subjects described a recent personal potentially violent encounter with a client; 49% were rated high potential (3) or violent (4) on the Likert scale.

One-way ANOVA tests performed showed role group differences in five of the six simulated situations. Significant F scores at the .01 level were found in situations 3 and 5 and at the .05 level of significance for situations 2, 4, and 6. Two-way ANOVA tests were performed to test the interaction of the 13 independent demographic variables, role group affiliation, and violence ratings. Analyses showed the main effect of self-assessed competency significant at the .01 level in situation 3. Other significant differences found for the main effects and interactions with demographic variables, by situation, were as follows:

1. Situation 2: Number of violent encounters per week interacted with role group differences at the .01 level of significance and with age, preparation for predicting violence, self-assessed competency, and marital status at the .05 level of significance.
2. Situation 3: The main effect of self-assessed competency was found significant at the .01 level; interactions at the .01 level were found for age, number of encounters per week, and self-assessment of competency. At the .05 level, preparation for predicting violence and basic nursing program were significant. All other demographic variables had .05 levels of significance, indicating strong role group response differences.
3. Situation 4: Role group differences were significant at the .01 level for age, marital status, and self-assessment of competency; .05 level of significance for number of violent encounters per week was found.
4. Situation 5: No significant tests for the main effect or interactions of the variables were found. Significant findings for role group differences were for age, education, marital status, self-assessment of competencies, and preparation for violence prediction at the .05 level of significance.
5. Situation 6: Role group differences at the .01 level of significance were found for marital status, years of experience, age, and prediction for violence preparation.

Chi-square analysis of cross tabulations showed within- and between-group differences. Significant differences at the .05 level were found in situations 2, 3, and 5.

Cues used by respondents in assessing a person's potential for violence in the simulated situations were reported within the broad conceptual categories used for data analysis. According to Hoffman, Slovic, and Rarer (1968), configurations involve two- and three-element patterns, thus only the total pattern configuration is relevant. The 135 subjects had five options for the six situations, and a cue category could possibly be listed 810 times. With these constraints in mind, the cues used by the subjects are as follows (the number of times the cue was used is given in parentheses):

1. Category II—verbal cues (637)
2. Category V—purposeful motor behaviors (497)
3. Category VI—nonpurposeful motor behaviors (325)
4. Category I—personal background information (38)

Comparisons of cue categories used by subjects in scaling responses to the six situations and subject-elicited salient cues given in response to the open-ended questions showed consistency in cue reliance. The number of subjects listing the cue categories is noted in parentheses:

1. Nonpurposeful motor actions of increasing tension (75)
2. Hostile, threatening verbalizations (67)
3. Body language (36)
4. Level of awareness (36)
5. History of past violent behavior (33)

The frequency distribution of a subject's use of cue categories does not indicate the importance (saliency) given the cue category. To ascertain the importance given a specific cue, cue category saliency scores were computed for data analysis. One-way ANOVA tests were performed to determine if there were significant differences in the cue category saliency scores assigned by the six role groups. Findings were as follows:

1. Two F scores significant at the .05 level were found in situation 5. The state mental hospital group gave the least saliency to verbal cues, and the correctional agency group gave the highest saliency to verbal cues. The verbal saliency scores were significantly higher for private than for municipal emergency room groups.
2. In situation 4, nurses from correctional agencies assigned a statistically significant higher saliency score (.05) to nonpurposeful motor actions (category VI) than subjects in other groups.

Using a reduced denominator contingent on a subject's use of the cue category, a second series of ANOVA tests were computed for role group differences in assigning saliency to cue categories. Significant (.05) findings were that state hospital nurses assigned high saliency to category X (social history) whereas the public health and municipal emergency room nurses assigned low saliency to the same category. The number and percentage of public health nurses using this category was very high, thus they relied on it consistently, yet assigned it low saliency. Conversely, state mental hospital nurses used social history frequently and assigned it great importance in diagnostic formulations of violence potential.

The F scores found statistically significant in the one-way ANOVA tests of cue category saliency and role groups were not considered to be of sufficient distinction for additional role group differentiation. Responses of the six role groups were combined as total sample data for the analysis of cue category saliency scores and violence ratings. One-way ANOVA tests were performed using the reduced denominator, which excluded subjects not using the cue category. Six differences significant at the .05 level were found:

1. Situation 3: Significant differences were found for violence ratings, category II saliency scores (medical history), and category V (purposeful motor actions). Inspection of the differences in the means indicated that when medical history was inferred highly salient, potential for violence was judged low. The two categories appear influential in vio-

lence ratings in this situation. If purposeful motor actions were given high saliency, potential for violence was high; if medical history was given high saliency, potential for violence was low.

2. Situation 5: Medical history (category II), level of awareness (category IX), and social history (category X) were statistically significant. Inspection of the differences in the means indicated that subjects rating the client nonviolent gave high saliency to cues in categories II and IX and low saliency scores to cues in category X; the reverse was true for high violence potential inferences.

The final ANOVA tests were performed on cue category saliency scores and violence ratings, using the reduced number of scores contingent on use of the cue category. Four saliency scores at the .05 level and one at the .01 level of significance were found:

1. Situation 1: Violence ratings were found significantly different in cue category VIII saliency scores assigned labile states. Inspection of differences in the means indicated that as saliency for category VIII increased, inferences of violence increased.

2. Situation 3: Inspection of differences in the means indicated that the less importance given verbal cues (category III), the lower the violence ratings. The reverse was true for purposeful motor actions (category V) and labile emotional states (category VIII). As saliency scores for these categories increased, violence ratings decreased.

3. Situation 4: Cue category saliency scores decreased for nonpurposeful motor behaviors (category VI) as inferences of potential for violence increased. The reverse was found for medical history (category II): the higher saliency given medical history, the higher the inferences of potential for violence.

The configurations of these analyses indicate that inferences of potential for violence generally vary according to the assigned cue category saliency rather than cue category usage in each situation. An important finding was that cues nurses relied on most for assessment of potential for violence were those occurring below the client's level of awareness, the autonomic nervous system changes resulting in nonpurposeful motor activities and physical reactions such as pupil changes, uncontrolled shaking, and tone of voice. For example, chalk-faced (pale) clients were rated more dangerous than red-faced clients (who have passed the body's stress peak symptom).

The consistency in the responses within each group could be a result of learning cues found reliable in specific practice settings, since perceptual sets tend to become intensified when relied on automatically or when the nurse is in intense and/or potentially violent situations. While highly refined perceptual sets are very productive in one practice setting, they can produce a rigidity of response that could be disastrous in another practice setting. The finding suggests that the transfer of learning from one practice setting could inhibit productive performance when practice settings are changed.

The cues nurses used in assessing a person's potential for violence in this study were holistic, reflecting appraisal of the client's various domains. Cue usage was configural, and patterns discerned were specific to role group affiliation.

DISCUSSION

The major focus of this presentation has been to illustrate a technique interfacing sociologic and statistical methodology. The inductive method for discovering grounded theory set forth by Glaser and Strauss (1968) has been viewed by many nurses as a "less than scientific" nursing research methodology (Ludemann, 1979). Deductive methods have also been a preferred method for developing nursing diagnoses. But suggested frameworks for inductive approaches were included in Gebbie and Lavin (1975). Nurses involved in the development of clinical science together with nursing diagnoses, for the most part, support the widely held belief that deductive methodologies are more rigorous, thus more valid and reliable.

During the past few years there has been increased interest and acceptance of grounded theory in nursing, as seen in the number of articles published on the topic (Ludemann, 1979; Simms, 1981; Stein, 1980). This perspective can be attributed, in part, to the number of publications that provide nurse researchers with convincing rationales for broadening research methods to include multiple research methodologies. For example, Newman (1979) articulated the need to search for holistic methods of inquiry and suggested the use of action research for theory development. Ludemann (1979) reinforced the position that the nurse researcher's proclivity for deductive methodology impedes development of the knowledge base needed for holistic care. Kritek (1978) has taken the position that nurse theorists have bypassed the first step in theory development, the level one step that generates descriptive data. This stepskipping has created the current dilemma of the inability of extant prescriptive nursing theories to synthesize holistic concepts at the diagnostic juncture (Kritek, 1978).

The recent publications on grounded theory have given considerable attention to the method and rationale for its use. Limited overviews, because of space limits, may reinforce the idea that the research method is simplistic. At this time, when some nurse researchers are being "introduced" to grounded theory methodology, the method is being expanded and explored by many anthropologic researchers who are discussing the interface between anthropologic and psychologic research methods (Guthrie, 1977; Harrington, 1977).

Of the recent publications on grounded theory, Stein's article (1980) provides an overview of previous grounded theory research that has had considerable impact on nursing and medical management of clients and that has contributed to improving the quality of care. Fagerhaugh and Strauss (1977) and Glaser and Strauss (1965) have made major contributions that involve several clinical specialty areas, are holistic, and illustrate the value of grounded theory methodology. Wilson's use of grounded theory (1977), which identifies limiting intrusion as a way of preserving autonomy, also has applicability to all areas of nursing, although the research was generated from community psychiatric settings. For those nurse researchers not yet convinced, review of these works should validate the credibility and contribution of grounded methodology to holistic diagnosis development.

At the time this violence research was completed, there was a tremendous lack of behavioral science literature on violence. A recent review of literature on violence reveals that there has been a marked increase in theorizing and little advance in the state of knowledge. One of the most comprehensive summaries of the 15 theories of violence and the distinctive contributions of each theory has been set forth by Gelles and Strauss (1979). Although the 15 theories are not new, the authors' idea that a theory of violence should integrate the complementary and interacting factors identified by all the theories, is a new perspective in contrast to the many efforts to prove or disprove a specific theory.

A recent publication in the nursing literature (Babich, 1981) indicates that many nurses involved in violence predictions are ready to progress beyond the level one descriptive data generation. Babich (1981) suggests that future research might do well to shift from studying variables that predict potentially violent behaviors to investigations of interventions that defuse violence potential. Materials presented by Babich relating to assessment behaviors provided no new cues or categories to those generated by this research.

When this descriptive research was completed in 1975, the cue categories could not be conceptualized further, given the limitations of extant nursing theories and the limitations of violence theory. The development of the unitary man/human model (Kim and Moritz, 1982), provided the means for further study (Table 1). The fit of the data generated in the descriptive study and the unitary man/human framework provides for using the conceptual factor language for propositional statements. It is possible to order the unitary man/human factors with the statistically significant findings and generate directional statements for future research. Several tentative statements are as follows:

1. If action levels increase and levels of awareness decrease, there is an increased potential for violence.
2. If action levels decrease and levels of awareness remain unchanged, there is a decrease in the potential for violence.
3. Increased interactions decrease violence potential.

TABLE 1 Comparison of the unitary man/human framework and potential violence behavior cue categories

Characteristics of unitary man/human framework for classification of nursing diagnoses[*]	Cue categories derived from nurse subjects[†]
Factor I: Interaction	
Exchanging	II. Medical history: Presence or absence of disease, injury, drugs, and/or alcohol; physical status includes physical characteristics such as body build, height, and appearance of attire
Communicating	III. Verbalizations (verbal cues): Content of speech, what is said
Relating	XI. (Peer) relationships: Interpersonal relations with others—family, employer, staff, provocative victims; also "nonspecific discomfort" of nurse; intuitive "feelings" about the person that (nurse) subject could not define verbally
Factor II: Action	
Valuing	X. Social history: History of past violence, personality and behavioral changes, goals, interests, and pursuits
Choosing	I. Background factors: Age, sex, nationality, marital status, occupation, area of residence, religion
Moving	V. Purposeful motor actions: Goal-directed behavior within person's control; aggressive gestures such as pounding fists, throwing things
Factor III: Awareness	
Waking	VI. Nonpurposeful motor actions and responses: Physiologic autonomic manifestations inferred as cues of increasing or fluctuations in tension outside control of person; involuntary muscular reactions such as tremors, jerky movements, postural and facial expressions
	IV. Verbalizations: How words are said; quality, rate, tone such as shouted, whispered; inferences by nurse of intensity or emotionality such as "angrily," "fearfully," or threats
Feeling	VII. Affective states of sustained or pervasive quality: Depression, paranoia, repressed anger, characteristic temperament, and dynamics
	VIII. Labile emotional reactions: Emotional reactivity, instability, and signs of weakening ego control shown in fluctuations in responses
Knowing	IX. Level of awareness: Cognitive indications of disequilibrium such as altered levels of consciousness and reality assessment; confusion, noncompliance, inability to follow requests, respond to expectations of others

[*]From Kim, M.J., and Moritz, D.A., eds.: Classification of nursing diagnoses: proceedings of the third and fourth national conferences, New York, 1982, McGraw-Hill Book Co.
[†]From Clunn, P.: Nurses' assessment of a person's potential for violence, doctoral dissertation, New York, 1975, Teachers College, Columbia University.

Reservations about these statements stem from a pervasive finding in the violence literature regarding the impact of the role group affiliation on the rating of violence potential. Significant role group differences were found for five of the six simulated situations; violence ratings were a function of role group membership rather than demographic variables of the subject. However, cue usage and cue saliency were relatively similar. The difference was that role groups were found unique in their ratings, using comparable cues for ranking.

A feasible explanation for this difference was that each agency served a specific cultural or subcultural group that resides in "pockets" in New York and seeks medical care from health agencies whose values are similar to theirs and compatible with their cultural expectations. It was hypothesized that nurses employed in the various agencies had developed a set of behavioral expectations consistent with the unique cultural repertoire of the clients for whom they provided care.

The findings emphasized the need for more concise theory development in the realm of cultural differences in response to health alterations. Thus although grounded research methodology has contributed to holistic constructs concerning pain, death, and autonomy, there is a great need to use this level one methodology to discern cultural group (in lieu of role group) differences.

The limitations of the violence research conceptual categorization was perceived after completion of the research and resulted from the lack of a clearly specified cultural category, which includes more than the "valuing" factor of the unitary man/human framework. Although culture-specific behaviors are emphasized in extreme crisis states, they are also critical considerations in other "states of the patient." To date, it is known that these cultural variables include health beliefs and practices, locus of control, expectations of health care providers, and use of folk medicines, to mention a few. It seems likely that the nurse's reliance on the physiologic autonomic nervous system changes presented a cue-reliance that crossed cultures, since the "fight or flight" response is universal.

Several reports in the nursing education literature (Derdiarian, 1979; Roy, 1979) have discussed education as a way of theory development in nursing. Since baccalaureate programs specifically focus on teaching nursing clinical science, it seems likely that nurse educators could use the grounded theory methodology and through case studies and critical incidents generate nursing diagnoses that identify the body of knowledge related to cultural differences at the level one, descriptive point.

Based on the findings of this descriptive research, it seems that research describing holistic behavior without cultural qualifiers lacks diagnostic synthesis such as extant nursing theories. Thus it is suggested that the unitary man/human framework be expanded to include a factor specific to culture rather than subsuming it within the value context. Culture, in and of itself, is more than a set of values and beliefs. In the area of emotional/psychologic health alterations, it has been established that there are wide variations in cultural expressions and the psychopathology attributed to these variations. These findings have ramifications for other nursing diagnoses in the behavioral realm such as self-concept, pain, alterations in parenting, and thought disorders. The potential usefulness of nursing diagnoses depends on their cross-cultural applicability.

REFERENCES

Ackerman, N.: Comments. In Standal, S., and Corsini, R., eds.: Critical incidents in psychotherapy, Englewood Cliffs, N.J., 1959, Prentice-Hall, Inc.

Babich, R.S., ed.: Assessing patient violence in the health care setting, Boulder, Colo., 1981, Western Interstate Commission for Higher Education.

Bettelheim, B.: Violence: a neglected mode of behavior, Ann. Am. Acad. Polit. Soc. Sci. **34**:50, 1966.

Bruner, J.S., Goodnow, J.J., and Austin, G.A.: Study of thinking, New York, 1956, John Wiley & Sons, Inc.

Clunn, P.: Nurses' assessment of a person's potential for violence, doctoral dissertation, New York, 1975, Teachers College, Columbia University.

Derdiarian, A.: Education: a way to theory construction in nursing, J. Nurs. Educ. **18**:36, 1979.

Devons, E., and Gluckman, M.: Modes and consequences of limiting a field of study in closed systems and open minds, Chicago, 1964, Aldine Publishing Co.

Dickoff, J., James, P., and Wiedenback, E.: Theory in a practice discipline. I. Practice oriented theory, Nurs. Res. **17**:415, 1968.

Fagerhaugh, S., and Strauss, A.L.: Politics of pain management, Reading, Mass., 1977, Addison-Wesley Publishing Co., Inc.

Fleiss, J., Spitzer, R., and Burdock, E.: Estimating accuracy of judgment using recorded interviews, Arch. Gen. Psychiat. **12**:562, 1965.

Flynn, G.: Hostility in a mad, mad world, Perspect. Psychiatr. Care **4**:115, 1969.

Fortin, J.D., and Rabinow, J.: Legal implications of nursing diagnosis, Nurs. Clin. North Am. **14**:553, 1979.

Fromm, E.: The anatomy of human destructiveness, New York, 1973, Holt, Rinehart & Winston, Inc.

Gebbie, K.M., and Lavin, M.A.: Classification of nursing diagnoses, St. Louis, 1975, The C.V. Mosby Co.

Gelles, R.J., and Strauss, M.: Determinants of violence in the family: toward a theoretical integration. In Wesley, R., and others, eds.: Contemporary theories about the family, New York, 1979, The Free Press.

Glaser, B.G., and Strauss, A.L.: Awareness of dying, Chicago, 1965, Aldine Publishing Co.

Glaser, B.G., and Strauss, A.L.: The discovery of grounded theory, Chicago, 1968, Aldine Publishing Co.

Gordon, M.: Predictive strategies in diagnostic tasks, Nurs. Res. **29**:35, 1980.

Guthrie, G.: Problems of measurement in cross cultural research, Ann. N.Y. Acad. Sci. p. 131, 1977.

Hammond, K., and others: Clinical inference in nursing: use of information seeking strategies by nurses, Nurs. Res. **15**:330, 1966.

Hammond, K., and Summers, D.A.: Cognitive dependence on linear and non-linear cues, Psychol. Rev. **72**:215, 1965.

Hammond, K., and Summers, D.: Cognitive control, Psychol. Rev. **79:**58, 1972.

Harrington, C.: Methods and issues in cross-cultural research, Ann. N.Y. Acad. Sci. p. 89, 1977.

Hoffman, P., Slovic, P., and Rarer, L.: An analysis of variance model for the assessment of configural cue utilization in clinical judgment, Psychol. Bull. **69:**338, 1968.

Jick, T.D.: Mixing qualitative and quantitative methods: triangulation in action, Adm. Sci. Q. **24:**602, 1979.

Kelly, K.: Clinical inference in nursing. I. A nurse's viewpoint, Nurs. Res. **15:**23, 1966.

Kim, M.J., and Moritz, D.A., eds.: Classification of nursing diagnoses: proceedings of the third and fourth national conferences, New York, 1982, McGraw-Hill Book Co.

Kritek, P.B.: The generation and classification of nursing diagnoses: toward a theory of nursing, Image **10:**33, 1978.

LeCompte, W., Butts, S., and Busch, D.: Effects of training on behavioral observations by nurses, Nurs. Res. **21:**448, 1972.

Lesnick, M., and Anderson, B.: Nursing practice and the law, ed. 2, Philadelphia, 1955, J.B. Lippincott Co.

Ludemann, R.: The paradoxical nature of nursing research, Image **11:**2, 1979.

Newman, M.: Theory development in nursing, Philadelphia, 1979, F.A. Davis Co.

Roy, Sister C.: Relating nursing theory to education: a new era, Nurse Educ. p. 16, March-April, 1979.

Siegel, F.: Survey of five metropolitan New York mental hospital staff nursing personnel for continuing education program planning, Unpublished papers, New York, 1971, Teachers College, Columbia University.

Simms, L.: The grounded theory approach in nursing research, Nurs. Res. **30:**356, 1981.

Stein, P.: Grounded theory methodology: its uses and process, Image **12:**20, 1980.

Thomas, D.B., and Hansen, A.D.: Role group differences in assignment of priorities: a variable perspective interpretation, Nurs. Res. **15:**12, 1966.

Thomas, D.B., and Hansen, A.D.: Professionalization of priority decision judgments, Nurs. Res. **19:**343, 1970.

Wald, F.S., and Leonard, R.C.: Towards development of practice theory, Nurs. Res. **13:**309, 1964.

Wilson, H.S.: Limiting intrusion—social control of outsiders in a healing community, Nurs. Res. **26:**103, 1977.

ADDITIONAL READINGS

Bender, L.: Hostile aggression in children. In Garattini, S., and Skipp, E.B., eds.: Aggressive behavior, Amsterdam, 1969, Excerpta Medica Foundation.

Cole, M., Glick, O., and Sharp, D.: The cultural context of learning and thinking, New York, 1971, Basic Books, Inc., Publishers.

Dickoff, J., and James, P.: A theory of theories: a position paper, Nurs. Res. **17:**197, 1968.

Flanagan, J.C.: The critical incident technique, Psychol. Bull. **8:**327, 1954.

Glaser, B.G.: Theoretical sensitivity, Mill Valley, Calif., 1978, The Sociology Press.

Glaser, B.G., and Strauss, A.L.: The purpose and credibility of qualitative research, Nurs. Res. **15:**56, 1966.

Gordon, M., and Sweeney, M.A.: Methodological problems and issues in identifying and standardizing nursing diagnoses, Adv. Nurs. Sci. **2:**1, 1979.

Gottschalk, L., and Gleser, G.: The measurement of psychological states through content analysis of verbal behavior, Berkeley, 1969, University of California Press.

Hansen, A., and Thomas, B.: Role group differences in judging the importance of advising medical care, Nurs. Res. **17:**525, 1968.

Landa, L.: Algorithmization in learning and instruction, Englewood Cliffs, N.J., 1974, New Jersey Educational Technology Publications.

Lucas, W.: The case-survey method: aggregating case experience, Santa Monica, Calif., 1974, Rand Corp.

McCall, G.L., and Simmons, L.: Issues in participant observation, Reading, Mass., 1979, Addison-Wesley Publishing Co., Inc.

Reinharz, S.: On becoming a social scientist: from survey research and participant observer to experiential analysis, San Francisco, 1979, Jossey-Bass, Inc., Publishers.

Sarbin, T.: The scientific status of the mental-illness metaphor. In Plag, S., and Edgerton, R., eds.: Changing perspectives in mental illness, New York, 1969, Holt, Rinehart & Winston, Inc.

Taylor, J.B.: Rating scales as measures of clinical judgment: a method for increasing scale reliability and sensitivity, Educ. Psychol. Measur. **28:**747, 1968.

Toby, J.: Violence and the masculine ideal: some qualitative data, Ann. Am. Acad. Polit. Soc. Sci. **34:**20, 1966.

Critical indicators for the nursing diagnosis of disturbance in self-concept

ANNE MARIE CHENEY, R.N., M.S.N.

The nursing process, as it is currently conceptualized, consists of five steps: assessment, diagnosis, planning, intervention, and evaluation. The relatively recent addition of diagnosis to the traditional four-step approach is essential to the development of nursing as a science (Gordon and Sweeney, 1979). According to Gordon (1976, p. 1298), "nursing diagnoses . . . describe actual or potential health problems, which nurses, by virtue of their education and experience, are capable and licensed to treat." She sees nursing diagnoses "as a short hand way of referring to a cluster of signs and symptoms that occur as a clinical entity . . . in which the responsibility for therapeutic decisions can be assumed by the professional nurse" (Gordon, 1976, p. 1299).

Identifying and labeling the problem accurately is the first step in the diagnostic process. The Fourth National Conference on the Classification of Nursing Diagnoses issued a list of currently accepted nursing diagnoses (Kim and Moritz, 1982). Included in that list is the diagnosis of *disturbance in self-concept*. Changes in the health state challenge a person's self-concept. Persons deal with this challenge with varying degrees of success. Nursing's ability to diagnose that struggle would significantly affect the care that an individual receives. Clients who are managing the challenge with some success could be identified and supported, making alteration of self-concept possible with a miniumum of distress. Early diagnosis of disturbance in self-concept would also identify ineffective management of that threat by the client. Strategies could then be implemented that would assist the client in making those modifications in the self-concept imposed by the health state.

Gordon (1976, p. 1300) states that "the process of clinical diagnosis involves: collecting, clustering, weighing and validating information." The ability to recognize and label the patterns that emerge depends on well-established criteria for any given diagnosis or pattern. These criteria, or critical indicators, are the signs and symptoms that must be present if the diagnostic category is to be used. Nursing as a profession is beginning to undertake the task of developing these critical indicators.

Identification of the critical indicators begins during the assessment process as data are collected on the state of the client. Isolated facts and observations, the signs and symptoms, are identified. These signs and symptoms are collected and clustered into groups of related data. Applying clinical knowledge and judgment allows the nurse to organize these clusters into meaningful patterns. Those signs and symptoms that lead to the recognition of the pattern are the critical indicators for that diagnosis.

An initial attempt to identify critical indicators for the nursing diagnosis of *disturbance in self-concept* is presented in this paper. The data were drawn from a client population of four men and two women ranging from 42 to 75 years of age. All the clients had cardiovascular disease. The methodology involved a retrospective review of the documentation of the clinical practice of the author as a graduate student in nursing. The Bonham-Cheney model for concept of self provided the conceptual framework (Table 1) (Bonham and Cheney, 1982). Each client was reviewed for both subjective and objective data pertinent to the various model categories. The critical indicators were then abstracted from the supportive data available in each category (Table 2).

Drawing from a population of cardiovascular clients, critical indicators for the nursing diagnosis of *threatened concept of self* have been identified. Using the Bonham-Cheney model for concept of self, criteria for each of the categories have been developed. For any particular client, it is unlikely that every criterion in each category will be present. However, at this level of concept development it is not yet possible to determine the number of critical indicators that must be present to justify the diagnosis. It may be that the presence of one of the critical indicators is sufficient to alert the nurse to a potential problem area for which nursing intervention would prove helpful.

TABLE 1   **Bonham-Cheney model for concept of self**

| | Self-perspectives | | | | | |
| | Self-image | | Self-esteem | | Self-in-action | |
Personal identity	**Critical indicators**	**Supportive data**	**Critical indicators**	**Supportive data**	**Critical indicators**	**Supportive data**
Intellectual self	S		S		S	
	O		O		O	
Physical self	S		S		S	
	O		O		O	
Moral/ethical self	S		S		S	
	O		O		O	
Emotional self	S		S		S	
	O		O		O	

KEY: S = subjective, O = objective.

TABLE 2   Critical indicators for diagnosis of disturbance in self-concept

Category	Critical indicators	Supportive data
Intellectual self	**Self-image**	
	Subjective	
	Verbalizations regarding:	
	Educational experience	"I never did graduate from high school."
	Cognitive functioning, e.g., Memory	"My memory just isn't what it used to be."
	Attention span	"I just can't seem to concentrate."
	Imagination	"I try to imagine different ways of handling it."
	Objective	
	Observation of cognitive functioning	Ability to ask pertinent questions.
		Data pertaining to cognitive functioning, e.g., memory, attention span, educational level.
	Self-esteem	
	Subjective	
	Verbal indications of level of satisfaction with intellectual ability	"I'm self-taught. I'm proud of that."
	Objective	
	Behavioral indications of level of satisfaction with intellectual ability	Tries to cover up lack of education.
	Self-in-action	
	Subjective	
	Verbalizations of the use of intellectual ability, e.g.,	
	Job	"I can hold my own against those college boys."
	Recreation	"I read a lot."
	Problem solving	"I like to tackle the hardest part of the problem first."
	Objective	
	Behavioral demonstrations of the use of intellectual ability	Able to imagine potential sources of family conflict during convalescence and possible ways to deal with it.
		Choice of recreational activities: reading, crossword puzzles, T.V.

TABLE 2 **Critical indicators for diagnosis of disturbance in self-concept—cont'd**

Category	Critical indicators	Supportive data
Physical self	*Self-image*	
	Subjective	
	Verbalization regarding the body: Structure	"The bottom of my heart is dead."
		"They've operated on my heart. What's left?"
		"Every time I feel a pain, I think there goes another piece."
	Function	"I was testing the bypass to see if it was still working."
		"I'm aware now of every little twinge. I never used to pay any attention."
		"I'm afraid I'll become a hypochondriac, always worrying about how I feel."
	Appearance	"They've marked up my beautiful body."
		"I can always tell when people are looking at my scar."
	Statements denoting level of integration of the health state into the self-concept	"My heart attack."
		"My heart surgery."
		"They say I had a heart attack."
	Objective	
	Observation of the structure, function, and appearance of the body	Presence of scars.
		Energy level.
		Presence of symptoms, e.g., cyanosis, tobacco stains on hands and teeth, clubbing of fingers.
	Observation of the level of ability to integrate the health state into the self-concept	Absence of statements denoting integration, e.g., unable to say "my heart attack."
		Noncompliance with treatment plan.

Continued.

Category	Critical indicators	Supportive data
	Self-esteem	
	Subjective	
	Statements relating to the ability to control the functioning of the body	"I have to be able to move around. I can't stay still."
		"I got to find a way to get some energy. I've got to keep going."
	Statements relating self-worth to the body:	
	Structure	"I know I look awful inside."
	Function	"Even if all the tests are negative, I know something is wrong."
	Appearance	"I can't go grocery shopping with her because I can't carry the bags and so people will look at me funny."
	Objective	
	Behavioral demonstrations of level of pride in appearance	Level of grooming.
		Posture.
		Ability to maintain eye contact.
		Hides presence of a scar.
	Observation of over-identification with altered health state, i.e.,	
	Self	Excessive interest in every detail of altered health state.
	Disease	Development of "rotating symptoms"; i.e., nursing attention to one symptom will find the client switching to another.
	Self-in-action	
	Subjective	
	Verbalizations regarding congruence of role expectation	"I just want to be able to do the things I'm used to—a little dusting, a little gardening."
		"Being dependent on others, that's the hardest part."
	Objective	
	Demonstrated ability or inability to alter life style	Gave up smoking.
		Lost 30 lbs.
		Poor compliance with treatment plan.
	Behavioral manifestations of the level of ability to maintain role functions	Demonstrated desire to keep active and functioning, e.g., continues to be involved with business during hospitalization; continues to participate in family decision making.

Category	Critical indicators	Supportive data
Moral/ethical self	**Self-image**	
	Subjective	
	Statement identifying a personal belief system	"Maybe the Lord sends sickness to test me."
	Objective	
	Behavioral manifestations of a personal belief system	Data pertaining to personal belief system, e.g., identifies self as a Baptist.
	Self-esteem	
	Subjective	
	Statements referring to level of satisfaction with personal belief system	"My life is in God's hands."
		"I get a lot of help from prayer."
		"Everybody tells me I have to change and think of myself more, but isn't that just selfish?"
	Objective	
	Behavioral manifestations of level of satisfaction with personal belief system	Appears to draw support from practice of belief system, e.g., visits from minister, use of rosary.
	Self-in-action	
	Subjective	
	Statements regarding the practice of the personal belief system	"Maybe this is a time for me to rethink my values."
		"I was going to try for church this week, but the doctor nixed that."
	Objective	
	Behavioral manifestations of level of compliance with personal belief system	Use of prayer as a coping strategy.
		Incorporation of religious practices into daily life.
Emotional self	**Self-image**	
	Subjective	
	Statements regarding the feeling state; client may or may not be able to identify the feeling	"There's no way out. I'm like a rat in a cage."
		"Usually, I'm an optimist, but this time, I don't know."
		"I might die before they can do something."
		"You just have to lie here and take it."
		"If anything happens to me—get an autopsy."
	Objective	
	Behavioral manifestations of feeling state	Data pertaining to feeling state, e.g., input of significant others; also sees critical indicators for anxiety, depression.

Continued.

TABLE 2   Critical indicators for diagnosis of disturbance in self-concept—cont'd

Category	Critical indicators	Supportive data
	Self-esteem	
	Subjective	
	Statements denoting the level of acceptability of feeling state	"I keep everything inside."
		"I'm a terrible person. I don't like myself."
		"I'm not a worrier. Worry doesn't do any good."
		"When I'm nervous, I move around a lot."
	Expressions of guilt or shame	"I've been taking everything out on the wife. I shouldn't do that."
	Objective	
	Behavioral manifestations of the level of acceptability of the feeling state	Use of humor as an outlet for anger.
		Substituting the word "upset" for "angry."
		Denies anxiety but requests an increase in sedation.
	Self-in-action	
	Subjective	
	Statements regarding the impact of feelings on roles	"I couldn't take a desk job—too much tension."
		"I'd rather retire or go on relief than change jobs."
		"I don't trust anybody."
	Statements regarding level of ability to cope with feelings	"I have to learn how to handle anger better."
		"I was afraid if I started to talk, I'd cry, so I wrote notes."
		"Just laying here gives me too much time to think."
	Objective	
	Level of ability to identify and use support systems	Able to draw strength from a supportive family.
		Refuses support of significant others.
	Behavioral manifestations of the emotional impact of the altered health state	Inability to cope with the downward trajectory of the disease, e.g., blames medication for loss of energy rather than disease.
		Able to use relaxation techniques for stress management.

REFERENCES

Bonham, P., and Cheney, A.M.: Concept of self: a framework for nursing assessment. In Advances in nursing theory development, Rockville, Md., 1982, Aspen Systems Corp.

Gordon, M.: Nursing diagnosis and the diagnostic process, Am. J. Nurs. **76**(8):1298, 1976.

Gordon, M., and Sweeney, M.A.: Methodological problems and issues in identifying and standardizing nursing diagnosis, Adv. Nurs. Sci. **2**(1):1, 1979.

Kim, M.J., and Moritz, D.A., eds.: Classification of nursing diagnoses: proceedings of the third and fourth national conferences, New York, 1982, McGraw-Hill Book Co.

Poster presentation

A framework to analyze a taxonomy of nursing diagnoses

MARGARET LUNNEY, R.N., M.S.N.

The National Conference Group for the Classification of Nursing Diagnoses is meeting for the fifth time to continue development of its system of language, the taxonomy of nursing diagnoses. It is expected that the systematic use of the taxonomy will facilitate both the provision of quality care by nurses and the process of developing nursing science. The taxonomy is developing slowly because of the complexity of formulating a system of names or labels for the situations that nurses treat. Three factors that contribute to the complexity are as follows: (1) nursing has been using other language systems to guide its practice, for example, medical and psychiatric diagnoses, (2) developing a system of any kind requires careful selection of all the interrelated parts so that consistency allows the system to operate as a whole, and (3) language systems are formulated to reflect thinking processes, yet nursing consists of many different conceptual models that guide thinking processes. It is possible, however, to reduce the complexity of the task by identifying the basic standards that must be met by a diagnostic system.

The standards I have been using to analyze the fit of diagnostic statements were formulated from the literature of the last 30 years. They evolved from descriptions of how nursing diagnoses are supposed to function by leaders such as Abdellah (1969), Chambers (1962), Gebbie (1976), Gordon (1976), Johnson (1959), Komorita (1963), and Roy (1976). For 15 to 20 years before beginning the organization of a taxonomy of nursing diagnoses, nurses were developing an awareness of how it should function, which is consistent with the development of other organized systems in that function precedes the development of structure (Guttman, 1964). In the case of nursing diagnoses, the words and phrases of the system constitute the structure of the system and must serve the overall function of the system. Therefore the knowledge of how diagnostic statements are supposed to function should be the primary guide for both the formulation and the analysis of the structure of a diagnostic system. The knowledge comes from the themes that can be identified in the literature on nursing diagnosis.

Many reasons for using nursing diagnosis have been cited, but the major function is that of a communication tool. It is the language by which nurses can (1) express a focus that is specific to the discipline, (2) communicate accurate interpretations of health assessment, and (3) indicate the elements of a treatment plan. As with other types of tools, a language system for nursing must be consistent and clear if it is to serve the purposes for which it was designed; all parts of the structure must interrelate to form an organized system.

Recognition that the system must function in a certain way is not sufficient, however, as a framework for development. If the tool is to communicate the focus of nursing, it must also address what nursing is and address the situations that nurses treat that are different from those of other disciplines. The situations are described in various conceptual models for nursing (Riehl and Roy, 1980). Although these models can be used to develop clear and consistent diagnostic systems that would function as expected, each system that was developed would be different from the others. For example, a diagnosis using Johnson's behavioral systems model might be *maladaptive affiliative behavior*, and one using Roger's science of man model might be *desynchronous mother/child interaction*. Nurses who use the language of one of these models might have difficulty in communicating with other nurses who do not use the model or do not believe in the model. The difficulty is compounded when nurses try to communicate a specific focus to clients, other health care professionals, and the public. I am proposing that instead of using each of the models that Riehl and Roy describe, we should use the concepts and philosophic ideas that are consistent among the models.

Similarities among conceptual models have been identified (Donaldson and Crowley, 1978; Fawcett, 1978; Flaskerud and Halloran, 1980; Yura and Torres, 1975). These similarities outline the boundaries of the discipline and provide the basic standards of expectation for a nursing diagnosis. The four concepts of nursing have also been identified as health, person, environment, and nursing. Inherent in the term *person* is the assumption that nurses are concerned with individuals, families, and communities. In this paper, client and person have the same meaning. Fawcett (1982) referred to the four concepts as a "metaparadigm," that is, a general model for the focus of the discipline, when she gave support for the position that nursing is advancing as a science. Although the relationships among the concepts are viewed somewhat differently within each model, there are enough similarities to recognize a nursing perspective.

Nurses agree, for instance, that persons concepts of health depend on their own values and beliefs and that the health status of an individual, family, and community is judged in the context of values and beliefs. They also agree that health is achieved by the client and not by the health professional. Diagnostic statements, then, should illustrate that nurses assess a client's health-regulatory behaviors and judge the behaviors with the client, using past patterns and the client's expectations and potentials as a guide. Diagnoses that fit this philosophy would consist of concepts representative of daily behaviors that keep people healthy, for example, nutrition, elimination, parenting, communication, and thought patterns. The concepts can be prefaced by a phrase such as "alteration in" when there is a change from usual healthy patterns. A client's current behavioral patterns are judged against past patterns rather than in terms of an idealistic norm. When a nurse judges that even past patterns do not meet the client's expectations or potentials, a different qualifying phrase could be used, such as "dysfunction in." In either case, nurses assess for certain indications of health that should be the concepts of nursing diagnosis.

Since persons define health according to their own values and beliefs, a nurse participates with a client in interpreting health status, which is a theme in the various conceptual models. Collaborative determination of health status is one aspect of the nursing process that has been difficult to put into action because of the profession's previous use of medical and psychiatric models. Other health care models tend to be more authoritarian and paternalistic than mutually participatory.

The philosophy of mutual participation is consistent with nursing's traditional interest in holistic care. Historic research substantiates that the philosophy evolved from nursing's continued focus on the health/functioning of individuals, families, and communities as well as the parts that might be diseased. Nursing's difficulty in expressing its interest in the whole as opposed to only the parts of the client is not surprising, since the prevailing scientific approach until after the 1930s was concerned with reducing items to small parts for understanding. Nursing, as other groups, needs support from the general community for growth and development. Nursing has that support, since science recognizes that the whole is more than the sum of the parts and values the effort to understand the whole in addition to the parts.

In trying to understand the client as a whole, nurses have always considered the relationship between clients' interactions with the environment and their health status. Identifying and modifying environmental factors that interfere with health have been part of nursing since its inception by Florence Nightingale. The emphasis on creating a healthy environnment can be noted in nursing sources throughout history. For example, if one wanted to explain how a nurse helps a person who is isolated because of a contagious disease, both the management of asepsis (nonpersonal environment) and the provision for social support (interpersonal environment) would be emphasized. Nurses have developed a strong role in institutional settings as managers of the enviroment. When environmental situations are identified by nurses as factors that must be modified for the promotion, maintenance, or restoration of health, the elements of a treatment plan become evident. For example, nurses in intensive care units prevent and treat diagnoses such as *alteration in thought process related to lack of meaningful stimuli*. The treatment plan for the diagnosis involves providing meaningful stimuli, such as talking about home and family, to help the person restore optimum thought processes.

USING THE FRAMEWORK

The beliefs common to nursing and the expected function of diagnostic statements have been combined to form a framework for analyzing a taxonomy (Figure 1). The framework was outlined in 1978 (Greene and Lunney) and has been used to formulate a diagnostic system (Lunney, 1982). It has been invaluable as a guide for choosing diagnostic statements that are consistent with a nursing philosophy. Although the National Conference Group for Classification of Nursing Diagnoses is awaiting the conceptual model being designed by the Theorist Group (Gordon, 1979), members may want to consider this framework as a guide for organization of present and future systems. If so, the following implications seem to apply.

First, diagnostic labels should illustrate nursing's concern for the person, who is, by nature, whole (Krieger, 1981). Although nurses help people with disruptions in parts of a system, for example, airway clearance or skin integrity, they do so because the disruptions affect health functioning. If diagnostic statements refer to only parts of a system, they do not reflect nursing's unique focus on the whole person.

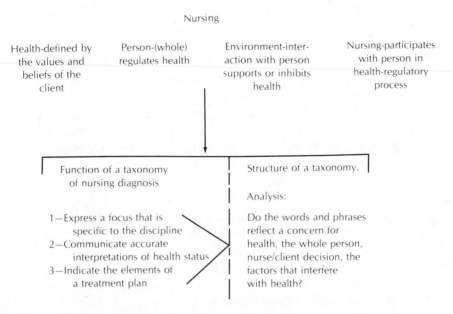

FIGURE 1   Framework for analyzing a taxonomy.

Second, statements should show that nurses help persons to promote, maintain, or restore their own health. Since the regulation of health is achieved through patterns of daily living, the nurse identifies the health-regulatory patterns that are not optimum, for example, activity/rest, coping, and parenting. Concepts such as fear, grieving, injury, rape, trauma, and violence do not meet this criterion.

Third, qualifying phrases should indicate that the behaviors of persons are being judged against their own personal optimum. Using "alteration in" works well in this situation. Another phrase, "dysfunction in," is needed when a person's behaviors are chronically less than optimum. Phrases that characterize permanent disabilities are not needed. If a person has emphysema, for instance, he remains labeled with the disease name. But if a carefully planned regimen is being followed and there is nothing else related to the illness or other functioning that nurses can do anything about, the person should not have *impaired oxygenation* as a diagnosis. When there is no nursing treatment, there is no nursing diagnosis.

Fourth, nursing diagnoses should be two-part statements (Mundinger and Jauron, 1975). The first part communicates the overall focus of the nurse, and the second part states the specific focus of the nurse (Box 1, pp. 408 and 409). A two-part statement makes it possible for diagnoses to be accurate and to indicate exactly which behaviors, specific and general, the nurse will be treating. The method works the same as the National Conference Group method of designating the problem and the etiology, except that both parts are considered to be the diagnosis.

Fifth, since the "person" or client" concept of nursing can refer to individuals, families, or communities, different diagnostic statements for families, such as ineffective family coping, may not be necessary. If the concepts being used are holistic, for example, coping and communication, they should be applicable both to individuals and to groups. Community assessment can be done, for example, using the same diagnostic concepts as for an individual assessment (Table 1). When it is obvious from the data who the client is, it is redundant to state it again in the diagnostic statement.

Sixth, it is possible for any health-regulatory behavior to change from its usual optimum. Therefore every concept could be preceded by "potential" when a person is at risk for moving away from optimum, for example, potential alteration in oxygenation related to decreased mobility. The term *actual* should be understood when potential is not used.

These recommendations were developed from the use of this framework to analyze and structure diagnostic statements for consistency in depicting the health situations nurses treat. The framework reflects the work of many nurse scientists in addition to those cited. Consistency in the positions nurses are assuming with respect to nursing science indicates a readiness to develop a taxonomy that will be universally accepted.

TABLE 1   **Assessment tool for nursing diagnosis of community health status**

Diagnosis	Data
Activity/rest	Mobility of children, adults, elderly adults; transportation resources; accommodations for handicapped; elevators, accessibility of food stores, banks, recreation, senior citizen centers; crime rate
Comfort	Mood of community, mortality and morbidity levels, common complaints, for example, fear of crime
Communication	Verbal and nonverbal to outsiders, network in community, for example, newpapers, government officials, mode-language, ethnicity
Coping	Support systems—family, churches, health agencies, particularly crisis intervention centers, senior citizen centers, peers, volunteers, government; information centers—political, economic, health, recreation, religious; usual mechanisms—community strengths, stressors, for example, crime, inadequate housing, absent landlords, poor self-image; ways of dealing with stressors, for example, community organizations, newsletters, denial, hopelessness; resources—mental health centers
Elimination	Management of debris, waste disposal, water drainage
Growth and development	Boundaries of community—political, geographic, social; land use—open spaces, parks, undeveloped space, type and quality of housing, commercial space (private, public), industrial space, quality of roads
Independence/dependence	Strength of group identity, perceived need for other communities, gaps in services
Learning	Education—elementary, secondary, college; pupil-teacher ratio, reading levels, levels of education, responsiveness of schools to community needs, opportunities for adult education
Life-style	Day, week, year balance of work, social, recreation
Management of health	Definition and meaning of health, health behaviors for prevention—exercise, nutrition, use of health resources, immunizations, hygiene, drug abuse, crime, juvenile delinquency; economic resources, quality of work opportunities
Management of illness	Medical resources—private, public; institutions—acute, chronic; community support systems—outpatient services, home care services; patterns of responsibility—consumer, providers; accountability—consumer, provider
Nutrition	Cultural beliefs, knowledge related to health, availability of quality meats, fruits, vegetables, water, cost relative to other communities
Oxygenation	Air quality, industrial risk areas, smoking habits
Parenting	Family patterns, standards, routines—infancy, adolescence, adulthood, aging; counseling services—marriage, child abuse, school
Protection	Police, fire, emergency medical services; institutional protection patterns
Relationships	Social and recreational patterns, openness/attitudes toward strangers, evidence of level of trust, family and community attachment/separation, inclusion of elderly in community affairs
Self-concept	Positive/negative views of community, specific groups; stigmas
Sexuality	Prevailing views of male/female roles; relatedness between sexes, acceptance of sexuality in young and old, birth rate, contraception
Sleep/wake	Prevailing biorhythms
Thought	Sensory deprivation, overload; evidence of mental incompetence

BOX 1   **Two-part nursing diagnosis examples**

Diagnoses being treated in psychiatric inpatient units[*]

Alteration or dysfunction in:

Protection related to delusions, hallucinations

Coping related to extreme hostility, panic

Comfort related to moderate/severe anxiety; hopelessness; self-injury; violent outbursts; refusal to provide self-care; withdrawal; extremes of somatic symptoms; disoriented × 3; low self-esteem; refusal to take medications; family conflict; grieving; anger; suspiciousness; insomnia; social isolation; attention-seeking behaviors

Relationships related to isolation of self; anger; sexual preoccupation; loneliness; lack of trust; dependent patterns; childlike behaviors; attention-seeking behavior

Self-concept related to depersonalization; feelings of guilt; responsibility, powerlessness

Activity/rest related to insomnia; withdrawal; fear of sleeping; isolation of self; self-medication patterns

Nutrition related to anorexia; refusal to eat

Diagnosis that nurses prevent and treat

Schizophrenia

Alteration in thought related to disturbance in reality testing; fear of others; decreased self-esteem

Alteration in relationships related to decreased interpersonal skills; anxiety; feelings of alienation, depersonalization, persecution

Dysfunction in self-concept related to feelings of powerlessness; disturbed body image; decreased self-esteem

Dysfunction in independence/dependence related to inability to provide self-care; perception of role; family patterns

Cardiovascular accident

Alteration in activity/rest related to hemiplegia; anxiety; sensory deprivation; knowledge with deficit about safe mobility

Alteration in independence/dependence related to decreased ability to provide self-care; knowledge deficit about transfer techniques; perception of sick role; frustration about difficulty of tasks; grieving for losses

Potential alteration in protection related to decreased mobility; partial paralysis of throat; decreased sense of balance; impaired touch and pain sensations; visual disturbances; perceptual disturbances; contractures

Alteration in elimination related to memory lapses; inability to communicate needs; decreased mobility or hydration; changes in diet patterns; incontinence

Alteration in communication related to aphasia; fear of failure; knowledge deficit about alternative methods

Heart disease

Alteration in oxygenation related to decreased tolerance of usual patterns (mobility, social); lack of knowledge or misconception about cardiac status; fear of activity, death; feelings of helplessness

Alteration in management of illness related to lack of knowledge about drugs; nonacceptance of limitations; decreased support systems

Alteration in self-concept related to change in role; change in body image

Alteration in relationships related to care of disabled family member; conflict about roles; projection of anger; unresolved grieving

---

[*]Permission to use this material may be obtained from: Margaret Lunney, 310 Willowbrook Road, Staten Island, New York 10314.

BOX 1   Two-part nursing diagnosis examples—cont'd

Head injury
  Alteration in protection related to inadequate respiratory exchange; fluid
    and electrolyte imbalance; decreased level of consciousness;
    susceptibility to aspiration; shock; infection; increased intracranial
    pressure; spinal injury; decreased mobility; restlessness
  Alteration in comfort related to pain, restlessness; excess environmental
    stimulation; decreased mobility; disorientation
Cancer
  Alteration in coping related to feelings of loneliness, hopelessness; grieving,
    unresolved grieving; decreased support systems; anxiety; fear of isolation
    or abandonment; lack of meaningful stimuli; difficult acceptance of
    limitations
  Alteration in protection related to risk of infection, fluid and electrolyte
    imbalance; fractures; cell destruction; bleeding
  Alteration in self-concept related to change in body image; alopecia
Hospitalization/bed bound at home
  Alteration in protection related to open area of skin (specify); decreased
    mobility; perception of reality; risk of infection (intrusive therapies, bone
    marrow depression); sensory deprivation or overload; inability to provide
    self-care
  Alteration in coping related to decreased support systems; lack of
    knowledge about hospital routines, treatment regimens; feelings of
    helplessness; misconceptions about illness
  Alteration in independence/dependence related to expectations of others;
    decreased ability for self-care; lack of knowledge about possible activities
  Alteration in self-concept related to change in body image; change in role
Diabetes mellitus
  Alteration in management of illness related to lack of knowledge about
    illness; fear of rejection, disability, feelings of helplessness; decreased
    support systems
  Alteration in self-concept related to misconceptions about illness
  Alteration in coping related to decreased support systems; lack of
    knowledge about management, prognosis
  Alteration in nutrition related to decreased utilization of glucose; lack of
    knowledge about diet management, balance between diet, exercise,
    insulin
  Potential alteration in protection related to lack of knowledge about
    complications; susceptibility to infection, vascular degeneration
  Alteration in protection related to fluid and electrolyte imbalance;
    hypoglycemia, hyperglycemia
Depression
  Alteration in coping related to loss of loved one; change in body image;
    loneliness; decreased support systems; fear of terminal illness
  Alteration in relationships related to social isolation; decreased
    interpersonal skills; unrealistic expectations of others
  Alteration in protection related to feelings of hopelessness; loss of impulse
    control
  Alteration in activity/rest related to anxiety; withdrawal from others
  Dysfunction in life-style related to feelings of failure, rejection, of
    worthlessness

REFERENCES

Abdellah, F.G.: The nature of nursing science, Nurs. Res. **18**:390, 1969.

Chambers, W.: Nursing diagnosis, Am. J. Nurs. **62**:102, 1962.

Donaldson, S.K., and Crowley, D.M.: The discipline of nursing, Nurs. Outlook **26**:113, 1978.

Fawcett, J.: The "what" of theory development. In National League for Nursing, ed.: Theory development: what, why, how, New York, 1978, The League.

Fawcett, J.: Paper presented at New York University for the Doctoral Students' Organization Research Day, March 20, 1982.

Flaskerud, J.H., and Halloran, E.J.: Areas of agreement in nursing theory development, Adv. Nurs. Sci. **3**:1, 1980.

Gebbie, K.M.: Development of a taxonomy of nursing diagnosis, In Walters, J.B., Purdee, G.P., and Molbo, D.M., eds.: Dynamics of problem-oriented approaches: patient care and documentation, Philadelphia, 1976, J.B. Lippincott Co.

Gordon, M.: Nursing diagnosis and the diagnostic process, Am. J. Nurs. **76**:1298, 1976.

Gordon, M.: The concept of nursing diagnosis, Nurs. Clin. North Am. **14**:487, 1979.

Greene, M.A., and Lunney, M.: Unpublished framework, 1978.

Guttman, H.: Structure and function, Genet. Psychol. Monogr. **70**:3, 1964.

Johnson, D.E.: A philosophy of nursing, Nurs. Outlook **7**:198, 1959.

Komorita, N.I.: Nursing diagnosis, Am. J. Nurs. **63**:83, 1963.

Krieger, D.: Foundations for holistic health nursing practices: the renaissance nurse, Philadelphia, 1981, J.B. Lippincott Co.

Lunney, M.: Nursing diagnosis: refining the system, Am. J. Nurs. **82**:456, 1982.

Mundinger, M.O., and Jauron, G.D.: Developing a nursing diagnosis, Nurs. Outlook **23**:94, 1975.

Riehl, J.P., and Roy, Sister C.: Conceptual models for nursing practice ed. 2, New York, 1980, Appleton-Century-Crofts.

Roy, Sister C.: The impact of nursing diagnosis, Nurs. Digest **4**:67, 1976.

Yura, H., and Torres, G.: Today's conceptual frameworks within baccalaureate nursing programs, In National League for Nursing, ed.: Faculty, curriculum development. Part III. Conceptual framework—its meaning and function, New York, 1975, The League.

Patterns for teaching the diagnostic process

SHEILA LaFORTUNE-FREDETTE R.N., M.S.

Nursing diagnosis, although not new terminology in the nursing literature, has recently emerged as a national movement that will have implications for nursing in future years. Since the First National Conference on the Classification of Nursing Diagnoses in 1972, the applicability of nursing diagnosis to clinical practice has begun a slow but steady acceleration. Many clinical agencies are implementing the use of nursing diagnosis, often in conjunction with a problem-oriented recording system. Recent literature gives credence to the fact that nurses are successfully using nursing diagnosis in clinical practice (Bruce, 1979; Dalton, 1979; Feild, 1979; Gordon, Sweeney, and McKeehan, 1980). Increasing number of nurses are requesting information about nursing diagnosis and are seeking educational programs to guide them in learning how to adapt the concept to their particular clinical area. It seems that methods and systems for teaching nursing diagnosis must be devised by nursing educators, since they are the logical professionals to respond to the need.

BASIS FOR DEVELOPING TEACHING METHODS

As we began the task of teaching the diagnostic process, three questions seemed paramount. How do practicing nurses make nursing diagnoses? Can the particular cognitive processes involved be altered or taught? What specific educational methods can be used to teach diagnosis in the most feasible and successful manner?

The complex question of what cognitive processes nurses use in diagnosing has been explored by Gordon (1980) and by Matthews and Gaul (1979). Matthews and Gaul (1979), using the Watson-Glaser Critical Thinking Appraisal (Watson and Glaser, 1964), reported no overall relationship between the ability to think critically and the ability to derive nursing diagnoses. Gordon (1980), when studying the effect of higher inferential ability (as measured by the Miller Analogies Test or Verbal Aptitude Subtest of the Graduate Record Examination) and the diagnostic task, discovered that those subjects with higher inferential ability neither used a more complicated form of multiple hypothesis testing nor had greater accuracy of diagnosis.

Although further corroborative research into the cognitive aspects of the diagnostic process is needed, there is an urgent message for nursing education in the conclusions of these researchers. Both reports imply that nurses have to be taught to think in a nursing diagnostic mode. The researchers also imply that skill in making an accurate diagnosis may be more strongly influenced by the learning environment than by the learner's already attained level of critical thinking or inferential ability. Gordon (1980) urges that nurses be taught a network of propositional inferences that can be retrieved from memory along with the relationships and variables that influence high-risk states. Matthews and Gaul (1979) believe that the ability to make nursing diagnosis is related to the nurse's application of theory to clinical practice; that is, the nurse must be able to interpret, evaluate, categorize, and infer from cues derived from the client. It seems essential that educators, while awaiting further research on cognitive processing, move ahead using whatever data are available to generate strategies for teaching the diagnostic process.

TEACHING NURSING DIAGNOSIS

Fredette and O'Connor (1979) taught nursing diagnosis for several years and described how the concept was incorporated into their theoretic and clinical teaching. They indicated that baccalaureate nursing students do learn how to use the diagnostic process. After teaching nursing diagnosis for the past 8 to 10 years to both baccalaureate and registered nurse students, I am convinced that diagnostic skills can be taught. Although diagnosis does require a particular kind of intellectual process (the ability to access that intellectual process is unique to each person), my experience has shown that growth in diagnostic processing skills can occur. Each nurse will diagnose at a different level of sophistication that seems to hinge on factors such as intellect, memory, theoretic background, general problem-solving ability, motivation, and experience. Nevertheless, each nurse can grow through the use of specific educational methods and clinical practice guided by an educator with diagnostic expertise. The purpose of this paper is to share classroom methods for teaching the diagnostic process.

Theoretic concepts

The nursing process, professional nursing's scientific problem-solving methodology, forms the foundation for any diagnostic development. The *ANA Standards of Nursing Practice* (1973), *Nursing: A Social Policy Statement* (ANA, 1980), and Nurse Practice Acts in most states clearly delineate the nursing process as the systematic approach to be used in the practice of nursing. Nursing curricula must include both theory and practice in teaching the nursing process.

What is a nursing diagnosis? Where does it come from? How does it differ from patient problem, concern, or need? It has been my experience that all students must proceed through an initial phase of learning about nursing diagnosis. The introduction, which can be included in teaching the nursing process, consists of three parts:

1. Basic ideas about the concept of nursing diagnosis: What is it? How is it defined? What are some synonyms? How does it fit into the nursing process?
2. A history of nursing diagnosis obtained from the literature: When did it begin? How do nursing professionals conceptualize it? What does professional literature say about it?
3. A history of the work of the National Conference on the Classification of Nursing Diagnoses: What is this group? How are nursing diagnoses decided on? What happens at each national conference? Who can go? How is the work proceeding?

Most of this introductory material can be gleaned from a review of the literature. Educators can develop a command of the subject matter and structure classes around the fundamental concepts. Various classroom methods can be used to model patterns for clinical decision making: (1) using case studies and films, (2) structuring lectures around each nursing diagnosis, and (3) demonstrating the relationship of nursing diagnosis to medical diagnosis.

Case studies and films

Once the general theory of process and diagnosis has been presented, the use of case studies and films is a nonthreatening way of increasing comfort with diagnosing. Original case studies or case study books can be used. Students can study the case independently, identify meaningful data leading to a diagnostic statement, write objectives, and cite nursing interventions. The exercise reinforces the nursing process, integrates nursing diagnosis as one step of the process, and encourages the student to think in a diagnostic mode. Further learning occurs when the independent endeavors are shared in small groups sessions. Films that depict clinical patient situations can be used in the same manner to spin off nursing diagnoses. Two such films are "The Mastectomy Patient" and "Childhood Leukemia," both available free of charge from the American Cancer Society.

Structuring lectures around accepted nursing diagnoses

To assist students to think in terms of nursing diagnosis, lectures can be developed focusing on each accepted diagnosis. Nursing diagnosis, the language of professional practice, fits into any curriculum conceptual framework. An outline using problem, etiology, and signs and symptoms (the PES format used by the National Conference Group for developing each diagnosis) can be adapted to didactic material in any course. The following example (Box 1) demonstrates how one diagnosis, *sensory-perceptual alteration*, can be taught in this manner.

BOX 1   *Sensory-perceptual alteration*—a class outline

I. Objectives: At the completion of class and assigned readings, the student will be able to:
   A. Identify nursing and other scientific research related to the study of sensory-perceptual alterations
   B. Understand how the reticular activating system mediates the sensory process
   C. Define terminology specific to sensory-perceptual alterations
   D. Identify patients at risk for developing sensory-perceptual alteration
   E. Perform a nursing assessment for sensory-perceptual alterations
   F. Use the nursing diagnosis of sensory-perceptual alterations appropriately with clients who have a variety of pathophysiologic and psychosocial etiologies
   G. State the defining characteristics of sensory-perceptual alterations
   H. Use specific nursing intervention as preventive to or treatment for a client exhibiting sensory-perceptual alteration.
II. Class content
   A. The sensory process (a review)
   B. Sensory alteration research (nursing and related fields)
   C. Definition of terms
   D. Etiology
      1. Environmental factors
         a. Therapeutically restricted environments (isolation, intensive care, confining illnesses, incubator)
         b. Socially restricted environments (institutionalization, aging, chronic illness, dying, infant deprivation, mental illness)
      2. Altered sensory reception, transmission, and integration
         a. Neurologic disease, trauma, or deficit
         b. Altered visual, olfactory, tactile, auditory, or gustatory status
         c. Inability to communicate, understand, speak, or respond
         d. Aging process
         e. Sleep deprivation
         f. Pain
      3. Chemical alteration
         a. Endogenous (electrolyte imbalance, elevated BUN or ammonia, hypoxia)
         b. Exogenous (central nervous system stimulants or depressants, any mind-altering drugs)
      4. Psychologic stress (narrowed perceptual fields created by anxiety)
   E. Signs and symptoms
      1. Behavioral changes (lack of concentration, daydreaming, hallucinations, self-stimulation, noncompliance)
      2. Affective changes (anxiety, fear, depression, rapid mood swings, irritability, anger, exaggeated emotional responses)
      3. Cognitive changes (poor concentration, disordered thought sequencing, bizarre thinking)
      4. Perceptual changes (visual and auditory distortions, numbness, hallucinations, motor incoordination, feelings of body floating)

BOX 1   *Sensory-perceptual alteration—a class outline—cont'd*

   F. Nursing assessment (a combination of the following two parts)
      1. Knowledge of etiology cues alertness to the types of clients who are at risk for developing sensory-perceptual alteration
      2. Knowledge of signs and symptoms gives the clues of what to look for in the client who is at risk
   G. Selected nursing intervention
      1. If patient is verbal, legitimize the experience by talking about it, decrease anxiety through validation of the alteration as a common happening for persons in the same situation
      2. Assist person to cope with and understand the experience
      3. Use available sounds, sights, and smells for reality orientation
      4. Alter environment to decrease sensory overload or monotony
      5. Give explanations of sounds and sights
      6. To increase sensory stimulation, position by window, change setting, use mirrors, clocks, posters, calendar, pictures
      7. Use of self: read, look at books, talk
      8. Have family alternate visiting hours
      9. Use physical and tactile stimulation: range of motion, back and foot rubs, isometric exercises
    10. Make referral to occupational therapist
    11. Make extra use of touch during physical care
    12. Plan staggered visits by nursing staff
    13. Evaluate pathophysiologic sources of sensory disturbances (hypoxia, drugs, electrolytes)

Nursing diagnosis related to medical diagnosis

Although the nursing diagnostic taxonomy is professional nursing's statement of autonomy, nursing for the most part still exists in a cooperative practice situation with medicine. The majority of nurses practice their profession in hospitals and clinics in which clients are being treated under a medical diagnosis. The nurses have an urgent need for visible models after which to pattern their diagnostic conceptualization and documentation. Little and Carnevali (1976) believe that ways of integrating medical diagnostic labels and concepts into nursing diagnoses and plans of management must be made explicit. They cite several ways in which the medical diagnosis articulates with and influences the nursing diagnosis: as a stressor, as an explanation of coping deterrents, and as a genesis of nursing diagnosis.

The National Conference Group for Classification of Nursing Diagnoses, in an apparent urgency to identify what is unique and different about professional nursing practice, has understated the link that nursing will always have with medicine. Although this position is understandable, it has left

BOX 2   **Selected nursing diagnoses and interventions for the patient receiving antineoplastic drugs**

Problem 1—Alteration in nutrition
S   States has been unable to eat for several days because of nausea, vomiting, and painful sores in mouth
O   Vomited during interview, 20 pounds weight loss with 5 occurring during last week
A   Nutritional deficit related to nausea, vomiting, anorexia, stomatitis
P   Interventions for stomatitis
Use distraction, meditation, relaxation
Dry crackers, small frequent feedings
When a drug protocol restarted, give drugs during evening
Antiemetics and sedatives per physician protocol
Calorie count
Observe for evidence of fluid and electrolyte deficits
Monitor parenteral fluids and hyperalimentation if ordered
Problem 2—Discomfort related to stomatitis
S   "I have been having difficulty swallowing, and my mouth feels raw and sore."
O   Swollen, irritated mucous membrane visible in mouth and throat
A   Discomfort related to stomatitis secondary to antineoplastics
P   Observe all orifices: mouth, vagina, stoma, rectum
Mouthwash of equal parts of hydrogen peroxide and saline solution
Mouth care every 2 to 3 hours
Soft toothbrush or water spray
Avoid extreme hot or cold foods, spices, and citrus fruits
Avoid alcohol and smoking
Soft or liquid diet and food supplements
Referral to nutritionist
Ointments to lips
Analgesics (local or systemic) per physician order
Bacteriostatic mouth washes per physician order
Parenteral, tube, or hyperalimentation feedings if ordered
Problem 3—Alteration in self-concept related to alopecia, weight loss, and cancer
S   "I have been so discouraged. I am no good for anything. I am getting worse rather than better. I can't even take care of my house.
O   Alopecia, physically debilitated, main role of housewife has been lost because of weakness
A   Alteration in self-concept as a result of several factors associated with the cancer
P   Use of wigs, scarves, eyebrow pencil, and false eyelashes
Encourage verbalization of feelings
Assess further for level of grieving/depression
Visit a minimum of 15 minutes every shift to establish relationship

From Fredette, S.L., and Gloriant, F.: Am. J. Nurs. **81**:2013, 1981.

BOX 3   **Selected nursing diagnoses and interventions related to acute hepatic failure**

Problem 1—Inadequate tissue perfusion and potential impairment of skin integrity
- S   "My stomach seems so bloated, it is getting larger every day."
- O   Increased abdominal girth, weight gain, visible edema in feet and ankles, decreased capillary refill time, decreased hematocrit and hemoglobin levels
- A   Data shows inadequate tissue perfusion and potential impairment of skin integrity, needs preventive nursing care
- P   Position to relieve discomfort (elevate head, use pillow to support intercostals when in side-lying position)
        Daily abdominal girth and ankle measurements
        Accurate intake and output
        Pressure-relieving measures: turn every 2 hours, alternating pressure mattress
        Observation of all skin surfaces for tissue breakdown
        Auscultation for pulmonary edema preventive respiratory interventions
        Observe for action of diuretics

Problem 2—Discomfort, pruritus related to bile salt deposits in skin
- S   "I can't stand this itching. Can't you do something?"
- O   Restlessness, scratching, rubbing arms and legs on bed linen, jaundiced skin, elevated bilirubin, light-colored stools
- A   Jaundiced tissue is irritated
- P   Tepid water, emollient baths, emollient lotions
        No soap
        Cut nails short; if comatose, wrap hands to avoid skin damage
        Observe urine, stool, skin, and sclera for color changes
        Assess need for administration of pre-antihistamines

Problem 3—Altered thought processes related to acute liver failure
- S   Evidence of any of the following: forgetfulness, confabulation, hallucinations, disorientation to time, place, or person
- O   Any variation on a mental assessment scale from confusion to coma wandering around aimlessly, combative behavior, anxiety, diminished response to pressure or pain, elevated blood ammonia levels
- A   Impairment in cognition resulting from elevated ammonia levels
- P   All nursing intervention related to neurologically damaged patient, that is, assessment of degree of coma, measures to raise level of consciousness, protective devices

From Fredette, S.L.: Nursing diagnosis for the person in acute hepatic failure, Manuscript accepted for publication, Am. J. Nurs.

many nurses unable to identify how to use nursing diagnoses in their particular job situations. Several authors (Fisk, Fredette, Sjoberg, all to be published; Tilton and Maloff, 1982) have demonstrated how the theory of nursing diagnosis can be used in the care of patients who are being treated for medical problems. In each instance, the client's pathophysiology, clinical symptoms, reactions to illness, reactions to medical treatment, and the many independent nursing diagnoses and interventions have been merged into a problem-oriented method of documenting nursing practice. Excerpts from two of the articles are given in Boxes 2 and 3.

CONCLUSION

Several inadequacies make the organization of class content around nursing diagnosis difficult: incomplete development of each diagnosis, lack of assigning the critical defining signs and symptoms, absence of research examining each diagnosis, and insufficient literature about each diagnosis. Therefore the teacher must search the literature, organize the material, and explain that nursing diagnosis is in its infancy. An annotated bibliography for each diagnosis developed by the Northeast Task Force Group should provide some assistance for educators and students. The task will become easier as more literature becomes available. In the interim, if we expect student nurses to think "nursing process and nursing diagnosis," we must begin to structure our classroom materials following that mode of thought.

REFERENCES

American Nurses' Association: ANA standards of practice, Kansas City, Mo., 1973, The Association.

American Nurses' Association: Nursing: a social policy statement, Kansas City, Mo., 1980, The Association.

Bruce J.A.: Implementation of nursing diagnoses: a nursing administrator's perspective, Nurs. Clin. North Am. **14:**509, 1979.

Dalton, J.: Nursing diagnoses in a community health setting, Nurs. Clin. North Am. **14:**525, 1979.

Feild, L.: Nursing diagnoses in clinical practice, Nurs. Clin. North Am. **14:**497, 1979.

Fisk, N.: Nursing diagnoses for the alcoholic, Manuscript accepted for publication, Am. J. Nurs.

Fredette, S.L.: Nursing diagnosis for the person in acute hepatic failure, Manuscript accepted for publication, Am. J. Nurs.

Fredette, S.L., and Gloriant, F.: Nursing diagnosis in cancer chemotherapy: in theory and in practice, Am. J. Nurs. **81:**2013, 1981.

Fredette, S., and O'Connor, K.: Nursing diagnoses in teaching and curriculum planning, Nurs. Clin. North Am. **14:**541, 1979.

Gordon, M.: Predictive strategies in diagnostic tasks, Nurs. Res. **29:**39, 1980.

Gordon M., Sweeney, M.A., and McKeehan, K.: Nursing diagnosis: looking at its use in the clinical area, Am. J. Nurs. **80:**672, 1980.

Little, D., and Carnevali, D.: Nursing care planning ed. 3, Philadelphia, 1976, J.B. Lippincott Co.

Matthews, C.A., and Gaul, A.L.: Nursing diagnosis from the perspective of concept and attainment and critical thinking, Adv. Nurs. Sci. **2:**17, 1979.

McKeehan, K.: Nursing diagnoses in a discharge planning program, Nurs. Clin. North Am. **14:**517, 1979.

Sjoberg, E.: Nursing diagnosis for the person in the community with chronic lung disease, Manuscript accepted for publication, Am. J. Nurs.

Tilton, C., and Maloff, M.: Diagnosing the problems in stroke, Am. J. Nurs. **82:**596, 1982.

Watson, G., and Glaser, E.: Watson-Glaser critical thinking appraisal, New York, 1964, Harcourt Brace Jovanovich, Inc.

Exploring nursing diagnoses with baccalaureate nursing students: practice in nursing science

MARY A. KELLY, R.N., Ed.D.

This paper reports on a project that focused on developing understanding of the nursing diagnosis process and terminology in baccalaureate nursing students. The report will present phases of the project plan and activity in relation to nursing science and an innovation-decision process model. The project was conducted in a baccalaureate program in which students have used (since 1976) terminology approved by the National Conference Group for Classification of Nursing Diagnoses. Teaching related to the nursing diagnosis process and introduction to the terminology has been a focus for third-year students. They are expected to use nursing diagnosis in clinical practice and in writing nursing care plans. The goal of the faculty was to foster the adoption of a nursing diagnosis framework in the clinical practice of students after graduation.

The process by which people accept and use or reject new ideas was explored by Rogers and Shoemaker (1971), who identified a process by which individuals adopt innovations. The stages of this innovation-decision process model are as follows:

Stage One: Knowledge function—development of awareness and gaining information about the idea

Stage Two: Persuasion function—forming a favorable or unfavorable impression through confirmation of beliefs about the idea

Stage Three: Decision function—trial on a probationary basis, activities leading to a decision to adopt or reject the idea

Stage Four: Confirmation function—seeking reinforcement of the decision

Faculty tended to focus on the knowledge function when seeking to bring about behavior change and adoption of innovative ideas by students. Faculty involved in this project furnished the students with opportunities to engage in behaviors that assisted in knowledge and decision functions through classroom teaching and clinical practice application of the nursing diagnosis framework. They did not address the persuasion function as it is described by Rogers and Shoemaker (1971).

Approval by the National Conference Group (Kim and Moritz, 1982) of a new listing of nursing diagnoses was a catalyst for faculty in development of the nursing diagnosis exploration project. This project provided the students with an opportunity to explore and seek confirmation of their ideas of nursing diagnoses, which are needed behaviors during the persuasion function phase of the innovation-decision process model.

Instances of the confirmation stage were observed occasionally as former students contacted faculty members for partial or complete replacement of a faculty-prepared manual of nursing diagnoses. These students had found reinforcement for their decision to adopt the nursing diagnosis framework by continuing to use this manual and sharing it with other nurses.

PURPOSE AND OBJECTIVES

The general purpose of the project was to foster the idea of persuasion. The following objectives were identified by the faculty:
1. Exploration of nursing diagnoses through use of knowledgeable sources
2. Enhancement of observation and decision-making skills
3. Production of a student manual of nursing diagnoses

These objectives, in addition to fostering the idea of persuasion, provided students with the opportunity to experience involvement at an elementary level in nursing science. Jacobs and Huether (1978, p. 66) have described nursing science as "the process, and the result, or ordering and patterning the events and phenomena of concern to nursing." Theory formation is the eventual goal of nursing science, and the exploration of nursing diagnoses can be related to the first level, or factor-isolation, theory according to the Dickoff and James (1968) schema of situation-producing theory. Gordon and Sweeney (1979) have identified as a primary step in building a clinical science the activity of describing health problems diagnosed and treated by nurses. As students engaged in exploring activities described later in this paper), they became involved in the nursing science of exploring and describing events that are identified as phenomena of concern to nurses.

Jacobs and Heuther's definition of nursing science (1978) describes a dual nature in science—the process and product. The production of the student manual of nursing diagnoses is the product.

PROCESS: NURSING SCIENCE

Teacher preparation of students for the project consisted of three activities: creating awareness, providing knowledge, and identifying objectives and guidelines for the exploration project. Before engaging in activities, students were informed about the nursing diagnosis framework through classroom lectures and discussion. Nursing diagnosis as an activity was defined, and the independent, autonomous nature of the activity was emphasized. *Nursing diagnosis* was defined by faculty as identification and labeling of an undesirable or unhealthful situation (from the client's or nurse's view) that can be prevented, corrected, or mitigated by nursing activity for which a physician's order is unnecessary. The last was included to prevent restatement by the student of the physician's diagnosis as the nurse's diagnosis, for example, restatement of diabetes as altered nutrition. This mistake seems to be common among students beginning to use nursing diagnosis terminology.

To further delineate the independent nature of nursing diagnostic activity, nursing functions were placed in two categories: (1) planning and implementing a nursing regimen and (2) assisting with a medical regimen. Activities in the first category were described as (1) observation, monitoring, data gathering, (2) intervention, prevention, correction, mitigation, (3) support, nurturing, emotional support, and (4) guidance, teaching, counseling, exploring. Activities in the second category were described as (1) observation of medical outcomes, (2) performing procedures and treatments, (3) administering medications and (4) communicating with and for physicians.

The students were also given instruction in making a diagnosis, including identification of a set of characteristics and a diagnostic label.

Student activity in the project was related to the first-level practice of nursing science. Jacobs and Huether (1978) identified four steps in the process of nursing science. The first two steps involve defining and operationalizing the concepts of interest. The final steps involve linking the concepts into relationships and verifying these links. Activities of the students in the project fell within the range of the first two steps. Guidelines for the student activities established by the faculty included four steps:

1. Formation of small work groups and the selection of a diagnosis for exploration
2. Investigation of the diagnosis through review of related literature, interviewing of nurses, and observation of clients
3. Comparison of findings with previous knowledge of the diagnosis
4. Preparation of a new listing of the diagnosis, with a definition and a list of characteristics

The project was conducted in the spring of 1981; 59 students participated. Most students chose to work in groups of three; several worked individually. Students selected 22 diagnoses for exploration from the list approved at the Fourth National Conference on the Classification of Nursing Diagnoses (Kim and Moritz, 1982).

Students conducted library searches for related books and nursing literature. Descriptions and terminology for a list of characteristics were taken from these resources and were used in client assessment. Staff nurses, head nurses, clinical specialists, and faculty were consulted by students for discussion of their experience and knowledge of the diagnoses.

The nursing diagnoses adopted by the National Conference Group were experientially derived. The link between theory and practice in nursing science results from selection of concepts derived from practice. These concepts are expected to have unique components based on individual experiences and common elements (Jacobs and Huether, 1978).

In most instances students were able to collect data during nursing care activities in clinical laboratory sessions. Some diagnoses chosen by students, however, could not be observed in clients during the time of the project, for example, rape trauma syndrome, spiritual distress, and potential for violence.

In his work on the science in clinical examinations performed by physicians, Feinstein (1967) explored clinical judgment mathematically and called it *enumerational measurement.* In this measurement "the entity to be assessed is already a unit, and the measurement consists of finding a particular category in which the unit is to be counted (Feinstein, 1967, p. 62). To classify the unit into a subgroup, the different attributes are identified and then compared with attributes of other units in the subgroup. Critical features of this scientific enumeration are observation of the attributes and the criteria used for their classification as part of a subgroup. Jacobs and Huether (1978, p. 69) call these attributes *empirical referents*, which must be "behavioral manifestations or clinically available physiological indicators."

Students in the project attempted to identify verbal, nonverbal, physical, psychologic, and emotional characteristics of the diagnosis. After collection of the data, students examined their findings for duplication of characteristics obtained from the various sources and compared them with any characteristics listed by the National Conference Group. Once the data were compared, the students prepared a new listing of the diagnoses to be included in the student manual. The listing contained the diagnostic label, subcategories, definitions, and a list of characteristics. Literature sources used were compiled into a bibliography for each diagnosis.

PRODUCT: NURSING SCIENCE

Listings prepared by the students and those diagnoses not chosen by students for exploration but that had previously been prepared by faculty were collected into the Student Manual of Nursing Diagnosis. This manual also contains the bibliographies prepared by the students. The manual has been in continuous use by junior and senior students in the baccalaureate program since that time. It has become a valuable reference for the nursing students in all clinical courses. Students invariably discuss client health problems using nursing diagnoses terminology.

Jacobs and Huether (1978) have commented that a poorly developed process and product tend to inhibit further growth of science, but once begun the process tends to increase and sustain development of the product. It was believed that some evidence for the perpetuation of the student involvement in the nursing science activity might be observed by comparing activity of individual students in the project with their activity the following year in a nursing research course. In this course, students prepare a proposal for a research project in a nursing area of interest. When variables of projects designed by 36 of the students (topics and variables for the other 23 students were unavailable) were examined for their relationship to the nursing diagnosis chosen for the exploration project, seven students had used nursing diagnosis terminology to indicate variables to be studied. Six students had chosen as variables concepts directly related to the chosen diagnosis used in the exploration project. For example, one student proposed to investigate the relationship of stress and orientation in clients in an intensive care unit. In the nursing diagnosis exploration project, she had chosen ineffective individual coping. Only two students had used the same nursing diagnosis terminology in the research proposal and the exploration project.

Problems experienced by the students in the project were believed to be the result of lack of sufficient time for data collection (2 weeks were allowed) and lack of interest on the part of faculty involved in the clinical laboratory experiences with the students. The project was an activity in a course that has no clinical component.

REFERENCES

Dickoff, J., and James, P.: A theory of theories: a position paper, Nurs. Res. **17**:197, 1968.

Feinstein, A.R.: Clinical judgment, Huntington, New York, 1967, R.E. Krieger Publishing Co., Inc.

Gordon, M., and Sweeney, M.A.: Methodological problems and issues in identifying and standardizing nursing diagnoses, Adv. Nurs. Sci. **2**:1, 1979.

Jacobs, M.K., and Huether, S.E.: Nursing science: the theory-practice linkage, Adv. Nurs. Sci. **1**:63, 1978.

Kim, M.J., and Moritz, D.A.: Classification of nursing diagnoses: proceedings of the third and fourth national conference, New York, 1982, McGraw-Hill Book Co.

Rogers, E.M., and Shoemaker, F.F.: Communication of innovations: a cross-cultural approach, ed. 2, New York, 1971, The Free Press.

Development of a nursing diagnosis health assessment tool

SALLY TRIPP, R.N., M.S.

Faculty of baccalaureate schools of nursing need tools to enhance the teaching of nursing diagnosis and the diagnostic process. Fundamental to analysis of data to derive nursing diagnoses is the collection of patient data that systematically identifies a broad range of empirical indicators. In teaching sophomore and junior students, it is essential that faculty assist students to learn to categorize data in a manner that enhances clustering of empirical patient cues to reveal relationships. For a nursing conceptual framework to be relevant and useful to students, it is also essential that teaching methodologies be designed to assist students in operationalizing the abstract concepts of the framework in concrete clinical practice situations. Students also need to learn ways to implement the ANA Standards of Practice, Social Policy Statement, and Quality Assurance Model as an integral part of clinical professional nursing practice. The development, utilization, and testing of a health assessment tool for collecting subjective and objective patient data, as the first step in the nursing process linked to the conceptual framework of the nursing program, may be one answer to these learning needs of students.

PROBLEM

In the 1980-1981 academic year the faculty of the Division of Nursing, University of Massachusetts recognized and acknowledged a problem common to many settings. We did not have a defined data base assessment tool to utilize in teaching students to collect empirical client cues from which nursing diagnoses could be derived and nursing care plans could be designed and implemented. It was decided to develop such a tool.

BACKGROUND

When faculty acknowledged the problem, sophomore, junior, and senior students were taught the nursing process (data collection and diagnosis, planning, implementation, and evaluation) by using different data collection tools and nursing care plan formats at each level of the curriculum. Individual faculty designed or selected the data collection tool to use in each course. These tools ranged from those organized around the medical model and body systems to those organized around primarily psychosocial nursing histories for specialty practice areas. Faculty had differing beliefs, knowledges, and skills related to patient data collection, nursing diagnosis, and clinically based application of the nursing process. A majority of faculty, however, agreed that one data collection tool and one nursing care plan format should be taught and used at all three levels of the curriculum. These faculty also believed that one data collection tool and one nursing care plan format would facilitate identification of the breadth and depth of patient data and nursing interventions taught at each curriculum level.

Concurrently, the Curriculum Committee was rewording and refining our conceptual framework so that it would give increased guidance in curriculum decision making and organization of learning experiences. The faculty recognized the weak articulation of the eclectic conceptual framework with its discrete clinically applicable subconcepts and skills for student teaching/learning experiences. Several faculty, however, expressed interest, skill, and commitment in articulating our conceptual framework in teaching nursing process and in improving our teaching methodologies to assist students in learning relationships between and among subconcepts taught at each level of the curriculum. Some faculty were committed to the work of the National Conference Group for Classification of Nursing Diagnoses.

METHODOLOGY

Three faculty task force groups were formed: Nursing Care Plan Format, Conceptual Framework Refinement, and Health Assessment Tool. Recommendations of each task force were presented to the Curriculum Committee. Curriculum Committee recommendations, based on each task force's work, were shared with the faculty for discussion. The Curriculum Committee then revised their recommendations, if indicated, based on faculty input. Finally, Curriculum Committee recommendations for each task force were presented to the Faculty Assembly vote for implementation.

PROCESS AND OUTCOMES
Nursing care plan format

Because development of a nursing care plan format was perceived by faculty as a priority, it was developed first. The decision was made by the task force to use nursing diagnosis as the organizing focus and to define the terms used in the format to enhance consistency by faculty in teaching. The format is shown in Box 1. Nursing diagnosis initially was defined based on the wording of our conceptual framework. The format and definition of terms were accepted by the Faculty Assembly for trial. The outcome was the implementation of the problem–etiology–signs and symptoms (PES) nursing diagnostic statement of Gordon (1976), which served as the basis for developing nursing care plans throughout the curriculum. Recently the Curriculum Committee has accepted a revised definition of nursing diagnosis based on refinement of the conceptual framework, which will be presented to the Faculty Assembly. This definition states that nursing diagnosis is a classifying statement that designates an actual or potential disruption in the ordered relationship of person/environment that nurses are licensed to treat.

Conceptual framework refinement

The task force reworded and refined the conceptual framework of the curriculum. It is still an eclectic framework, and an attempt has been made to avoid use of words that might be interpreted as relating to the work of any one specific nursing theorist. A schematic drawing of the conceptual framework that was accepted by the Faculty Assembly is given in Box 2.

Health assessment tool

In development of the health assessment tool, the following steps were undertaken primarily in the order indicated, but often with movement back and forth:

1. Examination of the conceptual framework for direction in data collection. As can be seen in Box 2, data needed to be collected related to all the subconcepts of person/environment and health.
2. Identification of empirical client indicators that would be representative of each subconcept.
3. Categorization of the nursing diagnoses approved by the Fourth National Conference (Kim and Moritz, 1982) into the 11 patterns shown in Box 3 for use in clustering of empirical data.
4. Organization of identified empirical client cues into subjective and objective data under each of the 11 client patterns with consideration given to client characteristics recommended for validation under approved nursing diagnoses, clinical practice experience, expertise of faculty, and subconcept definitions of our conceptual framework.
5. Development of a format for recording all empirical data collected that would also give direction for what data to collect. At this step it was found that some empirical data identified previously did not seem to fall under the category patterns. Therefore these categories were added: demographic, health promotion/illness prevention practices, medical illness data, and belief/value and environmental patterns.
6. Data to be collected was divided into subjective/history and objective/examination. A comprehensive health history and examination tool was then designed. The final format was reviewed and revised by selected faculty to ensure that it was applicable to clients of all ages.
7. Faculty informally chose to test the health assessment tool in all Level I and II nursing courses for the year. Feedback and revision will take place later before bringing the tool to the Faculty Assembly.

Informal, ongoing feedback from both students and faculty has already provided suggestions for modification and revision of the tool. Comments

BOX 1   **Nursing care plan format**

Nursing diagnosis: (problem and etiology)

Subjective data: Objective data:

Long-term goal:

Client objectives	Nursing intervention	Rationale	Evaluation

BOX 2   **Curriculum conceptual framework model**

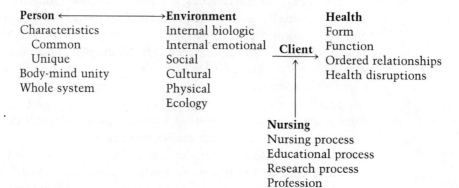

Person ⟵————————⟶**Environment**   **Health**
Characteristics   Internal biologic   Form
  Common   Internal emotional   **Client**   Function
  Unique   Social   ————⟶   Ordered relationships
Body-mind unity   Cultural   Health disruptions
Whole system   Physical
                    Ecology

Nursing
Nursing process
Educational process
Research process
Profession

Goal of nursing: Promote ordered relationships of person/environment

BOX 3	**Pattern categories identified**

1. Nutrition
2. Elimination
3. Activity/exercise
4. Rest/sleep
5. Sensory
6. Cardiorespiratory
7. Skin integrity

8. Sexuality
9. Cognition/perception
10. Self-concept
11. Role/relationship
Added later:
12. Belief/value
13. Environment

from both faculty and students have indicated that the tool is achieving its purpose. Most significantly, an increased number of faculty have become interested and committed to developing and testing nursing diagnosis concepts and the diagnostic process as the pivotal step in nursing process. Ideas have been generated for articulating our conceptual framework in clinical nursing practice.

RESULTS

In less than 2 years, the following have been achieved by faculty at the Division of Nursing, University of Massachusetts:

1. A single, comprehensive health assessment tool (Box 4) linked to our curriculum conceptual framework and nursing diagnosis is being implemented and tested by sophomore and junior students and faculty.
2. A single nursing care plan format based on nursing diagnoses is being implemented throughout the curriculum with definition of terms based on our conceptual framework.
3. Breadth and depth of faculty and student understanding and knowledge of nursing diagnosis has taken place with resultant changes in course content and teaching methodologies related to the nursing diagnostic process.
4. There is increased consistency across curriculum levels and in individual courses in teaching all steps of the nursing process with beginning clearer identification of breadth and depth of concepts and skills taught at each level.
5. Increased operationalization of our conceptual framework in teaching clinical nursing practice throughout the curriculum is in the process of evolving.

The faculty believes that these efforts represent a beginning step in the development of a scientific assessment guide for nursing as urged by Mallick

BOX 4   **Comprehensive health assessment tool**

Patient's name: _____   Student's name: _____
                                                  Date completed: _____

General appearance:

Nutrition pattern status:
    Weight _____   Height/length _____
    Head circumference: Infant _____
    Skin turgor/mobility:
    Skin moisture:
    Adipose tissue distribution:
    Mouth:
        Lesions   Condition of teeth/gums:
        Fit of dentures   Condition of lips:
        Tongue: (C.N.VII)   Pharynx/tonsils (C.N.IX and X)
Elimination pattern status:
    Abdominal percussion: Abdominal tenderness:
    Bowel sounds:
    Hernias: Palpable abdominal masses:
    Anus/rectum: Occult blood test (type and result):
    Urine appearance:
Activity/exercise pattern status:
    Posture and gait:
    Joint—tenderness, swelling:
    Joint ROM:
    Spine:
Cardiovascular pattern status:
    Thorax/lung:
        Structure/movement:
        Respirations:
        Breath sounds/adventitious sounds:
    Heart:
        P.M.I.:
        Apical rate and rhythm:
        Heart sounds (aortic, pulmonic, erbs point, tricuspid and mitral areas):
    Peripheral vascular:
        Pulses:

	Brachial	Radial	Femoral	Popliteal	Posterior tibia	Dorsalis pedis
R						
L						

Extremities—temperature, color, condition of nails:
    Hands:
    Feet:

BOX 4   **Comprehensive health assessment tool—cont'd**

Blood pressure:
    Sitting/lying _____ R _____ L
    Standing _____ R _____ L
Sensory pattern status:
    Eyes:
        Acuity (C.N.II):   E.O.M.'s (C.N.III, IV and VI):
        Conjunctiva/sclera: Visual fields:
        Pupils (C.N.II):
    Ears:
        Acuity (C.N.VIII):   External lesions:
        Position: Canals/drums:
    Nose:
        Smell (C.N.I.):   Nasal mucosa:
        External nares: Sinuses:
    Tactile:
        Light/deep touch:
        Response to pin prick:
Sexuality patterns:
    Breasts
        Size/symmetry:
        Masses:
    External genital (pubic hair distribution, symmetry of structures, discharge,
        lesions):
Cognitive/perception patterns:
    Mental status:
        Consciousness/mood:
        Thought processes/content:
        Orientation (person, place, time):
        Abstract thinking:
        Memory (recent and remote):
    Cranial nerves not previously tested:
        V Trigeminal (jaw movement):
        VII Facial (movement-expression symmetry):
        XI Spinal (strength and contraction of muscles):
    Speech:
Environmental patterns:
    Immediate physical environment:
        Convenience
        Safety
        Sensory level
    Interactions with social environment:
        Family members:
        Staff and others:
Other examination data (Romberg, Homan's sign, liver size, lymph nodes,
    temperature as appropriate for patient):
Developmental observations (Denver, Draw a Person done by you):

(1981), enhancement of teaching students to use and test nursing diagnosis in clinical practice, and movement of faculty toward teaching baccalaureate nursing students from the perspective of a nursing model. The development of this assessment guide must be duplicated by other nursing education and service settings. The process has been time consuming and thought provoking in raising additional questions and ideas but holds promise for advancing the scientific practice of nursing.

REFERENCES

Gordon, M.: Nursing diagnosis and the diagnostic process, Am. J. Nurs. **76**(8):1298, 1976.

Kim, M.J., and Moritz, D.A., eds.: Classification of nursing diagnoses: proceedings of the third and fourth national conferences, New York, 1982, McGraw-Hill Book Co.

Mallick, M.J.: Patient assessment-based on data, not intuition, Nurs. Outlook **29**(10):600, 1981.

Strength-oriented nursing diagnoses

SUE POPKESS-VAWTER, R.N., Ph.D.

As nursing grows and evolves as a profession, several trends can be observed. Traditionally nursing has followed directives for care given it by other professionals or has borrowed other models on which to base nursing practice. Currently nursing is becoming an autonomous, decision-making profession regarding specific nursing intervention for the client. Nurses are now more frequently initiating collaboration with other health care professionals instead of ritualistically following orders.

Another growing trend in the nursing profession is the recognition of a person's holism. Care for a person as a biologic, psychosocial, and spiritual being is the core of holistic nursing practice. In developing a taxonomy of nursing diagnoses, I believe that nurses must provide a holistic classification of nursing diagnoses. Presently the Fourth National Conference listing of nursing diagnoses is problem oriented. It is my belief that nursing diagnoses, unlike medical diagnoses, should include positive, strength-oriented diagnoses to be consistent with the holistic approach that we profess in caring for our patients.

The purpose of this paper is to present a rationale and examples of positive, strength-oriented nursing diagnoses. Specifically, an historic overview will be presented to clarify the present diagnostic process. The value of assessing patient strengths and problems and implications for nursing practice will be reviewed. A potential process for generating positive nursing diagnoses will be discussed.

HISTORIC OVERVIEW

The POMR, a logical, simplified approach for organizing medical data, was developed in 1964 (Weed, 1964). The POMR set an example for nursing to follow for reorganizing nursing data. Identification of patient problems and the organization of the problem list were the basis for the problem-oriented record. Nurses began to develop problem lists but at the same time had concern about making medical diagnoses. Physicians diagnose to cure disease; nurses diagnose to care more effectively for the patient. Because medical and nursing diagnoses are frequently difficult to separate, unrest and confusion developed among physicians and nurses alike.

In 1973 the First National Conference on the Classification of Nursing Diagnoses was held for the purpose of developing a common diagnostic classification system to identify the patient problems that underlie therapeutic interventions (Gebbie and Lavin, 1975). Much searching, questioning, and clarification has occurred during each of the four conferences. The nursing diagnosis is viewed as the end product of nursing assessment and may also be found as a subproblem related to a medical diagnosis (Kim and Moritz, 1982). For example, a traumatic amputation of the right leg is the medical diagnosis for Dennis, a 23-year-old man involved in a motorcycle accident (Popkess, 1981). On the other hand, the nursing diagnoses for this man might include:

1. Mobility, impaired physical
2. Skin integrity, impairment of: actual/potential
3. Self-concept, disturbance in: body image
4. Grieving, dysfunctional
5. Breathing patterns, ineffective: potential for
6. Comfort, alterations in: pain: actual/phantom

Nursing diagnoses describe the patient's health problems for which nurses are responsible. In other words, nurses will directly care for Dennis' immobility, grieving, and pain related to his amputation. Nurses will assist with range of motion, turning, and positioning, lend support through his grieving process, and explore methods for relieving the pain. Gordon (1976, p. 1299) defined nursing diagnoses in the following manner: "Clinical diagnoses made by professional nurses describe actual or potential health problems which nurses, by virtue of their education and experience are capable and licensed to treat."

A problem frequently encountered is whether to include separate listings of medical diagnoses and nursing diagnoses in the patient's record. I believe that separation of medical and nursing diagnoses potentiates fragmentation of patient care. When the patient is fragmented, or symbolically broken down into parts, the holistic approach becomes impossible. Clearer delineation of medical and nursing diagnoses and understanding of how these diagnoses relate can preserve the holistic approach to patient care. Therefore a combined problem list enables all members of the health care team to perceive the whole patient and to know what problems are their primary focus.

THE VALUE OF STRENGTH-ORIENTED DIAGNOSES AND IMPLICATIONS FOR NURSING

Throughout the historic process of developing nursing, a vital element seems to be missing from the diagnostic process. Have the positive aspects of the patient been assessed? What strengths does the patient have? Dennis, the 23-year-old man with a traumatic amputation of the right leg, has multiple strengths even though he has experienced a devastating alteration in life-style

(Popkess, 1981). The nursing history revealed that Dennis has several potential positive nursing diagnoses: a devoted wife, group life insurance with disability coverage, an understanding boss who assures his job as soon as he is ready to go back to work, and a strong faith in God. These potential positive diagnoses can be added to complete the strengths portion of his problems and strengths list. These strengths might be used to help Dennis more successfully rehabilitate and adjust. The question then remains: How does one state these positive nursing diagnoses and further develop them to parallel problem nursing diagnoses?

NURSING IMPLICATIONS

Both the assessment and the identification of problems and strengths are primary nursing responsibilities (Popkess, 1981). Without a strengths list, nursing care is planned in isolation; there is no recycling of patient energy back into his system to revitalize his recovery process. Without assessing the patient's strengths, the nurse is second-guessing what would be a therapeutic approach to care for the patient's problems.

In the following section, the four steps for determining nursing diagnoses will be discussed to demonstrate how strengths assessment can be viewed as an integral part of the nursing process. Implications for the use of strengths assessment or positive nursing diagnoses include every area of nursing practice, whether it is based in the hospital setting, in the clinic, or in the community. Strengths diagnoses are made about the client regardless of clinical setting. Weed (1964) suggested that patients should have a permanent, computerized listing of their problems that could be retrieved by any health care professional by the simple input into the computer of the patient's name or hospital number. A similar ongoing list of strengths could be recorded as baseline data for each client. Then as the client moves frome home throughout the community, as a patient in the hospital, or as an outpatient in a clinic, his strengths list would accommpany him. Regardless of where they practice, nurses could then use that patient's strengths to help counterbalance the problem diagnoses.

Other implications for nursing practice include schools of nursing. If nursing students began early in their careers to assess strengths as well as problems for patients, the holistic approach could be implemented more easily. Communication skills that nursing students learn could be incorporated to assess and validate strengths of the client. Furthermore, nursing students could learn to explore with clients how they believe their strengths might be used to help manage their problems. Students would then have thorough nursing plans that considered the patient's input directly. The success of those plans would most likely be greater because the patients were allowed to have direct input into them. The remainder of the nursing process falls logically into sequence; the implementation, evaluation, and revision phases would include the patients' input regarding the success of the mutual plans. Students could identify more quickly the components of nursing process with this commonsense approach rather than performing many of the academic exercises that students are forced to experience in nursing education today.

PROCESS FOR GENERATING POSITIVE NURSING DIAGNOSES

Gebbie and Lavin (1975), Gordon (1976), and Price (1980) have discussed the process by which nursing diagnoses are made. I believe that the same process for making problem-oriented nursing diagnoses can be used in making strength-oriented nursing diagnoses. For example, Price (1980) recommended the following four steps in determining a diagnostic statement:

1. Data collection: validating objective and subjective data from the patient, family, health record, physical and psychosocial assessment, and consultation with other health team members
2. Data analysis: sorting out the data in appropriate categories: physiologic, sociologic, spiritual, or psychologic
3. Organization of data, synthesis of diagnosis: determining patterns that exist within the data, rather than using a single clue to formulate a diagnosis; a diagnostic category may be chosen that clearly describes the health problem; the pattern within a diagnostic category outlines the characteristics of the health problem identified
4. Validation: reviewing the data base to determine if synthesis of the data pattern includes signs and symptoms that identify the health problem; ensuring that the diagnosis is based on scientific knowledge and clinical expertise, has independent nursing actions indicated, and is most likely the same diagnosis that 50% of other qualified practitioners would make

These four steps for making nursing diagnoses are an integral part of initiating the nursing process. To be holistic, the positive aspects of the patient must be assessed in addition to the problems. Therefore I am suggesting that each of the steps listed be applied to generate strength-oriented nursing diagnoses. To each of the four steps could be added the phrase *health problems and patient strengths*. Nurses would then begin assessing strengths in the initial step of the nursing process, thereby ensuring a holistic assessment. Box 1 contains a listing of potential sources of patient strengths-oriented nursing diagnoses (Popkess, 1981). The potential sources from which strengths diagnoses can be made can be elicited from the nursing history. Basic psychosocial, and physical assessment, can be generated from the basic nursing history. The same sources from which problem-oriented diagnoses are derived contain data regarding strengths diagnoses. To demonstrate this process, strength-oriented nursing diagnoses have been paralleled for most of the problem-oriented nursing diagnoses accepted at the Fourth National Conference (Box 2).

It should be noted that one positive nursing diagnosis has been accepted by the Fourth National Conference (Kim and Moritz, 1982). *Coping, family: potential for growth* is a strength-oriented nursing diagnosis. This diagnosis has the same PES format describing etiology and defining characteristics as do the problem-oriented diagnoses.

Another example of how the PES format can be applied to a positive nursing diagnosis is the diagnosis of *self-care deficit: feeding, bathing/hygiene, dressing/grooming, toileting.* This diagnosis consists of levels of ability ranging from "completely independent (level 0)" to "dependent, does not participate in activity (level 4)" (Kim and Moritz, 1982). A positive nursing diagnosis, *self-care, adequate,* could specify level 0 for each activity to describe the patient's strengths. Other positive diagnosis examples are given in Box 3.

I believe that numerous positive diagnoses could be made for many moderately healthy patients. Listing every positive diagnosis for every patient would soon become very unwieldy. Nurses must use their judgment and experience as a guide to determine which are the most pertinent positive diag-

---

BOX 1   **Potential sources of strength-oriented nursing diagnoses**

 1. Age
 2. Family, significant others
 3. Support systems, that is, owns home, religion
 4. Job, work, vocation, position
 5. Financial status
 6. Insurance
 7. Exercise
 8. Proper weight for height, diet habits
 9. General health status
10. Hobbies, leisure activities
11. Self-care practices, that is, health habits
12. Education, training
13. Intelligence, knowledge, special aptitudes
14. Organizational, imaginative, and creative abilities
15. Humor, zest for living, attitudes, willingness to participate

---

From Popkess, S.: Nursing **81**:34, 1981.

BOX 2   **Potential positive nursing diagnoses**

Airway clearance, effective
Bowel elimination, regular, healthy
Breathing patterns, effective
Cardiac output, adequate for body needs
Comfort, pain-free
Communication, effective verbal
Coping, effective individual
Coping, effective family
Coping, family: potential for growth
Diversional activity, adequate
Fear, freedom from
Fluid volume, adequate
Gas exchange, adequate
Grieving, appropriate, effective
Home maintenance management, adequate
Injury, prevention activities
Knowledge, adequate (specify)
Mobility, physical adequate (specify)
Compliance (specify)
Nutrition, adequate to meet body requirements
Parenting, effective
Self-care, adequate (specify level: feeding, bathing/hygiene, dressing/grooming, toileting)
Self-concept, healthy (specify)
Sensory perception, appropriate
Sexual function, adequate
Skin integrity, healthy
Sleep pattern, healthy
Spiritual faith (specify)
Thought processes, appropriate
Tissue perfusion, adequate
Urinary elimination, adequate

BOX 3   **Examples of positive nursing diagnoses**

Coping, effective individual

DEFINITION: Use of adaptive behaviors and problem-solving abilities in meeting life's demands and roles

Etiology	Defining characteristics
Situational crises	Verbalization of ability to cope or ability to ask for help*
Maturational crises	Ability to meet role expectations
Personal vulnerability	Ability to meet basic needs
	Ability to problem solve*
	Adaptation in social participation
	No destructive behavior toward self or others
	Appropriate use of defense mechanisms
	Use of usual communication patterns
	No verbal manipulation
	Regaining illness-free and accident-free life-style

Home maintenance management, adequate

DEFINITION: Ability to independently maintain a safe growth-promotion immediate environment

Etiology	Subjective defining characteristics
Lack of individual/family member disease or injury	Household members express no difficulty in maintaining their home in a comfortable fashion*
Sufficient family organization or planning	Household members request no assistance with home maintenance*
Sufficient finances	Household members describe adequate financial situation*
Familiarity with neighborhood resources	**Objective defining characteristics**
	Orderly surroundings
Adaptation in cognitive or emotional functioning	Washed and available cooking equipment, clothes, or linen*
	No accumulation of dirt, food wastes, or hygienic wastes*
Adequate knowlede	No offensive odors
Adequate role modeling	Appropriate household temperature
Adequate support systems	Rested, coping family members*
	Necessary equipment or aids
	Absence of vermin or rodents
	No excessive hygienic disorders, infestations, or infections*

*Critical defining characteristic.

noses that could be used in planning to help with patient problems. A similar judgment is seen when the nurse determines which potential problem nursing diagnoses might be pertinent for the patient. Noting every potential problem for every patient would soon yield an overwhelming list.

SUMMARY

In summary, this paper has reviewed the development of classification systems for patient problems. Specifically, the National Conference on the Classification of Nursing Diagnoses has generated many problem-oriented nursing diagnoses, with little regard for strengths-oriented nursing diagnoses. However, the exact opposite of each problem diagnosis might be used to describe and classify strengths diagnoses. Other sources for strengths diagnoses can be obtained from the strengths elicited from the nursing history of each patient. The last step of problems and strengths identification is using the strengths to help manage the problems, which leads directly to the nursing care plan and through the remaining steps of the nursing process in a holistic manner.

"Without assessment of patient strengths, nursing practice dwells upon the negative aspects of patients problems" (Popkess, 1981, p. 37). Soon these negative aspects generate negative attitudes toward patient care. If nurses begin to focus on the strengths of patients, attitudes may in turn become more positive and hope in the future will be emphasized for every patient for whome they care.

REFERENCES

Gebbie, K., and Lavin, M.: Classification of nursing diagnoses, St. Louis, 1975, The C.V. Mosby Co.

Gordon, M.: Nursing diagnosis and the diagnostic process, Am. J. Nurs. **76:**1298, 1976.

Kim, M.J., and Moritz, D.A., eds.: Classification of nursing diagnoses: proceedings of the third and fourth national conferences, New York, 1982, McGraw-Hill Book Co.

Popkess, S.: Diagnosing your patient's strengths, Nursing **81:**34, 1981.

Price, M.: Nursing diagnosis: making a concept come alive, Am. J. Nurs. **80:**668, 1980.

Weed, L.: Medical records, patient care, and medical education, Ir. J. Med. Sci. **462:**271, 1964.

A personal viewpoint of the relevance of organic brain syndrome

PATRICIA D. BARRY, R.N., M.S.N.

In 1980 the Fourth National Conference on the Classification of Nursing Diagnoses presented a list of 42 nursing diagnoses to be used in clinical nursing practice, education, and research. In reviewing the possible etiologies under each diagnostic heading, there is a common potential cause that has been omitted in a majority of the categories. I believe that organic brain syndrome (OBS) can be an etiologic factor in most of the diagnostic categories. Changes in neurologic status from either a primary neurologic disease or a systemic sequela of another condition can result in changes in physiologic functioning in brain structures. Whenever brain physiology is disrupted, a subtle to severe alteration in mental status occurs. This changes in mental status can be observed in the patient's behavioral functioning. Decreased coping ability and many other types of psychosocial dysfunctions included in the diagnostic list can be caused by OBS. Conditions that can result in temporary or permanent organic brain changes include (Goldberg, 1980; Kaplan and Saddock, 1981; Lishman, 1978):

Metabolic disorders*
  Changes in endocrine gland functioning
  Electrolyte disturbances
Electrical disorders
  Various types of epilepsy
Neoplastic disease
  Benign or malignant tumors
Degenerative diseases
  Multiple sclerosis
  Lupus erythematosus
  Alzheimer's disease
Arterial disease
  Cerebrovascular accidents
  Arteriosclerotic cerebral artery disease
Mechanical (structural) changes
  Head trauma
  Subdural hematoma
  Normal pressure hydrocephalus

---

*Note that the first letters of each category form the mnemonic MEND A MIND (Goldberg, 1980).

TABLE 1   Two types of organic brain syndrome

Symptom	Delerium	Dementia
Onset	Usually rapid: waxes and wanes abruptly	Usually slow: 1 month or more
Level of awareness	Increased or decreased	Normal or decreased
Orientation	Disoriented to time, person, and place at constant or transient intervals (time should be charted)	Usually not affected until late in course
Appearance	May be comatose to markedly agitated	Carelessness in grooming
Behavior	On continuum from coma to psychotic and out of control	Dulled behavioral response or mildly atypical behavior
Speech and communication	Incoherence; degree of change based on severity of delerium	Usually slowed because of cognitive deficits
Mood	Labile; anxiety or panic common	Constricted affect or depression
Thinking process	Markedly altered; psychotic at constant or transient intervals (time should be charted)	Mildly altered; decreased intellectual ability
Memory	Partial or full loss of recent memory; remote memory intact	Partial loss of both recent and remote memory
Perception of surroundings	Usually markedly altered	Usually intact or mildly affected
Abstract thinking and social judgment	Markedly decreased	Mildly decreased
Sleep-wakefulness cycle	Disrupted	Not affected significantly
Treatment	Identify and treat underlying cause; symptomatic treatment	Symptomatic treatment
Prognosis	Reversible in most cases	Usually irreversible

Infections
  Encephalitis
  Meningitis
  Abscess in brain
  Systemic septicemia
Nutritional (vitamin) deficiencies
  B_{12}
  Folic acid
  Nicotinic acid
  Thiamine
Drugs
  Alcohol
  Hallucinogens
  Heavy metals
  Other drugs

The 24-hour monitoring of patients by nurses places them in a primary role in the recognition of a developing acute brain syndrome (delerium) or chronic brain syndrome (dementia). Many acute brain syndromes are reversible before they reach a delerium state. Reversal, however, depends on astute nursing assessment so that medical care givers are alerted and a change in medical regimen can treat the underlying cause. Often the symptoms of a developing OBS are overlooked by nursing and medical care givers. Severe levels of stress can be experienced by patients, families, and staff members when OBS reaches the delerium or dementia stage. The symptoms of the two types of OBS are give in Table 1 (Kaplan and Saddock, 1981; Langsley, 1979; Lipowski, 1979; Lishman, 1978; Solomon and Patch, 1974).

Utilization of nursing diagnosis requires that the nurse correctly identify the various etiologies of specific diagnoses to plan successful interventions. Although OBS requires medical intervention to diagnose and treat the underlying cause, without recognition by the nurse that the identified nursing problem(s) are a possible outcome of an undiagnosed OBS, the nursing process will be consistently frustrated because of incomplete assessment data.

REFERENCES

Goldberg, R.: Strategies in psychiatry for the primary care physician, Darien, Conn., 1980, Patient Care Publications, Inc.

Kaplan, H., and Saddock, B.: Modern synopsis comprehensive psychiatry/III, ed. 3, Baltimore, 1981, The Williams and Wilkins, Co.

Langsley, D.: The mental status examination. In Lewis, J., and Usdin, G., eds.: Psychiatry in general medical practice, New York, 1979, McGraw-Hill Book Co.

Lipowski, Z.: Delerium: acute brain failure in man, Springfield, Ill., 1979, Charles C Thomas, Publisher.

Lishman, W.: Organic psychiatry: the psychological consequences of cerebral disorder, Oxford, Eng., 1978, Blackwell Scientific Publications.

Solomon, P., and Patch, V.: Handbook of psychiatry, Los Altos, Calif. 1974, Lange Medical Publications.

Nursing diagnosis in the community: case management for the homebound elderly

WANDA B. RUTHVEN R.N., c., P.H.N., M.S.

The need to state the case for quality care through records has been addressed by several community health nurses and others through the years (Bonkowsky, 1972; Bower, 1982; Yura and Walsh, 1978). Concerned nurses are giving a great deal of thought to refining a communication tool using nursing diagnosis to provide clear written expressions of the needs and care events involving their patients. The goal of their work is to devise a method that is clear to each nurse, each physician, and each layperson (Campbell, 1978). According to the ANA (1973), records should be accurate, concise, and retrievable. Accuracy has been an area about which nurses agree; however, deciding on the best ways to make the nursing record concise and retrievable is another matter. Nurses as a group believe that recording (usually their own) demonstrates the uniqueness of nursing without sacrificing clarity. To others on the health care team, the average nursing record is not clear but often too lengthy and illegible, not always pertinent to the situation, and repetitious. Recording, undeniably, is a very personal matter, falling somewhere between religion and politics in its sensitivity rating. Yet an understandable, universal method is needed that allows common sense and technical expertise to coexist.

Bargaining teams from nursing organizations and individual nurses working in the private sector are concentrating their efforts toward equal pay for equal work in the health marketplace (Comparable worth, 1982). In some cases they are sacrificing their salaries and their time to bring about not just comparable worth but also lower care costs, better nurse-patient ratios, and more adequate health care settings. These are worthy goals, but it seems unrealistic, in one sense, to believe that such goals will be realized without an understandable and accessible record in the health care setting that can prove the worth of the nurse. It is not logical that patients paying such high costs for health care should take the nurses' views on faith and not have the right to know that care plans will be developed. It is the patient's right to know that documenting appropriate information in the record will communicate to the physician and to other staff his or her needs, plans for care, and evaluation procedures.

In the ideal health care situation, all nurses would use the vernacular of nursing diagnosis to identify problems that nurses can treat. Recording would be concise and logical and include a care plan. The nurse would most likely use Weed's SOAP structured format (1968) to plan and include the subjective, objective, and assessment components for better organization. A checklist would be used after a record is closed or a patient is discharged to ensure that the problems treated, their assessments, and their outcomes are individually entered, along with an evaluation of care goals specifying whether or not these problems were met. Each nurse would maintain current records and would participate in ongoing in-service programs to teach as well as to learn the refinements of record keeping. Nurses would be willing to be audited and at the same time be using continuous self-evaluation through the feedback system inherent in the problem-oriented medical record (POMR) (Weed, 1968).

The need for a recording system that is understandable to professionals and others and that offers quality control is recognized. Such a method would provide a means for communicating with physicians, nursing peers, and others. It would offer nurses ways to refine their skills and evaluate themselves in the process. The information gained could provide data for the improvement of care and for future health planning. This type of recording is also adaptable to the community health setting.

PURPOSE

The purpose of this paper is to describe a recording method that integrates nursing diagnosis and problem-oriented medical recording into a case management service program for the homebound elderly client.

DEFINITIONS

Terms used in this paper are defined as follows:

Case management: A coordinating and problem-solving function designed to ensure continuity of care and overcome system rigidity, misutilization, and inaccessibility. Case managers have the primary function for ensuring that the five case management activities are carried out: assessment, planning, linking, monitoring, and advocacy (Joint Commission, 1978).

Homebound elderly: A person over 60 years of age, unable to perform the activities of daily living without assistance, and cannot leave home or leaves home with difficulty.

Nursing diagnosis: An existing or potential health problem that nurses are qualified and licensed to treat (Price, 1980).

POMR: A record that consists of the identified data base, the complete problem list, the initial plans, and the progress notes.

Traditional record: A narrative type of recording format seen as informative but exhaustive in nature, is often too long and repetitious, has goals that are not stipulated, and has plans that are difficult to find.

THE POMR IN CASE MANAGEMENT

The POMR concept was introduced into the recording system of my health department–directed case management program. It used a brief, goal-oriented approach (Figure 1). Based on a modified form of Weed's method (1968), it was organized to encompass the components of the POMR and contained the following checklists and tools for scrutinizing the homebound elderly client's health status (Boxes 1 to 3):

1. Assessment: A multi-page form designed to evaluate all areas of health, that is, physical, social, and psychologic.
2. Risk categories: Items used to determine priorities of problems.
3. Nursing diagnoses: Items used to identify problems a nurse can treat.
4. Progress notes: The main body of the record.
5. Plan/worksheet: Form used for planning care and its outcomes.

Numerous weaknesses were found in the use of this model: (1) the completed records and the recording instructions were not easy to follow by non-nursing personnel such as physicians, social workers, and ancillary staff; (2) staff members had difficulty understanding the rationale behind the method when they did learn it; and (3) the method was not universal. Therefore a second model was developed and implemented in an effort to increase utility and understanding of record keeping in a case management work setting (Figure 2). *Text continued on p. 452.*

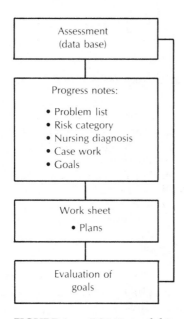

FIGURE 1   POMR model I.

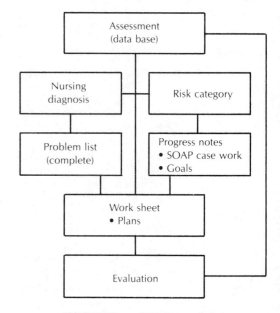

FIGURE 2   POMR model II.

BOX 1   **Assessment: health/medical**

Client: _____ Age: _____ Date of interview: _____
            name

Information to be provided by client/reliable source. Listed below are a
review of medical care, health history, review of systems, and some chronic
diseases/problems. If the client suffers from any of these diseases/problems,
please enter YES or NO in the space provided.

I. Chronic diseases/problems common to the elderly person:

	Yes or No	Handicapping	Not handicapping
A. Arthritis			
B. Diabetes			
C. Pulmonary			
1. Emphysema			
2. Chronic bronchitis			
3. Chronic cough			
4. Shortness of breath			
D. Cardiovascular			
1. Heart problem			
2. High blood pressure			
3. History of stroke			
E. Circulation/ extremities			
1. Leg pain with exercise			
2. Edema			
3. Leg ulcers			
4. Chronic phlebitis			
5. Varicose veins			
6. Arteriosclerosis			
F. Gastrointestinal			
1. Diverticulosis			
2. Hiatical hernia			
3. Constipation			
4. Acid stomach			
5. Other			

Continued.

BOX 1   **Assessment: health/medical—cont'd**

G. Eye
  1. Blindness
  2. Glaucoma
  3. Cataracts
  4. Retinal disease
  5. Other
H. Ear
  1. Deafness
  2. Nerve damage
  3. Other
I. Neurologic
  1. Dizziness
  2. Numbness
  3. Paralysis
  4. Parkinsonism
     (tremors)

J. Endocrine system
   (e.g., thyroid)

K. Cancer

L. Genitourinary
   system
  1. Incontinence
  2. Other
M. Musculoskeletal
   system
  1. Osteoporosis
  2. Nonunion of
     fracture
  3. Podiatry
N. Miscellaneous
   problems
  1. Dental
  2. Chronic pain
  3. Severe itching/
     burning
  4. Allergies
  5. Medication
     problem
  6. Poor nutrition
  7. Abuse/neglect
  8. Other

BOX 1   **Assessment: health/medical—cont'd**

Assessment: other problems affecting health

II. Functional
     1. Activities of living (ADL)
     2. Personal/ environmental safety

III. Financial problems

IV. Social resource problems

V. Psychosocial problems

VI. Medications
     Please list below all the medications the client is presently taking. Include over-the-counter medicines also:

Date filled	Rx physician	Medication/instructions/dose	Reason medication/Rx'd	Side effect to report to MD

VII. Allergies

Foods	Medication

VIII. Review of medical care
     Please enter date of last examination and physician's name in the space provided:
     a. GP/internist_____   e. Eye_____
     b. Skin_____   f. Podiatrist_____
     c. Dentist_____   g. Other_____
     d. Ear_____   h. Other_____

☐ Consent given (verbal) to contact physician

☐ Consent *signed* for release of medical information from physician/other

BOX 2   **Priority setting by risk category definitions**

At risk: emergency category

1. Abuse, neglect
2. Frequent falls, cause unknown: dizziness, blackouts, etc.
3. Client is disabled and care system collapses
4. Medication crisis (includes alcohol):
    a. Overdose: prescribed, accidental, or other
    b. Adverse drug reaction (compliant)
    c. Noncompliant drug reaction (e.g., stopped taking)
5. Suicide attempt/threat
6. Sudden physical collapse, disease
7. Sudden collapse, mental health problem
8. Client is newly bedfast more than 80% of the day
9. Client is newly bedfast with skin breakdown
10. Client is refusing to seek medical care in the face of serious injury or disease
11. Financial crisis:
    a. Risk of robbery/injury
    b. Loss of check, check did not come, bank foul-up, etc.
    c. No money, other reason
12. No food
13. No heat

High-risk: Potentially a life-threatening condition

1. Possible abuse
2. Noncompliant about medical recommendations
3. Sudden reduction in self-care.
4. Severe illness in last year especially with crisis intervention
5. Client takes three medications or more.
6. Possible drug overuse (includes alcohol)
7. Unable to perform the activities of daily living
8. Client suffered severe dizziness or falling in last year
9. Housekeeping has deteriorated (rotting food, etc.)
10. Spends excessive time in bed
11. Possible reduced mental capacity: client may communicate with difficulty, wander and become a nuisance to neighbors, forget things, lose belongings, hallucinate
12. Demonstrates poor nutrition: client may have poor nutrient intake in general, low level or imbalance of potassium, unexplained weight loss, gross obesity

Low-risk: People with the potential for becoming high risk, especially in view of how serious their disabilities are, but who are teachable, motivated toward better health, and act on knowledge acquired.

No-risk: People who are knowledgeable and able to cope with their problems, illnesses, and disabilities; basically seen as well elderly clients.

BOX 3   **Problems/conditions of the elderly that affect health: nursing diagnoses***

Physical health
  Chronic disease supervision, need
    for
  Conservation of energy, need for
  Mobility impaired
  Pain
  Fatigue
  Respiratory dysfunction
  Suffocation, potential for
  Cardiac output, alterations in
  Blood pressure, alterations in
  Fluid volume deficit
  Body fluids, alterations in
  Tissue perfusion, chronic abnormal
  Skin integrity, impairment of
  Digestion, impairment of
  Bowel elimination, alterations in
  Sensory-perceptual, alterations in
  Dentition, alterations in
  Level of consciousness, alterations
    in
  Verbal communication,
    impairment of
  Urinary elimination, impairment
    of
  Sexuality, alterations in
  Weakness, marked signs of
  Podiatry, dysfunctional signs of
  Vital signs, alterations in (specify)
  Sleep-rest pattern, dysrhythm of
  Abuse, possibility of
  Drug-related problem
  Health promotion, need for
  Nutrition, alteration in
Functional health
  Self-care activities, alterations in
  Trauma, potential for
Environment
  Home maintenance impaired
  Environment, inappropriate
  Environment, unsanitary (specify)
  Translocation shock, potential for
Social health
  Income assistance needed
  Social isolation
  Social interactions, need for

Psychosocial health
  Anxiety
  Cognition, dysfunction of
  Confusion/disorientation
  Coping patterns maladaptive,
    (individual)
  Coping, maladaptive family
  Family process inadequate
  Fear
  Fears of the aged: attack, illness,
    abandonment, etc.
  Grieving, acute or chronic
  Knowledge, need for (specify)
  Loneliness
  Manipulation
  Noncompliance (specify)
  Role disturbance
  Self-concept, alterations in
  Altered life-style
  Altered resource availability
  Spirituality, matters of (not just
    religious beliefs)
  Environmental barriers
  Culture, alterations in
  Health advocate, lack of
  Crime
  Poverty
  Housing
  Legislation
  Transportation, dysfunction of
  Demographic factors, alterations
    in: elderly ghettos, indigent
    elderly
  Losses of significance: widowhood,
    self-esteem, memorablia, health,
    etc.

*Some have been adapted from Nursing diagnoses (presenting problems), American Nurses' Association certification in gerontologic nursing practice test specification outline, 1979; Price, 1980.

PROCEDURE

The experiment using the second model of the POMR was conducted on a composite example of a typical elderly male client with a history of numerous health problems who might have been served by our agency. To improve the utility of the record as well as its understanding, two departures from the first model (Fig. 1) were necessary. All the basic tools and checklists were retained but (1) the master problem list was separated from the record, and (2) the progress notes incorporated Weed's developmental SOAP structure—subjective, objective, assessment, and plan.

The progress notes and the master problem list are developed concurrently and sequentially using the second model (Fig. 2) from the multi-page assessment, which identifies client expressed problems; from the list of nursing diagnoses, which identifies problems that a nurse can treat; and from the risk categories, which categorize both of these sets of problems for case work and for emergency status (Boxes 4 and 5). Each active problem is entered both on the master list of problems and on the progress notes as the assessment review progresses from health/medical problems to social and psychologic problems. Each problem assessed as needing immediate intervention is planned for and documented on the master problem list in the active column. Each problem and plan is entered as the nurse reviews the assessment form

---

BOX 4   **Problem list**

Problem	Date of onset	Active problem	Date of onset	Inactive problem
1	1/14/80	Chronic disease supervision, need for		
2			No date	Arthritis
3			No date	Prostate disease
4			4/1/80	Thrombectomy
5	1960	Aphasia: mild; post CVA; verbal communication impaired		
6	4/1/80	Podiatry: arteriosclerotic gangrene L two middle toes; tissue perfusion chronic abnormal		
7	4/1/80	Pain		
8	No date	Deaf, bilateral; sensory-perceptual, alterations in		
9	No date	Multiple medications		
10	No date	Nutrition, alterations in: no food available and no food preparation		

BOX 5   **Progress notes**

Problem	Date	Active problem	Inactive problem
	4/14/80	Client is an 85 y/o male with Hx of aphasia, post CVA, of 20 yr duration; lives with disabled wife in small house; recent episode involving an acute thrombectomy with aftermath of reduced physical and mental function now causing a threat to independent living (client expressed)	
1	4/14/80	Chronic disease supervision, need for	
2	No date		Arthritis
3	No date		Prostate disease
4	4/1/80		Thrombectomy
5	1960	Aphasia: mild, post CVA; verbal communication impaired	
6	4/1/80	Podiatry: arteriosclerotic gangrene, L two middle toes; tissue perfusion, chronic abnormal	
7	4/1/80	Pain	
8	No date	Deaf, bilateral; sensory-perceptual alterations	
9	No date	Multiple medications	
10	No date	Nutrition, alterations in: no food available and no food preparation	
1	4/14/80	*Subjective:* Expresses concern over gangrenous toes; pain; inability to hear; preparation of food; management of finances and other affairs	
		Objective: Observably anxious; stressed; tearful	
		Assessment: Problems 5-10 seen as acute; client "at risk" because of problems and general inability to function, particularly his lack of food	
		Plan: Develop care plan for each acute problem above with counseling goal that client will be able to regroup and subsequently cope with assistance in present situation	
10	4/14/80	*Subjective:* "We need a hot meal"; no food available to client; wife apparently unable to plan or prepare it	
		Objective: Wife confused and uncertain; unable to prepare food	
		Assessment: Adequate nutrition needed for both spouses	
		Plan: Arrange for Meals-on-Wheels via United Fund; will encourage client to assume expense as soon as able; will submit request for sliding scale payment for meals now; assist wife to accept above for self too if possible but definitely for client; coordinate with neighbor (who shops for couple lately) if necessary as wife seems to cue-in on preparing own meal when food is mentioned; attempt education about nutrition as appropriate	
6	4/14/80	Problems: Gangrene L (see above); skin integrity, impairment of; tissue perfusion, chronic abnormal	
		Subjective: Anger; denial that foot is improving	
		Objective: Grief; client tearful and uncomprehending; client cognitively intact, just *very* anxious	
		Assessment: Tissue perfusion drastically reduced; client blocking	
		Plan: Monitoring of part; observe for increased death of tissue, pain, and further reduced circulation; educate about nature of disease, MD recommendations and their bases; offer grief counseling; coordinate with MD, wife, visiting nurse, and supportive special neighbor	

until each one in need of work is completed. Goals are then stated in the record, and the daily case work begins. Subsequent documented case work or service in the form of telephone coordination or direct nursing treatment follows, and the progress of problem-solving activities is entered and dated appropriately.

The worksheet (Box 6), completed concurrently or just after the above portion of the record, is a synopsis of the problem-solving process carried out on behalf of the client. It also shows specific outcomes at the completion of the entire plan and service outcomes at the completion of the entire plan and service process. The worksheet's value is its function as a planning tool, its quick perusal qualities, its summation of care, and the availability of data to study problems and their solutions, care given, and so on.

BOX 6   Worksheet for second model

Problems/needs	Plans	Goals	Time limit	Implemented	Agency	Client	Outcome/response
4-14-80							
#1 Chronic Disease supervision, need for	Review all diseases with client as able: Nature of Disease Pain Medication Safety M.D. care	Maximum health and function	4-20-80	√	A	√	Client understands but still denying outcome will be positive
#10 Nutrition, alteration in	Set up meals (coordinate with wife, neighbor, funding agency) Monitor for adequacy	Adequate nutrient intake	4-14-80 4-14-80 4-14-80	√ √ √	A A A	√ √ √	Meals delivered as ordered Client's nutritional status improved— wt. gain, color and vigor improved
#6 Gangrene, tissue Perfusion Chronically Abnormal	Monitor for change Educate RE: Nature of disease management of pain M.D. recommendations	Restoration of function	4-15-80 4-15-80	√ √	A A	√ √	Visiting nurse cooperating with A; reinforcing teaching/ counseling as is M.D.
	Offer counseling RE: grief Coordinate with wife, visiting nurse	Resolution of grief	4-14-80 4-14-80	√ √	A A	√ √	Not receptive at present but appreciative They understand and are assisting as able

Client's name: <u>John Doe</u>   Risk cat./Date: <u>4-14-80</u> At risk Hi risk Lo risk No risk

RESULTS

The second model had the following strengths:
1. Provides a data base
2. More understandable to professional and others who undertake instruction in its use.
3. More useful because of the above strength
4. Provides validity for methods of care, assistance given, and the amount of time to spend by means of a cross section of the various professionals who work with the same client
5. Organizes data, therefore reducing the overwhelming feeling of professionals when faced with numerous and serious health problems in elderly clients
6. Strengthens nursing service and nursing care plans through better comprehension and utilization of nursing by other disciplines.

The second model had the following weaknesses:
1. As concise as it is, it can still be lengthy.
2. Learning this type of recording, like any other, takes commitment on the part of staff members to use it well.
3. It requires one more step than the first model because of the addition of the SOAP format.

CONCLUSIONS

This single recording experiment did facilitate a more comprehensive record. The problem list gave a quick reference to active problems and to nursing diagnoses. The SOAP format, though it added an extra step to the recording process, provided a more accurate picture of the client's feelings and individual views than the single-entry method. Although the total recording time was increased, the time and detailing needed to complete the worksheet was reduced, which tended to balance the effort expanded.

In general, this different approach to the POMR has clarified needs and increased the nurse's ability to treat the multiple problems of homebound elderly clients. Goals and time limits were more realistically set, which resulted in greater utility and efficiency and allowed more nursing time for creative care.

REFERENCES

American Nurses' Association: Standards of nursing practice, Kansas City; Mo., 1973, The Association.

Bonkowsky, M.L.: Adapting the POMR to community child health care, Nurs. Outlook **20**:515, 1972.

Bower, F.L.: The process of planning nursing care: a theoretical model, ed. 3, St. Louis, 1982, The C.V. Mosby Co.

Campbell, C.: Nursing diagnosis and intervention in nursing practice, New York, 1978, John Wiley & Sons, Inc.

Comparable worth, Calif. Nurs. **77:**1, 1982.

Joint Commission on the Accreditation of Hospitals: Perspectives on accreditation, Chicago, 1978, The Commission.

Nursing diagnoses (presenting problems), American Nurses' Association certification in gerontologic nursing practice test specification outline (1979). In American Nurses' Association: Division of gerontologic nursing practice: guidelines for documentation as a gerontologic nurse, Kansas City, Mo., 1980, The Association.

Price, M.: Nursing diagnosis: making a concept come alive, Am. J. Nurs. **80:**668, 1980.

Weed, L.L.: Questions often asked about the problem-oriented record: does it guarantee quality?, The Modular, Cambridge, Mass., April 1968, Harvard University Press, p. 51.

Yura, H., and Walsh, M.: The nursing process: assessing, planning, implementing, evaluating, ed. 3, New York, 1978, Appleton-Century-Crofts.

Nursing diagnosis: integral to standards of practice

CLAUDIA GAMEL-BENTZEL, R.N., B.S.N., C.C.R.N.

The American Association of Neurosurgical Nurses and the ANA are collaborating to revise the neurologic and neurosurgical standards of practice. The goal of the professional developers is to create standards that can be implemented readily in clinical practice settings through the use of the nursing process. The ANA's definition of nursing (1980, p. 9) serves as the framework for such revision: "the diagnosis and treatment of human responses to actual or potential health problems." Standards are being developed for human responses that are the focus of neurologic and neurosurgical nurses. Such standards incorporate frequently encountered nursing diagnoses and their associated outcome and process statements. This paper discusses the relevancy of standards of practice to nursing diagnosis and the methodology for development of neurologic-neurosurgical outcome-process standards and provides a draft of the standards for consciousness and for communication.

RELEVANCE

National standards of practice are "authoritive statements enunciated and promulgated by the profession by which the quality of practice, service, or education can be judged" (ANA, 1981, p. 1). Three types of standards exist: (1) structure, which focuses on the environment and resources, (2) process, which focuses on the delivery of (nursing) services, and (3) outcome, which focuses on measurable change in the recipient of (nursing) services. Nursing diagnosis and nursing process are fundamental concepts of nursing practice and as such are incorporated into standard statements and measurements of same. In the 1977 Standards of Neurological and Neurosurgical Nursing Practice, nursing diagnosis and nursing process were advocated but not operationalized. It was believed that the revised standards could be operationalized best by (1) naming frequently encountered nursing diagnoses, (2) formulating desired patient or family outcomes, and (3) specifying nursing interventions that engender the outcome.

METHOD

Standards are being developed for human responses that are the focus of neurologic and neurosurgical nurses. Review of those human responses identified by the ANA (1980, p. 10) led to the following list:

Self-care
Cognition
Communication
Consciousness

Elimination
Mobility
Nutrition
Protective mechanisms
Rest and sleep
Sensation
Sexuality
Behavioral manifestations: moving away, moving toward, moving against
Self-perception: body image, self-esteem, self-concept
Coping
Affiliative relationships

A standard statement is written and assessment factors are identified for each of the human responses. Nursing diagnoses are formulated for each standard. The structure of the nursing diagnosis statement includes the nursing observation followed by the defining characteristics. An outcome and process statement is written for each identified nursing diagnosis.

Text continued on p. 462.

Standards of practice for consciousness

Standard	The patient will attain, maintain, or regain his highest level of consciousness The family possesses the knowledge, attitude, and skills to interact with the patient with altered consciousness
Assessment	The nurse assesses, records, and reports the following:

Patient: Glasgow coma score

Pupillary size and reactivity (direct and consensual)

Eye movements

Presence and strength of movement

Brainstem reflexes (swallowing, cough, gag, and corneal)

Family: Perception of consciousness, coma, cognition

Preference for teaching-learning strategies

Readiness for learning

Nursing diagnosis	**Outcome**	**Process**
Inability to control or maintain human responses related to altered consciousness	Until patient regains control of human responses: 1. Elimination patterns are maintained as measured by daily record of fecal and urinary output 2. Nutritional requirements are maintained as measured by daily: intake/output, calorie counts, weights	Provides self-care patient would ordinary perform

Nursing diagnosis	Outcome	Process
	3. Sleep and rest are maintained as measured by daily periods of uninterrupted rest	Manipulates environment to minimize sources of sensory overload
	4. Mobility and skin integrity are maintained as measured by range of movement and absence of decubiti	
	5. Hygiene needs are met as measured by appropriate skin, hair, and mouth care and absence of odors	
	6. Communication and sensory input needs are met as measured by daily auditory, visual, tactile stimulation	
	Family verbalizes that patient has been cared for with respect for privacy and individuality	Controls environment to ensure privacy during patient interventions
		Uses patient's preferred name
Altered consciousness: coma as defined by no eye opening to any stimuli	Patient is involved in program of sensory stimulation	Coordinates program that includes tactile, gustatory, olfactory, visual, and auditory stimuli
High risk for death related to coma	Family verbalizes that patient experienced a dignified death	Supports family members in verbalizing their feelings
Change in pattern of family interaction with patient related to altered consciousness	Family participates in patient's care	Identifies verbal and nonverbal cues of desire to interact with and care for patient
		Supports and teaches family to care for patient
Lack of knowledge (family) of altered consciousness	Family distinguishes between:	Teaches meaning of the following behavioral responses:
	1. Comatose patient (who does not open eyes)	1. Eye opening
	2. Awake patient (who opens eyes)	2. Movement
	3. Aware patient (who opens eyes and follows commands)	3. Following commands
		4. Speech
		Teaches definition of terms and relates to behavioral responses
High risk for increased intracranial pressure or hernia-	Patient's consciousness is maintained at base level or improves	Assess, record, and report consciousness, specifically deterioration

Continued.

Standards of practice for consciousness—cont'd

Nursing diagnosis	Outcome	Process
tion syndrome related to altered consciousness		Avoid or minimize increased intracranial pressure by: 1. Controlling environmental stimuli 2. Positioning to avoid obstruction of brain vascular outflow 3. Implementing measures to prevent increased intrathoracic pressure 4. Maintaining normothermia 5. When ordered, restricting fluids and free water

Standards of practice for communication

Standard The patient will attain, maintain, or regain his maximum communication ability

The patient and family possess the knowledge, attitude, and skills to acknowledge the communication disability and to promote communication ability

Assessment The nurse assesses, records, and reports the following:

1. Ability to recognize and interpret spoken language
2. Ability to recognize and interpret written language
3. Ability to repeat
4. Ability to name
5. Ability to produce spontaneous speech
6. Mass, tone, and strength of face, arm, and hand musculature
7. Motor coordination of speech structures, arms, and hands
8. Presence of auditory agnosias or auditory neglect syndrome
9. Presence of speech apraxia or apraxia involving the arm and hand

Nursing diagnoses	Outcome	Process
Impaired verbal communication as defined by altered ability to: 1. Repeat 2. Name 3. Produce spontaneous speech	Patient begins to establish a method of communication Patient initiates and participates in communication with others	Anticipate patient needs until effective method of communication is developed For impaired verbal or written communication; collaborate with speech therapist to introduce patient to assistive devices such as:

Standards of practice for communication—cont'd

Nursing diagnoses	Outcome	Process
Impaired written communication as defined by altered ability to write with pen or pencil		1. Eye blinks 2. Communication board 3. Word printers 4. Hand gestures 5. Sign language
Impaired written language comprehension related to altered vision and inability to follow commands Impaired spoken language comprehension related to altered hearing	For impaired written or spoken language comprehension, collaborate with speech therapist to develop method of comprehension 1. Pictures 2. Words 3. Gestures	
Lack of knowledge (patient and family) of nature of communication disability and measures to promote communication ability	Patient and family state nature of communication disability Patient and family identify measures to maximize communication ability rather than communication disability	Teach nature of communication disability Teach, by role modeling, measures to promote communication ability: 1. Allot daily time and opportunity for practice of communication and use of assistive devices 2. Plan successful experience for conclusion of each practice session 3. Remove and reduce environmental distractions 4. Adjust length of session to complement patient's attention span If consciousness decreases, prepares for any of the following: 1. Administration of medications 2. Hyperventilation 3. Insertion of intracranial monitoring device 4. Withdrawal of cerebrospinal fluid 5. Induction of barbiturate therapy 6. Removal of bone or infarcted brain or mass lesion

SUMMARY

The goal of the professional developers is to create standards that can be implemented readily in clinical practice settings. It is our belief that this goal will be realized by the previously described method of standards development. Neurologic and neurosurgical nurses throughout the United States and Canada are writing and critiquing the proposed standards. The opinions and comments of nurses with a nonneurologic clinical focus are also being sought. The drafts of standards for consciousness and communication are provided for review and comment.

REFERENCES

American Nurses' Association: Nursing: a social policy statement, Kansas City, Mo., 1980, The Association.

American Nurses' Association: Guidelines for development and revision of standards of nursing practice, Kansas City, Mo., 1981, The Association.

Implementation of a nursing diagnosis to increase autonomy and accountability

NAOMI DAVENPORT, R.N., M.N.
MARGARET D. McCOMB, R.N., B.S.

Using nursing diagnosis implies the acceptance of the responsibility to assess and treat problems independently in the scope of nursing practice. This paper reports on a clinical project in which the implementation of a single nursing diagnosis created an organizational expectation that authorized such independent action.

CLINICAL PROBLEM

This project was developed in response to an increase in decubitus ulcers among patients on a long-term care (LTC) ward of a state psychiatric hospital. Of the 32 patients on the ward, 15 had decubitus ulcers. Additional factors considered in developing the project included the following.

Ward population

The primary need of the LTC ward residents is for skilled nursing care. However, the nature and extent of their psychiatric problems precludes placement in nursing homes. Most are elderly and confused, eat poorly, are sedentary or bedridden, and are incontinent.

Staffing

Typical staffing for the ward is:

1. Day: two registered nurses and four psychiatric aides
2. Evening: one registered nurse and four psychiatric aides
3. Night: 0.5 FTE registered nurse and two psychiatric aides

The turnover rate among the aide staff has been high, and the training of the group is focused primarily on psychiatric care. New staff or staff "floated" from other units are often not as attuned to the particular needs of this patient group as are the "regular" ward staff.

Resources

There were significant resources on which to draw. The unit RN staff was stable. The nursing and hospital administration were mobilized by the situation and in support of the project. Both the clinical specialist and the quality assurance nurse were assigned to the project. "Networking" contacts permitted the clinical specialist to draw on the professional wisdom of colleagues in rehabilitation and LTC facilities. The hospital librarian assisted in a literature search.

Existing nursing practice and policy

Nursing autonomy can be seen as the authority to make and act on clinical decisions within the scope of nursing practice. Nursing autonomy and accountability are enhanced when there are explicit or formal expectations of performance in nursing policies and/or standards of practice that include both the responsibility and the authority to make and act on clinical decisions. There were no such explicit, formal expectations of vigilance in identifying the potential for skin breakdown or for initiating the tedious and time-consuming preventive nursing measures. Nor were there significant informal reinforcements (for example, attention and praise).

In addition, psychiatric facilities have moved toward a great emphasis on the "multidisciplinary team" at a time when nursing is placing emphasis on the identification of its own contributions and area of practice. Nursing diagnosis is seen as unnecessary by some, who say the multidisciplinary focus of the DMS-III removes the need for a nursing nomenclature. Yet the failure of nursing to identify and treat a nursing problem with sufficient consistency had led to a significant problem. Since the clinical specialist's focus is one of enhancing nursing practice within the agency, it was decided to use this assignment to address the nursing practice issues as well.

PROJECT OBJECTIVES

The project objectives were to (1) decrease the number of decubitus ulcers among the LTC population and (2) develop a program that would authorize and formalize nursing assessment and identification of the at risk patient as well as authorize an independent nursing treatment response.

METHODOLOGY

The quality assurance nurse developed a data base by investigating the existing situation. The area of specialization of the clinical nurse specialist was psychiatric/mental health nursing, so professional colleagues were contacted for assistance and consultation. They and the literature search reaffirmed our suspicion that no substitute had been developed for the early identification of patients liable to develop decubitus ulcers and for the institution of appropriate preventive measures (Berencek, 1975; Horsley, 1981; Norton, McLaren, and Exton-Smith, 1962). Scrupulous attention to the nursing component supersedes any other treatment and/or product.

The rehabilitation unit at Emanuel Hospital in Portland, Oregon, was using an assessment form adapted from Norton, McLaren, and Exton-Smith (1962). In this assessment the high-risk patient received a higher rather than a lower score, as in the Norton scale. This scale seemed helpful and was further modified. The mental status categories seemed out of order conceptually ("confused" rated a higher score than "apathetic") and were not consistent with clinical observations of our patients, so they were revised. More direction and clarification were added to the form, which was then pretested by several nurses. Of special concern was interrater reliability and the predictive validity of the tool. In response to staff feedback, another item was added in the mental status column to provide a full range of choices. A page of definitions was prepared to train raters and to have available on the ward for clarification. The nursing diagnosis, *potential for impaired skin integrity*, was introduced because the potential for the development of a decubitus ulcer is something nurses diagnose and treat (Box 1).

A protocol for a preventive treatment regimen was developed. If a nurse assesses that a patient is at high risk, the preventive treatment is initiated. The nurse then signs and dates a protocol form and places it in the medical record, making the implementation of the nursing treatment a formal pro-

---

BOX 1 **Nursing assessment tool: potential for impaired skin integrity**

Dammasch State Hospital
Nursing assessment tool: potential impaired skin integrity

A General* condition	B Mental state	C Activity	D Mobility	E Incontinence
__0 Good	__0 Alert	__0 Ambulates	__0 Full	__0 Continent
__1 Fair	__1 Confused	__1 Walks with help	__1 Slightly limited	__1 Occasional (urine or stool)
__2 Poor	__2 Apathetic	__2 Chair-fast	__2 Moderately to very limited	__2 Usually (urine or stool)
__3 Bad	__3 Stuporous	__3 In bed all day	__3 Immobile	__3 Incontinent of both urine and stool
	__4 Comatose			
_____Score	_____Score	_____Score	_____Score	_____Score

_____Total score†

Patient at high risk for skin impairment?   Yes_____
                                             No_____

_____/_____
R.N. Signature   Date

*This rating takes into account the patient's general state of health, especially hydration and nutrition and impaired peripheral circulation as indicated by color, temperature, and pulses.
†Total score of 5 or more mandates the nursing diagnosis *high risk for impaired skin integrity*.

Adapted from Nursing Standards, Emanual Hospital, Portland, Ore.

TABLE 1   **Percentage of occurrence of decubitus ulcers**

	Before implementation (N = 32)*	Nine months after implementation (N = 30)*	Twelve months after implementation (N = 22)*
LTC patients with decubitus ulcers	47	7	0
LTC patients without decubitus ulcers	53	93	100

*N = Actual ward census at the time surveyed and therefore differs with each survey.

cess. Related policies and procedures were developed by the clinical specialist and the quality assurance nurse as part of the project. All patients on the LTC ward are assessed for the potential for impaired skin integrity. Because the base rate is so low in the rest of the general psychiatric setting, other patients are assessed only if the nurse assesses problems of incontinence and/or immobility.

Evaluation consists of ongoing weekly data collection (number of patients at high risk, number of patients with decubitus ulcers, number of patients admitted with decubitus ulcers, number of patients developing decubitus ulcers *not* assessed as high risk). These data are summarized periodically by the quality assurance nurse. An audit of compliance with the new procedures was also done by this nurse.

RESULTS

Over half the patients on the LTC ward have been assessed at high risk, using the nursing assessment tool for *potential for impaired skin integrity* (60% and 59% at 9 and 12 months postimplementation, respectively). Before implementation, 47% of the patients had decubitus ulcers. This number decreased to 7% in 9 months and to 0% 12 months after implementation (Table 1).

In addition, the organizational changes (policies, procedures, and evaluation) created the formal expectation and reinforcement for independent nursing actions in the asssessment and treatment of the potential for impaired skin integrity (Table 2).

DISCUSSION

Norton, McLaren, and Exton-Smith (1962) suggest that some patients are at risk only at certain times, usually at night. This group will not be scored at high risk and, as such, presents a predictive liability with this assessment. The 9- and 12-month audits revealed that staff nurses had corrected for this deficit by overrating such patients, thus using their clinical judgment ("I don't care what the rating says, this patient *is* at high risk") to compensate for the form's deficiency. What we lost in predictive validity, we have gained

TABLE 2   Organizational issues before and after implementation

Issue	Before implementation	After implementation
Accountability	Informal expectation of nursing responsibility to institute preventive measures	Formal expectation that nursing will assess need and institute preventive measures
	No nursing policy/procedures regarding assessment of at risk population	Explicit in policy statement that "nursing staff are expected to assess the potential for impaired skin integrity using a standardized assessment tool
	No distinct nursing policy regarding preventive measures	Nursing policy/procedure for implementing preventive measures
	No routine audit	Ongoing data collection summarized at intervals; chart and Kardex audits done by quality assurance nurse
Autonomy	No formal or informal authority or reinforcement for independent action	Policies/procedures give nurses authority to act independently within scope of practice

in autonomous nursing practice. However, refinement of the form may be indicated.

The use of this form with long-term psychiatric patients has not been previously reported. It is hoped that a center with a larger population will undertake more comprehensive validity testing, revising the form, if indicated. At this time the LTC nursing staff has not had any patients develop decubitus ulcers who are not assessed at high risk.

The initial policy for the agency does not require periodic reassessment, so patients whose condition changes subtly may move into high risk status without detection. Ideally, patients should be assessed at regular intervals and whenever their condition changes. The frequency of reassessment may vary with the setting.

REFERENCES

Berencek, K.H.: Treatment of decubitus ulcers Nurs. Clin. North Am. **10:**171, 1975.

Horsley, J.: Preventing decubitus ulcers: CURN project, New York, 1981, Grune & Stratton, Inc.

Norton, D., McLaren, R., and Exton-Smith, A.N.: Pressure sores. In Norton, D., et al., eds.: An investigation of geriatric nursing problems in hospitals, London, 1962, The National Corporation for the Care of Old People.

ADDITIONAL READING

Exton-Smith, A.N., and Sherwin, R.W.: The prevention of pressure sores: significance of spontaneous bodily movements, Lancet **2:**1124, 1961.

CHAPTER 6

Approved nursing diagnoses and small group work on diagnostic labels

This chapter is organized in four sections. The first section presents the listing of those nursing diagnosis labels that have been approved by the National Conferences to date. Only those eight new nursing diagnoses approved at the Fifth National Conference give etiology and defining characteristics. The *Pocket Guide to Nursing Diagnoses,* which accompanies this *Proceedings,* includes the etiologies and defining characteristics of previously approved nursing diagnoses. The second section includes the report of small group work on diagnostic labels. The process, tasks completed, and output are self-explanatory. Needless to say, the work of the groups played the major role in providing the list of nursing diagnoses for the Task Force members to approve. The third section includes a list of the defining characteristics associated with patterns of unitary man/human. The defining characteristics are listed under each nursing diagnosis whenever the relationships were said to exist by the small groups. The fourth section presents issues, researchable questions, and references for approved nursing diagnoses.

Perhaps this chapter reflects the nature of this conference most vividly, since one major emphasis has been to use the research data base in making decisions about the fate of any nursing diagnosis. The majority of participants were asked to examine the current nursing diagnoses, to generate issues and researchable questions, and to provide references for each nursing diagnosis. Specific suggestions as to the etiologies or defining characteristics were incorporated into the new diagnoses in the *Pocket Guide* whenever appropriate. Some suggestions that needed further clarification remained as issues. A small number of participants who suggested new nursing diagnoses formed a group to examine the content and the format in the usual manner.

Questions raised for each diagnosis need to be addressed in terms of philosophic, theoretic, clinical, and research perspectives. Our commitment to generation of nursing knowledge by the study of nursing diagnoses has been simply reaffirmed by this effort and the direction the conference took.

Section I   **Approved nursing diagnoses**

List of new approved nursing diagnoses

Activity intolerance*
Activity intolerance, potential*
Airway clearance, ineffective
Anxiety*
Bowel elimination, alteration in: constipation
Bowel elimination, alteration in: diarrhea
Bowel elimination, alteration in: incontinence
Breathing pattern, ineffective
Cardiac output, alteration in: decreased
Comfort, alteration in: pain
Communication, impaired: verbal
Coping, family: potential for growth
Coping, ineffective family: compromised
Coping, ineffective family: disabling
Coping, ineffective individual
Diversional activity, deficit
Family process, alteration in*† (formerly Family dynamics)
Fear
Fluid volume alteration in: excess*†
Fluid volume deficit, actual
Fluid volume deficit, potential
Gas exchange, impaired
Grieving, anticipatory
Grieving, dysfunctional
Health maintenance, alteration in*
Home maintenance management, impaired
Injury, potential for: (poisoning, potential for; suffocation, potential for;
    trauma, potential for)
Knowledge deficit (specify)
Mobility, impaired physical
Noncompliance (specify)

Etiology and defining characteristics of nursing diagnoses are listed in the *Pocket Guide,* which is a companion to this *Proceedings.*
*Addition from 1982 conference.
†Moved from TBD list.

Nutrition, alteration in: less than body requirements
Nutrition, alteration in: more than body requirements
Nutrition, alteration in: potential for more than body requirements
Oral mucous membrane, alteration in*
Parenting, alteration in: actual
Parenting, alteration in: potential
Powerlessness*
Rape trauma syndrome
Self-care deficit: feeding, bathing/hygiene, dressing/grooming, toileting
Self-concept, disturbance in: body image, self-esteem, role performance, personal identity
Sensory-perceptual alteration: visual, auditory, kinesthetic, gustatory, tactile, olfactory
Sexual dysfunction
Skin integrity, impairment of: actual
Skin integrity, impairment of: potential
Sleep pattern disturbance
Social Isolation*†
Spiritual distress (distress of the human spirit)
Thought processes, alteration in
Tissue perfusion, alteration in: cerebral, cardiopulmonary, renal, gastrointestinal, peripheral
Urinary elimination, alteration in patterns
Violence, potential for: self-directed or directed at others

---

*Addition from 1982 conference.
†Moved from TBD list.

New diagnoses accepted for clinical testing at the Fifth National Conference

ACTIVITY INTOLERANCE

Etiology

Bed rest/immobility
Generalized weakness
Sedentary life-style
Imbalance between oxygen supply/demand

Defining characteristics

Verbal report of fatigue or weakness*
Abnormal heart rate or blood pressure response to activity
Exertional discomfort of dyspnea
Electrocardiographic changes reflecting arrhythmias or ischemia

ACTIVITY INTOLERANCE, POTENTIAL

Etiology

To be developed
Defining characteristics
History of previous intolerance
Deconditioned status
Presence of circulatory/respiratory problem
Inexperience with the activity

ANXIETY

Definition

A vague, uneasy feeling the source of which is often nonspecific or unknown to the individual.

Etiology

Unconscious conflict about essential values/goals of life
Threat to self-concept
Threat of death
Threat to or change in health status
Threat to or change in socioeconomic status
Threat to or change in role functioning
Threat to or change in environment
Threat to or change in interaction patterns
Situational/maturational crises
Interpersonal transmission/contagion
Unmet needs

---

*Critical defining characteristic.

Defining characteristics

Subjective

Increased tension

Apprehension

Painful and persistent increased helplessness

Uncertainty

Fearful

Scared

Regretful

Overexcited

Rattled

Distressed

Jittery

Feelings of inadequacy

Shakiness

Fear of unspecific consequences

Expressed concerns re: change in life events

Worried

Anxious

Objective

Sympathetic stimulation—cardiovascular excitation, superficial vasoconstriction, pupil dilation*

Restlessness

Insomnia

Glancing about

Poor eye contact

Trembling/hand tremors

Extraneous movement (foot shuffling, hand/arm movements)

Facial tension

Voice quivering

Focus "self"

Increased wariness

Increased perspiration

FAMILY PROCESS, ALTERATION IN

Etiology

Situation transition and/or crisis

Development transition and/or crisis

Defining characteristics

Family system unable to meet physical needs for its members

Family system unable to meet emotional needs of its members

Family system unable to meet spiritual needs of its members

Parents do not demonstrate respect for each other's views on child-rearing practices

Inability to express/accept wide range of feelings

Inability to express/accept feelings of members

Family unable to meet security needs of its members

Inability of family members to relate to each other for mutual growth and maturation

---

*Critical defining characteristic.

Family uninvolved in community activities
Inability to accept/receive help appropriately
Rigidity in function and roles
Family does not demonstrate respect for individuality and autonomy of its members
Family inability to adapt to change/deal with traumatic experience constructively
Family fails to accomplish current/past developmental task
Unhealthy family decision-making process
Failure to send and receive clear messages
Inappropriate boundary maintenance
Inappropriate/poorly communicated family rules, rituals, symbols
Unexamined family myths
Inappropriate level and direction of energy

FLUID VOLUME, ALTERATION IN: EXCESS

Etiology

Compromised regulatory mechanism
Excess fluid intake
Excess sodium intake

Defining characteristics

Edema
Effusion
Anasarca
Weight gain
Shortness of breath, orthopnea
Intake greater than output
S_3 heart sound
Pulmonary congestion: chest x-ray examination
Abnormal breath sounds: crackles (rales)
Change in respiratory pattern
Change in mental status
Decreased hemoglobin and hematocrit
Blood pressure changes
Central venous pressure changes
Pulmonary artery pressure changes
Jugular vein distention
Positive hepatojugular reflex
Oliguria
Specific gravity changes
Azotemia
Altered electrolytes
Restlessness and anxiety

HEALTH MAINTENANCE, ALTERATION IN

Definition

Inability to identify, manage, and/or seek out help to maintain health.

Etiology

Lack of, or significant alteration in, communication skills (written, verbal and/or gestural)

Lack of ability to make deliberate and thoughtful judgments

Perceptual/cognitive impairment

Complete/partial lack of gross and/or fine motor skills

Ineffective individual coping

Dysfunctional grieving

Unachieved developmental tasks

Ineffective family coping: disabling spiritual distress

Lack of material resources

Defining characteristics

Demonstrated lack of knowledge regarding basic health practices

Demonstrated lack of adaptive behaviors to internal/external environmental changes

Reported or observed inability to take responsibility for meeting basic health practices in any or all functional pattern areas

History of lack of health-seeking behavior

Expressed client interest in improving health behaviors

Reported or observed lack of equipment, financial, and/or other resources

Reported or observed impairment of personal support system

ORAL MUCOUS MEMBRANE, ALTERATION IN

Etiology

Pathologic conditions—oral cavity radiation to head and/or neck

Dehydration

Trauma

Chemical, e.g. acidic foods, drugs, noxious agents, alcohol

Mechanical, e.g. ill-fitting dentures, braces, tubes endotracheal/nasogastric, surgery of oral cavity

NPO—greater than 24 hours

Ineffective oral hygiene

Mouth breathing

Malnutrition

Infections

Lack of or decreased salivation

Medication

Defining characteristics

Oral pain/discomfort

Coated tongue

Xerostomia (dry mouth)

Stomatitis

Oral lesions or ulcers

Lack of or decreased salivation
Leukoplakia
Edema
Hyperemia
Oral plaque
Desquamation
Vesicles
Hemorrhagic gingivitis
Carious teeth
Halitosis

POWERLESSNESS

Definition

The perception of the individual that one's own action will not significantly affect an outcome. Powerlessness is a perceived lack of control over a current situation or immediate happening.

Etiology

Health care environment
Interpersonal interaction
Illness-related regimen
Life-style of helplessness

Defining characteristics

Severe
Verbal expressions of having no control or influence over situation
Verbal expressions of having no control or influence over outcome
Verbal expressions of having no control over self-care
Depression over physical deterioration that occurs despite patient compliance with regimens
Apathy
Moderate
Nonparticipation in care or decision making when opportunities are provided
Expressions of dissatisfaction and frustration over inability to perform previous tasks and/or activities
Does not monitor progress
Expression of doubt regarding role performance
Reluctance to express true feelings fearing alienation from care givers
Passivity
Inability to seek information regarding care
Dependence on others that may result in irritability, resentment, anger, and guilt
Does not defend self-care practices when challenged
Low-passivity
Expressions of uncertainty about fluctuating energy levels

SOCIAL ISOLATION

Definition

Condition of aloneness experienced by the individual and perceived as imposed by others and as a negative or threatened state.

Etiology

Factors contributing to the absence of satisfying personal relationships, e.g.,

Delay in accomplishing developmental tasks
Immature interests
Alterations in physical appearance
Alterations in mental status
Unaccepted social behavior
Unaccepted social values
Altered state of wellness
Inadequate personal resources
Inability to engage in satisfying personal relationships

Defining characteristics

Objective

Absence of supportive significant other/s: family, friends, group
Sad, dull affect
Inappropriate or immature interests/activities for developmental age/stage
Uncommunicative, withdrawn, no eye contact
Preoccupation with own thoughts, repetitive, meaningless actions
Projects hostility in voice, behavior
Seeks to be alone or exists in a subculture
Evidence of physical/mental handicap or altered state of wellness
Shows behavior unaccepted by dominant cultural group

Subjective

Expresses feelings of aloneness imposed by others
Expresses feelings of rejection
Experiences feelings of difference from others
Inadequacy in or absence of significant purpose in life
Inability to meet expectations of others
Insecurity in public
Expresses values acceptable to the subculture but unable to accept values of the dominant culture.
Expresses interests inappropriate to the developmental age/stage

Small group work on diagnostic labels

Report of the small group work on diagnostic labels
KRISTINE M. GEBBIE, R.N., M.N.

Participants in these national conferences, have come to expect that at least a portion of their time will be devoted to discussion and decision making in small group settings; the Fifth National Conference was no exception. The historic basis for the inclusion of small group work is supported by the following rationale: In a working conference of 100 or more nurses, work groups of less than the whole are needed to give each participant a fair chance to have direct involvement in discussions and decisions. The participants of the First National Conference were assigned to 10 groups that were heterogeneous as to specialty, level of preparation, and work role. Each group was asked to consider a human system (such as cardiovascular) in its broadest possible perspective and generate any possible diagnostic labels. From that rough begining, the process has become more precise and group products more sophisticated.

At the first three national conferences, the small groups generated ideas. The conferences as a whole were decision-making bodies determining whether or not a given diagnostic label would be included on the published list of accepted diagnostic labels. At the Fourth and Fifth National Conferences, the small groups generated ideas and made recommendations, but the conferences as a whole had no role in decision making regarding specific diagnoses. The Task Force, which has provided interconference structure to the diagnostic development process, has reserved the right to review the recommendations of small groups and further edit the number of diagnoses to be published. The review was based on whether or not the following criteria were met: (1) the diagnosis was clearly expressed; (2) the existence of the phenomenon was adequately supported with statements of etiology, defining characteristics, and scientific references; (3) the diagnosis could be influenced by nursing; and (4) the diagnosis was useful to the practitioner or the scholar. Diagnoses recommended by small groups that were not approved by the Task Force have been mentioned in this text and earlier ones to acknowledge the work done and to encourage further work by interested nurses. In some cases, the small group made the direct recommendation that a label be considered "to be diagnosed" (TBD) for similar reasons.

The list of accepted diagnostic labels from the preceding national conference provided the basis for small group assignments at the last three national conferences. In the process of registering as a participant, nurses were given a list of the diagnostic labels, grouped by apparent similarity or relatedness, and asked to express a preference. With few exceptions, participants were assigned to a first or second choice grouping, which in most instances was directly related to the participants' clinical specialization, patient case load, or teaching/research area. Awareness of assignments in advance of actual arrival at the conference was intended to encourage participants to review literature and personal materials and to bring needed materials to the conference so that the discussions would be above an anecdotal level of discussion or debate. Although the less formal level may have been fruitful at the outset of the process, it was no longer consistent with the profession's need for disciplined and scholarly progress.

To facilitate discussion in each small group and to free participants from the burden of taking notes during the discussions each group was assigned a group leader and a group recorder. The individuals were recruited from several sources: faculty from St. Louis University and other schools of nursing, graduate students from St. Louis University and elsewhere, practicing nurses who had previously been a leader or recorder while a faculty member or student, and colleagues of individuals active in the national group who wished to participate in some way in furthering the conference. The names of these individuals are listed in Appendix F. Special credit must be given to Mary Woods, R.N., M.S., of St. Louis University who handled the work of recruiting these individuals and organizing the diagnoses into workable clusters.

A major difference in small group work at this Fifth National Conference was the invitation to nurses to submit research and clinical papers about specific diagnoses, either existing or proposed, for consideration. The submitted papers appear elsewhere in this publication and deserve careful attention because they added to the scholarly nature of the conference. Each was the product of advance work, in some cases involved extensive research, and provided careful documentation of source material. Participants were thus challenged in discussion within each topical area. Work to date has not been equally distributed among the diagnostic labels, however, so that some groups heard more than one submitted paper, and others, none. This variation had an effect on the time available for subsequent discussion, and in some cases, on the sophistication with which a given small group handled its work. That variability will probably never be entirely eliminated, although it should become more balanced.

Group leaders and conference participants were instructed in three main tasks for small group work:

1. Hear and critique any paper presented. If the paper contains a proposal

for a new diagnosis, consider the diagnosis and reach a decision about recommending that label to the Task Force for inclusion in the regular listing, or on the TBD list.

2. Consider all previously listed diagnoses assigned to the group and generate researchable questions and issues deserving further consideration by individual nurses or by subsequent conferences. Although the group might raise the question of removing a listed diagnosis or moving it to the TBD list, the Task Force would make no such decision but would publish the complete list of issues, suggestions, and researchable questions along with the diagnosis as previously listed. The publication of this list provides continuity for practitioners, especially those working with automated record systems programmed around the work from the Fourth National Conference while making the full range of considered possibilities readily available to practitioners, students, and researchers.

3. Identify any general issues, questions, or recommendations that should be widely considered by any nurse interested in nursing diagnoses. These are included, with little editorial alteration, at the end of this chapter.

After the main tasks of the small groups were outlined, the Nurse Theorist Group requested that the small groups consider the defining characteristics of the established diagnosis in relation to the patterns of unitary man/human presented by the theorists. The interest was multiple: Is it possible for any one defining characteristic to be identified with a single one of the patterns? Will there be consistency in that identification if done by more than one nurse? Can something be learned about the patterns by examining, across multiple diagnoses, the characteristics assigned to a given pattern? The theorists also asked participants to identify any characteristics that fit no pattern or multiple patterns and to identify any additional patterns that might suggest themselves. The raw data of responses to the multiple questions were returned to Sister Callista Roy, chairperson of the Nurse Theorist Group. One item of information is included in the materials on individual diagnostic labels. If a clear majority of participants working on any one diagnosis indicate that a given defining characteristic is associated with one pattern, the pattern name is indicated in parenthesis after the characteristic. This listing is added for the information of the nurse who may be attempting to use the unitary man/human materials in practice or in theoretic consideration about the diagnostic process and for the value it may have in clarifying the relationship between the very abstract work of the theorists and the pragmatic work of the small groups. One small group did not fit the pattern of work as presented thus far. This group attempted to move from the theorists' work and other possible frameworks into a true taxonomy of the diagnostic labels. The work produced by this group is presented in Chapter 2 ("Report of the group work on taxonomies").

A final note is needed about the process of translating notes of a small group recorder into a formal publication. The group recorders were provided with a specific format for submitting new diagnostic labels for consideration. All other information was recorded in narrative notes, often summarized on a daily basis, and reviewed with group leaders. The content has been edited to present *issues, researchable questions* and *references* when available so that they clearly appear with the diagnosis to which they refer. If specific, very little of the exact query or suggestion has been altered, and the reader will quickly identify the wide variation in level of sophistication among the products. This fact does not represent a "better" or "worse" small group, but simply that some diagnoses have been studied more or were of greater interest to the individuals in attendance at the conference. Some diagnoses are better prospects for all nurses to engage in the joint professional task of defining that which we treat in our patients, using our experience but more particularly our scholarly skills. The ideas contained in the issues and questions can provide the basis for generation of research center projects, theses and dissertations, and clinical studies in practice settings. Each student of nursing diagnosis, at whatever stage of professional career, can benefit from consideration of the listings and can contribute to the process of creating a professional diagnostic nomenclature and taxonomy.

Some general issues and questions arose in slightly different form in more than one small group and have been combined here for ease of reading.

1. The diagnostic materials do not deal consistently with individuals, family groups, and community. More community diagnoses must be developed.
2. The language used in diagnoses must have more consistency.
3. The taxonomy of nursing diagnosis is now at several levels of abstraction. Should the list be at one level? If so, at what level?
4. Regarding etiology:
   a. Review and define the characteristics of each known etiology.
   b. The etiologies published thus far are not all inclusive. Additional publications are needed, especially for students and practitioners attempting to use them.
   c. Decide whether or not a label can be used as etiology for another diagnosis.
   d. Does an etiology legally need to suggest intervention by a nurse?
   e. Does an etiology need to be a guide for intervention?
   f. Can we call something an etiology when it is used with a "potential for" diagnosis, since etiology denotes a specific illness or entity? Would "risk factor" be more appropriate?

5. Regarding risk factors:
   a. How many risk factors, on the average, lead to identification of a problem?
   b. Is it possible to separate more clearly defining characteristics from risk factors?
   c. For all diagnoses: Identify individuals who are at high risk; identify methods of making differential diagnoses.
   d. Design categories so that there may be an "absence of risk factors," since that helps define the wellness of the client.
6. Define health problem versus human response.
7. Rejection of proposed new diagnoses was based on a number of reasons including: the material was not submitted according to the guidelines, which left the group without clear information regarding etiology, characteristics, and references; a proposed diagnosis was covered adequately in an existing or new diagnosis; it was a statement of a care plan rather than a diagnosis; or it could not be changed by nursing actions. Examples of proposed diagnoses that were rejected are altered mucous membranes, altered bowel function, care of the child with graft vs. host disease, altered urinary function, and alteration in waste product elimination: bilirubin.
8. Regarding the process:
   a. The collective efforts of nurses using automated data systems must be extended.
   b. More time must be allotted for small group work, with fewer tasks assigned, so that the quality of the work produced can improve.
   c. More small group work should be done on the taxonomy itself.
   d. Continuing efforts should be made to keep all specialties in nursing involved in identifying nursing diagnoses.
   e. Can the nursing researchers involved in nursing diagnosis provide a system to disseminate validated tools for use with nursing diagnoses?
   f. Consider a presentation at the next conference on methods of developing tools or an annotated bibliography of tools.
9. What are the ethical and legal issues related to nursing diagnoses? What is the problem the nurse is solving?
10. Keep reminding all of us that nursing diagnoses are made for the care of the patient by the ordinary practicing nurse: IMPERATIVE!!

Section III **Defining characteristics associated with patterns of unitary man/human***

AIRWAY CLEARANCE, INEFFECTIVE
Defining characteristics
> Abnormal breath sounds (rales [crackles], rhonchi [wheezes])—(exchanging)
> Cyanosis—(exchanging)

BOWEL ELIMINATION, ALTERATION IN: CONSTIPATION
Defining characteristics
> Hard, formed stool—(exchanging)
> Palpable mass—(exchanging)

Other possible defining characteristics
> Abdominal pain—(exchanging)
> Appetite impairment—(exchanging)

BOWEL ELIMINATION, ALTERATION IN: DIARRHEA
Defining characteristics
> Abdominal pain—(perceiving)
> Loose, liquid stools—(exchanging)

BREATHING PATTERN, INEFFECTIVE
Defining characteristics
> Shortness of breath—(exchanging)
> Abnormal arterial blood gas—(exchanging)
> Cyanosis—(exchanging)
> Assumption of three-point position—(moving)
> Use of accessory muscles—(moving)
> Altered chest excursion—(moving)

CARDIAC OUTPUT, ALTERATION IN: DECREASED
Defining characteristics
> Oliguria, anuria—(exchanging)
> Decreased peripheral pulses—(exchanging)
> Cold, clammy skin—(exchanging)
> Restlessness—(moving)

---

*Only those defining characteristics that had relationships identified with patterns of unitary man/human are listed here. For the complete list of nursing diagnoses, etiologies, and defining characteristics, refer to the *Pocket Guide to Nursing Diagnoses*, which is a companion to this *Proceedings*.

Other possible defining characteristics

Shortness of breath—(exchanging)

Frothy sputum—(exchanging)

COMFORT, ALTERATION IN: PAIN

Defining characteristics

Communication (verbal or coded) of pain descriptors—(communicating)

Guarding behavior, protective—(moving)

Narrowed focus (altered time perception, withdrawal from social contact, impaired thought process)—(perceiving)

Alteration in muscle tone (may span from listless to rigid)—(moving)

COMMUNICATION, IMPAIRED VERBAL

Defining characteristics

Unable to speak dominant language—(communicating)

Does not or cannot speak—(communicating)

Stuttering, slurring—(communicating)

Dyspnea—(exchanging)

COPING, INEFFECTIVE INDIVIDUAL

Defining characteristics

Verbalization of inability to cope or inability to ask for help—(communicating)

Inability to meet role expectations—(relating)

Alteration in social participation—(relating)

Change in usual communication patterns—(communicating)

Verbal manipulation—(communicating)

DIVERSIONAL ACTIVITY, DEFICIT

Defining characteristic

Boredom—(feeling)

FLUID VOLUME DEFICIT, ACTUAL (2)

Defining characteristics

Decreased urine output—(exchanging)

Concentrated urine—(exchanging)

Output greater than intake—(exchanging)

Sudden weight loss—(exchanging)

Hemoconcentration—(exchanging)

Increased serum sodium—(exchanging)

Other possible defining characteristics

Increased pulse rate—(exchanging)

Decreased skin turgor—(exchanging)

Decreased pulse volume/pressure—(exchanging)

Change in mental state—(perceiving)

Increased body temperature—(exchanging)

Dry skin—(exchanging)

Dry mucous membranes—(exchanging)

Weakness—(moving)

GAS EXCHANGE, IMPAIRED

Defining characteristics

> Confusion—(perceiving)
> Somnolence—(perceiving)
> Hypercapnea—(exchanging)
> Hypoxia—(exchanging)

GRIEVING, ANTICIPATORY

Defining characteristics

> Guilt—(feeling)
> Anger—(feeling)
> Sorrow—(feeling)
> Choked feelings—(feeling)
> Alterations in: activity level—(moving)
> Altered libido—(feeling)
> Altered communication patterns—(communicating)

GRIEVING, DYSFUNCTIONAL

Defining characteristics

> Verbal expression of distress at loss—(communicating)
> Expression of guilt—(feeling)
> Anger—(feeling)
> Sadness—(feeling)
> Crying—(communicating)
> Difficulty in expressing loss—(communicating)
> Alteration in: activity level—(moving)
> Alteration in: libido—(feeling)
> Idealization of lost object—(valuing)
> Labile affect—(feeling)

KNOWLEDGE DEFICIT (SPECIFY)

Defining characteristics

> Verbalization of the problem—(communicating)
> Inadequate performance of test—(knowing)

MOBILITY, IMPAIRED PHYSICAL

Defining characteristics

> Inability to purposefully move within the physical environment, including bed mobility, transfer, and ambulation—(moving)
> Reluctance to attempt movement—(choosing)
> Limited range of motion—(moving)
> Decreased muscle strength, control, and/or mass—(moving)
> Imposed restrictions of movement, including mechanical, medical protocol—(moving)
> Impaired coordination—(moving)

NONCOMPLIANCE (SPECIFY)

Defining characteristic

> Failure to keep appointments—(choosing)

NUTRITION, ALTERATION IN: MORE THAN BODY REQUIREMENTS

Defining characteristics

        Sedentary activity level—(moving)

        Concentrating food intake at end of day—(choosing)

RAPE TRAUMA SYNDROME

A. Rape trauma

Defining characteristics

        Anger—(feeling)

        Embarrassment—(feeling)

        Fear of physical violence and death—(feeling)

        Humiliation—(feeling)

        Sleep pattern disturbance—(perceiving)

        Changes in life-style—(choosing)

            Changes in residence—(choosing)

            Dealing with repetitive nightmares and phobias—(perceiving)

            Seeking family support—(relating)

            Seeking social network support—(relating)

B. Compound reaction

Defining characteristic

        Reliance on alcohol and/or drugs—(choosing)

C. Silent reaction

Defining characteristics

        Increase in nightmares—(perceiving)

        Increasing anxiety during interview, that is, blocking of associations, long periods of silence, minor stuttering, physical distress—(feeling)

SELF-CARE DEFICIT

A. Self-feeding deficit

Defining characteristic

        Inability to bring food from a receptacle to the mouth—(moving)

B. Self-bathing/hygiene deficit

Defining characteristic

        Inability to wash body or body parts—(moving)

D. Self-toileting deficit

Defining characteristics

        Unable to get to toilet or commode—(moving)

        Unable to sit on or rise from toilet or commode—(moving)

        Unable to manipulate clothing for toileting—(moving)

        Unable to carry out proper toilet hygiene—(moving)

        Unable to flush toilet or empty commode—(moving)

SELF-CONCEPT, DISTURBANCE IN
A. Body image, disturbance in

Defining characteristics
>Verbalization of change in life-style; fear of rejection or of reaction by others; focus on past strength, function, or appearance; negative feelings about body; feelings of helplessness, hopelessness, or powerlessness—(communicating)

B. Self-esteem, disturbance in

Defining characteristics
>Lack of follow-through—(choosing)
>Nonparticipation in therapy–(choosing)
>Not taking responsibility for self-care (self-neglect)—(valuing)

C. Role performance, disturbance in

Defining characteristics
>Change in self-perception of role—(perceiving)
>Denial of role—(choosing)
>Conflict in roles—(valuing)
>Lack of knowledge of role—(knowing)

SENSORY-PERCEPTUAL ALTERATION: VISUAL, AUDITORY, KINESTHETIC, GUSTATORY, TACTILE, OLFACTORY

Defining characteristics
>Altered abstraction—(knowing)
>Altered conceptualization—(knowing)
>Change in problem-solving abilities—(knowing)
>Reported or measured change in sensory acuity—(perceiving)
>Anxiety—(feeling)
>Apathy—(feeling)
>Restlessness—(moving)
>Irritability—(feeling)
>Altered communication patterns—(communicating)

Other possible defining characteristics
>Complaints of fatigue—(feeling)
>Alteration in posture—(moving)
>Change in muscular tension—(moving)

SEXUAL DYSFUNCTION

Defining characteristics
>Alterations in achieving perceived sex role—(perceiving)
>Seeking confirmation of desirability—(relating)

SLEEP PATTERN DISTURBANCE

Defining characteristics

        Verbal complaints of difficulty falling asleep—(communicating)

        Verbal complaints of not feeling well rested—(communicating)

        Restlessness—(moving)

        Slight hand tremor—(moving)

        Expressionless face—(communicating)

        Thick speech with mispronunciation and incorrect words—(communicating)

        Changes in posture—(moving)

SPIRITUAL DISTRESS (DISTRESS OF THE HUMAN SPIRIT)

Defining characteristics

        Anger toward God (as defined by the person)—(feeling)

        Verbalizes concern about relationship with deity—(communicating)

        Questions moral/ethical implications of therapeutic regimen—(valuing)

        Displacement of anger toward religious representatives—(communicating)

        Alteration in behavior/mood evidenced by anger, crying, withdrawal, preoccupation, anxiety, hostility, apathy—(communicating)

THOUGHT PROCESSES, ALTERATION IN

Defining characteristics

        Inaccurate interpretation of environment—(knowing)

        Memory deficit/problems—(knowing)

        Egocentricity—(valuing)

        Hyper/hypovigilance—(perceiving)

Other possible defining characteristics

        Inappropriate nonreality–based thinking—(knowing)

URINARY ELIMINATION, ALTERATION IN PATTERNS

Defining characteristics

        Frequency—(moving)

        Nocturia—(exchanging)

VIOLENCE, POTENTIAL FOR: SELF-DIRECTED OR DIRECTED AT OTHERS

Defining characteristic

        Increased motor activity, pacing, excitement, irritability, agitation—(moving)

Other defining characteristics

        Increasing anxiety level—(feeling)

        Fear of self or others—(feeling)

        Inability to verbalize feelings—(communicating)

        Repetition of verbalizations: continues complaints, requests, and demands—(communicating)

        Anger—(feeling)

        Depression (specifically active, aggressive, suicidal acts)—(feeling)

Section IV   # Issues, research suggestions, and references for approved nursing diagnoses* and diagnoses to be developed

ACTIVITY INTOLERANCE

Issues

1. Look at level of intolerance/tolerance and classification of signs in each class or level.
2. Consider a rating system for characterizing the activity so that when the diagnosis is used, one can look at the specific activities.
3. Are there other etiologies, such as "sedentary life-styles"?
4. Consider the effect of bed rest or prolonged immobility.
5. Consider the problem of valuing, if the client does not value activity. Is there a new diagnosis, "value conflict"?

References

Brammell, H.L., and Niccoli, A.: A physiologic approach to cardiac rehabilitation, Nurs. Clin. North Am. **11**:223, 1976.
Gordon, M.: Assessing activity tolerance, Am. J. Nurs. **76**:72, 1976.
Louis, M.C., and Provse, S.M.: Aphasia and endurance: considerations in the assessment and care of the stroke patient, Nurs. Clin. North Am. **15**:265, 1980.
Schmitt, Y., and others: Armchair treatment in the coronary care unit: effect on blood pressure and pulse, Nurs. Res. **18**:114, 1969.

AIRWAY CLEARANCE, INEFFECTIVE

Research suggestions

1. How often does pulmonary inflammatory process occur in patients with this diagnosis?
2. How often is "fever" used as a defining characteristic for this diagnosis?

ANXIETY

Issues

1. Reestablishing anxiety as a nursing diagnosis was discussed and supported by the following rationale:
   a. Kim and associates reported that *anxiety* as a specific diagnosis was reported 30 times in 158 cardiovascular patients.
   b. The study by Jones and Jacob, Phase 3: in 33% (427) of the patients, *anxiety* was identified and validated by three separate nurses as being present during assessment.

---

*Etiology and defining characteristics of nursing diagnoses are listed in the *Pocket Guide*, which is a companion to this *Proceedings*.

c. The 11 members of the small group described nurses in clinical practice differentiating *anxiety* from *fear*, which has been in the published list. At times each is used as a distinguishing characteristic of the other.

d. *Ineffective coping* is sometimes too broad a category. *Anxiety* may have *ineffective coping* as an etiology, since the interventions used are primarily concerned with decreasing anxiety.

Research suggestions

1. What are the reported indicators from the patients' view?
2. What are the indicators observed by the nurse?
3. What is the correlation of the findings of questions 1 and 2?
4. After identifying the defining characteristics that led to the diagnosis *anxiety* in a specific client, validate these with the client.
5. What physiologic and behavioral traits distinguish *fear* from *anxiety?*
6. What are the cultural manifestations of *anxiety?*
7. Can the definition of *anxiety* be refined?

BOWEL ELIMINATION, ALTERATION IN: CONSTIPATION

Research suggestions

1. Replicate phases one and two and complete phase three of the study by McLane, McShane, and Sliefert.
2. Study nursing protocols for this diagnosis to predict prevention and treatment.
3. Add cost-effectiveness to all studies when possible to identify savings to family or hospital with prevention.
4. Identify the effect parents have on a child's view of bowel habits.
5. Study patient outcomes when the treatment is managed by nurses.
6. Study variations in normal bowel elimination with varying circadian rhythms.
7. Confirm or deny the suggested etiologies.

BOWEL ELIMINATION, ALTERATION IN: DIARRHEA

Research suggestions

1. Which of the defining characteristics are critical?
2. How does one predict *diarrhea* and initiate prevention?

BOWEL ELIMINATION, ALTERATION IN: INCONTINENCE

Research suggestions

1. Identify from clinical practice if this diagnosis is an entity, a subcategory, or a sign of another condition.
2. What frequency of involuntary passage of stool constitutes a diagnosis?
3. Conduct clinical studies to generate additional defining characteristics.

BREATHING PATTERN, INEFFECTIVE

Research suggestions

1. How often does pulmonary inflammatory process occur in patients with this diagnosis?
2. How often does decreased lung expansion occur in patients with this diagnosis?
3. How often does tracheobronchial obstruction occur in patients with this diagnosis?

CARDIAC OUTPUT, ALTERATION IN: DECREASED

Research suggestions

1. Conduct regional replication of the study, "Nursing Diagnosis in Acute Cardiovascular Nursing," conducted by Kim and coworkers.
2. Separate the independent, interdependent, and dependent nursing actions for *decreased cardiac output* related to altered preload, altered afterload, and altered contractility.
3. Separate the independent, interdependent, and dependent nursing actions for *decreased cardiac output* related to altered rate, altered rhythm, and altered conduction.
4. Identify the incidence of use of structural etiology in arriving at this diagnosis.
5. Does the use of mechanical, electrical, or structural etiologies make a difference in the selection of nursing actions for patients with this diagnosis?
6. How often are blood chemistries used as defining characteristics?
7. Which changes in mental status are most frequently identified as defining characteristics in patients with this diagnosis?
8. Is there value in knowing how the defining characteristics are clustered by nurses in the following nursing areas: critical care, general medical-surgical, and community health?
9. Determine the validity of identifying two distinct nursing diagnoses and their defining characteristics: *acute decrease in cardiac output* and *chronic decrease in cardiac output.*

COMFORT, ALTERATION IN: PAIN

Issues

1. Suffering is as important as *pain.* Is it the same or different?
2. Should this nursing diagnosis deal only with that which nursing can assist or treat independent of other health care workers?
3. Clarify the etiology. Can it be a medical diagnosis (surgical incision)? Does it direct the plan of care? How does "related to" differ from "etiology"?
4. Define "pain" and "comfort."

Research suggestions

1. Using a rating scale of 0 to 10, what is a level of pain with which an individual can cope in an acute or chronic situation?
2. Identify the kinds of tools people are using to measure the helpfulness of intervention.
3. How does *alteration in comfort* relate to a patient's perceived locus of control?
4. What is the relationship of this diagnosis to others? Is the experience of *pain* sensation or perception?
5. How is *pain* endured or dealt with differently if it is known to be temporary?
6. Study the myths of *pain.*
7. Which objective characteristics do nurses use to make the diagnosis?
8. Which are the most important indicators using different frameworks?
9. Given all indicators, how do different nurses view *pain* in the same patient?
10. Replicate research done by Silver and co-workers that crying is not an indicator of pain.

References

Copp, L.: The spectrum of suffering, Am. J. Nurs. **3:**491, 1974.

Graham, L., and Conley, E.: Evaluation of anxiety and fear in adult surgical patients, Nurs. Res. **20**(2):113, 1971.

McCafferey, M.: Nursing management of the patient with pain, Philadelphia, 1972, J.B. Lippincott Co.

McLachlan, E.: Recognizing pain, Am. J. Nurs. **3:**496, 1974.

Melzack, R.: The puzzle of pain, New York, 1973, Basic Books, Inc., Publishers.

Melzack, R.: Pain, the McGill pain questionnaire: major properties and scoring methods, Amsterdam, 1975, North-Holland.

Melzack, R., and Torgerson, W.S.: On the language of pain, Anesthesiology **34:**50, 1971.

Melzack, R., and Wall, P. D.: Psychophysiology of pain, Int. Anesthesiol. Clin. **8:**3, 1970.

Merskey, H.: The perception measurement of pain, J. Psychosom. Res. **17:**251, 1973.

Moss, F.T., and Mayer, B.: The effects of nursing interaction upon pain relief in patients, Nurs. Res. **15:**303, 1966.

Munleg, M.J., and Keane, M.C., eds.: Impressions of pain: a nursing diagnosis, Nurs. Clin. North Am. **12**(4):609, 1977.

Nursing the patient having a problem resulting from disorders in regulation: neural regulation. In Beland, I., and Passos, J.: Clinical nursing, ed. 3, New York, 1975, Macmillan Publishing Co., Inc.

Pilowsky, I., and Bond, H.R.: Pain: its management in malignant disease elucidation of staff-patient transactions, Psychosom. Med. **31:**400, 1969.

Strauss, A., Fagerhaugh, S., and Glaser, B.: Pain: an organizational-work-interactional perspective, Nurs. Outlook **22**(9):560, 1974.

Weisenburg, M.: Pain: clinical-experimental perspectives, St. Louis, 1975, The C.V. Mosby Co.

Wolfer, J., and Davis, C.: Assessment of surgical patients' preoperative emotional condition with postoperative welfare, Nurs. Res. **19**(4):402, 1970.

COMMUNICATION, IMPAIRED: VERBAL

Issues

1. Consider reorganizing the etiology into three categories:
   a. Anatomic-structural
      (1) Physical barrier (tracheostomy, intubation)
      (2) Loss of anatomic structures: tongue, larynx, cleft palate
   b. Neurologic-functional
      (1) Physical barriers, for example, tumor, CVA
      (2) Physiologic barriers—toxic (alcohol, drugs, chemicals), weak muscles, shortness of breath
      (3) Psychologic barriers—disorientation, overload, psychoses, lack of stimuli, controlling others, anxiety
   c. Language
      (1) Cultural differences
      (2) Development or age related

References

Johnson, J.H., and Cryon, M.: Homonymous hemianopsia: assessment and nursing management, Am. J. Nurs. **79:**2131, 1979.

Mahoney, E.K.: Alterations in cognitive functioning in the brain-damaged patient, Nurs. Clin. North Am. **15:**283, 1980.

Norman, S.: Diagnostic categories for the patient with a right hemisphere lesion, Am. J. Nurs. **79:**2126, 1979.

Norman, S., and Baratz, R.: Understanding aphasia, Am. J. Nurs. **79:**2135, 1979.

COPING, FAMILY: POTENTIAL FOR GROWTH

Issues

1. Should this category be included under the new heading *family process, alteration in?*
2. Are the defining characteristics of this diagnosis overlapping with those of *family process, alteration in?*

References

Iles, J.P.: Children with cancer: healthy siblings' perceptions during the illness experience, Cancer Nurs. **2:**371, 1979.

Levin, L.S.: Patient education and self-care: how do they differ? Nurs. Outlook. **26:**170, 1978.

Maslow, A.H.: Toward a psychology of being, ed. 2, New York, 1968, Van Nostrand Reinhold Co.

Norris, C.M.: Self-care, Am. J. Nurs. **79:**486, 1979.

Smith, D.W.: Survivors of serious illness, Am. J. Nurs. **79:**440, 1979.

Weisman, A.D.: Coping with cancer, New York, 1979, McGraw-Hill Book Co.

COPING, INEFFECTIVE FAMILY: COMPROMISED

Issues

1. Should this category be included under the new heading *family process, alteration in?*
2. Are the defining characteristics of this diagnosis overlapping with those of *family process, alteration in?*

COPING, INEFFECTIVE FAMILY: DISABLING

Issues

1. Should this category be included under the new heading *family process, alteration in?*
2. Are the defining characteristics of this diagnosis overlapping with those of *family process, alteration in?*

COPING, INEFFECTIVE INDIVIDUAL

Issues

1. Should this diagnosis be replaced with the diagnosis *life stress response (chronic), maladaptive?*
2. Could "catastrophic events" be included under etiology?
3. Are there any other defining characteristics that are critical?

Research suggestions

1. What is the effectiveness/ineffectiveness of usual coping mechanisms?
2. What is the relationship between social life changes and *ineffective individual coping?*
3. Does the personality style of an individual contribute to *ineffective individual coping?*
4. Does the person's normal coping style change with the threat of illness?
5. What are the patterns of coping?
6. Are there cultural differences in manifestations of ineffective coping?
7. What is the conceptual relationship of *fear, anxiety, and ineffective individual coping?*

References

Hambrua, D.A., and Adams, J.: A perspective on coping behavior, Arch. Gen. Psychiatr. **17**:277, 1967.

Lipowski, Z.J.: Physical illness: the individual and the coping processes, Psychiatr. Med. **1**:91, 1970.

Murphy, L.B., and Moriary, A.E.: Vulnerability, coping and growth from infancy to adolescence, New Haven, Conn., 1976, Yale University Press.

DIVERSIONAL ACTIVITY, DEFICIT

Issues

1. Is this a diagnosis, a treatment, an etiology, a defining characteristic of another diagnosis, or a problem?
2. Consideration should be given to distinguishing between recreation (considered therapeutic) and diversion (not necessarily therapeutic).
3. Careful definition of "diversion" is needed.

Research suggestions

1. How often is this diagnosis used in the clinical setting?
2. Why is this diagnosis perceived as useful?
3. Concurrent or retrospective audit:
   a. Which signs and symptoms do nurses use to identify this diagnosis?
   b. How do nurses decide which activities are appropriate?
4. How is this diagnosis related to the developmental stage of the client?

FAMILY PROCESS, ALTERATION IN

Issue

1. Three categories have been suggested as diagnostic categories in working with families: *boundary maintenance, interaction,* and *decision making* (Hayes). Are these diagnostic categories or are they assessment parameters?

Research suggestions

1. What criteria are needed to differentiate what is adequate from what is potentially inadequate and from what is inadequate?
2. Does the use of systems theory have as its outcome a more holistic perspective for nurses as compared with other theories?
3. What is the relationship among community, group, family, and individual diagnoses?
4. Consider the merits of descriptive, retrospective, concurrent, or prospective studies of individual, family, and community at high risk for this diagnosis.
5. When is the presenting system indicative of a family problem and when of an individual problem?
6. What is the appropriate time to focus on an individual as the unit of intervention and when the family?
7. What are the criteria for choosing the individual unit as the system of study?
8. What are the criteria for choosing the family unit as the system of study?

References

Briar, S.: The family as an organization: an approach to family diagnosis and treatment. Soc. Serv. Rev. **38:**247, 1964.

Hall, J.E., and Weaver, B.R., eds.: Distributive nursing practice: a systems approach to community health, Philadelphia, 1977, J.B. Lippincott Co.

Mimichen, P.: Marriage and family development, ed. 5, New York, 1977, J.B. Lippincott Co.

Otlo, H.: Criteria for assessing family strengths, Fam. Process **2:**329, 1963.

Satir, V.M.: Conjoint family therapy: a guide to theory and technique, Palo Alto, Calif., 1967, Science & Behavior Books.

Satir, V.M.: Peoplemaking, Palo Alto, Calif., 1972, Science & Behavior Books.

VonBertalanfy, L.: General systems therapy, New York, 1968, George Braziller, Inc.

Watzlawick, P., Beavin, J.H., & Jackson, D.D.: Pragmatics of human communication: a study of interactional pattern, pathologies, and paradoxes, New York, 1967, W.W. Norton & Co., Inc.

FEAR

Research suggestions

1. Are there cultural differences in the manifestations of *fear?*
2. How do nurses differentiate between *fear* and phobia?

FLUID VOLUME, ALTERATION IN: EXCESS

Issue

1. Should the following be considered risk factors?
   a. Extremes of age
   b. Altered regulatory mechanisms
   c. I.V. therapy
   d. High sodium intake
   e. Response to injury, for example, surgery, burn, trauma

References

Kim, M.J., and others: Clinical use of nursing diagnosis in cardiovascular nursing. In Kim, M.J., and Moritz, D.A., eds.: Classification of nursing diagnoses: proceedings of the third and fourth national conferences, New York, 1982. McGraw-Hill Book Co.

FLUID VOLUME DEFICIT, ACTUAL AND POTENTIAL

Research suggestions

1. Test the defining characteristics of fluid volume loss, no matter what the etiology, across all age groups (pediatric to geriatric) to identify commonalities in characteristics.
2. Assuming question 1 is answered, identify whether or not interventions differ with different etiologies.

GAS EXCHANGE, IMPAIRED

Research suggestions

1. For each proposed new etiology, how often is this present in a patient with *impaired gas exchange?*
2. To clarify whether there is overlap between this and other respiratory diagnoses *airway clearance, ineffective; breathing pattern, (ineffective)*, conduct a clinical validation of the defining characteristics for each diagnosis.

GRIEVING, ANTICIPATORY AND DYSFUNCTIONAL

Issue

1. Consider using as definitions:
    a. Anticipatory grieving—grieving before an actual loss
    b. Grief—response to actual/potential loss
    c. Dysfunctional grieving—delayed or exaggerated response to a perceived actual or potential loss

Research suggestions

1. Are hopelessness, helplessness, powerlessness, and lack of trust related to grieving? If so, how?
2. What are the common somatic manifestations of grieving? Do they differ with different etiology?

HEALTH MAINTENANCE, ALTERATION IN

Issues

1. Does the value system of the client influence the defining characteristics?
2. This diagnosis is different from *self-care deficit* but is associated with it. How should they be distinguished?

References

American Nurses' Association: Guidelines for continuing education in development disabilities, Kansas City, Mo., 1978, The Association.

American Nurses' Association: Nursing: a social policy statement, Kansas City, Mo., 1980, The Association.

Chang, B.L.: Evaluation of health care professionals in facilitating self-care: review of the literature and a conceptual model, Adv. Nurs. Serv. **3:**43, 1980.

Curry, J., and Peppe, K., eds.: Mental retardation: nursing approaches to care, St. Louis, 1980, The C.V. Mosby Co.

Given, B.: Patient participation. In American Nurses' Association: Nursing influence on health policy for the eighties: 1978 scientific session of the American Academy of Nursing, Kansas City, Mo., 1979, The Association.

Joseph, L.S.: Self-care and the nursing process, Nurs. Clin. North Am. **15:**131, 1980.

Maloney, M., and Ward, M.: Mental retardation and modern society, New York, 1979, Oxford University Press.

McNelly, P.: Quality assurance in residential settings. In Curry, J., and Peppe, K. eds.: Mental retardation: nursing approaches to care, St. Louis, 1980, The C.V. Mosby Co.

Orem, D.: Nursing: concepts of practice, ed. 2, New York, 1980, McGraw-Hill Book Co.

Peret, K., and Stachowiak, B.: Health maintenance dependency: conceptual base, etiology, and defining characteristics. In Kim, M.J., McFarland, G.K., and McLane, A.M.: Classification of nursing diagnoses: proceedings of the fifth national conference, St. Louis, 1984, The C.V. Mosby Co.

INJURY, POTENTIAL FOR: POISONING, SUFFOCATION, TRAUMA

Research suggestion

1. How effective are safety "mechanisms" used to treat this diagnosis?

KNOWLEDGE DEFICIT (SPECIFY)

Issues

1. "Inaccurate," "inadequate," and "inappropriate" are too value laden to use as defining terms and must be examined.
2. Possible definition—lack of specific information.
3. Possible diagnostic labels and definitions:
   a. Knowledge deficit: state of health. Definition—lack of specific information regarding level of function.
   b. Knowledge deficit: factors influencing state of health. Definition—lack of specific information regarding phenomena possibly affecting level of function.
   c. Knowledge deficit: health maintenance measures. Definition—lack of specific information regarding activities sustaining level of function.
   d. Knowledge deficit: preventive health measures. Definition—lack of specific information regarding activities decreasing risk of impaired level of function.
   e. Knowledge deficit: Restorative measures. Definition—lack of specific information regarding activities that move the individual toward an optimal level of function.

Research suggestions

1. What is the definition of knowledge deficit?
2. Explore the concept "readiness to learn" as etiology and define relevant characteristics.
3. What are the characteristics seen in patients' readiness or lack of readiness to learn that would lead to different interventions?
4. Is there a perceivable difference in outcome criteria when teaching style of the nurse differs from patient's learning style?
5. How do nurses determine what patient's learning needs are?
6. Which learning theory is most effective with different levels of acuity?
7. What are the variables involved in the generalizability or transfer of learning (for example, context, degree of illness)?
8. What are the factors considered and methods used in drawing conclusions from assessment data to define *knowledge deficit?*
9. Examine *knowledge deficit* as an etiologic factor in other diagnoses.
10. Examine the effectiveness of learning and outcomes of various interventions derived from learning theories.
11. Does basing educational content on patient's perceived needs affect learning or outcomes?
12. Identify variables that predict successful resolution of *knowledge deficit.*

MOBILITY, IMPAIRED PHYSICAL

Issues

1. How useful is this diagnosis in the clinical setting?
   a. Is it more useful in a long-term care facility because progress that has occurred can be evaluated using a coding system?
   b. There are problems in an acute care setting because the levels change so quickly.
   c. Determining progress using a coding system is useful for accreditation purposes.
2. Do other disciplines such as physical therapy use a coding system in clinical practice?

Research suggestions

1. What are the assessment factors or guidelines for assessment related to impaired mobility?
2. Is there congruence between a patient's view of the diagnosis and a nurse's view?
3. Are clients' goals similar to nurses' goals?

NONCOMPLIANCE (SPECIFY)

Issue

1. The etiologies stated are not clear-cut and inclusive.

Research suggestions

1. Identify alternative label for noncompliance, one that is less value laden. Recommended methodology—Delphi study to identify best way to use term or alternate label.
2. What is the effect of nurse's diagnosing *non-compliance* on patient's behavior?
3. How are nurses' behaviors affected by this label?
4. Explore the validity of *noncompliance* as a defining characteristic of other diagnoses.
5. Explore the quality of client-nurse interaction as it influences or is a predictor of or an etiologic factor for *noncompliance.*
6. Explore patient involvement in goal setting and lack of mutual goal setting as a defining characteristic.
7. What is the relationship of this diagnosis to the degree that nurses encourage patients to maintain self-care?
8. Test a variety of interventions and approaches based on current literature: locus of control, health/belief model, support system, provider, reactant's theory, attribution theory, intentionality.
9. How do nurses decide when patients become noncompliant, and when is the label removed?

NUTRITION, ALTERATION IN: LESS THAN BODY REQUIREMENTS

Issues

1. Consider identifying information about a diagnosis as "risk factors," "etiology," and "defining characteristics."
2. If the preceding is accepted, information about *alteration in nutrition*, subcategory decreased caloric intake, would be presented as:
   a. Risk factor: low body weight, "yo-yo dieting," gastric bypass
   b. Etiology: inadequate intake, ineffective processing of nutrients
   c. Defining characteristics: may overlap with etiology and must be developed further.
3. The suggested sequence is important and is perceived as leading from the general to the specific. In the minds of some, risk factors are more psychosocial. Defining characteristics are fewer in number and more measurable.

References

Green, M.L., and Harry, J., eds.: Nutrition and contemporary nursing practice, New York; 1981, John Wiley & Sons, Inc.

Krause, M., and Mahn, L.K.: Food, nutrition, and diet therapy, ed. 6, Philadelphia, 1979, W.B. Saunders Co.

NUTRITION, ALTERATION IN: MORE THAN BODY REQUIREMENTS (POTENTIAL FOR)

Issue

1. It is possible to have excess and decreased intake simultaneously (for example, excess caloric intake and decreased protein intake). The specific increase or decrease would then be a subcategory with identified risk factors, etiology, defining characteristics.

ORAL MUCOUS MEMBRANE, ALTERATION IN:

Research suggestions

1. Evaluate and summarize studies to verify current diagnostic label.
2. Test current treatment protocols, for examples, Toothettes, Water Pik, sodium bicarbonate rinse.

References

Ariaudo, A., and others: How frequently must patients carry out effective oral hygiene procedures in order to maintain gingival health, J. Periodont. **42:**309, 1971.

Beck, S.: Impact of systematic oral care protocol on stomatitis after chemotherapy, Cancer Nurs. **2:**185, 1979.

Bruya, M., and Maderia, N.: Stomatitis after chemotherapy, Am. J. Nurs. **75:**1349, 1975.

Daeffler, R.: Oral hygiene measures for patients with cancer, Cancer Nurs. Part I, **3:**347, 1980; Part II, **3:**427, 1980; Part III, **4:**29, 1981.

Dewalt, E.: Effect of timed hygienic measures on oral mucosa in a group of elderly subjects, Nurs. Res. **24:**104, 1975.

Dewalt, E., and Haines, S.: Effects of specific stressors on health oral mucosa, Nurs. Res. **18:**22, 1969.

Ginsbery, M.: A study of oral hygiene nursing care, Am. J. Nurs. **61:**67, 1961.

Ginsbery, M., and Yonder, A.: The effects of some traditional methods of oral hygiene nursing care, J. Periodont. **35:**513, 1964.

Greene, J., and Vermillen, J.: The oral hygiene index: a method for classifying oral hygiene status, J. Den. Assoc. **61:**172, 1960.

Kloch, J., and Seidduth, A.: Oral hygiene instruction and plaque formation during hospitalization, Nurs. Res. **18:**124, 1969.

Lovelock, D.J.: Oral hygiene for patients in hospitals, Nurs. Mirror **61:**39, 1973.

Moses, R.: A comparison of oral hygiene agents, Unpublished master's thesis, College Park, Md., 1975, University of Maryland.

O'Leary, T.J.: Oral hygiene agents and procedures, J. Periodont **41:**625, 1970.

Passos, J., and Brand, L.: Effects of agents of oral hygiene, Nurs. Res. **75:**196, 1966.

Reitz, M., and Pope, W.: Mouth care, Am. J. Nurs. **73:**1728, 1973.

Suomi, J.D., and others: The effects of controlled oral hygiene procedures on the progression of periodontal disease in adults, results after third and fourth year, J. Periodont. **42:**152, 1971.

Van Drimmelen, J., and Rollins, H.: Evaluation of a commonly used oral hygiene agent, Nurs. Res. **18:**327, 1969.

Wiley, S.: Why lemon and glycerol? Am. J. Nurs. **69:**342, 1969.

PARENTING, ALTERATION IN: ACTUAL OR POTENTIAL

Issue

1. Defining characteristics need additional attention. The definition given for parenting is in positive terms, but the defining characteristics of the definition are negative. The terms refer to both parent and child but do not include the relationship or the interaction.

Research suggestions

1. Is parenting an environment that you create or a relationship?
2. How far does parenting go?
3. Are sociopsychologic growth–fostering behaviors the same as intellectual growth–fostering behaviors?
4. Is "abuse" an *alteration in parenting* or is *child abuse/neglect* a separate diagnosis?
5. What is the domain of parenting? Social? Physical?
6. What developmental groupings might emerge from question 2?
7. Do the parenting problems that nurses treat change along developmental stages?
8. Does parenting reflect coping?
9. Is this an environmental deficit, in which case the nurse should focus on the child, or a skill deficit, in which case the nurse should focus on the mother?
10. How does the developmental stage of the parent affect parenting?
11. Can the norms for parenting be defined by asking parents what it is "to parent," or "what is parenting"?
12. Study the nursing assumption that the mother's immediate postpartum concern is child interaction. Perhaps other concerns are more important, such as appearance.
13. Can the same norms applied to "parenting" be applied to any significant care giver?
14. What are the cultural variations in components of parenting?
15. Is this a diagnosis affected by the nurses making it?
16. What variables of parenting are affected by changing women's roles?
17. What are the differences in parents among those with prior information about child care, those who get child care information in the hospital (bath demonstration, feeding), and those who get child care information at home?
18. Are there clusters of symptoms or specific nursing diagnoses that are associated with medical diagnoses such as "failure to thrive"?
19. How is *alteration in parenting* related to *home maintenance management*?
20. Have current reports had an effect on the terms used in defining parenting or the etiology of alterations?
21. Which of the many characteristics are the critical defining variables?
22. Are there means of measuring the critical characteristics that are reliable and valid?
23. Is the mother's ability to pick up cues from the child a critical characteristic? Does this change with a new child, a developing child, a first child? How significant is the clarity of the child's cues?
24. What is the child's responsibility in the parenting process?
25. How does the child's behavior, such as hyperactivity, affect the parent?
26. What are the needs of the child who receives care from multiple care givers? Does the child seek out one individual to meet needs?
27. What is an effective parenting role model?
28. What are parenting, behaviors in an abuse situation as compared with a nonabuse situation?
29. What would be the indicators of sexual abuse?
30. Is child abuse/neglect always a component of *parenting, alteration in*? Are there characteristics of a child that evoke abusive behavior in an adult?
31. Since the definition of parenting focuses on the parent, how is change measured over time? Is the mother a good or improving mother because the child gains weight?

References

Affonso, D.: The newborn's potential for interaction, JOGN Nurs. **5**:9, 1976.

Anthony, E.J., and Therese, B., eds.: Parenthood: its psychology and pathophysiology, Boston, 1970, Little, Brown & Co.

Ballard, W., and Gold, E.: Medical and health aspects of reproduction in the adolescent, Clin. Obstet. Gynecol. **14**:338, 1971.

Barnard, M.U.: Supportive nursing care for the mother and newborn who are separated from each other, Matern. Child Nurs. **1**:107, 1976.

Barnett, C.R., and others: Neonatal separation: the maternal side of interactional deprivation, Pediatrics, **45**: 197, 1970.

Bell, S.M., and Ainsworth, M.D.: Infant crying and maternal responsiveness, Child Dev. **43**:1171, 1976.

Cannon, R.B.: The development of maternal touch during early mother-infant interaction, JOGN Nurs. **6**:28, 1977.

Clark, A.L.: Recognizing discord between mother and child and changing it to harmony, Matern. Child Nurs. J. **1**:100, 1976.

Clark, A.L., and Affonso, D.: Childbearing: a nursing perspective, Philadelphia, 1976a, F.A. Davis Co.

Clark, A.L., and Affonso, D.: Infant behavior and maternal attachment: two sides to the coin, Matern. Child Nurs. J. **1**:94, 1976b.

Cropley, C., Lester, P.A., and Pennington, S.: Assessment tool for measuring maternal attachment behaviors. In McMall, L.K., and Galeener, J.T., eds.: Current practice in obstetric and gynecologic nursing, St. Louis, 1976, The C.V. Mosby Co.

Daniels, A.: Reaching the unwed adolescent mothers, Am. J. Nurs. **69**:332, 1969.

Dubois, D.R.: Indications of an unhealthy relationship between parents and premature infant, JOGN Nurs. **4**:21, 1975.

Duenhaelter, J., and Jiminez, J.H.: Pregnancy performance of patients under fifteen years of age, Obstet. Gynecol. **46**:(1):49, 1975.

Ehrman, M: Sex education for the young, Nurs. Outlook **23**(8):583, 1975.

Erickson, E.: Childhood and society, ed. 2, New York, 1963, W.W. Norton & Co., Inc.

Fischman, S.H.: The pregnancy-resolution decisions of unwed adolescent, Nurs. Clin. North Am. **10**(2):217, 1975.

Goldmeier, H.: School-age parents in Massachusetts, Boston, 1975, Massachusetts Committee on Children and Youth.

Gollober, M.: A comment on the need for father-infant postpartal interaction, JOGN Nurs. **5**:17, 1976.

Heald, F., ed.: Adolescent gynecology, Baltimore, 1966, The Williams & Wilkins Co.

Hurd, J.M.L.: Assessing maternal attachment: first step toward the prevention of child abuse, JOGN Nurs. **4**:25, 1975.

Iorio, J.: Parent-child relationship: implication for nursing. In Clark, A., Bunnell, M., and Hennings E., eds.: Parent-child relationships: role of the nurse, New Brunswick, N.J., 1968, Rutgers Univeristy Press.

Kelly, J.S.: The school and unmarried mothers, Children, **10**:60, 1963.

Klaus, M.H., and Kennell, J.H.: Maternal-infant bonding, St. Louis, 1976, The C.V. Mosby Co.

Klaus, M.H., and others: Human maternal behavior at first contact with her young, Pediatrics, **46**:187, 1970.

Klaus, M.H., and others: Maternal attachment: importance of the first post-partum days, New Engl. J. Med. **286**:460, 1972.

Klein, C.: The single parent experience, New York, 1973, Avon Books.

Klerman, L.V., and Jekel, J.F.: Services for teenage mothers: what do we need to know? Conn. Heath Bull. **84**:219, 1970.

Klerman, L.V., and Jekel, J.F.: School-age mothers: Problems, programs, and policy, 1973, The Shoe String Press, Inc.

Kuhr, M.: Fatalism in ghetto adolescents (editorial), Pediatrics, **55**(3):443, 1975.

Leonard, S.W.: How first-time fathers feel toward their newborns, Matern. Child Nurs. J. **1**:361, 1976.

Lieberman, F.: Sexual liberation and the adolescent girl, Birth Fam. J. **2**(2):51, 1975.

Maier, H.W.: Three theories of child development, ed. 2, New York, 1967, Holt, Rinehart & Winston, Inc.

Maslow, A.: Toward a psychology of being, ed. 2, New York, 1968, Van Nostrand Reinhold Co.

McAnarney, E.: Adolescent pregnancy: a pediatric concern, Clin. Pediatr. **14**(1):19, 1975.

Mercer, R.T.: Postpartum illness and acquaintance-attachment process, Am. J. Nurs. **77**:1174, 1977.

Morris, M.: Maternal claiming: identification processes, their meaning for mother-infant mental health, In Clark, A., Bunnell, M., and Hennings, E., eds.: Parent-child relations: role of the nurse, New Brunswick, N.J., 1968, Rutgers University Press.

Nadelson, C.: Abortion counseling: focus on adolescent pregnancy, Pediatrics **54**(6):765, 1974.

Nursing Clinics of North America, 7(4), 1972. Entire volume on adolescent, body image, psychologic impact of pregnancy on adolescent, and related topics.

Oppel, W.: Teenage births: some social, psychological, and physical sequelae, Am. J. Public Health **61**:751, 1971.

Osofsky, J.F.: The pregnant teenager, Springfield, Ill., 1968, Charles C Thomas, Publisher.

Pannor, R.: The teenage, unwed father, Clin. Obstet. Gynecol. **14**:466, 1971.

Porters, C.: Maladaptive mothering patterns: nursing intervention, ANA Clinical Sessions, 1972.

Raugh, J., and Johnson, L.B.: The reproductive adolescent, Pediatr. Clin. North Am. **20**(4):1005, 1973.

Robson, K.S., and Moss, H.A.: Patterns and determinants of maternal attachment, J. Pediatr. **77**:976, 1970.

Rubin, R.: Binding in the postpartum period, Matern. Child Nurs. J. **6**:67, 1977.

Sommers, J.P., and Lamers, W.M., Jr.: Teenage pregnancy, Springfield, Ill., 1968, Charles C Thomas, Publisher.

Stein, O.C., and others: School leaving due to pregnancy in an urban adolescent, Am. J. Public Health, **54**:1, 1964.

Thomas, A., and Chess, S.: Temperament and development, New York, 1977, Brunner/Mazel, Inc.

Towle, C.: Common human needs, New York, 1957, National Association of Social Workers.

Woodbury, R.: Help for high school mothers, Life, p. 34, Apr. 2, 1971.

Zackler, J., and Branstadt, W.: The teenage pregnant girl, Springfield, Ill., 1975, Charles C Thomas, Publisher.

POWERLESSNESS

Research suggestions

1. Can dependence be either voluntary or involuntary?
2. Does *powerlessness* arise from the dependence or from the feelings generated as a result of the dependence, for example, irritability, resentment, anger, guilt?

References

Miller, J.: Development and validation of a diagnostic label: powerlessness. In Kim, M.J., McFarland, G.K., and McLane, A.M.: Classification of nursing diagnoses: proceedings of the fifth national conference, St. Louis, 1984, The C.V. Mosby Co.

Miller, J.: Powerlessness: coping with chronic illness, Philadelphia, 1982, F.A. Davis Co.

RAPE TRAUMA SYNDROME

Issues

1. How do you separate this diagnosis from other related ones, such as genital injury?
2. Is *rape trauma syndrome* a distinct category, or is rape an etiology of one or more diagnoses?

Research suggestions

1. Does the event rape equal *rape trauma syndrome?*
2. How do incest victims differ from rape victims?

3. What are the variations of *rape trauma syndrome?*
4. Are the characteristics the same in cases of rape of men or of children?

References

Burgess, A.W., and Holmstrom, L.L.: Rape trauma syndrome, Am. J. Psychiatr. **131**:981, 1974.
Holmstrom, L.L., and Burgess, A.W.: Development of diagnostic categories: sexual trauma, Am. J. Nurs. **75**:1288, 1975.

SELF-CARE DEFICIT: FEEDING, BATHING/HYGIENE, DRESSING/GROOMING, TOILETING

Issues

1. In identifying the etiology/etiologies of a *self-care deficit,* how specific should they be?
2. Is there congruence between the use of "self-care" according to Orem and *"self-care deficit"* according to the national conference?
3. Are the defining characteristics different for the various types of *self-care deficit?*
4. There is a need for more specific criteria for each level of *self-care deficit.*

Research suggestions

1. Differentiate between patients not performing self-care and patients not capable of performing self-care. Are the defining characteristics different?
2. In a pediatric population, identify normal self-care behavior congruent with the developmental level and then identify the characteristics of a deficit.
3. What are the etiologies of *self-care deficit?*

References

Buchwald, E.: Activities of daily living: general classification, physical rehabilitation for daily living, New York, 1952, McGraw-Hill Book Co.
Jones, E., and others: Patient classification for long-term care: users' manual, HEW Pub. No. HRA-75-3107, Washington, D.C., 1974, DHEW.
Katz, S., and Akpom, A.: A measure of primary sociobiological functions, Int. J. Health Serv. **6**:493, 1976.

SELF-CONCEPT, DISTURBANCE IN: BODY IMAGE, SELF-ESTEEM, ROLE PERFORMANCE, PERSONAL IDENTITY

Research suggestions

1. Study should be done longitudinally of specific individuals' self-concepts over time.
2. Are "critical indicators" listed actually etiology? What is the terminology used by clinicians?
3. Study *self-concept* as a construct with other categories as subconcepts.
4. Is knowledge of etiology necessary for intervention? Is etiology always identifiable?
5. Specifically regarding *body image:*
   a. What are the changes in a patient's perceptions of actual or perceived changes over time?
   b. Which scale is appropriate for identifying body image?
   c. How long is denial effective as a coping mechanism? When is a patient ready for nursing intervention in relation to a body image change?
   d. Develop a nonverbal behavior tool for assessing body image.

6. Specifically regarding self-esteem:
   a. "Negative self-talk" must be researched as a defining characteristic.
   b. What are the critical defining characteristics?
   c. On a continuum of negative and positive self-talk, is there a point at which we can identify self-esteem, disturbance in?
   d. What is "lack of follow-through" as a defining characteristic?
   e. Through interview of significant others of patients, determine premorbid level of self-esteem, looking for correlation or predictability with decreased self-esteem associated with the current illness.
   f. Identify the ethical issues of using data from significant others for nursing intervention.
   g. At what point do nurses decide that intervention is necessary?
   h. Do we intervene to change the presentation of self or to help develop self-insight?
   i. Study the reported feeling "unworthy or reluctant to ask for help" as a possible defining characteristic.
   j. What is the relationship of "help-seeking behavior" to self-esteem? Is control over one's internal and external environment a control issue in one's self-esteem? Does loss of control place an individual at high risk for loss of self-esteem?
7. Specifically regarding *role performance, disturbance in:*
   a. How does it differ from *role disturbance,* listed on the TBD list?
8. Specifically regarding *personal identity, disturbance in:*
   a. Is there a difference between identity and self-concept based on established research?
   b. Is the inability to distinguish between "self" and "not self" related to body image?
   c. Is identity a constant core, with self-concept always changing with feedback from others and the environment?
   d. If a broader definition of self-concept is used (based on Bonham and Cheney), would *personal identity, disturbance in* be dropped as a diagnosis?

References

Berscheid, E., Walster, E., and Bohrnstedt, G.: Body image: a psychology today questionnaire, Psychol. Today **6**:58, 1972.

Bonham, C., and Cheney, A.M.: Concept of self: a framework for nursing assessment, In Chinn, P., ed.: Advances in nursing theory and development, Rockville, Md., 1983, Aspen Systems Corp.

Fisher, S., and Cleveland, S.E.: Body image and personality, New York, 1968, Dover Publications, Inc.

Gruendemann, B.J.: The impact of surgery on body image, Nurs. Clin. North Am. **10**:635, 1975.

McCloskey, J.C.: How to make the most of body image theory in nursing practice, Nursing '76 **6**(5):68, 1976.

Murray, R.L., ed.: Symposium on body image change, Nurs. Clin. North Am. **7**:597, 1972.

Polivy, J.: Psychological effects of mastectomy on a woman's feminine self-concept, J. Nerv. Ment. Dis. **164**:77, 1977.

Ritchie, J.: Schilder's theory of the sociology of the body image, Matern. Child Nurs. J. **2**:143, 1973.

Secord, P.F., and Jourard, S.M.: Appraisal of body cathexis and the self, J. Consult. Psychol. **17**:343, 1953.

Shontz, F.C.: Body image and its disorders, Int. J. Psychiatry Med. **6**:461, 1974.

Smith, E.C., Liviskic, S.C., and McNemar, A.: Re-establishing a child's body image, Am. J. Nurs. **77**:445, 1977.

SENSORY-PERCEPTUAL ALTERATION: VISUAL, AUDITORY, KINESTHETIC, GUSTATORY, TACTILE, OLFACTORY

Research suggestions

1. Which of the defining characteristics serve as critical indicators?
2. Are the characteristics used to define *sensory-perceptual alteration* measurable? If not, can they be replaced with lower-level terms that are measurable?

SEXUAL DYSFUNCTION

Issue

1. This diagnosis was originally labeled *sexuality*. Which label is more valid?

Research suggestion

1. Study nonverbalization of the problem versus verbalization of the problem as a defining characteristic.

SKIN INTEGRITY, IMPAIRMENT OF: ACTUAL

Issues

1. Consider recombining *actual* and *potential skin integrity, impairment of.*
2. Provide consistency between the two diagnoses by:
   a. Add to etiology: "excretions/secretions."
   b. Use "immunologic" not "immunologic deficit."
   c. Move "psychogenic" to actual etiologies.
   d. Change "altered sensation" to "decreased sensation."
   e. Change "altered circulation" to "decreased circulation."
3. Consider removing the separation of "external" and "internal" etiology.
4. Add "edema" to etiology.

SKIN INTEGRITY, IMPAIRMENT OF: POTENTIAL

See discussion under *Skin integrity, impairment of, actual*

SLEEP PATTERN DISTURBANCE

Issues

1. Define sleep.
2. What outcomes can the nurse reasonably expect from interventions?
3. How does this diagnosis differ from the medical label "insomnia"?

Research suggestions

1. What are the long-term effects of not sleeping well?
2. If this is more than one diagnosis, how do the interventions differ?
3. Can additional etiologies be identified?

SOCIAL ISOLATION

Issues

1. High-risk factors include being elderly, female, member of an ethnic/racial minority, disadvantaged educationally or economically, handicapped, and suffering physical, mental, or chronic illness. Should *social isolation (potential)* be considered a diagnostic label?

2. Social isolation must be differentiated from solitude, which has no negative connotations for the individual, and loneliness, which is not perceived as imposed by others.

Research suggestions

1. Is "expression of feelings of aloneness imposed by others" a necessary and sufficient characteristic of the diagnosis *social isolation?*
2. This diagnosis describes an altered state of wellness. Is this repetitive of a statement of the population at risk?

SPIRITUAL DISTRESS (DISTRESS OF THE HUMAN SPIRIT)

Issues

1. Consider that *spiritual distress* may be an etiology for *sleep pattern disturbance.*
2. Consider *spiritual distress related to forgiveness* as a diagnostic label.
   A. Relationship with God characterized by:
   (1) Distance/separation/absence
   (2) Lack of belief
   (3) Uncertainty
   (4) Fear
   b. Lack of forgiveness experienced by:
   (1) Inability to feel God's forgiveness
       (a) Feels illness is a punishment for a real or imagined wrongdoing
       (b) Feels God only forgives if a person has demonstrated worthiness in some way
       (c) Believes God judges and expects more than what he/she has done
       (d) Feels God as being judgmental and demanding rather than gracious, loving, kind, and forgiving
   (2) Inability to forgive self
       (a) Is unable to accept self as is
       (b) Feels need to reach some level of perfection to be okay
       (c) Punishes self psychologically or physically for real or imagined wrongdoings
       (d) Engages in self-blame or, at the other extreme, denies all responsibility for problems
   (3) Inability to forgive others
       (a) Blames other people or things for circumstances as they are
       (b) Is unable to see other people or their actions realistically/objectively
       (c) Holds onto real or imagined injustices of other people
       (d) Feelings of being judged by others
3. Consider *spiritual distress related to love* as a diagnostic label.
   a. Relationship with God characterized by:
   (1) Distance/separation/absence
   (2) Lack of belief
   (3) Uncertainty
   (4) Fear
   b. Lack of loving relationships characterized by:
   (1) Lack of a healthy loving relationship with God or a transcendent power
       (a) Lack of belief in God or a higher power
       (b) Lack of love of God

          (c) Childlike, immature love of God, dependent type of love (expectations of God to magically take care of problems)

          (d) Feelings of distance or separateness from God

          (e) Unusual distress during normal trials of life

     (2) Lack of healthy self-love

          (a) Poor self-esteem and self-confidence

          (b) Inability to realistically accept self as worthwhile individual with strengths and weaknesses

          (c) Sees mostly weakness in self

          (d) Demonstrates false pride and selfishness

          (e) Inability to believe that "I am okay just because God loves me"

          (f) Feels unworthy of love of God or others

     (3) Lack of ability to give and receive love with others

          (a) Uses and manipulates others to get what is wanted

          (b) Feels others do not love them as they are, always must be something or do something for another to earn his love

          (c) Is able to love only those who meet his needs

          (d) Seldom able to experience closeness to another

4. Consider *spiritual distress related to hope* as a diagnostic label.

  a. Relationship with God characterized by:

     (1) Distance/separation/absence

     (2) Lack of belief

     (3) Uncertainty

  b. Lack of hope characterized by:

     (1) Sense that life is overwhelming

     (2) Feelings of futility

     (3) Feels no one, no higher being, nothing can or will help

     (4) Inability to provide self with even the smallest gratification

     (5) Feels loss of control over everything

     (6) Lacks belief in a future

     (7) Lacks vision of possible alternatives

     (8) Lacks belief that somehow the future could still be okay

     (9) Lacks belief in a transcendent purpose of being

     (10) Value of life placed on external things or individuals

     (11) Inability to experience love, caring, or trust in God, self, and others

     (12) Lacks motivation to help self and often refuses help of others

     (13) Wishes for lack of existence and even death

5. Consider *spiritual distress related to trust* as a diagnostic label.

  a. Relationship with God characterized by:

     (1) Distance/separation/absence

     (2) Lack of belief

     (3) Uncertainty

     (4) Fear

  b. Lack of trust characterized by:

     (1) Lack of openness with God or a higher being

     (2) Lack of faith in a transcendent power

     (3) Fear of God's intentions

     (4) Inability to find solace in difficult times

     (5) Uncomfortableness with awareness of self

(6) Gullibility

(7) Either total reliance on self or overdependence on others, little interdependence

(8) Little faith in self

(9) Feels need to be perfect before accepted by God and others

(10) Feelings of alienation and loneliness

(11) Inability to be open with others

(12) Manipulative relationships with others

(13) Feelings that only certain people and places are safe

(14) Fears and avoids new situations and new people

(15) Expects people to be unkind and undependable unless they have demonstrated to the contrary

(16) Wants prompt gratification, not being able to trust enough to wait

(17) Is less accepting of others, especially those who deviate from his ways of thinking, feeling, and behaving

6. Consider *spiritual distress related to meaning and purpose in life* as a diagnostic label.

   a. Relationship with God characterized by:

     (1) Distance/separation/absence

     (2) Lack of belief

     (3) Uncertainty

     (4) Fear

   b. Lack of meaning and purpose in life characterized by:

     (1) Lack of reason for living

     (2) Inability to find meaning in life's struggles

     (3) Inability to cope with life's struggles

     (4) Inability to know and thus act out one's true values

     (5) Lack of goals in life

     (6) Feelings of meaninglessness of life

     (7) Feelings of inner emptiness

     (8) Existential vacuum

       (a) Addictions

       (b) Juvenile or adult delinquency

       (c) Rampant sexual libido

     (9) A life goal of power

       (a) Goal of power through money

     (10) A life goal of pleasure

     (11) Complaints of dissatisfaction with marriage, vocation, and/or depression

     (12) Setting only one all-important goal to direct all activities

     (13) Trying to reach unattainable goals (for example, perfection)

     (14) Unclear values, beliefs, and goals

     (15) Conflicting values

     (16) Incongruence of life-style and true values

     (17) Lack of commitment

     (18) Conflict of beliefs with those of significant others

Research suggestions

1. What are the degrees of *spiritual distress?*

2. Do degrees of *spiritual distress* require different intervention?

3. What are the coping mechanisms one uses to "prevent" *spiritual distress* or maintain spiritual well-being?

4. Do a factor analysis of the identified critical indicators of *spiritual distress*. What are the psychologic responses to these indicators?
5. Is there a possibility of different definitions, that is, religious vs. spiritual?
6. What do other disciplines see as the nurse's role in spiritual needs?
7. What are patient's perceptions of the nurse's role in meeting spiritual needs?
8. Conduct case studies to document behavior in measurable terminology.

References*

Allport, G.: The individual and his religion, New York, 1950, Macmillan.

Baskerville, N.T.: Another dimension of care: spiritual consolation. American Cancer Society: Proceedings of national conference on cancer nursing, New York, 1974, The Society.

Byrne, M., and Thompson, L.: Key concepts for the study and practice of nursing, St. Louis, 1972, The C.V. Mosby Co.

Campbell, C.: Nursing diagnosis and intervention in nursing practice, 1978, John Wiley & Sons, Inc.

Carlson, C.E.: Behavioral concepts and nursing intervention, Philadelphia, 1970, J.B. Lippincott Co.

Clemance, M.: Existentialism: a philosophy of commitment, Am. J. Nurs. **66**:500, 1966.

Dickinson, C.: The search for spiritual meaning, Am. J. Nurs. **75**(10):1789, 1975.

Draper, E., and others: On the diagnostic value of religious ideation, Arch. Gen. Psychiatry **13**:202, 1965.

DuGas, B.W.: Introduction to patient care: A comprehensive approach to nursing, ed. 3, Philadelphia, 1977, W.B. Saunders Co.

Duncan, F.D.: Pastoral care of disabled persons. In Oates, W.E., and Lester, A.D., eds.: Pastoral care in crucial human situations, Valley Forge, Pa., 1969, Judson Press.

Fish, S., and Shelley, J.A.: Spiritual care: the nurse's role, Downers Grove, Ill., 1978, Inter-Varsity Press.

Frankl, V.E.: Man's search for meaning: an introduction to logotherapy, New York, 1963, Washington Square Press.

Gebbie, K.M.: Classification of nursing diagnoses: summary of the second national conference. St. Louis, 1976, Clearinghouse-National Group for Classification of Nursing Diagnoses.

Gruendemann, B.J.: Hospital chaplain: the "now" member of the health team, RN **37**(10):38, 1973.

Henderson, V., and Nite, G.: Principle and practice of nursing, ed. 6, New York, 1978, Macmillan Publishing Co., Inc.

Hubert, M.: For every patient, J. Nurs. Educ. **2**(2):9, 1963.

Hulme, W.E.: Dialogue in despair, Nashville, Tenn., 1968, Abingdon Press.

James, W.: The varieties of religious experience, New York, 1929, Random House, Inc.

Journard, S.M.: The transparent self, Princeton, N.J., 1964, Van Nostrand Reinhold Co.

Jung, C.G.: Modern man in search of a soul, New York, 1931, Harcourt Brace Jovanovich, Inc.

Jung, C.G.: Psychology and religion, New Haven, Conn., 1964, Yale University Press.

Kelly, L.Y.: Dimensions of professional nursing, ed. 3, New York, 1975, Macmillan Publishing Co., Inc.

Kiening, M.M.: Spiritual needs of the psychiatric patient. In Dunlap, L., ed.: Mental health concepts and nursing practice, New York, 1978, John Wiley & Sons, Inc.

Kinget, G.M.: On being human: a systematic view, New York, 1975, Harcourt Brace Jovanovich, Inc.

Manfreda, M.L.: Psychiatric nursing, ed. 9, Philadelphia, 1973, F.A. Davis Co.

Maslow, A.H.: New knowledge in human values, Chicago, 1959, Henry Regnery Co.

Maslow, A.H.: Toward a psychology of being, ed. 2, New York, 1968, Van Nostrand Reinhold Co.

Maslow, A.H.: The farther reaches of human nature, New York, 1971a, The Viking Press, Inc.

Maslow, A.H.: Religions, values and peak experiences, New York, 1971b, The Viking Press, Inc.

*Provided in 1978.

McGreeby, A., and Van Heukelem, J.: Crying: the neglected dimension, Can. Nurse **72**(1):19, 1976.

Medicine and Religion Committee: Religious aspects of medical care: a handbook of religious practices of all faiths, Rochester, Minn., 1976, Zumbro Valley Medical Society.

Meininger, K.: Whatever became of sin? New York, 1973, Hawthorn Books, Inc.

Murray, R., and Zentner, J.: Nursing concepts for health promotion, Englewood Cliffs, N.J., 1975, Prentice-Hall, Inc.

Naugle, E.H.: The difference caring makes, Am. J. Nurs. **73**:1890, 1973.

Niklas, G.R., and Stafanice, C.: Ministry to the hospitalized, New York, 1975, Paulist Press.

Oates, W.E., and Lester, A.D., eds.: Pastoral care in crucial human situations, Valley Forge, Pa., 1966, Judson Press.

Paige, R.L., and Looney, J.F.: Hospice care for the adult, Am. J. Nurs. **77**(11):1812, 1977.

Peipgras, R.: The other dimension: spiritual help, Am. J. Nurs. **68**(12):2610, 1968.

Perrine, G.: Needs met and unmet, Am. J. Nurs. **71**(11):2128, 1971.

Powell, J.: A reason to live! a reason to die! Niles, Ill., 1975, Argus Communications.

Pumphrey, J.B.: Recognizing your patients' spiritual needs, Nursing '77 **7**(12):64, 1977.

Recognizing your patients' spiritual needs, Nurs. Update **6**(7):3, 1975.

Rines, A., and Montag, M.: Nursing concepts and nursing care, New York, 1976, John Wiley & Sons, Inc.

Southard, S.: Religion and nursing, Nashville, Tenn., 1959, Broadman Press.

Stallwood, J., and Stoll, R.: Spiritual dimensions of nursing practice. In Beland, I.L., and Passos, J.Y., eds.: Clinical nursing, New York, 1975, Macmillan Publishing Co., Inc.

Torres, G., and Yura, H.: Today's conceptual framework: its relationship to the curriculum development process, Nat. League Nurs. Pub. 15:1529, 1974.

Tournier, P.: The healing of persons, New York, 1965, Harper & Row, Publishers.

Travelbee, J.: Interpersonal aspects of nursing, Philadelphia, 1966, F.A. Davis Co.

Vaillet, M.C.: Hope: the restoration of being, Am. J. Nurs. **70**(2):270, 1970.

White House Conference on Aging: Spiritual well-being, Washington, D.C., 1971, U.S. Government Printing Office.

Wygant, W.E.: Dying, but not alone, Am. J. Nurs. **67**(3):572, 1967.

Research projects*

A list of unpublished Master's theses related to the spiritual needs of patients, all by nurses. These resources may prove useful to students who wish to conduct further study.

Blecke, J.R.: Development of a tool for determining appropriate nursing actions in meeting spiritual needs of patients in selected situations, Seattle, 1963, University of Washington.

Byles, L.S.: A survey of pediatric hospitals in the United States to describe the available facilities, personnel, programs, policies, and activities designed to meet the spiritual needs of hospitalized children, Seattle, 1961, University of Washington.

Chance, J.P.L.: Nurses' responses to patients' spiritual needs, Loma Linda, Calif., 1967, Loma Linda University.

Fish, S.A.: Man and his needs in the presence of illness, Rochester, N.Y., 1973, University of Rochester.

†Flesner, R.: Development of a measure to assess spiritual distress in the responsive adult, Milwaukee, 1981, Marquette University.

Kealey, C.: The patients' perspective on spiritual needs, Columbia, Mo., 1974, University of Missouri-Columbia.

Kramer, P.: A survey to determine the attitudes and knowledge of a selected group of professional nurses concerning spiritual care of the patient, Portland, 1957, University of Oregon.

---

*Compiled from Fish, S., and Shelly, J.A.: Spiritual care: the nurse's role, Downers Grove, Ill., 1978, Inter-Varsity Press.

†Content from this work served as basis for developmental work on diagnosis labels related to spiritual distress at the Fifth National Conference.

Lewis, J.E.: A resource unit on spiritual aspects of nursing for the basic nursing curriculum of a selected school of nursing, Seattle, 1957, University of Washington.

Nelson, B.E.: How graduate nurses in maternal child care health (MCH) perceive their role in the spiritual dimension of nursing care: a survey, Boston, 1976, Boston University.

THOUGHT PROCESSES, ALTERATION IN

Issues

1. The previous diagnosis list (1980), *conciousness, altered level of,* cannot be subsumed under the diagnosis *thought processes, alteration in,* which is on the TBD list.
2. *Thought processes, alteration in* is a separate diagnosis with defining characteristics of disorientation to time, place, or person; alteration in attentiveness (distractibility, altered ability to follow commands); alteration in motor response (voluntary or involuntary); absence of any meaningful response to stimulation; and altered reflex response to stimuli (increased and decreased, pupillary, gag/swallow, cough, corneal). The etiology may be neurologic, functional, or chemical.

Research suggestions

1. Are the characteristics used to define this diagnosis measurable? If not, can they be replaced with more concrete terms that are measurable?
2. What is the relationship between levels of awareness and ability to engage in specified thought processes?
3. Which of the defining characteristics for impaired thought processes and lower levels of consciousness are critical for use of the diagnostic label? Can the defining characteristics be ranked from the critical to those that might be present?

TISSUE PERFUSION, ALTERATION IN: CEREBRAL, CARDIOPULMONARY, RENAL, GASTROINTESTINAL, PERIPHERAL

Issue

1. Consider dividing this diagnosis into four categories: cerebral, cardiopulmonary, renal, and gastrointestinal.

Research suggestion

1. For each of the new categories proposed above, ask: What are the etiologies of this diagnosis? What are the defining characteristics?

References

Brantigan, C.O.: Hemodynamic monitoring: interpreting values. Am. J. Nurs. **82**:86, 1982.

Campbell, C.: Nursing diagnosis and intervention in nursing practice, New York, 1978, John Wiley & Sons, Inc.

Lamb, L.: Think you know septic shock. Nursing '82 **12**(1):34, 1982.

URINARY ELIMINATION, ALTERATION IN PATTERNS

Issue

1. Consider adding an additional diagnosis *Urinary elimination, alteration in: alteration in urine formation.*

Research suggestion

1. Review currently available research and use for validation studies of etiology and characteristics.

VIOLENCE, POTENTIAL FOR: SELF-DIRECTED OR DIRECTED AT OTHERS

Issues

1. This diagnosis has some relationship to the TBD diagnosis *self-harm, potential for*. *Violence* has a stronger meaning than *self-harm*, which includes acting with the intent of self-destruction, or the outcome of self-destruction, including self-neglect and suicide.
2. The diagnosis *self-harm, potential for* is easier to share with a patient than the diagnosis *violence, potential for*.
3. Develop the diagnosis *violence, potential for: self-directed* separate from the diagnosis *violence, potential for: directed at others*.
4. As an alternative, use the label *self-harm: potential for* instead of *violence, potential for: self-directed*.
5. The rationale for the alternatives listed above includes the fact that the small group discussing this diagnosis could not deal clearly with etiologies and defining characteristics that would fit *both* self-directed and other-directed violence.
6. Practitioners have identified that both the defining characteristics and the interventions are different for self-directed and other-directed violence.

Research suggestions

1. What are the anthropologic differences in cultural backgrounds that would indicate *violence, potential for?*
2. Is there a difference between the potential for self-directed violence and violence directed at others? Does this extend beyond the definition to differences in etiology, defining characteristics, and nursing interventions?
3. Is the diagnosis viable, valid in practice?
4. What is the relationship of *fear* to *violence, potential for?*
5. What is the relationship of anger to *violence, potential for?*
6. What level of anxiety is present with this diagnosis?
7. What level of patient awareness is present with this diagnosis?
8. What are the etiologies and defining characteristics for *violence, potential for* and/or *suicide, potential for?*
9. Is there a difference between *self-harm, potential for* and *violence, potential for: self-directed?*

References

American Psychiatric Association: Diagnostic and statistical manual of mental disorders, ed. 3, Washington, D.C., 1980, The Association.

Bandura, A.: Aggression: a social learning analysis, Englewood Cliffs, N.J., 1973, Prentice-Hall, Inc.

Diagnoses to be developed

This section provides available work on these diagnoses except Rest-activity pattern, ineffective, and Role disturbance, which were not examined at this conference. The materials are presented to stimulate inquiry and movement toward more specific action at a later conference. Although the materials are extensive, the contents have not been reviewed adequately for approval by the conference participants.

Aggressive coping mode*

Aggressive responsive state*

Cognitive dissonance†

Consciousness, altered levels of*

Decision making, impaired/ineffective

Dependent coping mode*

Depleted health potential*

Impulse-dominated state*

Impulsive coping mode*

Manipulative coping mode*

Memory deficit†

Rational anger state*

Rest-activity pattern, ineffective

Role disturbance

Self-harm*

Self-exhaltation state*

Social network support, alteration in*

Subtle obstructive mode*

Victim abuse syndrome*

AGGRESSIVE COPING MODE

Etiology

Lacks theoretic consensus. Several psychologic theories offer different explanations for individuals who, over a long period, develop a pattern of aggressive responses to problem-solving behaviors.

Defining characteristics

One or more of the following four patterns:

History of repeated assaultiveness

History of property destruction

History of using force to achieve wants/goals

Patterned, repetitive inappropriate aggression

Improverished ability to resolve anger through discussion

Hostility

---

*Addition from 1982 conference.

†Suggested deletion.

Perceptually distorted world view
Impaired judgment
Impaired reality testing
Impaired concentration
Limited self-insight
Rejecting toward intervention
Physically tense
Unpredictable
Long-standing tumultuous family relationships
Grandiosity
Sullen facial expression
Resentful manner
Rationalization of own actions
Projection of responsibility
Restlessness
Disregard for realistic consequences
Easily irritated
Lacking in compliance/cooperation

Comment

Low to moderate amenability to independent nursing therapy

Reference

See *aggressive responsive state*

AGGRESSIVE RESPONSIVE STATE

Etiology

A perceived threat to personal security
Acting-out defense for internal conflict
Overresponding to frustration or general emotional arousal
Transference reactions
Physiologic factors such as hormonal and biochemical alterations, temporal lobe or anterior hypothalamic brain pathology, hypoglycemia, food, drug, or substance allergies, and toxic brain states

Defining characteristics

Temporary state
Verbal threats of harming others
Physical aggression such as hitting, throwing objects, biting
Agitation
Argumentative
Verbally abusive, sarcastic, belittling
Irrational behavior
Hostility
Impaired judgment
Impaired reality testing
Limited self-insight
Rejects attempts at intervention
Physically tense
Perceptually distorted world view
Rationalization of own actions
Projection of responsibility

Perception of goal conflict or blockage
Impoverished ability to resolve anger through discussion
Excessive concern with inconsequential ideas
Sullen expression
Resentful
Unpredictable

Comment

Low to high degree of amenability to independent nursing therapy, depends on etiology

References

Brown, M., and Fowler, G.: Psychodynamic nursing, ed. 3, Philadelphia, 1966, W.B. Saunders Co.

Bursten, B.: The manipulator: a psychoanalytic view, New Haven, Conn., 1973, Yale University Press.

Carney, F.: Treatment of the aggressive patient. In Madden, D., and Lion J., eds.: Rage, hate, assault and other forms of violence, New York, 1976, Spectrum Publications, Inc.

Clunn, P.: Potential for violence, a handout sheet at the Fourth National Conference on the Classification of Nursing Diagnoses, 1980.

Coleman, J.: Abnormal psychology and modern life, ed. 4, Glenview, Ill., 1972 Scott, Foresman & Co.

Cuthbert, B.: Switch off, tune in, turn on, Am. J. Nurs. **69:**1206, 1969.

Gordon, M: Historical perspective: the national conference group for classification of nursing diagnoses. In Kim, M.J., and Moritz, D.A., eds: Classification of nursing diagnoses: proceedings of the third and fourth national conferences, New York, 1982, McGraw-Hill Book Co.

Group for the Advancement of Psychiatry: Toward therapeutic care, ed. 2, New York, 1970, The Group.

Gruber, K., and Schniewind, H.: Letting anger work for you, Am. J. Nurs. **76:**1450, 1976.

Karshner, J.: The application of social learning theory of aggression, Perspect. Psychiatr. Care. **16:**223, 1978.

Kiening, M.: Hostility. In Carlson, C., ed.: Behavioral concepts and nursing intervention, Philadelphia, 1970, J.B. Lippincott Co.

Kutash, I., and others, eds.: Violence: prespectives on murder and aggression, San Francisco, Calif., 1978, Jossey-Bass, Inc. Publishers.

Kyes, J., and Hofling, C.: Basic psychiatric concepts in nursing, ed. 3, Philadelphia, 1974, J.B. Lippincott.

Loomis, M.: Nursing management of acting-out behavior, Perspect. Psychiatr. Care **8:**168, 1970.

Luetje, V.: The person whose behavior is abusive. In Murray, R., and Huelskoetter, M., eds.: Psychiatric-mental health nursing: giving emotional care, Englewood Cliffs, N.J., Prentice-Hall, Inc. (In Press.)

Matheney, R., and Topalis, M.: Psychiatric nursing, ed. 4, St. Louis, 1965, The C.V. Mosby Co.

Mereness, D., and Karnash, L.: Essentials of psychiatric nursing, ed. 7, St. Louis, 1966, The C.V. Mosby Co.

Moritz, D.A.: Understanding anger, Am. J. Nurs. **78:**81, 1978.

Moyer, K.E.: The physiology of aggression and the implication for aggression control. In Singer, J., ed.: The control of aggression and violence, New York, 1971, Academic Press, Inc.

Rogers, C.: Characteristics of a helping relationship, Can. Ment. Health. **27**(suppl.):1, 1962.

Rouslin, S.: Developmental aggression and its consequences, Perspect Psychiatr. Care **8:**170, 1975.

Scherer, K.R., Abeles, R., and Fischer, C.: Human aggresion and conflict, Englewood Cliffs, N.J., 1975, Prentice-Hall, Inc.

Sundeen, S., and others: Nurse-client interaction: implementing the nursing process, St Louis, 1976, C.V. Mosby Co.

Wolfgang, M.: Violence in the family. In Kutash, I., and others, eds.: Violence: perspectives on murder and aggression, San Francisco, Calif. 1978, Jossey-Bass, Inc., Publishers.

CONCIOUSNESS, ALTERED LEVELS OF

Etiology
>Neurologic
>Functional
>Chemical

Defining characteristics
>Disorientation to time, place, or person
>Alteration in attentiveness
>>Distractibility
>>Altered ability to follow commands
>Alteration in motor response
>>Voluntary
>>Involuntary
>Absence of any meaningful response to stimulation
>Altered reflex response to stimuli: increased or decreased
>>Pupil
>>Gag
>>Cough
>>Corneal

DECISION MAKING: IMPAIRED INEFFECTIVE

Etiology
>Stress
>Anxiety
>Unachieved developmental tasks
>Toxic substances
>Addiction
>Lack of elimination of toxins
>Chemical imbalance
>Crisis
>Ambiguity of choice
>Life changes
>Life-style
>>Cognitive problems
>>Economics
>>Resources
>Developmental level/maturity

Defining characteristics
>Inability to identify alternatives
>Inability to choose from alternatives
>Fails to take decisive action

Issues
>Consider changing label to lack of ability to make decisions

DEPENDENT COPING MODE

Etiology
>1. Response to dysfunctional early parenting
>2. Regression under severe stress or chronic illness

Defining characteristics

Resistance to self-care
Repetitive statements of helplessness
Clinging manner
Overt anxiety
Unverifiable somatic complaints
Frequent demands on staff
Inappropriate "sweet" behavior
Attention seeking
Extreme compliance

Comment

Moderate amenability to independent nursing therapy

Reference

See *aggressive coping mode*

DEPLETED HEALTH POTENTIAL

Definition

Depleted health status that interferes with one's ability to grow or change (as defined by client)

Defining characteristics

Verbalizes a decreased perceived health status
Verbalizes a high level of stress
Mobility and exercise
Problem solving
Social contact characterized by tension
Nutritional status inadequate

Comments

1. Concept must be explored.
2. Useful in ambulatory setting.
3. Definition of depleted: can restore or improve to a new balance.
4. There is little difference between "depleted" and "altered."

References

Anderson, M.: A psychosocial tool for ambulatory health care clients: a pilot study of validity, Nurs. Res. **29**:347, 1980.

Belloc, N., and Breslow, L.: Relationship of physical health status and health practices, Prev. Med. **1**:409, 1972.

Breslow, L.: Risk factor intervention for health maintenance, Science **200**:908, 1978.

Breslow, L., and Enstrom, J.: Persistance of health habits and their relationship to mortality, Prev. Med. **9**:469, 1980.

Claus, K., and Bailey, J., eds.: Living with stress and promoting well-being: a handbook of nurses, St. Louis, 1980, The C.V. Mosby Co.

Evans, S.: Descriptive criteria for the concept of depleted health potential, Adv. Nurs. Sci. **1**:67, 1979.

Giordano, S., and Everly, J.: Controlling stress and tension, Englewood Cliffs, N.J., 1979, Prentice-Hall, Inc.

Hollen, P.: A holistic model of individual and family health based on a continuum of choice, Adv. Nurs. Sci. **3**:27, 1981.

Jalowiec, A., and Powers, M.: Stress and coping in hypertension and emergency room patients, Nurs. Res. **30**:10, 1981.

Newman, M.: Theory development in nursing, Philadelphia, 1979, F.A. Davis Co.

Pelletier, K.: Mind as healer: mind as slayer, New York, 1977, Delacorte.

Pesznecker, B., and McNeil, J.: Relationship among health habits, social assets, psychological well-being, life change, and alterations in health status, Nurs. Res. 24:442, 1975.

Rogers, M.: Nursing: a science of unitary man. In Riehl, J., and Roy, Sister C., eds.: Conceptual models for nursing practice, ed. 2, New York, 1980, Appleton-Century-Crofts.

Schwerin, H., and others: Food eating pattern and health: a reexamination of the Ten-State and HANES I survey, Am. J. Clin. Nutr. 34:568, 1981.

Shaw, S.: Health education for the public: stress and stress management, Top. Clin. Nurs. 1:53, 1979.

Sutterly, D.: Stress and health: a survey of self-regulation modalities, Top. Clin. Nurs. 1:1, 1979.

Travis, J.: Wellness workbook, Mill Valley, Calif., 1977, Wellness Resource Center.

Wan, T.: Predicting self-assessed health status: a multivariate approach, Health Serv. Res. 11(4): 464, 1976.

Wan, T.: Health people, The Surgeon General's Report on Health Promotion and Disease Prevention, U.S. Department of Health, Education and Welfare, Pub No. 79-55071, Washington, D.C., 1979, U.S. Government Printing Office.

IMPULSE-DOMINATED STATE

Etiology

Ego insufficiently regulating instincts or drives, related to organic and/or psychologic states

Defining characteristics

Temporary state
Excitable beyond cultural range of acceptability
Fearful of others or of external environment
Behavior that disregards realistic consequences
Labile affect
Low tolerance for frustration
Lacking in compliance/cooperation
High overall activity level
Restlessness
Unpredictable
Impaired concentration
Impaired judgment
Impaired reality testing
Indirect aggression
Passively resistant
Inability to verbalize frustration
Perception of goal conflict or blockage
Rejecting toward intervention
Exposes self or others to harm or danger

Comments

Low to high amenability to independent nursing therapy dependent on etiologic factors

References

See *aggressive coping mode* and Luetje's presentation at Fifth National Conference.

IMPULSIVE COPING MODE

Etiology

Perceptual and/or learning disabilities
Nutritional imbalances, food allergies
Dysfunctional parenting styles

Defining characteristics

History of hasty, heedless actions
Childhood history of nonviolent disciplinary problems
History of sudden and multiple school or job changes
Lack of meaningful friendships
High overall activity level
React to momentary concerns
History of sudden geographic relocations
History of many romantic liaisons
Inability to adequately verbalize frustration
Low tolerance for frustration
Long-standing tumultuous family relationships
Indirect aggression
Passive resistance
Makes frequent demands on staff
Overtly anxious
Unverifiable somatic complaints
Labile

Comments

Low to moderate amenability to independent nursing therapy once the mode is established; potentially high amenability to independent nursing therapy in a preventive or very early treatment situation

References

See *aggressive coping mode*

MANIPULATIVE COPING MODE

Etiology

Lacks theoretic consensus. Several psychologic theories offer different explanations for individuals who adapt this pattern over time.

Defining characteristics

Pattern and repetitive use of others to own advantage
Perceived goal conflicts with others
Conscious intent to influence other person
Conscious deception and insincerity
Feeling of "having put something over" on another
Inability to adequately verbalize frustration
Apparent lack of fear of sensitivity to others/environment
Excessively concerned with inconsequential ideas
Resentful
Rationalization of own actions
Projection of responsibility
Procrastination

Intentional failures
Indirect expression of aggression
Passive resistance
Extreme compliance

Comments

Low amenability to independent nursing therapy

Reference

See *aggressive coping mode*

RATIONAL ANGER STATE

Etiology

Health-appropriate needs and desires frustrated by external factors.

Defining characteristics

Temporary state
Direct expression of anger
Degree of manifested anger is reasonable to assist in relation to provoking stimulus
Anger is expressed in a manner that is reasonable to the assessor in relation to ethnic
    mores of the client and prevailing community
Behavior is goal directed
Mental alertness
Oriented
Angry facial expression
Organized thinking
Physically tense
Sudden expression
Restlessness

References

See *aggressive coping mode*

SELF-HARM

Definition

The act or potential to act with the intent of self-destruction or the outcome of self-destruction. Behaviors include a wide range of intensity from self-neglect to an active suicide attempt.

Etiology

Impaired impulse control
Impaired judgment
Chronic or acute illness
Pain
Life change, positive or negative
Crisis from life change, situational or transition
Collapse of support systems
Low self-esteem
Limited or ineffective decision making
Unable to generate alternatives
Signs of depression, for example, decreased intake
Noncompliance with medical regimen

Defining characteristics

Current self-harm behavior
Verbal statement of intent, desire of plan to harm self
Previous behavior, attempt
Self-derogatory statements
Signs of depression
Decreased self-care
Isolated/seclusive
Sudden/dramatic mood elevation
Egocentricity
Increased anxiety
Delerious
No future plans
Putting effects in order
Verbal expression of helplessness and hopelessness
Feeling of "can't take it"
Delusive-vigilant fears
Deliberate noncompliance with medical regimen

Comment

Seen as different from *violence, potential for*

References

Batchelor, I.R.C.: Suicide in old age. In Farberow, N., and Schneidman, E., eds.: Cues to suicide, New York, 1957, McGraw-Hill Book Co.

Dorpat, T., and others: The relationship of physical illness to suicide, In Resnik, H.L.P., ed.: Suicidal behaviors: diagnosis and management, Boston, 1968, Little, Brown & Co.

Gage, F.B.: Suicide in the aged, Am. J. Nurs. **71**:2153, 1971.

Hart, N., and Keidel, G.: The suicidal adolescent, Am. J. Nurs. **79**:81, 1979.

Litman, R., and Farberow, N.: Emerging evaluation of self-destructive potentiality. In Farberow, N., and Schneidman, E., eds.: The cry for help, New York, 1961, McGraw-Hill Book Co.

Schneidman, E.: Preventing suicide, Am. J. Nurs. **65**:111, 1965.

Tabachnick, N., and Farberow, N.: The assessment of self-destruction potential. In Farberow, N., and Schneidman, E., eds.: The cry for help, New York, 1961, McGraw-Hill Book Co.

Weiss, J.: Suicide in the aged. In Resnik, H.C.P., ed.: Suicidal behaviors: diagnosis and management, Boston, 1968, Little, Brown & Co.

Westercamp, T.: Suicide, Am. J. Nurs. **75**:260, 1975.

SELF-EXHALTATION STATE

Etiology

Possible genetic and/or biochemical alterations
Defensive coping maneuvers of denial and overcompensation

Defining characteristics

Temporary state
Pervasive grandiose thinking
Impaired judgment
Impaired insight
Impaired reality testing
Irritability

Extreme verbosity
Excitable
Resentful
Agitated
Projection of responsibility
Lack of intentional deception or insincerity

Comment

Low to moderate amenability to independent nursing therapy

Reference

See *aggressive coping mode*

SOCIAL NETWORK SUPPORT, ALTERATION IN

Definition

Personal social network—a system of social interactions an individual has that functions to provide support, affirmation, validation, and information about one's environment and/or material assistance. It is generally stable and reciprocal and is maintained through interaction. The network is described in family patterns, neighboring patterns, or friendship patterns.

Etiology

Change in the network
    Alteration in structure (loss of member, relocation)
    Alteration in availability (decreased frequency of interaction)
    Decreased ability of network to continue to meet demands of individual
Change in individual's situation without a reciprocal change in the social network
    Stressful event (illness, change in role)
    Institutionalization
    Decrease or increase in mobility
    Increased demands caused by chronic disease
    Decreased ability of individual to meet network demand

Defining characteristics

Inadequate or overload in number of members
Inadequate pattern of interaction (quality and quantity)
Traumatic role change within network
Lack of interconnectedness within the network
Inability of the network to meet the demands of the individual
Knowledge deficit regarding resources and functioning of network

Comments

Rating of independent nursing therapy involved in preventing, treating, or resolving the health problem: high degree

Issues

1. This is similar to *social isolation*; the difference is in the perspective of subculture information. The taxonomy should describe the relationship.
2. An additional diagnosis in this group that should be developed is *radical change in life situation resulting in no social network*, for example, moving from another country, moving to a new part of the country, radically altering social role.

Research suggestions

1. Study the effects of overload of network as an alteration.
2. Utilize literature and available studies to validate defining characteristics.
3. Restate a definition of the diagnosis itself, not just one term of the definition.

REFERENCES

Balkeland, F., and Lundwall, L.: Dropping out of treatment: a critical review, Psychol. Bull. **82:**738, 1975.

Cassel, J.: The contribution of the social environment to host resistance, Am. J. Epidemiol. **104:**107, 1976.

Cobb, S.: Presidential Address—1976, social support as a moderator of life stress, Psychosom. Med. **38**:300, 1976.

Dean, A., and Linn, N.: The stress-buffering role of social support: problems and prospects for systematic investigation, J. Nerv. Ment. Dis. **165**:403, 1977.

Finlayson, A.: Social networks as coping resources, Soc. Sci. Med. **10**:97, 1976.

Murawski, B., Penman, D., and Schmitt, M.: Social support in health and illness: the concept and its measurement, Cancer Nurs. **1**:365, 1978.

Norbeck, J.S.: Social support: a model for clinical research and application, Adv. Nurs. Sci. **3**:43, 1981.

Norbeck, J.S., Lindsey, A.M., and Carrieri, V.L.: The development of an instrument to measure social support, Nurs. Res. **30**:264, 1981.

SUBTLE OBSTRUCTIVE MODE

Definition

Pattern of using indirect measures to respond to autonomy, authority, and dependency conflicts

Etiology

TBD

Defining characteristics

Repeatedly fails to follow through on promises or agreements
Procrastinates
Seemingly intentional failures
Indirect aggression
Passively resistant
Extreme compliance
Perceived goal conflict with others
Lack of obvious irritability, anxiety, dismay, agitation, frustration, or anger

Comment

Moderate amenability to independent nursing therapy

Reference

See *aggressive coping mode*

VICTIM ABUSE SYNDROME

Etiology

TBD

Defining characteristics

Emotional reactions to assault
    Short-term:
        Helplessness
        Irritability
        Fear of returning to scene
        Feelings of resignation
        Sadness
        Depressed
        Anger
        Anxiety
        Shock

Apathy
Disbelief
Self-blame
Dependence
Long-term:
Fear
Anger
Anxiety
Social reactions to assault
Short-term:
Change in relationship with others
Difficulty in engaging in one's normal activities
Feeling sorry for person who assaulted
Feeling should have done something to prevent assault
Long-term:
Feeling sorry for person who assaulted
Biophysiologic reactions to assault
Short-term:
Startle response
Sleep pattern disturbance
Soreness
Headaches
Long-term:
Body tension
Soreness
Cognitive reactions to assault
Short-term:
Denial
Change in life-style
Long-term:
Anger with authority
Blaming authority

Research suggestion

1. What factors influence blame placement?
2. How do you teach nursing skills to deal with violent patients?

CHAPTER 7

State of the art of nursing diagnosis

The editors developed this chapter after the conference to provide up-to-date information on nursing diagnoses in the literature. McLane and Fehring provide a critical review of the nursing diagnosis literature. In addition, six books, including a manual, on nursing diagnosis are reviewed in a conventional manner to keep the readers abreast of the field and to encourage critical thinking that is required for the growth of the nursing diagnosis work.

Nursing diagnosis: a review of the literature

AUDREY M. McLANE, R.N., Ph.D.
RICHARD J. FEHRING, R.N., D.N.Sc.

More than 25 years ago, Abdellah (1957, p. 4) published an article in nursing's only research journal, *Nursing Research*, in which she defined a nursing diagnosis as ". . . a determination of the nature and extent of nursing problems *(presented)* by individual patients or families receiving care." She went on to define a nursing problem as ". . . a condition faced by the patient or family which the nurse can assist him or them to meet through the performance of her professional activities" (Abdellah, 1957, p. 4). One year earlier, Hornung attempted to define the term *nursing diagnosis*, but it is clear that she confused *a medical diagnosis made by a nurse* with a nursing diagnosis (Hornung, 1956).

A modification of Webster's dictionary definition of diagnosis was used by Chambers (1962, p. 102) to develop a definition of nursing diagnosis: "A working definition of nursing diagnosis is a careful investigation of the facts to determine the nature of the nursing problem." Chambers' most significant contribution to early discussions of nursing diagnosis was her insistence that nursing diagnoses be limited to those areas legally defined as being the province of the professional nurse.

Komorita attempted to lay to rest nurses' concerns about invading the medical domain by stating unequivocally that nurses do indeed make diagnoses, that is, "they recognize and identify the nature and extent of their patient's need for nursing care." She defined a nursing diagnosis as ". . . a conclusion based on a scientific determination of an individual's nursing needs . . ." (Komorita, 1963, pp. 83-84). The focus on individual needs as the *prime element* in the process of diagnosis was shared by others, such as Rothberg (1967), Soares (1978), and Yura and Walsh (1967).

With the exception of Komorita, the preceding definitions, most of which span a period of about 10 years, demonstrate a concern more for the *diagnostic process* than for the *outcome of the diagnostic process*, that is, the label or problem statement.

In 1966 Durand and Prince spelled out the diagnostic process in detail with emphasis not only on the diagnostic process and the actual diagnoses but also on the complex thinking processes that are required to make a diagnosis. Of particular historic significance was their calling attention to the importance of *pattern recognition* to arrive at a nursing diagnosis. In addition, Durand and Prince differentiated a descriptive diagnosis from an etiologic diagnosis, with the former describing the state of the patient and the latter suggesting pertinent nursing care. A tentative diagnosis was viewed as an hypothesis "which structured and stimulated the nurse's search for more information" whereas an actual diagnosis established a "point of departure, a basis for nursing care" (Durand and Prince, 1966, p. 58).

PROBABLE ETIOLOGIES

The importance of locating probable cause(s), etiologies, is a recurring theme in the literature on definitions of nursing diagnosis. Referring to nursing diagnosis as a process of clinical inference (again a focus on process, not label), Aspinall (1976, p. 434) stated, ". . . if it (diagnosis) is arrived at accurately and intelligently, it will lead to identification of the possible causes of symptomatology." A two-part diagnostic statement was also proposed by Mundinger and Jauron (1975, p. 96) ". . . so that the unhealthful response and contributing factors are both identified." They encouraged use of a "related to" phrase to connect the clauses instead of "due to," since the former does not mean that one clause ". . . causes or is responsible for the other clause" (Mundinger and Jauron, 1975, p. 97). However, later in the same article in a discussion of possible and potential diagnoses, they refer to etiology as causal: "If the causal factor is suspected or known and only the response is questioned, the diagnosis will have two clauses" (Mundinger and Jauron, 1975, p. 98). About the same time, Gordon (1976, p. 8) proposed a definition stating that nursing diagnoses ". . . describe actual or potential health problems which nurses, by virtue of their education and experience, are capable and licensed to treat." Although Gordon (1976, p. 7) seems to subscribe to the idea of treating the "health problem," she emphasized the importance of differentiation among possible etiologies ". . . because each may require different therapy." The importance of etiology was given further impetus with the development of a structural definition of a nursing diagnosis. The structural components described by Gordon were problem, etiology, and signs and symptoms, the PES format. "There may be multiple etiologic subcategories for a particular problem . . ." (Gordon, 1979a, p. 490).

The idea of etiology/cause as the key element in the diagnostic statement gained acceptance rapidly and is reflected in Derdiarian's admonition (1977, p. 19): "Until we till the field in this fashion, by classifying nursing diagnoses in some manner related to their causal factors, nursing interventions cannot be prescriptive since their intended outcomes will not yet have been identified."

Soares extended the notion of focusing on causality by emphasizing the importance of defining both direct and indirect causes of problems and of isolating *repetitive patterns* of *problem-etiologies*. She defined a nursing diagnosis as an altered pattern of human functioning, which is arrived at by assessing the patient's needs. "A nursing diagnosis is a statement about a health problem and its underlying causes" (Soares, 1978, p. 274). The problem statement is a description of a conflict between two or more needs.

PATTERN RECOGNITION

The importance of *pattern recognition* as the principle element in the diagnostic process, which received initial emphasis from Durand and Prince (1966), was shared by others who attempted to conceptualize nursing diagnosis both as process and product: ". . . a statement of a conclusion resulting from a recognition of a *pattern*" (Durand and Prince, 1966, p. 52). ". . . potential or actual disturbances in life processes, *patterns*, functions, or development" (Gordon, 1976, p. 8). ". . . altered *patterns* of human functioning" (Soares, 1978, p. 271). ". . . *patterns* of unitary man" (Kim and Moritz, 1982, p. 219). ". . . normal variations and altered *patterns* (actual or potential) of human functioning" (McLane, 1979, p. 33). The idea of pattern recognition in these definitions suggests that many patterns are manifested by a single individual, for example, a pattern of bowel elimination, a pattern of sleep/rest, and a pattern of activity, not a *total pattern* of the individual as described by Newman (1979) who views a *total pattern* of an individual as primary and existing before manifestations of health (with health conceptualized as a synthesis of disease and nondisease).

A typology of 11 functional health patterns, representing traditional and contemporary ideas of nursing practice, was proposed by Gordon (1982) to unify basic areas of client assessment regardless of the model of the client used by a nurse. The 11 functional health patterns are used as an organizing framework for the diagnoses "accepted" by the National Group for Classification of Nursing Diagnoses and for diagnoses suggested by Gordon. The unitary man/human framework suggested by the nurse theorists working with the National Group is also a framework of patterns, patterns of unitary man, designed to organize the accepted diagnoses.

POSITIVE DIAGNOSES VS. PROBLEMS

Concern about the problem focus of the proposed taxonomy was expressed verbally at the national conferences as well as in the periodical literature. Community health nurses raised questions about the absence of positive diagnoses on the accepted list. Since much of their time is spent in reinforcing positive health behaviors, they viewed the absence of positive diagnoses as an indication of a devaluing of preventive health care. McKay (1977, p. 223) expressed a need for a list of positive health states or conditions to make "an exclusion decision re need for nursing care. . . ." She subscribed to the idea that "a decision that nursing care was needed, would require a problem, need, or deficiency identification even if it were for health maintenance or prevention" (McKay, 1977, p. 223). McKay's view is shared by most authors, for example, nursing diagnoses are as follows: patient problems or concerns (Gebbie and Lavin, 1974; Roy, 1975); the problems that nurses diagnose and treat (Gordon, 1978); unhealthful responses, negative statements (Mundinger, 1978). Looking at the patient as a collection of problems without recognizing strengths would result in interventions based on educated guesses according to Popkess (1981). Gleit and Tatro (1981) also promoted use of positive nursing diagnoses based on a wellness model of the phases of disease. The emphasis on patient strength and wellness in developing plans of care is consistent with many nursing practice models. However, the complex conceptual issues involved in adding positive health states or wellness diagnoses to the taxonomy are not resolved by equating patients' strengths with positive diagnoses. The ANA's definition of nursing as the diagnosis and treatment of human responses may provide a way out of the conceptual dilemma imposed by the multiple definitions of nursing diagnosis and the concern for wellness. The proposed definition is similar to one used by Jones (1979, p. 68), that defined a nursing diagnosis as ". . . a statement of a person's response to a situation or illness which is actually or potentially unhealthful and which nursing intervention can change in the direction of health."

TAXONOMY DEVELOPMENT

In the year following the First National Conference on the Classification of Nursing Diagnoses, the conference's codirectors focused the profession's attention on taxonomy development with the following statement: "The classification of nursing diagnoses represents nothing less than the systematic description of the entire domain of nursing" (Gebbie and Lavin, 1974, p. 250). Brown suggested an epidemiologic approach to the development of diagnoses and a classification system and proposed five criteria for evaluating a taxonomy (Brown, 1974). Roy (1975, p. 91) proposed a definition of a taxonomy as a ". . . set of classifications which are ordered and arranged on the basis of a single principle or of a consistent set of principles . . ." and rules of categorization. Roy (1975, p. 90) also emphasized the importance of clarifying ". . . the nature of the phenomena with which nursing is concerned." Bircher described a 10-step process for the development of a taxonomy of nursing diagnoses (Bircher, 1975). Although Roy and Bircher visualized the taxonomy as a classification of summary statements of patient problems, it is important to remember that Soares and Derdiarian saw such a classification as incomplete. For them, diagnoses were patterns of "problem-etiologies," and a taxonomy would therefore be a classification of statements of problem-etiologies, not problems alone (Derdiarian, 1977; Soares, 1978).

It is interesting to note that the Committee on Taxonomy of the International Association for the Study of Pain has proposed an axes classification system of pain syndromes that ". . . moves from region, through system, to the description of the pain, and to the chronicity and severity of the pain, concluding with etiology" (Merskey, 1983, p. 48). Although Merskey sees many problems with the approach, he suggests that there would be many more if etiology were placed first, since the cause of many pain syndromes is unknown. In the same article the ICD-9 classification of pain is viewed as in a state of disarray with overlapping categories the rule rather than the exception. Since the study of pain and pain syndromes antedates recorded history, our failure to agree on an ordering principle for the diagnostic categories developing during a period of less than 2 decades seems consistent with the emerging nature of the work of describing the domain of nursing.

A proposal to refine the taxonomy was made by Lunney (1982) who suggested a two-part statement different from the now familiar problem-etiology format. The first part of the statement identifies the behaviors that can be improved by nursing, and the second part specifies the factors that must be "worked with" to improve the behavior. The terms used in part one ". . . represent functional behaviors that promote, maintain and restore health" (Lunney, 1982, p. 456). According to Lunney, each behavior represents both a pattern and a process, and hence the terms *pattern* and *process* do not appear in the proposed system, for example, sleep/wake replaces sleep pattern disturbance. Lunney believes that the system meets the criterion of wholeness, since the focus is on such "holistic concepts" as oxygenation rather than on concepts that refer to parts of the human body, for example, skin integrity. The connection between health and some of the diagnoses accepted by the National Conference Group has not been demonstrated according to Lunney (1982, p. 459), who prefers to use broad categories, for example, nutrition and parenting, that ". . . represent the person's pattern of attaining, using, and managing the system's needs."

The unitary man/human framework that was proposed by the nurse theorists working with the National Conference Group was described in detail by Kim and Moritz (1982), and a progress report is included in this publication (p. 26). The patterns of unitary man/human proposed by the theorists and the 11 functional health patterns developed by Gordon bear a striking resemblance to one another, which is not surprising when viewed from the perspective of the interplay between the two major activities of the participants of the national conferences: generation and refinement of diagnoses and classification of the diagnoses into an ordered category system. Douglas and Murphy (1981, p. 55) remind us that an ideal classification system is not needed to make progress and encourage use of emerging taxonomies in an Hegelian manner to synthesize a new direction and to generate hypotheses, ". . . raising questions about, as well as adding categories to, nursing diagnoses."

THEORY AND TAXONOMY

The relationships between taxonomy and theory development in nursing were addressed by Kritek (1978) and McKay (1977). Both viewed the process of identification of the phenomenon of concern to nursing, nursing diagnoses, as a theory-building activity and subscribe to Dickoff, James, and Wiedenbach's idea of a factor-isolating theory. In the ANA Social Policy Statement, the position is taken that theory is needed to understand both the nature of problems and their causes when known. "Diagnosis of phenomena leads to application of theory to explain the condition and to determine actions to be taken—otherwise, diagnosis is mere labeling" (ANA, 1980, p. 16).

The ANA Social Policy Statement can be viewed as confirming the work of the National Conference Group for Classification of Nursing Diagnoses. The definition of nursing as the diagnosis and treatment of human responses to actual and potential health problems and the identification of nursing diagnoses as the core of nursing have set the stage for (1) an unprecedented period of scientific activity in nursing, (2) change in the conceptualization of the focus of day-to-day nursing practice, (3) utilization of more precise interactions, (4) clearer specifications of the outcomes of nursing care, and (5) greater accountability for clinical decision making. Some of the knowledge-building and knowledge-using articles related to nursing diagnosis are reviewed later in this paper.

IMPLEMENTATION AND APPLICATION

Although Lash (1981) reported a gap in the use of nursing diagnoses because of misunderstanding the term and narrow application, articles on implementation have been published, including a symposium, edited, and reviewed by Gordon (1979a, 1979b). One of the key articles in the symposium was written from the perspective and experience of a practitioner and change agent. Feild used principles of change theory to design strategies to reduce resistance to the use of nursing diagnoses and to guide implementation activities, including intraprofessional and interprofessional communication (Feild, 1979). In contrast to Feild, Bruce (1979) addressed implementation of nursing diagnoses from the perspective of an administrator, highlighting their importance in focusing quality assurance activities and increasing quality of care. The roles of various administrative levels in implementing nursing diagnoses and a pilot test of implementation were also discussed.

Four articles gave accounts of implementation or application of nursing diagnoses within acute care settings. Mahomet (1975) described operating room nurses' use of nursing diagnoses in preoperative, postoperative, and interoperative observation and gave an example of diagnosing and treating preoperative anxiety. McKeehan (1979) and LaMontagne and McKeehan (1975) reported on the development and use of nursing diagnoses within an acute care referral system. In a related study (Gordon, Sweeney; and McKeehan, 1980), the frequencies of nursing diagnoses made on 163 OB/GYN patient referrals were categorized as nonacceptable (199) and acceptable (241). The need for a common language for nurses was frequently cited in these articles.

Leslie (1981) compared the frequency of nursing diagnoses (1521) with the frequency of medical diagnoses (237) in a long-term care facility. Nurses in the agency used the First National Conference list of accepted diagnoses, which was described as "more useful" than recent lists. The introduction of nursing diagnoses in a community health setting was described by Dalton (1979), who maintained that use of nursing diagnoses enhanced the independence of community health nurses. Weber (1979) gave a more personal view of implementation of nursing diagnoses within a private psychiatric nursing practice. She described nuances and dynamics of the diagnostic process, use of referral and record systems, and implication of nursing diagnoses for reimbursement.

Fredette and O'Connor (1979) described implementation of nursing diagnoses in a generic program of nursing education and illustrated the development of students' diagnostic capabilities. Nursing diagnoses were implemented in a hospital-based continuing education program by Morris (1982), who described improvement of nursing care subsequent to the program.

The next series of articles are more reflective of the "how to" aspect of making a nursing diagnosis. Mundinger and Jauron (1975) described common mistakes in writing diagnostic statements such as reversal of clauses, statements of needs, statements with legal implications, environment-based rather than person-based diagnoses, and medically oriented diagnoses. Their article seems to have served as a prototype for one by Dossey and Guzzetta (1981) and another by Hausman (1980), which include case presentations illustrating use of nursing diagnoses and instructions on writing diagnostic statements. The latter activity was also described by Price (1980) and Shoemaker (1979) with emphasis on the diagnostic process. Aspinall, Jambruno, and Phoenix (1977) focused on the process of differential diagnoses and demonstrated the differential diagnostic process with two case studies.

The legal issues related to making nursing diagnoses were clarified by Fortin and Rabinow (1979). They cited the absence of a legal requirement to make nursing diagnoses and suggested that inclusion of diagnostic ability in future nurse practice acts would increase legal accountability for diagnostic statements.

CLINICAL NURSING DIAGNOSES

The articles in this section include nursing diagnoses that are common to a given population of patients. Mundinger (1978) developed three broad categories of nursing diagnoses identified in patients with cancer during treatment periods: voluntary physical, involuntary physical, and psychologic responses. Diagnoses common to cancer patients' families were also delineated. Some of the diagnoses most common to cancer patients were pain, nausea and anorexia, malnutrition, skin breakdown, depression, anxiety, and drug use. In all, 26 nursing diagnoses were identified. Fredette and Gloriant (1981a) described 25 nursing diagnoses, potential responses to cancer drug toxicity. The 25 diagnoses were grouped according to body systems, for example, diagnoses of sensory alterations and impaired physical mobility were placed in the neurologic system. The article included a chart that listed common drugs, drug mechanisms, nursing interventions, and common medical measures related to each of the 25 nursing diagnoses. In another article, Fredette and Gloriant (1981b) presented a case study of a 52-year-old woman with nausea and vomiting related to chemotherapy. They presented descriptions of assessments of functional health patterns and SOAP notes for eight nursing diagnoses.

Four articles published in 1979 dealt with common nursing diagnoses related to specific medical diagnoses and had the general theme that nursing diagnoses help focus nursing care. Demers (1979) discussed assessment of functional patterns and treatment of lack of knowledge and maladaptive individual coping diagnosed in a patient with endocarditis. Fluid volume deficit, alterations in nutrition, inability to perform self-care, and alterations in socialization were described for a patient with malnutrition (Price, 1979). Fuhs (1979) described respiratory dysfunction and severe anxiety that occurred in a patient with chronic obstructive pulmonary disease (COPD). The strength of the article was in the description of the diagnostic investigation process. Gerber (1979) described the diagnosis of "metabolic imbalance related to dietary noncompliance" in a 58-year-old patient with "diabetes out of control." Validation of the nursing diagnosis and use of contracting as a treatment measure were also included.

Several authors developed nursing diagnoses common to the medical diagnosis of stroke. Tilton and Maloof (1982) identified seven nursing diagnoses and suggested appropriate nursing interventions and outcomes. Franklin (1978) also generated seven nursing diagnoses common to stroke. It is interesting to note, however, that only one diagnosis made by Franklin, impaired mobility, was similar to a diagnosis made by Tilton and Maloof. In a related article, Norman (1979) grouped behavioral changes common to patients with a right hemisphere cerebrovascular accident (RCVA) under four major nursing diagnoses: visual-spatial misperception, body scheme disturbances, impaired cognitive processes, and alteration in emotional sensitivities. Interviews were conducted with four patients with RCVA to identify common signs and symptoms for the diagnoses.

Using a case presentation of a 14-year-old boy with a spinal cord injury, Giubilato (1982) described problems encountered immediately after a spinal cord injury: respiratory system alterations, disturbances in cardiovascular reflexes, temperature control changes, and elimination problems. Giubilato proposed a list of 29 nursing diagnoses common to spinal cord injury.

Nursing diagnoses related to cardiovascular problems were described by Rossi and Haines (1979), who emphasized the importance of using nursing diagnoses to clarify the role of nurses in critical care settings. Seven nursing diagnoses common to patients with myocardial infarction were developed. One of the diagnoses, alteration in cardiac output, was given an alternate label, activity intolerance, because of the controversy about labels treatable by a limited number of independent nursing interventions. Seven nursing diagnoses related to hypertension and their possible etiologies were suggested by Randolph and Silberstein (1982).

Several articles have discussed nursing diagnoses common to respiratory problems. Chrisman (1974) suggested that dyspnea was a nursing diagnosis and elaborated on levels of dyspnea, common signs and symptoms of dyspnea, related medical diagnoses, precipitating conditions, and nursing interventions. Sjoberg (1983) discussed four diagnoses commonly found in patients with COPD: activity intolerance, sleep-pattern disturbance, noncompliance, and ineffective coping. Nurse members of The American Thoracic Society (Abraham, and others, 1981) published standards of care based on nursing diagnoses for patients with COPD. A pulmonary assessment guide and 12 nursing diagnoses with etiologies, signs and symptoms, nursing interventions, and outcome criteria were described. The standards could serve as a prototype for nurses specializing in other areas of practice.

Review of a symposium on nursing diagnoses related to pain (Munley and Keane, 1977) showed that only two articles included discussions of pain from the perspective of nursing diagnosis. *Alteration in comfort: pain*, an accepted diagnosis on the National Conference list, was not discussed. Mahoney (1977) emphasized the importance of nursing diagnoses in focusing care of patients with pain and included examples of potential diagnoses, for example, susceptible to pain related to bowel distention. Pain management problems related to daily wound irrigations of a 10-year-old boy were conceptualized by Cowherd (1977) as resistance related to fear of mutilation and anxiety related to loss of self-control to deal with the boy's responses to irrigations.

Nursing diagnoses related to spiritual matters have been discussed in several articles (Fleeger and Heukelem, 1977; Stoll, 1979; Wallace, 1979). Fleeger and Heukelem (1977) used three case studies to relate spiritual needs to the diagnosis of *alterations in faith*, which was accepted at the First National Conference on the Classification of Nursing Diagnoses. Stoll (1979) mentioned spiritual diagnoses in a discussion of spiritual assessment. Wallace (1979) referred to "matters of spirituality" approved by participants of the Third National Conference (Kim and Moritz, 1982). O'Brien (1982) developed the concept of spiritual integrity (conceptualized as a spiritual need) and used her spirituality assessment tool to demonstrate spiritual diagnoses in brief case presentations. The spiritual diagnoses presented, however, (for example, spiritual pain) are not on the National Conference list of accepted diagnoses.

Miscellaneous specific nursing diagnoses were also discussed in several articles. A list of 2517 nursing diagnoses generated by 57 nurses was used by Jones and Jakob (1981) to determine frequencies of diagnostic categories. Using definitions of *fear* (ranked third) and *anxiety* (ranked fourth), Jones and Jakob reviewed the diagnoses and revised 41 of them to fear. All but two of the revised *fear* diagnoses were originally labeled *anxiety*. Jones and Jakob believe that anxiety is a preliminary diagnosis to fear and emphasize the importance of diagnostic accuracy. LeSage, Beck, and Johnson (1979) analyzed the nursing diagnosis of drug incompatibility and illustrated diagnoses of problems stemming from drug therapy in a case example of drug incompatibility. Body image change, as a response to surgery, was discussed by Gruendemann (1975). Although Gruendemann did not analyze alterations in body image from the standpoint of a nursing diagnosis, she did believe that nurses would eventually establish a nursing diagnosis related to states of altered body image.

RESEARCH AND VALIDATION

Few research articles on nursing diagnoses have been published. Perry's review of nursing diagnoses research (1982) included background information and rationale for using nursing diagnoses but few articles on research studies. Most of the articles dealt with nursing diagnoses from a conceptual or application point of view. With two exceptions (Kim and others and Castle), this section is limited to research not included in published proceedings of national conferences. The articles include frequency studies, validation studies, research on the actual diagnostic process, and studies of specific nursing diagnoses.

Several studies have investigated frequency and patterns of nursing diagnoses in various settings (Gordon, Sweeney, and McKeehan, 1980; Jones and Jakob, 1981; Leslie, 1981; Roberts, 1982). Leslie (1981) reported on frequency of nursing diagnoses in long-term settings and compared them to medical diagnoses made in the same setting. Gordon, Sweeney, and McKeehan (1980) described diagnostic patterns made on discharge referrals from a hospital. Jones and Jakob (1981) reported on the frequency of diagnoses made by 57 nurses in an article differentiating anxiety and fear. Roberts (1982) used a different approach and rationale for reporting the frequency of nursing diagnoses made by professional nurses. Roberts was interested in differences in perception of problems identified by patients and nurses. In a pilot study, the number and type of diagnoses made by patients and their respective nurses were compared. The nurses used a list of diagnoses that included many from the National Conference list. The patients had a similar list to choose from that described the diagnoses (problems) in common language. There was a 19.53% agreement between patients and nurses.

Gordon (1980a) reviewed medical diagnoses, nursing models, and nursing diagnoses as potential sources for evaluation and research topics but placed major emphasis on nursing diagnoses. In a pilot study of five patients, Guzzetta and Forsyth (1979) investigated the nursing diagnosis *psychophysiologic stress.* Categories of stresses applicable to an intensive care unit environment and a measurement tool were developed from their conceptualization of a stress response. They recommended replication of the study and classification of stress into five levels, from low to extreme stress. Jones (1979) reported an in-progress study of diagnostic encounters of more than 50 volunteer practicing nurses from various practice settings. The goal was to collect a minimum of 2000 nursing diagnoses derived from the diagnostic encounters. The nursing diagnosis *maternal attachment* was proposed by Avant (1979), who described a seven-step approach for formulating a nursing diagnosis. The proposed seven-step approach is actually a validation process.

Gordon and Sweeney (1979) described three models for identifying and validating nursing diagnoses: a retrospective identification model, a clinical model, and a nurse validation model. The retrospective model was used as a method for identifying nursing diagnoses at the first four National Conferences on the Classification of Nursing Diagnoses. A pilot project to train raters for the nurse validation and clinical models was also described. Two researchers reported use of validation models in national conference proceedings. Kim and others (1982) studied pairs of baccalaureate nursing students who independently assessed and identified nursing diagnoses using a prepared list of diagnostic labels. The diagnoses were then compared for validation. Castle (1982) used a clinical identification model and demonstrated the difficulty in identifying nursing diagnoses in an intensive care setting. Holmstrom and Burgess (1975) used a similar participant-observation method to identify three nursing diagnoses related to sexual trauma.

Research studies of the diagnostic process were reported by several authors. Aspinall (1976, 1979) studied accuracy in making nursing diagnoses. In one study, 187 nurse subjects were given a case study and were instructed to identify patient problems. On the average, they were able to identify 3.4 problems out of 12. In a second study, Aspinall demonstrated that use of a decision tree enabled nurses to increase significantly their diagnostic accuracy when compared with nurses who did not use the decision tree. Hamdi and Hutelmyer (1970) also attempted to increase nurses' diagnostic effectiveness. They hypothesized that use of a systematic assessment tool would help nurses to identify problems. Although the nurse subjects who used the tool did not identify significantly more patient problems, they did identify a greater number of valid problems.

The effects of inferential ability and information conditions on the diagnostic accuracy, diagnostic confidence, and hypothesis-scanning strategies of 60 graduate nurses were studied by Gordon (1980b). Unrestrictive information and predictive hypothesis testing were associated with greater diagnostic accuracy in a postoperative general surgical patient situation. Inferential ability was not found to be a factor in diagnostic accuracy.

Two master's theses were reported by Matthews and Gaul (1979), who studied effects of critical thinking and concept attainment on diagnostic abilities of nursing student. Both of the studies used case studies to measure nurses' diagnostic abilities. One study used a case example of a patient with emotional disturbance and impaired elimination; the other study used a case presentation of mental confusion. There were no clear hypotheses for the study, and there was no relationship between cue perceptions and concept mastery among graduate student subjects. Matthews and Gaul, however, did find some significant positive relationships between diagnostic cues made by undergraduate students and concept mastery. One major implication of the study was that ability to derive accurate nursing diagnoses depends on identifying discriminating cues.

Using three criteria (client centered, reflect client concerns, and amenable to maintenance or change by nursing), DeBack (1981) analyzed 200 nursing care plans to determine the impact of curriculum models on senior nursing students' ability to formulate nursing diagnoses. Only 28% of the diagnoses formulated met all the criteria, and 35% met none of the three criteria. DeBack's hypothesis that curriculum models would predict students' relative ability to formulate diagnoses was not supported.

SUMMARY AND RECOMMENDATIONS

This section illustrates several points about research on nursing diagnosis: few diagnoses have been validated; diagnostic accuracy has not been demonstrated; strategies to increase diagnostic accuracy have yet to be devised; and the limited diagnostic skills of students, graduate and undergraduate, are a reflection of the skills of our practitioners and teachers.

The authors' attempt to do a general review of the literature on nursing diagnosis (excluding books and national conference proceedings) is consistent with the state of the art/science: there are not sufficient conceptual and research articles in one area to warrant a focused review. The lack of consensus about "what is a nursing diagnosis" can be viewed as a persistent problem or as part of a natural evolutionary process that carries with it opportunities for dialogue, debate, and unrestrained scientific effort. The ANA's statement that nursing is the diagnosis and treatment of human responses to actual or potential health problems represents yet another step in the evolution of nursing as a profession and a scientific discipline. The statement must not be viewed as a capstone on the richness and diversity of the many conceptualizations of nursing and nursing diagnosis.

The paucity of nursing diagnosis research, especially diagnostic validation studies and inquiries into the diagnostic process, is a cause for great concern. These two areas should be the profession's first priorities in the 1980s. Without valid diagnostic labels and skill in the diagnostic process, our interventions and outcomes are moot. Loomis and Wood's proposal (1983) that "cure" is the potential outcome of nursing care directed at treating human responses in six human response systems lends additional support to the importance of clear specification of human response/human response pattern to be treated and precision in the diagnostic process used to make the diagnosis. The ANA Social Policy Statement (1980) and Loomis and Wood's future-oriented conceptualization (1983) of nursing's potential, cure, may be the catalysts that focus researchers' attention on validation of diagnoses and strategies to improve diagnostic accuracy.

REFERENCES

Abdellah, F.G.: Methods of identifying covert aspects of nursing problems, Nurs. Res. **6**:4, 1957.

Abraham, M., and others: Standards for nursing care of patients with COPD, Am. Thorac. Soc. News p. 31, Summer 1981.

American Nurses' Association: Nursing: a social policy statement, Kansas City, Mo., 1980, The Association.

Aspinall, M.J.: Nursing diagnosis—the weak link, Nurs. Outlook **24**:433, 1976.

Aspinall, M.J.: Use of a decision tree to improve accuracy of diagnosis, Nurs. Res. **28**:182, 1979.

Aspinall, M.J., Jambruno, N., and Phoenix, B.S.: The why and how of nursing diagnosis, Matern. Child Nurs. J. **2**:354, 1977.

Avant, K.: Nursing diagnosis: maternal attachment, Adv. Nurs. Sci. **2**:45, 1979.

Bircher, A.: On the development and classification of nursing diagnoses, Nurs. Forum **14**:10, 1975.

Brown, M.: Epidemiologic approach and study of clinical nursing diagnosis, Nurs. Forum **13**:346, 1974.

Bruce, J.A.: Implementation of nursing diagnosis: a nursing administrator's perspective, Nurs. Clin. North Am. **14**:509, 1979.

Castle, M.R.: Interrater agreement in the use of nursing diagnosis. In Kim, M.J., and Moritz, D.A., eds.: Classification of nursing diagnoses: proceedings of the third and fourth national conferences, New York, 1982, McGraw-Hill Book Co.

Chambers, W.: Nursing diagnosis, Am. J. Nurs. **62:**102, 1962.

Chrisman, M.: Dyspnea, Am. J. Nurs. **74:**643, 1974.

Cowherd, M.: One child's reaction to acute pain, Nurs. Clin. North Am. **12:**639, 1977.

Dalton, J.M.: Nursing diagnosis in a community health setting, Nurs. Clin. North Am. **14:**525, 1979.

DeBack, V.: The relationship between senior nursing students' ability to formulate nursing diagnoses and the curriculum model, Adv. Nurs. Sci. **3:**51, 1981.

Demers, B.: How nursing diagnosis helps focus your care beyond endocarditis, RN **42**(12):51, 1979.

Derdiarian, A.: Roles and directions in cancer nursing education. In American Cancer Society: Proceedings of the second national conference on cancer nursing, St. Louis, 1977, The Society.

Dossey, B., and Guzzetta, C.E.: Nursing diagnosis, how to define the problem can be half the solution, Nursing '81 **11**(6):34, 1981.

Douglas, D.J., and Murphy, E.K.: Nursing process, nursing diagnosis, and emerging taxonomies. In McClosky, J.C., and Grace, H.C., eds.: Current issues in nursing, Boston, 1981, Blackwell Scientific Publications.

Durand, M., and Prince, R.: Nursing diagnosis: process and decision, Nurs. Forum **5:**50, 1966.

Feild, L.: The implementation of nursing diagnosis in clinical practice, Nurs. Clin. North Am. **14:**497, 1979.

Fleeger, R., and Heukelem, M.S.: The patient's spiritual needs—a part of nursing diagnosis, *Nurses Lamp* **28**(4):1, 1977.

Fortin, J.D., and Rabinow, J.: Legal implications of nursing diagnosis, Nurs. Clin. North Am. **14:**553, 1979.

Franklin, D.R.: Nursing assessment and nursing diagnosis of the client with a cerebrovascular accident, Va. Nurse Quar. **46**(2):7, 1978.

Fredette, S.L., and Gloriant, F.S.: Nursing diagnosis in cancer chemotherapy: in theory, Am. J. Nurs. **81:**2013, 1981a.

Fredette, S.L., and Gloriant, F.S.: Nursing diagnosis in cancer chemotherapy: in practice, Am. J. Nurs. **81:**2021, 1981b.

Fredette, S.L., and O'Connor, K.: Nursing diagnosis in teaching and curriculum planning, Nurs. Clin. North Am. **14:**541, 1979.

Fuhs, M.: How nursing diagnosis helps focus your care—it seems like acute respiratory dysfunction, RN **42**(10):51, 1979.

Gebbie, K., and Lavin, M.A.: Classifying nursing diagnoses, Am. J. Nurs. **74:**250, 1974.

Gerber, F.: How nursing diagnosis helps focus your care—diabetes out of control, RN **42**(9):65, 1979.

Giubilato, R.T.: Acute care of the high-level quadriplegic patient, J. Neurosurg. Nurs. **14**(3):128, 1982.

Gleit, C.J., and Tatro, S.: Nursing diagnosis for healthy individuals, Nurs. Health Care **2:**456, 1981.

Gordon, M.: Nursing diagnosis and the diagnostic process, Am. J. Nurs. **76:**1298, 1976.

Gordon, M.: Classification of nursing diagnoses, J.N.Y. State Nurses Assoc. **9:**5, 1978.

Gordon, M.: The concept of nursing diagnosis, Nurs. Clin. North Am. **14:**487, 1979a.

Gordon, M.: Symposium on the implementation of nursing diagnosis, Nurs. Clin. North Am. **14:**384, 1979b.

Gordon, M.: Determining study topics, Nurs. Res. **29:**83, 1980a.

Gordon, M.: Predictive strategies in diagnostic tasks, Nurs. Res. **29:**39, 1980b.

Gordon, M.: Nursing diagnosis: process and application, New York, 1982, McGraw-Hill Book Co.

Gordon, M., and Sweeney, M.A.: Methodological problems and issues in identifying and standardizing nursing diagnoses, Adv. Nurs. Sci. **2:**1, 1979.

Gordon, M., Sweeney, M.A., and McKeehan, K.: Nursing diagnosis: looking at its use in the clinical area, Am. J. Nurs. **80**:672, 1980.

Gruendemann, B.J.: The impact of surgery on body image, Nurs. Clin. North Am. **10**:635, 1975.

Guzzetta, C.E., and Forsyth, G.L.: Nursing diagnostic pilot study: psychophysiologic stress, Adv. Nurs. Sci. **2**:27, 1979.

Hamdi, M.E., and Hutelmyer, C.M.: A study of the effectiveness of an assessment tool in the identification of nursing care problems, Nurs. Res. **19**:354, 1970.

Hausman, K.A.: The concept and application of nursing diagnosis, J. Neurosurg. Nurs. **12**(2):76, 1980.

Holmstrom, L.I., and Burgess, A.W.: Development of diagnostic categories: sexual traumas, Am. J. Nurs. **75**:1288, 1975.

Hornung, G.: The nursing diagnosis—an exercise in judgment, Nurs. Outlook **4**:29, 1956.

Jones, P.E.: A terminology for nursing diagnoses, Adv. Nurs. Sci. **2**:65, 1979.

Jones, P., and Jakob, D.F.: Nursing diagnosis: differentiating fear and anxiety, Nurs. Papers (Can.) **13**(4):20, 1981.

Kim, M.J., and Moritz, D.A., eds.: Classification of nursing diagnoses: proceedings of the third and fourth national conferences, New York, 1982, McGraw-Hill Book Co.

Kim, M.J., and others: The effect of using nursing diagnosis in nursing care planning. In Kim, M.J., and Moritz, D.A., eds.: Classification of nursing diagnoses: proceedings of the third and fourth national conferences, New York, 1982, McGraw-Hill Book Co.

Komorita, N.: Nursing diagnosis, Am. J. Nurs. **63**:83, 1963.

Kritek, P.: The generation and classification of nursing diagnoses: toward a theory of nursing, Image **10**:33, 1978.

LaMontagne, M.E., and McKeehan, K.M.: Profile of a continuing care program emphasizing discharge planning, J. Nurs. Admin. **5**(10):22, 1975.

Lash, A.A. Nursing diagnosis: some comments on the gap between theory and practice. In McClosky, J.C., and Grace, H., eds: Current issues in nursing, Boston, 1981, Blackwell Scientific Publications.

LeSage, J., Beck, C., and Johnson, M.: Nursing diagnosis of drug incompatibility: a conceptual process, Adv. Nurs. Sci. **1**(2):63, 1979.

Leslie, F.M.: Nursing diagnosis: use in long-term care, Am. J. Nurs. **81**:1012, 1981.

Loomis, M.E., and Wood, D.J.: Cure: the potential outcome of nursing care, Image **15**:4, 1983.

Lunney, M.: Nursing diagnosis: refining the system, Am. J. Nurs. **82**:456, 1982.

Mahomet, A.D.: Nursing diagnosis for the OR nurse, AORN J. **22**:709, 1975.

Mahoney, E.A.: Some implications for nursing diagnoses of pain, Nurs. Clin. North Am. **12**:613, 1977.

Matthews, C.A., and Gaul, A.L.: Nursing diagnosis from the perspective of concept attainment and critical thinking, Adv. Nurs. Sci. **2**:17, 1979.

McKay, R.P.: What is the relationship between the development and utilization of a taxonomy and nursing theory? Nurs. Res. **26**:222, 1979.

McKeehan, K.M.: Nursing diagnosis in a discharge planning program, Nurs. Clin. North Am. **14**:517, 1979.

McLane, A.M.: A taxonomy of nursing diagnoses: toward a science of nursing, Milw. Prof. Nurse **20**:33, 1979.

Merskey, H.: Development of a universal language of pain syndromes, In Bonica, J.L., et al., eds.: Advances in pain research and therapy: proceedings of the third world congress on pain, vol. 5, New York, 1981, Raven Press.

Morris, J.L.: Nursing diagnosis—a focus for continuing education, J. Contin. Educ. Nurs. **13**(3):33, 1982.

Mundinger, M.O.: Nursing diagnosis for cancer patients, Cancer Nurs. **1**:221, 1978.

Mundinger, M.O., and Jauron, G.D.: Developing a nursing diagnosis, Nurs. Outlook **23**(2):94, 1975.

Munley, M.J., and Keane, M.C.: Symposium on impressions of pain: nursing diagnosis, Nurs. Clin. North Am. **12**:609, 1977.

Newman, M.: Theory development in nursing, Philadelphia, 1979, F.A. Davis Co.

Norman, S.: Diagnostic categories for the patient with a right hemisphere lesion, **79:**2126, 1979.

O'Brien, M.E.: The need for spiritual integrity. In Yura, H., and Walsh, M.B., eds.: Human needs and the nursing process, New York, 1982, Appleton-Century-Crofts.

Perry, A.G.: Nursing diagnosis research, J. Neurosurg. Nurs. **14**(2):108, 1982.

Popkess, S.A.: Diagnosing your patient's strengths, Nursing '81 **11**(7):34, 1981.

Price, M.R.: How nursing diagnosis helps focus your care: the patient is starving—but why? RN **42**(11):45, 1979.

Price, M.R.: Nursing diagnosis: making a concept come alive, Am. J. Nurs. **80:**668, 1980.

Randolph, S.A., and Silberstein, C.: Planning for the hypertensive employee in industry, Occup. Health Nurs. **30**(7):19, 1982.

Roberts, C.S.: Identifying the real patient problems, Nurs. Clin. North Am. **17:**481, 1982.

Rossi, L.P., and Haines, V.M.: Nursing diagnoses related to acute myocardial infarction, Cardiovasc. Nurs. **3:**11, 1979.

Rothberg, J.S.: Why nursing diagnosis? Am. J. Nurs. **67:**1040, 1967.

Roy, Sister C.: A diagnostic classification system for nursing, Nurs. Outlook **23:**90, 1975.

Shoemaker, J.: How nursing diagnosis helps focus your care, RN **42**(8):56, 1979.

Sjoberg, E.L.: Nursing diagnosis and the COPD patient, Am. J. Nurs. **83:**245, 1983.

Soares, C.A.: Nursing and medical diagnoses: a comparison of variant and essential features. In Chaska, N., ed.: The nursing profession: views through the mist, New York, 1978, McGraw-Hill Book Co.

Stoll, R.: Spiritual assessment, Am. J. Nurs. **79:**1574, 1979.

Tilton, C.N., and Maloof, M.: Diagnosing the problems in stroke, Am. J. Nurs. **82:**596, 1982.

Wallace, G.: Spiritual care—a reality in nursing education and practice, Nurses Lamp **31**(2):1, 1979.

Weber, S.: Nursing diagnosis in private practice, Nurs. Clin. North Am. **14:**533, 1979.

Yura, H., and Walsh, M.B.: The nursing process: assessing, planning, implementing, evaluating, ed. 3, New York, 1978, Appleton-Century-Crofts.

BOOK REVIEW

Nursing Diagnosis and Intervention in Nursing Practice by Claire Campbell. New York, 1978, John Wiley & Sons, Inc., 1928 pages.

The author has compiled a voluminous text that provides information for the nurse using the nursing process and writing nursing care plans for a variety of clients. The components of the nursing process, noted by the author, are assessment, possible etiology, nursing diagnosis, nursing plan, nursing intervention, and evaluation. Emphasis has been placed on the development and identification of nursing diagnoses and interventions.

This book may be used by the professional nurse in clinical practice or education and by the student who is learning the practice of nursing. The information is presented in four parts. Part I includes a brief discussion of Maslow's theory of human needs; describes a study by which nursing diagnoses, interventions, goals, and evaluation criteria were determined; and gives a general discussion of the nursing process using Maslow's needs as a framework. The last chapter in Part I explains how the book is to be used and provides a table associating data obtained from a physical examination with possible nursing diagnoses.

Part II lists 730 nursing diagnoses divided according to subject matter. Each diagnosis has related assessment data, possible etiology, planning information, and nursing interventions. The reader is directed to another part of the book for evaluation criteria. In Part III all nursing interventions mentioned in the previous part are listed.

They are arranged alphabetically in four chapters: nursing treatments, nursing observations, health teaching, and medical treatments performed by the nurse. Included with each intervention is a definition, a rationale, the needs resolved by that intervention, and, if appropriate, any contraindications. Parts II and III include many of the activities the nurse performs in the practice of nursing. Because of the vast amounts of information presented in these two parts, the reader may become overwhelmed initially. After continued use of the book, the process of obtaining the needed information becomes easier.

Part IV includes an extensive list of references and four indexes. Each nursing diagnosis and nursing intervention is indexed alphabetically and by subject.

Although Parts II and III have much information that may be helpful in using the nursing process, the book is not the quick, practical source of information for writing client care plans as noted by the author. After obtaining assessment data and determining the general subject heading of the client's problem, the reader must go to six or more different places in the book to compile all the information to complete the nursing process. Since there are various theories used in the practice of nursing, Maslow's theory, which has been integrated with the nursing process in this work, may not be an appropriate framework for all nurses.

The author addresses the problem of differentiating a nursing diagnosis from a medical diagnosis. She also notes the difference between medical diagnosis and medical terminology, which is an important consideration when reviewing the nursing diagnoses that have been listed. The list of nursing diagnoses consists of diagnoses related to human responses and resource limitations, some of which involve dual diagnoses (pertain to more than one professional domain). Readers must look at the listed diagnoses considering their own definition of a nursing diagnosis.

As the author states, the list of nursing diagnoses is a beginning. The concept of nursing diagnosis is in the initial stages of its development. This book can be helpful to the nurse who is struggling to incorporate nursing diagnoses into the nursing process and to write client care plans.

Ann Marie Becker, R.N., M.S.N.

BOOK REVIEW

Nursing Diagnosis by Judith H. Carlson, Carol A. Craft, and Anne D. McGuire. Philadelphia, 1982, W.B. Saunders Co., 258 pages.

The authors have compiled a volume on nursing diagnoses that includes historic and theoretic developments, the realities of formulating and using nursing diagnoses, and presentations of client models in which nursing diagnoses are used. The book serves as an orientation for undergraduate students to the general nature of nursing diagnosis, the diagnostic process, and the relationship of nursing diagnosis to the other components of the nursing process. Strengths and limitations encountered in using nursing diagnoses and a variety of practical client examples are presented.

The major criticism of this text is the limited emphasis given to the importance and use of the diagnostic labels and classification system developed at the five National Conferences on the Classification of Nursing Diagnoses. This national effort has made a concerted effort to develop a commonly accepted nomenclature or language by which nurses can communicate meaningfully on an international level with each other as well as with professionals from other disciplines. The orientation leaves the reader with the impression that nursing diagnoses can be developed readily—for pure convenience—without validation of the diagnostic label through research or at least deliberations among professional nurses. Multiple examples of such nursing diagnoses substantiating this criticism can be found throughout Section 3. In an earlier chapter, Resler states that the disadvantages of using published nursing diagnosis "include the fact that a published diagnosis is not tailored to the specific client or situation and for that reason may require one or more qualifying diagnosis" (p. 75). Granted, the organizing conceptual framework for this text is adaptation and an attempt is made to develop nursing diagnoses within this framework. The dilemma must then be raised, however, does the approach in this text contribute to the development of a standardized nomenclature that can be confortably used by *all* nurses regardless of their theoretic orientation?

Gertrude K. McFarland, R.N., D.N.Sc.

BOOK REVIEW

Nursing Diagnosis: Process and Application by Marjory Gordon. New York, 1982, McGraw-Hill Book Co., 387 pages.

Marjory Gordon has written a superb book on the daignostic process that undoubtedly will become a classic in the field and one that has the potential for bringing order to the chaos created by the proliferation of nursing practice frameworks with their competing views of the client and the goal of nursing. In this book, Gordon presents a typology of 11 functional health patterns that represent both traditional and contemporary health-related areas of information about clients needed to implement many of the nursing practice models. The 11 patterns are clearly defined in Chapter III, and a screening format for their assessment is included in Appendix C. It is the author's opinion that standardization of nursing's assessment structure is compatible with the diversity of nursing models and should be a priority for the profession.

Questions related to causality are addressed throughout the book. Etiologies are viewed as probabilistic and multiple. Readers are encouraged to search for causal explanations outside the functional health pattern within which a problem occurred but within another functional pattern. Although Gordon states that interventions are based on both problem and etiology, it is clear that she favors the latter. Her expressed opposition to naming a disease process as an etiology of a nursing diagnosis (nurses do not treat disease states) supports the preceding statement. Etiologic factors present in a client in the absence of health problems are referred to as risk factors that predispose a client to a potential health problem.

In a scholarly and practical discussion of the probabilistic nature of cues and cue clusters, Gordon clarifies the nature of a critical defining characteristic, that is a cue that is a highly valid and highly reliable indicator of a diagnosis. Cue-processing strategies and multiple hypothesis testing procedures required to make a precise diagnosis are described. After reading about the latter in Chapters V and VI, it will become evident to even the uninitiated that a high level of problem-solving ability is needed to make an accurate diagnosis.

Although the substance of the book is contained in Chapters III through VI, other chapters include valuable information about the use of nursing diagnoses to direct care activities, the relevance of nursing diagnosis to practice and professional issues, and nine appendixes.

A copy of this book in the hands of every professional nurse would go a long way toward implementing the ANA's *Standard of Nursing Practice* and improving the quality of health care. Faculty teaching in baccalaureate and graduate programs in nursing would be remiss if they failed to acquaint students with the contents of the book. All professional nurses reading the book will put it down with a new awareness of their own competence as diagnosticians and with renewed pride in nursing's movement toward becoming a scientific discipline.

Audrey M. McLane, R.N., Ph.D

BOOK REVIEW

Manual of Nursing Diagnosis by Marjory Gordon. New York, 1982, McGraw-Hill Book Co., 227 pages.

The author views the manual as a quick reference to diagnostic terms and their definitions, useful for learners and expert diagnosticians. With the exception of about 20 diagnoses, the diagnostic categories included in the manual are based on the work of the National Group for the Classification of Nursing Diagnoses. The 20 diagnoses that appear on shaded pages (to differentiate them from currently accepted diagnoses) were found useful for care planning according to Gordon. Some of the added diagnoses had appeared in earlier lists of accepted diagnoses, for example, anxiety, mild; anxiety, moderate; anxiety, severe. The nursing diagnosis of anxiety with all its subcategories was accepted again at the Fifth National Conference.

The use of a typology of functional health patterns to organize the diagnostic categories contributes to the unique character of the manual. However, it is the use of the structure of functional health patterns instead of a more traditional alphabetic listing that makes the manual difficult to use as a reference.

The book contains 227 pages, more than half of which are blank. Each diagnosis appears on the left page with a blank page on the right designed for taking notes. Although the idea of blank pages for notes is conceptually appealing, the additional bulk and costs for a manual that is outdated in 2 years must be questioned. Anyone seriously wishing to refine a diagnostic label will need more than a single page to collect data from a sufficient number of cases.

The manual's greatest usefulness would be as a companion to Gordon's book on the diagnostic process, *Nursing Diagnosis: Process and Application.*

Audrey M. McLane, R.N., Ph.D.

BOOK REVIEW

Handbook of Nursing Diagnosis by Nancy Lengel. Bowie, Md., 1982, Robert J. Brady Co., 192 pages.

This book does what it states. It is a quick, easy-to-read reference handbook of nursing diagnoses. However, it is difficult to evaluate the book because I have a basic philosophic difference to the approach of a statement of nursing diagnosis. The book seems to compound and multiply misconceptions that exist because the author uses the medical diagnosis as a part of the statement of a nursing diagnosis. I totally disagree with the use of any medical diagnosis as an etiologic factor or subcategory, since nursing intervention should be clearly directed toward the correction of the etiology to solve the health problem. Etiology must be amenable to nursing action. Consider, for example, her nursing diagnosis of "impairment of mobility related to quadriplegia." Certainly a nurse can do nothing independently about quadriplegia nor does this etiology direct the nursing intervention. Since nursing intervention is clearly going to be directed toward increasing mobility, I view mobility as the etiology and the problem as the specific situation generated in the client as a result of the immobility, for example, alteration in socialization, social isolation, and ineffective coping related to impaired mobility. The same approach of using medical diagnoses as etiologic factors appears throughout the book. To me this is a *gross* and *very serious error* in conceptualization.

Frances M. Lange, R.N., D.S.N.

BOOK REVIEW

Aids to Nursing Diagnosis, ed. 3, by Marie M. Seedor. New York, 1980, Teachers College, Columbia University, 379 pp.

This book presents basic principles related to the foundational elements of nursing techniques for the beginning student. However, it does not deal with the cognitive decision-making process that leads to a nursing diagnosis, as the book's title may lead one to expect.

While the programmed units may help students systematically discern reasons for different nursing actions, the format itself may fragment presentations of the core subject, nursing diagnosis. Often nursing diagnoses are not even related to the main text of each chapter. There are no clear examples of nursing diagnoses except in the form of indirect statements, such as elevated temperature, "fever." Considering the numerous articles written about nursing diagnoses and the proceedings of four National Conferences on Classification of Nursing Diagnoses, such an oversight is glaring.

The author stresses that nurses should be familiar with diagnostic techniques for nursing judgment which would enable the nurse to assist the physician in making medical diagnoses. These diagnostic techniques include vital signs, the electrocardiogram, observation, and laboratory tests and constitute four out of five chapters in the book. Each technique is presented at a level suitable for students who have had little prior knowledge of the subject matter. The simplicity of content can be appreciated best by some sample objectives: "Discuss, in your own words, the meaning of temperature," or "read a thermometer" (p. 26); "identify sites where the pulse may be taken" (p. 96); "define blood pressure" and "measure an arterial pressure" (p. 163); "define an electrocardiogram"; "calculate the heart rate from a rhythm strip" (p. 209); "define such terms as symptom and sign" (p. 288); and "describe where to find the results of laboratory tests" (p. 328).

It should be pointed out that the inferential abilities needed in making a nursing diagnosis are not developed by mastery of techniques. As the author clearly states (p. 289), making a nursing diagnosis is a very difficult function of a professional nurse. It requires an advanced theoretical knowledge base of all sciences contributing to nursing. Research to enhance information-seeking strategies and decision-making capabilities are badly needed, but the data base for such studies cannot be found in this book.

☐From Kim, M.J.: Res. Nurs. Health 5(1):48, 1982. Reprinted with permission.

In summary, the topic of the book is timely, considering the demand for implementing nursing diagnosis in clinical practice; but the book's content and level do not reflect the current understanding of nursing diagnosis and are limited to elementary technical aspects of nursing practice. One would benefit more if the book related to the state of the art of nursing diagnosis. The apparent gap between the diagnostic techniques and the making of nursing diagnoses may be filled best by a discussion of the cognitive process that utilizes the described techniques.

Mi Ja Kim, R.N., Ph.D.

CHAPTER 8

Conference events

The report of the Task Force Group was made by Gordon, who has been the chairperson of this group since 1973 when the First National Conference was held. She brings out the highlights of the group's activities between the Fourth and Fifth National Conferences and has added a report on the planning of the Fifth National Conference.

Carpenito and Becker provided a summary of the 1-day continuing education workshop that preceded the Fifth National Conference. As they reported, the feedback from participants was positive and there was a recommendation to offer the workshop again before the Sixth National Conference.

In an effort to capture the thoughts of participants about the conference program, process, and nursing diagnosis in general, McFarland and Kim obtained opinions of 25 nurses who volunteered to participate by questionnaire. Opinions expressed and information acquired from this survey should be useful for the growth of the North American Nursing Diagnosis Association (NANDA) and planning of the next conference.

Although several special interest groups (for example, Computer Group and Mental Health Group) held their meetings during the conference, only two reports from these groups are included. The Critical Care Group report was made by Wake, who also included a brief summary of the Critical Care Conference on nursing diagnosis, which was held after the national conference. Burke submitted a brief report of the Health-Oriented Group and indicated a need for further development of health-oriented diagnoses.

Finally, the historic document of the National Conference Group, the Bylaws, is presented as well as the discussion during the Forum on Bylaws. Both Gebbie and Haas put major work into finalizing the bylaws and reporting them for publication.

One cannot help but notice a parallelism between the work of the National Conference Group and acceptance of the Bylaws of the NANDA. If the work of the National Conference Group was to formulate the language for nursing profession, the acceptance of the Bylaws signals the official formulation of the NANDA. With proper structure, appropriate governance by the Bylaws, and strong leadership with vision, the work on nursing diagnosis will carry forward not only the NANDA but also the nursing profession.

Report of the Task Force Conference Group for Classification of Nursing Diagnoses

MARJORY GORDON, R.N., Ph.D., F.A.A.N.

The Task Force of the National Conference Group for Classification of Nursing Diagnoses was established in 1973. Its purpose was to continue developmental work on the identification and classification of nursing diagnoses in the years between national conferences. The members of the Task Force (Appendix A) are self-supporting and highly committed to the Task Force activities: (1) to promote information dissemination and exchange, (2) to promote education about nursing diagnosis at state, regional, and national levels, and (3) to promote research and development activities.

The 36 members of the Task Force are from 17 states and represent all regions of the United States, various nursing practice areas, and nursing positions in practice, education, research, and administration of nursing services. In 1980 through structural revision, the Task Force established Steering, Bylaws, and Nominating Committees to coordinate its activities (Appendixes B to D). As directed by the National Conference Group for Classification of Nursing Diagnoses, 1980, the Task Force prepared bylaws for presentation at the 1982 Fifth National Conference. Structural changes in the National Conference Group and bylaws were ratified in April 1982, and the name of the organization was changed to the North American Nursing Diagnosis Association, Inc.

Activities of the Task Force related to the identification and classification of nursing diagnoses were many and varied. These activities have supported the goals of the organization and assisted nurses in the use of diagnostic nomenclature accepted for clinical testing.

INFORMATION DISSEMINATION

The Clearinghouse for Nursing Diagnosis established in 1973 at St. Louis University continues to play a major role in the dissemination and exchange of information about nursing diagnoses on a national and international basis. The Clearinghouse, coordinated by Ann Marie Becker, R.N., M.S., and its publication *Nursing Diagnosis Newsletter,* edited by Ann Perry, R.N., M.S., and Patricia Potter, R.N., M.S., are valuable resources for nurses wishing information on current developments in nursing diagnosis. The newsletter permits nurses to raise questions, criticize activities, submit articles or reviews, and exchange information on the implementation of diagnoses in practice, education, and research. The Clearinghouse also maintains a speaker's bureau.

State conference groups on nursing diagnosis have been established in some states. The most long-standing groups are those of Wisconsin and Massachusetts. These and other state groups disseminate information, plan state or regional conferences, and encourage implementation and research at the local level. The Massachusetts group also prepares annotated bibliographies on nursing diagnoses distributed by the Clearinghouse. State groups also encourage nurses to identify diagnoses and submit them to the national biennial conferences.

Task Force members have also contributed to the literature on nursing diagnosis and its application in practice, education, and research. This contribution is considered an important means of disseminating information. In addition, members of the Task Force have edited the Proceedings of the Third and Fourth Conferences (Kim and Moritz, 1982) and the Fifth Conference (Kim, McFarland, and McLane, 1984).

INFORMATION EXCHANGE

It has always been considered important to maintain a liaison for information exchange with other nursing organizations in the United States and other countries. Of particular importance is the liaison with the American Nurses' Association. Information exchange has been possible since 1973 when Roberta D. Thiry (Kansas) was appointed by the ANA Congress for Nursing Practice as a liaison to the Task Force.

Following publication of *Nursing: A Social Policy Statement* (American Nurses' Association, 1980), a Steering Committee on Classification of Phenomena of Nursing Practice was established. This Committee has sought to establish a liaison with the NANDA. Two members of the Task Force are on the committee, Roberta D. Thiry (Kansas) and Marjory Gordon (Massachusetts).

A second important liaison for exchanging information has existed with Canadian nurses, who are implementing and testing diagnoses. With formation of the NANDA, Canadian and American nurses will be working together to identify and classify nursing diagnoses.

EDUCATIONAL ACTIVITIES

Knowledge about nursing diagnosis and the state of the art enables nurses to become involved in developing nomenclature and testing diagnoses in clinical practice. Educational programs at the local, regional, national, and international levels have been a high priority since 1973.

Task Force members have organized or participated in educational programs in various parts of the United States. Of particular note was the continuing education workshop that preceded the Fifth National Conference in St. Louis, 1982, designed and developed by Lynda J. Carpenito (Delaware).

The Task Force also presented a program at the American Nurses' Association Program on Nursing Diagnosis. This program was sponsored jointly by the Congress for Nursing Practice, Division of Medical-Surgical Nursing, and the National Conference Group for Classification of Nursing Diagnoses. A program submitted by the United States with the support of nurses in four other countries to the International Congress of Nurses, 1979, was not selected.

The Task Force, through the Clearinghouse, has also provided consultation or speakers for programs. State and regional groups, university continuing education departments, hospitals, and community nursing agencies have contributed to increasing nurses' knowledge of nursing diagnoses. Clearly, these efforts in the area of education have had an impact on the numbers of nurses using the nursing diagnoses approved for clinical testing by the association.

RESEARCH AND DEVELOPMENT ACTIVITIES

Nearly 10 years of sustained effort to identify and classify nursing diagnoses have passed. From a concept shared by a few in 1973, nursing diagnosis has become an integral part of nursing care delivery in the view of many practitioners. In planning the Fifth National Conference, the Task Force members reviewed previous efforts. They concluded that many nurses are committed to describing "what nurses do" from the perspective of nursing diagnoses (patient-client problems). This is a decided shift from previous decades when nursing was described as a set of tasks nurses did for patients. The issues identified by the Task Force in their review of the last decade were then translated into a program for the Fifth National Conference.

Nursing diagnoses are the *scientific concepts* used in developing clinical nursing science. The patient client conditions that diagnoses describe are the focus of concern in practice, education, and clinical research. They also serve to organize the body of nursing knowledge. For these reasons, the identification and classification of diagnostic concepts is a serious undertaking. Thus the Task Force decided that as this first decade of development draws to a close, it was advisable for the conference participants to review how classification systems are developed in sciences and professions. This review seemed appropriate for charting directions for the second decade of development that began with the Fifth National Conference.

Plans were made to examine the profession's Social Policy Statement (American Nurses' Association, 1980). Barnard (Washington), a member of the group that developed the statement, was invited to comment on implications of nursing's social policy for nursing diagnosis and the phenomena of concern discussed in the statement. Building on this commentary, Webster (Colorado) was asked to provide information on classification system development in general and its development in nursing in particular.

Classification requires an organizing framework or principle. In turn, the development of a framework raises questions about what the areas of concern in patient care are. The development of a framework was begun in 1977 by some of the major nursing theorists. They worked with the participants at each national conference. Following Webster's discussion of classification from a philosophic perspective, the Theorist Group was invited to present a progress report on the unitary man/human framework development.

The Task Force invited Kritek (Wisconsin) to review other efforts in classification of nursing diagnoses (Campbell, 1978; Jones, 1979; Simmons, 1980). Pertinent issues and overlaps were to be identified.

The Task Force considered conceptual issues in the definition of nursing diagnoses as pertinent to classification system development. Forsyth (Illinois) was invited to share ideas on the sense and value of the etiologic statement. Kim (Illinois) was asked to discuss issues surrounding physiologic diagnoses within the classification system. Both papers were to deal with issues considered controversial and thus pertinent to the work of the Fifth National Conference participants.

The conceptual issue of an operational definition of nursing diagnosis overshadows all nomenclature identification activities. If the operational definition is not clear, nomenclature can include diagnostic concepts at various levels of generality as well as different foci, the "apples and oranges" phenomenon. In planning the Fifth National Conference, the Task Force invited Shoemaker (Pennsylvania) to present her national study of the concept and definition of nursing diagnosis held by nurses.

The Task Force viewed the need for clinical validation of current nursing diagnoses as well as identification of other diagnoses as the most pressing issues for the next decade. Although it has increased in recent years, research on the diagnoses approved for clinical testing lags behind implementation in practice settings.

A diagnostic category label is merely a shorthand expression for a set of observable behaviors that occur repeatedly and are of therapeutic concern to nurses. The focus in clinical validation of nursing diagnoses is the cluster of defining characteristics (patient behaviors) of a diagnostic label. The Task Force invited Fitzmaurice (Massachusetts)to present a paper at the Fifth National Conference on methodology for identifying and clinically validating nursing diagnoses. The focus of the paper was to encourage clinical studies of diagnoses and to introduce methodology for this purpose.

Frequent changes in the diagnostic terminology during the last decade have been based on opinion rather than on clinical research. Realizing the difficulty frequent changes present to nurses in practice and in education, the Task Force implemented a new policy regarding the approved nomenclature at the Fifth National Conference. Changes in approved nursing diagnoses are to be based on clinical research, which does not negate adding new diagnoses.

When a diagnosis is sufficiently developed for clinical testing, it will be placed on the approved listing. Small group sessions focusing on specific diagnoses were also included in the program for the Fifth National Conference. Clinical papers on specific diagnoses were presented to the small group session participants. Poster presentations provided updates on current research and theory development related to nursing diagnosis.

SUMMARY

These activities of the Task Force represent increasing sophistication in the dissemination of information, promotion of education about nursing diagnosis, and facilitation of nomenclature and classification system development. The thoughtful consideration by the Task Force of work in the past decade and plans for the next decade is represented in the papers included in these *Proceedings*. As implementation of nursing diagnoses increases in practice settings and research clarifies currently "fuzzy" categories, new issues will arise. These issues will include the abstract as well as the concrete and, predictably, will range from ethical issues to reimbursement.

REFERENCES

American Nurses' Association: Nursing: a social policy statement, Kansas City, Mo., 1980, The Association.

Campbell, C.: Nursing diagnosis and interventions in nursing practice, New York, 1978, John Wiley & Sons, Inc.

Jones, P.E.: Terminology for nursing diagnoses, Adv. Nurs. Sci. **2**:65, 1979.

Kim, M.J., and Moritz, D.A., eds.: Classification of nursing diagnoses: proceedings of the third and fourth national conferences, New York, 1982, McGraw-Hill Book Co.

Kim, M.J., McFarland, G.K., and McLane, A.M., eds.: Classification of nursing diagnoses: proceedings of the fifth national conference, St. Louis, 1984, The C.V. Mosby Co.

Simmons, D.A.: Classification scheme for client problems in community health nursing, Pub. No. HRA 80-16, Hyattsville, MD., 1980, U.S. Department of Health and Human Services.

Continuing education program

I. PROGRAM SUMMARY

LYNDA J. CARPENITO, R.N., M.S.N.

To promote the use of the diagnostic categories, the Task Force of the National Conference Group for Classification of Nursing Diagnoses proposed that a continuing education program be offered before the Fifth National Conference convened. Participants would attend a 1-day educational program on nursing diagnoses and be invited to attend the first day of the Fifth National Conference as an introduction to the national group.

The Planning Committee consisted of Ann Marie Becker, R.N., M.S.N.; Lynda J. Carpenito, R.N., M.S.N. (Program Coordinator); Marjory Gordon, R.N., Ph.D., F.A.A.N.; and Mi Ja Kim, R.N., Ph.D., F.A.A.N. The program was designed for nurses who wish to obtain a beginning level of knowledge of nursing diagnoses. The program was divided into four content areas: (1) Historic etiology of nursing diagnoses, (2) Need for a taxonomy in nursing, (3) Nursing diagnosis–the concept, and (4) Deriving nursing diagnoses from case studies. The faculty for the program were Ann Marie Becker, R.N., M.S.N., Assistant Professor, St. Louis University School of Nursing, St. Louis, Missouri, and Lynda J. Carpenito, R.N., M.S.N., Nursing Consultant, Clinical Specialist in Nursing Process, Wilmington Medical Center, Wilmington, Delaware. The historic etiology of nursing diagnoses was presented by Becker (see the next paper). Carpenito presented the rest of the program.

The need for a classification system was based on nursing's historic search for a system to structure nursing knowledge. It was explained that nursing diagnoses can contribute to individual and professional autonomy and accountability by clearly differentiating nursing from other health professions, provide consistent terminology to improve the clarity and usefulness of communication, assist faculty and students to focus on nursing phenomena in curricula, and provide a framework for clinical investigation in nursing. A diagnostic classification system would give nursing an opportunity to be included in a computerized health care information system. Computerization would provide a system to retrieve client records using nursing rather than medical diagnoses. As a mechanism for reimbursement, nursing diagnoses can assist nursing in its quest for professional autonomy.

The term *nursing diagnosis* was traced from its introduction in 1953 to its present use as a classification system. The classifying process used at the national conferences was explained, contrasting an inductive aproach with a deductive approach. Various definitions of nursing diagnoses were presented and critiqued regarding their ability to clearly define and differentiate nursing diagnoses from other problems that nurses treat.

The participants were instructed on the components of a diagnostic category (label, defining characteristics, and etiologic factors), and the method for submitting new categories was reviewed. Guidelines for writing the diagnostic statement were presented with the focus on clarity and consistency. Common errors in diagnostic statements were presented.

The morning session concluded with the presentation of a nursing data base and care planning system using nursing diagnoses. The participants were divided into small work groups for the afternoon session. Each group, under the direction of an experienced group leader, developed nursing diagnoses from case studies. During the small group sessions, participants also had an opportunity to share their experiences with nursing diagnoses and to relate their plans for future involvement.

The group leaders for the small group work sessions were nurses who had participated as group leaders in nursing diagnoses workshops at the national or regional level. The group leders were Carol Ann Baer, West Roxbury, Mass.; Beverly Bartlett, Graby, Mass.; Frances Michelle Bockrath, Philadelphia, Pa.; Joanne Dalton,, Duxbury, Mass.; T. Audean Duespohl, Oil City, Pa.; Linda Freeman-Grilley, Wausau, Wis.; Sister Kathleen Krekeler, St. Louis, Mo.; Ruth McShane, Milwaukee, Wis.; Ann Reilly, Boston, Mass.; Marion Resler, St. Louis, Mo. and Mary Woods, St. Louis, Mo.

The program was evaluated by the participants as an excellent introduction to the concept of nursing diagnoses. The participants recommended that the workshops be lengthened and repeated at each national conference.

II. NURSING DIAGNOSES—HISTORY

ANN MARIE BECKER, R.N., M.S.N.

Nursing diagnosis cannot be considered in isolation. It is only useful to the client and the nurse as a component of the nursing process. To better understand the history of nursing diagnoses, we must look at the evolution of the nursing process. In the late 1950s and the early 1960s the process involved three steps and in the latter 1960s included four steps. At the time, diagnosis was not specifically listed as a component, but it was evident that decision making and judgment were parts of the process. In the 1970s diagnosis was listed as the second step in a five-step nursing process. In the 1980s "diagnosis" is used in the majority of definitions of the nursing process. The term *nursing diagnoses* has been used for only a short time, but the act of diagnosing has been evident since modern nursing began.

The act that nurses were performing for years is now a recognized function of the nurse. In the 1970s this recognition became evident when nursing diagnoses were included as a responsibility of the nurse in Nurse Practice Acts and Standards of Practice, the term was increasingly used in the literature, and the First National Conference on the Classification of Nursing Diagnoses was convened at St. Louis University School of Nursing. The conference began the task we continue: to plan for a classification system for nursing diagnoses. At that first conference in 1973, the National Conference Group for Classification of Nursing Diagnoses was formed. The National Conference Group, through the conferences and other activities, has identified nursing diagnoses; has encouraged the use of nursing diagnoses in education, practice, and research; has provided a forum for the discussion of a conceptual framework to be used in nursing diagnoses development; has established a clearinghouse for the dissemination of information; and has assisted with the formation of state and regional conference groups. It also publishes a quaterly newsletter. The activities of the National Conference Group will increase throughout the 1980s as other conferences are planned.

Nursing diagnosis is only 30 years old, but much has been accomplished in that time. Participation in the conferences is a participation in this history.

Analysis of view on issues and trends related to nursing diagnoses and the national conference

GERTRUDE K. McFARLAND, R.N., D.N.Sc.

MI JA KIM, R.N., Ph.D., F.A.A.N.

A selected number of conference participants were invited to respond to a questionnaire designed by the editors to give conference participants, especially those who were not presenting papers at the conference, an opportunity to share their views on nursing diagnoses and on the conference with the nursing community. Along with this selection factor, an attempt was made to select participants from all regions of the United States and practicing in different functional areas. Of the 42 nurses selected to participate, 25 completed the questionnaire.

Conference participants included 193 from the United States and 6 from Canada. When the 25 respondents were grouped according to 10 U.S. Department of Health and Human Services regions, the breakdown was as follows: Region I (Maine, Vermont, Massachusetts, Connecticut, Rhode Island, and New Hampshire) was represented by 5 out of 34 total conference participants, Region II (New York, New Jersey, Puerto Rico, and the Virgin Islands) by 2 out of 21, Region III (Pennsylvania, Delaware, District of Columbia, Maryland, Virginia, and West Virginia) by 2 out of 24, Region IV (Alabama, Florida, Georgia, Kentucky, Mississippi, North Carolina, South Carolina, and Tennessee) by 3 out of 9, Region V (Illinois, Indiana, Ohio, Minnesota, Michigan, and Wisconsin) by 5 out of 57, Region VI (Arkansas, New Mexico, Oklahoma, Texas, and Louisiana) by 2 out of 5, Region VII (Kansas, Iowa, Missouri, and Nebraska) by 3 out of 29, Region VIII (Colorada, Montana, South Dakota, North Dakota, Utah, and Wyoming) by 0 out of 0; Region IX (Arizona, California, Hawaii, Nevada, Guam, Trust Territory of Pacific Islands, and American Samoa) 2 out of 11, and Region X (Alaska, Idaho, Oregon, and Washington) 1 out of 4.

Questions 1 through 4 were analyzed as a group response. Representative individual responses for question 5 were selected to reflect the thinking of the respondents to the various questions and issues.

Question 1: How many times have you attended a National Conference on the Classification of Nursing Diagnoses?

The breakdown of data indicating attendance at national conferences is as follows:

Attended	Number of respondents
5 national conferences	1
4 national conferences	2
3 national conferences	4
2 national conferences	4
1 national conference	14

Question 2: What other experience have you had with nursing diagnoses?

Nursing diagnoses were used in direct clinical practice or in the management of nursing services by 10 of the respondents. In one patient care plan project, nursing diagnoses were used as the approach to the identification of patient problems. In another setting, charge nurses were consistently provided with educational experiences that introduced them to the use of nursing diagnoses within the nursing process, with the specific goal of improving continuity of care. One respondent noted that for many years she has been making clinical judgments in nursing practice that now are called nursing diagnoses.

Attendance and active participation in regional conference were mentioned by eight respondents. These regional conferences were held in the Northeast, Southeast, Northwest, and Midwest areas. Several attended workshops on the use of nursing diagnoses.

Research in the area of nursing diagnoses was conducted by four of the nurses, including one who reported participating in a funded study. Two reported publishing work on nursing diagnosis.

Many of the respondents (15) reported having prior background in nursing diagnoses through participation in workshops on nursing diagnoses, teaching continuing education classes on nursing diagnoses, or integrating nursing diagnoses in their undergraduate or graduate teaching. For example, one nurse teaches content nursing diagnoses to beginning undergraduate nursing students and assists them in developing nursing diagnoses for nursing home residents and clients in a health screening clinic. Another participant teaches content nursing diagnoses as part of a nursing assessment course in a baccalaureate in nursing science program for RN students. A third respondent reported on the inclusion of nursing diagnoses at the graduate level. Another respondent has taught nursing diagnoses and nursing process at both the undergraduate and graduate levels and uses the Kim and Moritz (1982) book as a required text at the graduate level. The majority of the 15 respondents who use nursing diagnoses in teaching report that they also conduct workshops on the topics, several on a state-wide basis.

Consultation with a variety of health care agencies was also reported by several respondents. In addition, one participant reported the development of a nursing theory along with a record system for nurses that includes the formulation of nursing diagnoses.

Question 3: Impressions of the Fifth National Conference on the Classification of Nursing Diagnoses.

a. Why attending conference?

The major reasons for attendance were congruent with the purposes of the conference: (1) to participate in the development of nursing diagnostic labels, nursing taxonomy, and a conceptual framework to define the domain of nursing; (2) to engage in dialogue with nurse colleagues interested in using nursing diagnoses in practice settings, educational arena, and research; and (3) to become more actively involved with decision making about nursing diagnoses at the national level. Many respondents indicated that their reason for attending the conference was to gain more knowledge about nursing diagnoses. Some of their learning needs were met through the nursing diagnosis workshop, which was conducted the day before the Fifth National Conference.

b. What other aspects should be available at future conferences?

All 25 respondents had ideas to share on this question. The majority of comments focused on the small work groups and special interest groups. Some of the key recommendations pertinent to program activities were:

1. Set up the group structure so that conference participants can choose to work on both the nursing diagnostic labels and the theoretic framework with the theorists.
2. Require expertise, rather than interest, as the basis for forming the small work groups.
3. Maintain a consistent core group of members of the small work groups from conference to conference. Identify other measures to provide for consistency.
4. Formalize and build into the conference schedule special interest groups; that is, allow for more time for special interest groups that does not lengthen the day.
5. Include reports from regional conferences.

Other suggestions related to future conference planning are:

1. Form more small groups, thus reducing group size.
2. Inform conference participants before the conference about the small group in which they will be placed.
3. Request that small group members review research paper before meeting to facilitate productive work groups.
4. Provide more direction to the participants before the conference so that they can prepare and the conference becomes more of a working session.
5. Send records of previous small groups to participants before their meeting.
6. Require clinical experience as basis for selecting group members.

Suggestions for the special interest groups were:
1. Provide more structure to special interest groups so participants can come prepared with specific concerns or "show-and-tell" materials.
2. Use a special interest group (on research) to develop research project(s) and pursue study with input from various geographic areas.

Several comments were related to the conference format in general. Two respondents suggested distributing a list of conference participants to the nurses during the meeting. Other suggestions included reducing the number of days the conference was held; initiating more publicity about the national conference; having more book displays and poster presentations; collating a bibliography from each diagnostic label; continuing the continuing education program held before the Fifth National Conference; continuing the presentation of research studies, including reports to the total group from regional conference groups; and providing information on establishing regional networks.

Content and topics that respondents would like to have addressed at future conferences are gerontology; holistic approaches in community health, health promotion, and nursing diagnoses; nursing diagnoses and interdependent practice; implementation of nursing diagnoses in clinical settings; findings regarding the unitary man/human framework; nursing diagnoses and quality assurance; use of nursing diagnoses in patient classification systems; and use of nursing diagnoses in risk management to reduce a hospital's liability.

This question specifically requested respondents to make suggestions for future conferences. These suggestions will continue to strengthen the development of a taxonomy of nursing diagnoses for use by the nursing profession. As one respondent summed it up: The quality of these National Conferences on the Classification of Nursing Diagnoses has been steadily improving. The presenters have been excellent during the conference. The content of this conference matches that of any other professional conference.

Nursing diagnoses must be used in conducting clinical studies. From all the diagnostic categories, many research questions can and will be generated. As one nurse commented, "The questions that were generated in the group work will provide a basis for research for many years to come." Some nursing diagnoses were conceptualized to the point that assessment tools and checklists can now be constructed to gather relevant data about the categories. In the words of another respondent, "The emphasis on the need for research in all these areas was well done." Another respondent commented, "All kinds of ideas have occurred to me with respect to research."

Other responses were related to the nursing profession. The relevance of nursing diagnoses is extremely high because this work is shaping the present as well as the future course of the nursing profession. Nursing diagnoses are critical and essential for the nursing profession. Nursing diagnoses deal with the essence of nursing as a professional endeavor. In summary, "nursing diagnoses," in the words of one respondent, "has the potential for being a unifying base for practice, education, and research. It gives direction for curriculum development, provides questions for research, and a mechanism for identifying and treating patient responses."

Question 4: Activities and attitiudes related to nursing diagnoses in your geographic area. (This question was examined in relation to the following components.)

a. Current activities in which you are involved, future commitment
b. Activities or projects in which your institution or other agency or group are involved, for example,
    1. Efforts in nursing administration related to nursing diagnoses
    2. Curriculum development projects related to nursing diagnoses
    3. Demonstration practice projects related to nursing diagnoses
    4. Research related to nursing diagnoses
    5. Activities or projects in specialty areas related to nursing diagnoses
c. Resources related to nursing diagnoses available in your area (for example, continuing education opportunities, organized nursing diagnoses groups)
d. Acceptance of nursing diagnoses in your geographic area

Representative activities from different regions of the United States are reported to indicate the general scope of involvement with nursing diagnoses.

In Region I some of the major activities and groups reported were an active Rhode Island Conference Group on Nursing Diagnoses; a Boston Nursing Diagnoses Group, and a New Hampshire Conference Group. Encouragement is being provided to nursing service administrators and schools of nursing in Rhode Island for implementing nursing diagnoses. In addition, diagnostic labels are being actively explored and developed within the clinical practice area. In Massachusetts, many conferences, programs, research activities, and publishing endeavors are occurring. In New Hampshire many health care agencies, especially Visiting Nurse Associations, are implementing nursing diagnoses. Nursing diagnoses are being incorporated into baccalaureate programs.

It is reported that the resources related to nursing diagnoses in Rhode Island are fairly good. Nurses involved in the State Conference Group are readily available to provide support and serve as a resource. Interstate support is received from conference groups in surrounding states. Boston College has an excellent resource library that also serves nurses in Rhode Island. Schools of nursing in Rhode Island are improving their resources relevant to nursing diagnoses. In addition, nursing diagnoses workshops and other continuing education activities are reported in this state. Many resources related to nursing diagnoses are present in the Boston area. In New Hampshire, conferences, workshops, and other activities are reported.

Adequate acceptance levels of nursing diagnoses were reported for Massachusetts. Acceptance of nursing diagnoses in Rhode Island was reported as uneven with areas of high acceptability and areas of total rejection. Since 1973, there has been a great improvement because several hospitals are now using nursing diagnoses and several agencies are beginning to use it. In New Hampshire the acceptance is viewed as moderately high and steadily growing. Optimism about the future use in New Hampshire is expressed.

Activities and groups reported for Region II include using nursing diagnoses in cardiac and cancer nursing, identifying new diagnostic labels related to specific population groups, establishing process and outcome standards for practice by using the diagnostic labels as a framework integrating content of nursing diagnoses in all nursing staff orientation programs, working with graduate nursing students with projects related to nursing diagnoses, and conducting workshops and defining nurse roles in joint practice situations. Continuing education programs on nursing diagnoses have been conducted in the New York City area; the attitude toward nursing diagnoses is generally one of acceptance.

Activities and projects reported for Region III were teaching graduate nursing students, conducting nursing research in this area, providing ongoing consultation, and developing a computerized nursing information system. Other activities and projects reported were integration of nursing diagnoses into the POMR format for computerization, development of a patient classification system, development of a risk management system, graduate nursing program curriculum revisions, integrating nursing diagnoses in all areas of the program, and conducting funded nursing research involving both faculty and graduate students. Resources that are reported include continuing education programs and the core group of experts in nursing diagnoses who serve as resource persons. At present, a regional conference group has not been organized, but thinking is moving in that direction. Acceptance of nursing diagnoses in the area is reported as variable. Implementation of nursing diagnoses is taking place in some hospitals. In one large hospital, it is reported that physicians will not accept the use of the term *nursing diagnoses.*

The involvement reported for Region IV included using nursing diagnoses as part of the nursing process in teaching junior nursing students, teaching nursing courses related to testing a nursing theory, teaching a graduate core course in which nursing diagnoses are covered within a cultural content, and identifying diagnostic labels. One continuing education program related to nursing diagnoses was reported as being offered in south Florida. Sporadic acceptance of nursing diagnoses is reported in the region.

Current activities and groups for Region V are Wisconsin Southeast Regional Group on Nursing Diagnoses, committee on nursing diagnoses of the Wisconsin Nurses Association, conducting workshops on nursing diagnoses for practicing nurses, implementing nursing diagnoses in 1000-bed hospital, developing standardized nursing care plans for several nursing diagnoses, conducting a research study on nursing diagnoses in cardiovascular nursing, implementing nursing diagnoses–based care planning on four units of a hospital, and using nursing diagnoses in clinical practice.

Other activities and projects reported were efforts of nursing administrators to make the transition to the use of nursing diagnoses in practice, efforts to study nursing diagnoses and their defining characteristics with certain categories of patients, networking among area hospitals to facilitate use of nursing diagnoses, implementation of nursing diagnoses and research in area hospitals, integration of nursing diagnoses in advanced nursing process course in developing BSN completion program, implementation of patient classification system, and initiation of standard nursing care plans based on nursing diagnoses. A state group on nursing diagnoses is being planned for Michigan. It is also anticipated that more continuing education offerings on nursing diagnoses will be held in this state. Continuing education offerings are reported in the region. Organized regional and state groups are reported in Wisconsin. In general, the region has geographic areas with high acceptance and use of nursing diagnoses. In these areas, it is reported that nursing diagnoses are accepted by many in practice as the essence and core of nursing. There is also a commitment in many educational institutions including the encouragement of research at the master's level.

Activities related to nursing diagnoses in Region VI are the integration of nursing diagnoses into the curriculum of a nursing service management course, the utilization of nursing diagnoses in critical care settings, the development of standardized care plans using nursing diagnoses, teaching beginning classes on nursing diagnoses by a hospital in-service department, and the conduction of research on nursing diagnoses in graduate schools of nursing. In general, however, the respondents believed that the acceptance of nursing diagnoses was not high primarily because of the lack of dissemination of information about it. The projection was made that it would take a lot of time to achieve improved acceptance.

Activities noted in Region VII include the design of a research study to analyze assessment tools with implications for a nursing diagnostic taxonomy; consultation with a hospital implementing new nursing care plans that incorporate nursing diagnoses; curriculum development related to nursing diagnoses; and organizing core courses at graduate level around the nursing process, including nursing diagnoses and teaching nursing diagnoses to beginning nursing students. Continuing education programs on the topic are offered in the area. Increasing interest and considerable use in certain areas of the region are reported.

No conference participants were from Region VIII, which includes Colorado, Montana, South Dakota, North Dakota, Utah, and Wyoming.

Although activities such as the implementation of nursing diagnoses in some service settings, the teaching of relevant content in some undergraduate programs, and the conduction of research on nursing diagnoses are taking place in Region IX, respondents reported limited and sporadic acceptance of nursing diagnoses.

In Region X a Northwest Regional Conference was noted. Activities that are related to nursing diagnoses in this area include revision of nursing documentation systems in which nursing diagnoses will be used in nursing care plans and in interdisciplinary progress notes. Acute care assessment tools are being revised to include Gordon's functional categories and patterns. Content analysis has been done on statements called *nursing diagnoses* which appear on care plans, as part of a quality assurance program. Skill in utilization of nursing diagnoses is expected of all primary care nurses. Although it is reported that nursing diagnoses are becoming more accepted in the Seattle area, the respondents noted that several nurse experts use approaches that are different from those of the National Conference Group, which does create some confusion but may eventually contribute to the development of the movement.

As previously stated, representative individual responses for question 5 were selected to reflect the thinking of the respondents to the various questions and issues.

Question 5a: Issues related to nursing diagnoses: (a) What are the key barriers/potentiators faced in the implementation of nursing diagnoses?

Joan Bruce: The key barrier which I have found in implementation is the resistance which normally appears when a change is taking place. The response is normal but it demands continuous work on the part of the implementor.

Dianne Christopherson: Key barriers to implementation include (1) verbiage of diagnoses i.e., convincing practitioners it is not a semantics game, (2) assisting practitioners to see positive and tangible benefits for patients, (3) general apathy or reluctance to try anything new, (4) coordinating numerous nursing research efforts about nursing diagnoses, (5) physician and hospital administrative skepticism and reluctance to change the status quo of the health care system, (6) major education effort that is needed within the profession, (7) major education effort needed with health care consumers and third party reimbursers regarding what a nursing diagnosis is and what it means to members.

Meg Gulanick: Barriers include: (1) limited number of participants in the national conference (less than 200), and hence, lack of broad participation providing open dialogue among large numbers of nurses so maximal voices are heard (not just select regions or practice settings); (2) need for more clinical nurses who can respond to application of labels and framework in practice settings as well as implement research studies; (3) lack of standardized nursing assessment tools which could clarify for nurses and other health professionals the areas of nurse accountability; (4) managers who only hold nurses accountable for implementation of medical orders; and (5) task-oriented "blue collar" nurses who only see their responsibilities as implementation of medical orders.

Jane Lancour: Barriers include: (1) diverse levels of preparation of staff nurses and therefore different knowledge bases, (2) varied commitments of the nurses, (3) monies are not always budgeted for necessary inservice, (4) lack of understanding of the role of nursing by some administrators, (5) impatience of practitioners in the learning process, (6) medicine's view of nursing, and (7) failure to see the broader picture in terms of the need to define nursing's unique contribution in the health care field so as to get third party payment. Potentiators include: (1) enthusiasm of young graduates, (2) nursing diagnoses being the basis of third-party payment, (3) framework for patient classification and staffing, (4) a means of evaluating practice of nurses, (5) clear differentiation of roles of RN and LPN, (6) basis for utilization of nursing process, (7) means of conveying nursing's unique contribution to patient care, (8) means of developing colleague relationship among nurses, and (9) basis for a sound quality assurance program for nursing.

Question 5b: Where do we go from here (i.e., what should be the future thrust of the nursing diagnosis movement)?

Patricia Ann Clunn: The greatest need for developing nursing diagnoses is exploring research methods that validate the defining characteristics. The data base generated for testing is being used as if its certitude has been established. For example, Toth presented an impressive use of nursing diagnosis as a basis for reimbursement, based on the assumption that the diagnoses were reliable and valid indices. While laudable, the use of the nomenclature, as if the validity has been established, underlies the seriousness of the need for concerted research efforts to validate the data generated by group work.

For the diagnoses to be useful in practice there has to be some clarification as to what cues are critical. The present lists are long and each defining characteristic needs listing and validation as to its relative importance. What are the necessary and sufficient cues to formulate a given nursing diagnosis? We need to identify critical factors needed for differential diagnoses. From my research, my hunch is that the differential indices are 3 or 4 cues, and we are a long way from that point in the process of diagnostic refinement. We need to know what is critical for a given nursing diagnosis to be established.

There is a need to identify the "lower" level concepts and how they relate to the "higher" level constructs. Perhaps the concepts need clear operational definitions before constructs at higher levels can be established. It seems our lack of conceptual clarity and consensus is a major problem. Perhaps we need a "nursing dictionary" comparable to the medical dictionary so we are at least using the same terms. Block (1974) and Vincent (1975) have had an interesting dialogue on these critical terms in nursing and my impression is that without a clear definition of terms we spin our wheels. Thus, we need to give specific definitions to our terms so the diagnoses can be tested and validated. I don't think attempting to get consensus before terms are clearly stated will help.

The conference group has generated a number of diagnoses. Perhaps we need to have a moratorium on new diagnoses in order to evaluate and research what we have. This is an appropriate level-one theory development strategy. There are a number of research strategies for this. The problem that seems to be emerging is that some "new diagnoses" are mere repetitions of what has been set forth, using different "words."

There are opportunities for researchers to identify their own "theoretical rationale." We need to have various research data to be able to evaluate the findings that "best fit" our practice parameters. In teaching, it is an interesting exercise to have graduate students validate the use of an "official diagnosis" with a theoretical rationale. Often it is found that the diagnosis "does not fit" a rationale supportive of interventions.

We need to begin looking at interventions to validate the reliability of the indices; some action research is needed to identify the theoretical rationale for the diagnoses. We need case studies and basic data from which to generate testable hypotheses.

Susan S. Labarthe (answering both 5a and 5b): Implementation of nursing diagnosis in a practice setting requires a complex change process at organizational, unit, and individual levels. One key barrier in this change process is the absence of frameworks for its implementation at several conceptual levels. Corollary implications for potentiators and for "where do we go from here" are that the existence of such frameworks would be powerful potentiators of implementation and that development of such frameworks is a crucial part of where we should go from here.

Several levels of framework development are necessary. An overall conceptual framework that can guide the development and organization of nursing diagnoses and their implementation and use in a rudimentary stage needs continuing work. The impact of this level of framework on implementation in clinical settings will be to guide planning and decision making, to achieve conceptual consistency, logical progression, and desired outcomes in the change process. Because of this important potential utility, it is essential that the conceptual framework be developed with consideration for, and empirical testing of, its congruence with the needs and patterns of clinical practice, practitioners, and their patients.

Taxonomy, another level of framework—that of organizing the names of diagnoses—also has implications for implementation, primarily in the organization of information. It will provide an ideal and much-needed tool for teaching and learning the concepts necessary for implementation. To be effective it must be developed in congruence with the developing conceptual framework, the content of existing diagnoses, and the needs and patterns of clinical practice. I suggest toleration of ambiguity in working at this from several different directions, i.e., working at alternative taxonomic frameworks with attention to congruence with one or two of these factors at a time and developing areas of convergence that would lead to the most effective outcomes.

Finally an operational framework (or frameworks) for the implementation and use of nursing diagnosis in practice needs to be developed. This is the level that all of us involved in implementation in the practice setting are engaged. It is the framework we need most, the one which most directly impacts and potentiates implementation of practice. It would be ideal to be able to base it on a fully developed conceptual framework and taxonomy. In the real practice world of 1982, we don't have those. So we put together what we individually see as valid from what is available.

When we achieve some degree of implementation, we have that degree of validation that our operational frameworks work. For this reason I suggest that those of us engaged in implementation in the here and now have an obligation to document the level of validity of our operational frameworks via research methods, and either to become involved or at least communicate our results to those involved in development of the conceptual framework and taxonomies. The reciprocal obligation of those involved in work on those other levels is apparent.

Where do we go from here? Development of conceptual, taxonomic, and operational frameworks are essential for implementation of nursing diagnosis. Congruence among these frameworks is as essential as their development. I suggest that while parallel work at all three levels will surely produce some ambiguity, frustration, and confusion, it can also produce conceptual richness and congruence. The conference has served the much-needed focus for achieving this convergence and one of its important tasks for the future should be to continue to do so.

Question 5c: What is the relevance of the nursing diagnosis movement practice?

Barbara Dossey: Nursing diagnosis has and continues to impact the quality of nursing practice. One of the major areas that must continue to be addressed is implementation into clinical practice. A nurse can be informed about nursing diagnoses and still not be able to work with it in the clinical setting. Practicing nurses need to understand that nursing diagnosis is a part of the nursing process and not a separate domain. As they become more aware of this, they will be able to integrate nursing diagnosis into standards of care throughout all specialty areas of nursing practice. The end result will be that nursing diagnosis helps nurses, in a logical way, define outcome criteria that can be evaluated in a systematic way. Unfortunately, too many nurses are still task oriented and do not put the nursing process into practice. Nursing diagnosis can take nursing practice to a very high professional level.

Mary Lee Kirkland: I see diagnosis aiding the quality of practice by helping the nurse cluster data and be more quickly able to arrive at a diagnosis. The diagnosis ultimately should give direction to the identification of specific, measurable patient outcomes and the selection of applicable nursing interventions as an independent nursing activity.

Elizabeth A. McFarlane: The relevance of nursing diagnosis to nursing practice comes through the potential impact that the use of nursing diagnosis can have in assuring a quality, holistic approach in the provision of nursing care. Nursing diagnosis is the pivotal point in the nursing process. The derivation of nursing diagnosis from data collected through an ongoing, comprehensive nursing assessment is a critical force in assuring that the process will move toward the identification of realistic achievable patient-oriented outcomes.

While the identified outcomes provide direction for planning nursing intervention and evaluating the effectiveness of the intervention, the validity and appropriateness of the identified outcomes are dependent on nursing diagnosis. Without nursing diagnoses, the process lacks a concrete linkage between assessment and the identification of outcomes.

The nursing diagnosis movement (i.e., the efforts to develop a framework for classification of nursing diagnoses; identify, define, and describe nursing diagnoses; support the use of nursing diagnoses by nurses in practice) is substantiating the essential links, nursing diagnosis, in the nursing process.

Suzanne Sikma: Nursing diagnosis is a key to identifying the unique contribution of nursing practice to health care. It enables the nurse to clarify the difference between independent nursing and dependent functions. I have repeatedly observed staff nurses becoming more energized and enthusiastic about practice when they become involved in identifying nursing diagnoses for their clients. Their self-esteem is enhanced by this activity because they are acknowledged as thinkers. Staff nurses frequently leave the nursing diagnoses workshops with the feeling that "this is what nursing is all about." Although they may become frustrated on occasion, the outcomes remain positive because the nurses know that none of this is written in stone and it is within their control to change.

Question 5d: What is the relevance of the nursing diagnosis movement to the nursing profession?

Imogene M. King: From the beginning of the nursing diagnosis movement, I believed that its relevance for the nursing profession is to lead us to a professional language for nursing. Every other profession has a language for communicating with all professionals and workers in an occupation.

Sr. Kathleen Krekeler: The nursing diagnosis movement: (1) encourages the individual nurse's accountability and increases gratification in nursing; (2) enhances autonomy of the profession by providing a body of knowledge, more practical use of the Code of Ethics, and holistic health care; (3) facilitates interaction with other professionals; (4) provides beginning frameworks for organizing teaching concepts; (5) suggests innumerable topics for research; (6) could provide for organizing groups of clients for nursing intervention, self-direction, and/or therapeutic self-help groups.

Joanne McCloskey: Nursing diagnosis is the key to the professional autonomy of nurses. Through the identification of the health problems that nurses treat, we are defining nursing. For the first time, our movement will be based on our own science and not come as an "add on" to medical diagnosis and treatment.

The prime danger to this movement is the premature closure of categories (diagnoses and levels of diagnoses). To get something that truly reflects what we do in practice, we need at this time in our history to live and work with a great deal of ambiguity. This is difficult, especially for a "doing" profession. Completeness and concreteness will come but it will take time.

The nursing diagnosis movement is moving along very well. In fact, the pace and accomplishments have been tremendous. It is good to have an organized group to spearhead such a movement and to get more and more nurses involved and knowledgeable.

Question 5e: What is the best method of achieving a consensus about nursing diagnosis?

Carolyn M. Crowell: To reach consensus for the taxonomy, it would be helpful to push for as many clinical research studies as possible, utilizing the diagnostic labels. Sigma Theta Tau, as part of its 10-year plan related to nursing scholarship, might consider using these diagnoses for research studies, which they would promote and/or fund. Another aspect of achieving consensus is to standardize assessment data tools. We need more research into what is an adequate data base to describe normal human responses.

Rosemary Y. Wang: The nursing profession has a long history of being a "house divided" and experiencing "lack of consensus." However, the time has come that the profession begins to focus on the issue at hand and recognize the need to work together in search of a common goal. The policy and procedures in the by-laws of the National Conference will facilitate the gaining of a consensus on the diagnoses. As more research is done on the diagnoses, the consensus of adopting a given diagnosis will be inevitable. Nurses are more educated, more sophisticated in their research, and increasingly articulate about their work.

Question 5f: What is the relevance of computers for nursing diagnosis?

Margaret E. Broidy: The relevance of computers for nursing diagnosis is present because computers are technical, scientific tools to be used to make work more efficient. I see computers saving tremendous time and energy in the area of data storage and retrieval, documentation, and data collection in the research process. I see them helping one nurse to cue into important patient data that may be missed due to human error. I see computers being able to collect the assessment data from the patient and family and be programmed to recognize weighted information. However, at no time do I see one computer being able to replace the judgmental, decision-making processes through which one nurse proceeds in order to make a statement about the person whom nursing can assist.

Again, computers are tools which can be of tremendous help in carrying out the nursing process and particularly nursing diagnoses (i.e., patient chart retrieval based on nursing diagnosis). But they are only as good as they are programmed. I see computers as essential as our body of knowledge regarding each part of the domain of nursing.

Karen A. Rieder: Computers are essential for documentation, storage, and retrieval of patient data and nursing interventions. Without the computer the process of identifying common problem areas and actions is too unwieldy and tedious to be useful. Computers offer a means for comparing nursing diagnoses across hospital and patient populations, for identifying common interventions and resultant outcomes of cases, and identifying gaps in nursing knowledge. At the present, one may be aware of a single instance or several instances of unsuccessful interventions. Through use of a computer whole patterns can be identified, variables can be selected and tested, and findings can provide a base for changing expanding nursing care.

Question 5g: What impact will the nursing diagnosis movement have on the autonomy of the nursing profession?

Joanne K. Farley: I believe the autonomy of the profession has increased directly proportionate to the diagnostic movement. Nurses are now able to say, "This is what we do. This is what makes us unique. This is what our business is all about." Utilization of nursing process, and nursing diagnosis particularly, has helped the nurse to move away from the medical model of care into the nursing model. It has helped nurses to deemphasize the carry-out-the-order-of-a-licensed-physician-or-dentist role of practice, and to expand the autonomous role of "assessing, diagnosing, planning, implementing and evaluating" patients.

The close link between the ANA's Social Policy Statement's definition of nursing and the diagnostic movement provides a firm foundation for autonomy in the profession.

Question 5h: What is the relevance of nursing diagnoses for third-party payment?

Wealtha Alex: When I talk with insurance executives about reimbursing for autonomous nursing service, they ask: (1) What did I do for the patient? (2) How much did the service cost? (3) Who decided the service was needed? The insurance people then say, nursing services are not covered and will not be until consumers demand such coverage. Nursing diagnoses are essential for answering the above questions. First, nurses need to determine their domain and tell the world about it in understandable terms. Then I could say, "I am a nurse. The patient and I decided he/she needed this nursing service." Having a nursing diagnosis would not only give me a diagnostic label but guide for effective intervention based upon research. Service cost per nursing diagnoses would open a whole field of economic possibilities. That is, knowing the cost of nursing diagnoses could enable prospective planning for nursing care delivery, productivity research on different levels and mix of nurse providers, and very importantly, the cost comparisons of treated versus untreated nursing diagnoses.

More clearly defining nursing via nursing diagnoses would unify the efforts of nursing in acute and community settings through longitudinal studies of resolution of nursing diagnoses.

Sylvia Weber: It is my belief that one of the reasons nurses have difficulty in receiving third-party payment for nursing services is because we have not made it clear what we do that's different and valuable from others. Of course there are many other reasons, including our lack of unity, other professionals feeling threatened, and our lack of control of the health care dollar. Nursing diagnoses will help us articulate this and present to third-party payors our independent functions. We can then establish a case for the need for nursing care, how it can impact on the health care system, how we can save health care dollars, and how nursing care can also lead to prevention of future illness. This is because our interventions for specific nursing diagnoses are not only illness oriented but also health and prevention oriented.

Question 5i: What is the relevance of nursing diagnosis for quality assurance programs?

Bernadine Cimprich: The use of nursing diagnoses can provide the basis for determining measurable standards of nursing care for specific patient/client populations. Long-term experience with specific patient populations shows that certain nursing diagnoses are made consistently when specific problems are present. Once nursing diagnoses are expertly identified and validated, both process and outcome standards may be developed, put in measurable terms, and agreed on by nurses in the setting. These standards can then be used in the quality assurance program to determine: (1) quality of individual care plans measured against existing standards, (2) quality of implementation of interventions, and (3) validity of stated outcomes in relation to stated interventions.

Wanda Ruthven: The relevant issues from my point of view regarding nursing diagnosis, quality control, and third-party payment are entertained with the inconsistencies most of us find in the existing use of nursing language to substantiate (a) roles, (b) valid records, and (c) evaluation processes.

Nurses do not know what other nurses deem primary in their practice roles. For example, the cardiovascular nurse in the acute setting does not fully comprehend the problems for such a nurse working in the home setting. Because we do not have a standard method of recording what we do so that others can comprehend, records seldom reflect the nurse's contribution to care.

Quality control using nursing labels to define nurse services given with structure (i.e., goals and outcomes) is necessary to substantiate the costs of nurses' salaries, since one of the major ongoing expenses within health care is this area. I believe that the vernacular of nursing, as "young" as it is, can facilitate communication and coordination in behalf of the patient. Third-party payment will be forthcoming more rapidly if nursing diagnoses are incorporated into the nursing record.

Question 5j: What is the relevance of nursing diagnosis for patient classification and the development of staffing patterns?

Mary Jo Aspinall: Patient classification systems and staffing patterns have to consider all the functions of the nurse, those medically delegated as well as nursing independent fuctions. Nurses eager to have the diagnoses utilized for staffing should exert care that their enthusiasm for nursing diagnoses does not increase the dichotomy between nurses working with the acutely ill (who work more extensively under medical protocols) and those working more independently in ambulatory care centers or primarily with the psychiatric population.

Question 5k: What should be considered regarding the nursing movement and fragmentation of patient care (i.e., introduction of another diagnosis) vs. the delineation of nursing practice and the provision of holistic nursing care?

Joseph T. Burley: Fragmentation is already occurring. I'm sure many staff nurses wonder how the magic 42 nursing diagnoses were developed. How are nursing diagnoses going to make the work of the staff nurse different? Will it be seen as just another task to do? Intensive education and careful movement of this concept in the practice environment is essential. Personally, I see it as an essential step in bringing enthusiasm back to the work setting.

Question 5l: Other comments?

Mary Marston-Scott: I am a little concerned with some of the nursing diagnoses in that they seem to place the nurse in the position of reacting to something which perhaps could have been avoided in the first place. An example comes from my own area of noncompliance. We need to further develop this area to take into account our knowledge of how to promote healthy behavior, even the following of a treatment regimen, before the patient decides against it. The patient should not be labeled as noncompliant if the nurse has not negotiated with the patient with regard to what the patient is willing to carry out and desires the assistance of the nurse in carrying through. In summary, (1) whenever possible, the nurse should validate the diagnoses with patients, which is not something we have emphasized; and (2) we need to continue to try to develop diagnoses that reflect needs for health promotion and disease prevention. I believe nursing diagnoses must not only address human responses to illness but also assist clients to help them improve health.

REFERENCE

Block, D.: Some critical terms in nursing: what do they really mean, Nurs. Outlook **22**(11):689, Nov. 1974.

Kim, M.J., and Moritz, D.A., eds.: Classification of nursing diagnoses: proceedings of the third and fourth national conferences, New York, 1982, McGraw-Hill Book Co.

Vincent, P.: Some crucial terms in nursing—a second opinion, Nurs. Outlook **23**(1):46, Jan. 1975.

Special interest group report: nursing diagnosis in critical care

MADELINE WAKE, R.N., M.S.N.

On April 15 and 16, 1982, a special interest group for critical care met to discuss concerns about developmental and utilization of nursing diagnoses in that area. Input from this group was given to individuals from Marquette University and the American Association of Critical-Care Nurses who were planning a cosponsored conference.

This conference was held March 17 and 18, 1983. Its purpose was to explore the evolution of nursing diagnosis and the issues related to using nursing diagnosis in critical care. Conference goals were to add to the current body of knowledge by refining established nursing diagnoses and promoting their validation and by clarifying issues concerning conceptualization and use of nursing diagnosis in critical care. Speakers for the conference included Audrey McLane, Mi Ja Kim, Cathie Guzzetta, Chris Tanner, and Jane Lancour.

Through their didactic presentations and group work, participants were enabled to (1) explain the vital position of nursing diagnosis in the evolution of nursing as a scientific discipline, (2) present various perspectives of at least two issues surrounding nursing diagnosis in critical care, (3) utilize a scientific approach to evaluate the process and product of nursing diagnosis and (4) identify a personal unique contribution to the development of nursing diagnosis.

Over 90% of the 270 participants believed the objectives were met. The majority committed themselves to specific projects including validation studies and implementation efforts. A complete report of the conference will be submitted to the NANDA.

Special interest group report: nursing diagnoses and the healthy client

BARBARA BURKE, R.N., M.S.N.

Nurses have some clients who do not have an identified problem. Examples may include clients from well-baby clinics, induction examinations at time of employment, public health newborn visits, and other occasions when nurses interact with clients who are not hospitalized.

Nursing diagnoses, using current definitions from the literature that all refer to a "problem," are not appropriate for these clients. A discussion of current practice may reveal information that is important for future development of nursing diagnoses.

Eight nurses who attended the Fifth National Conference on the Classification of Nursing Diagnoses participated in a special interest group on nursing diagnoses and the healthy client. They were from the eastern and midwestern United States, Hawaii, and Canada. Their functional areas were equally divided between education and clinical practice.

Current nursing practice includes identification of strengths of clients and families and reinforcement of those strengths. Nurses also support client behaviors that are already present, that are not associated with problems, and that enhance the life-style of the client. The accepted list of nursing diagnoses only provides for problem identification, actual or potential.

Some nurses are using nursing diagnoses from the national list and restating them in positive terms to direct their nursing actions. New diagnoses that are not on the current list are also being used. As the development of the new diagnoses progresses, they may be presented to the Sixth National Conference. Presently nurses in this area are experiencing a lack of interest and information.

Much work needs to be done in the area of nursing diagnoses when the client is "healthy" and problem identification is difficult. However, some of these diagnoses could be applicable to the client who also has problems, such as strength identification to best assess how to address the problem with the client.

The group states that eventually all of nursing practice will need to be addressed within a framework of nursing diagnoses to improve documentation and to facilitate reimbursement. The client who presents no problems but still benefits from interaction with the nurse is an area of nursing practice that must be included in an overall framework. Input from nurses practicing with such clients will be necessary for future development. This special interest group opens this area of nursing practice to the nursing community to encourage research, publication, or communication about practice that will, eventually, provide information for including the healthy client in the developing framework for nursing diagnoses.

Development of association bylaws

KRISTINE M. GEBBIE, R.N., M.N.
BARBARA HAAS, R.N., M.S.N.

The participants of the Fifth National Conference on the Classification of Nursing Diagnoses saw the formal creation of NANDA. After a decade of informal collaboration under the guidance of a spontaneously created task force and with the strong and very positive institutional help of St. Louis University, the professional nurses committed to the development of a diagnostic taxonomy voted to create a formal organizational structure. The bylaws that follow provide a management structure for the affairs of the Association, direction for the tasks of the Association, and a format for the formalization of diagnosis adoption.

The entire membership provides the final voting authority on most affairs of the association, including the final balloting on diagnoses. The general assembly, that is, those members participating in regularly scheduled meetings, provide a face-to-face forum for discussion of affairs of the association and clarification of issues. The board provides ongoing leadership, hires staff to do the work of the association, and appoints committees to assume specific responsibilities. Discussion and decisions about the bylaws are presented in Table 1.

The bylaws as adopted are different from those drafted and presented to the assembly in several respects. The Bylaws Committee (Kristine Gebbie, Oregon; Barbara Haas, Maine; Larry Sieck, Texas) proposed a national limitation, since the majority of active participants have been from the United States and it might be simpler to work with one country. The voting membership believed that the present level of activity from Canada was such that at least a North American designation would be appropriate.

NORTH AMERICAN NURSING DIAGNOSIS ASSOCIATION BYLAWS

Article 1. TITLE, PURPOSE, AND FUNCTION

Section 1. Title. The name of this association shall be the North American Nursing Diagnosis Association, Inc.

Section 2. Purpose. This association is organized to develop, refine, and promote a taxonomy of nursing diagnostic terminology of general use to professional nurses.

Section 3. Restrictions. The association is intended to qualify as a tax-exempt organization within the meaning of section 501 (c) (3) of the U.S. Internal Revenue Code of 1954, as amended. The affairs of the association shall be conducted in such a manner as to qualify for tax exemption under the provision. No substantial part of the activities of the association shall be the carrying on of propaganda or otherwise attempting to influence legislation; the association shall not participate in, or inter-

TABLE 1   **Discussion and decisions about the bylaws**

Meeting:	General Assembly of the Fifth National Conference on the Classification of Nursing Diagnosis	Topic:	Presentation and discussion of bylaws
		Presenting:	K. Gebbie
Date:	Saturday, April 17, 1982	Recording:	B. Haas
Place:	St. Louis, Missouri	Present:	71 Members

Topic	Discussion	Decision
Article I Section I Move to delete the word *National*	Omitting *National* might make scope more limited.	Accepted
Move to change Section I to include *North American* Nursing Diagnosis Association, Inc.	*North American* would include Canada but be restrictive to other nations.	Accepted
Article II Section Ia Move: as RN and who does not have license under suspension or revocation		Carried
Move: A member is one who has been granted a license to practice as an RN	Intent was not to exclude acceptable nurses because of terminology used in this section. Some areas do not have license but are professional nurses.	Defeated
and who does not have a license under suspension or revocation Move.	Perhaps best to refer to matter of definition to Board.	
Referred to Board to identify language for the intent	Suggestions: Exclude geography. Also needs to address Article IX, Section 2 for possible omission of word.	Approved
Article II Section Ib Delete Section Ib	None.	Approved
Article III Section 1 Move dues for members outside the U.S. be an additional $2.50 where the postage is greater than U.S. rate	Seconded. Administratively, it would be easier if there were no differences. Postage probably would not be excessive.	Defeated
Article IV Section 1 Move change of 6 directors to a treasurer and 7 (seven) directors	None.	Accepted

Continued.

TABLE 1   **Discussion and decisions about the bylaws—cont'd**

Topic	Discussion	Decision
Article VI Section 2a The program committee shall plan . . . to regional groups and *special interest groups* desiring. . . .	Interest groups may change.	Approved
Article VI Section 2h Add: Taxonomy Committee shall develop and regularly review a taxonomic system for the diagnoses and submit to Board for review and action; promote its use; and promote collaboration with groups supporting other established health-related taxonomies.	Board is final approval group.	Approved
Article VI Section 2b	This committee functions with approval of Board.	
Article VII Add Section I In addition to any other committees, the President shall appoint a chair and 2 members to a nominating committee. Two additional members shall be elected by the membership during the regular elections. At the first election, one elected and one appointed member will be given 2-year terms, and the remainder 4-year terms. All terms thereafter shall be 4 years.		Approved
Move-Accept		
Bylaws be accepted as amended.		Approved

vene in, any political campaign of any candidate for public office. (Needed only if formal incorporation takes place.)

Section 4. Equal Rights. The purposes of this association shall be unrestricted by consideration of nationality, race, creed, life-style, color, sex, or age.

Section 5. Functions. The function of the association shall be to develop and promote a taxonomy of nursing diagnoses, including, but not limited to:

a. Conducting conferences
b. Publishing documents
c. Facilitating research
d. Serving as an information resource

Article II. MEMBERSHIP

Section 1. Member. A member is one:

a. Who has been granted a license to practice as a registered nurse and who does not have a license under suspension or revocation, or

b. Whose dues are not delinquent.

Section 2. Associate Member. An associate member is one who does not qualify as a member, who shares an interest in the purposes of the association, and whose dues are not delinquent. Associate members do not have a vote but may actively participate in all other affairs of the association.

Section 3. The presentation to this association of completed application, as required by association policy or Bylaws, together with annual dues shall establish them as members or associate members of this association.

Section 4. Membership Year. The membership year shall be a period of twelve (12) consecutive months, beginning January 1 of each calendar year.

Article III. DUES

Section 1. Dues. The Dues of this association shall be as follows:

a. Member dues shall be $20 (U.S. dollars).

b. Associate member dues shall be half of the member dues.

Section 2. Change of Dues. No monies shall be refunded nor additional monies collected when a change of dues category is made within a membership year.

Article IV. OFFICERS AND DUTIES OF OFFICERS

Section 1. The officers of this association shall be a president, a vice-president, a secretary, a treasurer, and seven (7) directors who shall be elected as hereinafter provided.

Section 2. Officers shall perform the duties usually performed by such officers as specified in these Bylaws or designated by the Board.

Section 3. Term of Office. The term of office for all officers shall commence at the beginning of the association's fiscal year and shall continue until the expiration of their respective terms of office or until their successors are elected. No officer shall be eligible to serve more than two consecutive terms in the same office. A member who has served more than half a term shall be deemed to have served a term. The term of office shall be four (4) years. At this initial election only, the President, Secretary, and three Board members shall be elected for two (2) years, and all others for four (4) years.

Section 4. President. The President shall be chairman of the Board of Directors; shall be an ex officio member of all committees and task forces except the Nominating Committee; shall preside at all meetings of this association; shall appoint special committees or task forces as outlined by these Bylaws or the Board; shall serve as the association's representative; and shall perform all other duties of the office.

Section 5. Vice-President. The Vice-President shall assume the duties of the President in case of that officer's absence or inability to serve and shall chair the Diagnosis Review Committee.

Section 6. Secretary. The Secretary shall keep minutes of all proceedings of this association and the Board; shall report at meetings of this association or Board; and shall be familiar with procedures of the headquarters of this association relating to notification of elections or appointments, notices of time and place of meetings, records of members, and policies of the Board and the association. The Secretary shall perform such other duties as may be assigned by the Board.

Section 7. Treasurer. The Treasurer shall have custody of the funds and securities of this association; shall see that full and accurate financial reports are made to the Board and association meetings. The Treasurer shall perform such other duties as may be assigned by the Board.

Section 8. Compensation. Elected offices shall not receive any compensation for their services as such but may be reimbursed for their expenses.

Article V. BOARD OF DIRECTORS

Section 1. Composition. The officers of this association shall constitute the Board of Directors.

Section 2. Meetings. The Board of Directors shall meet at least annually during the fiscal year of the association.

Section 3. Special Meeting. Special meetings of the Board may be called by the President on ten (10) days notice to each member and shall be called by the President on like notice on the written request of four or more members of the Board.

Section 4. Automatic Vacancy of Office. If any member of the Board is absent from two regular meetings in succession, unless excused by the Board for valid reasons, the office shall automatically become vacant and the vacancy shall be filled as provided in these Bylaws.

Section 5. Powers of the Board. The Board of Directors shall have power and authority over the affairs and business of this association between regular association meetings, except that of modifying any action taken by the members. It shall perform the duties prescribed in these Bylaws and such others as may be delegated to it by the association. The Board in addition shall:

    a. Appoint an executive director and fix compensation for the position. The executive director shall serve at the pleasure of the Board with duties and responsibilities conferred by the Board.

    b. Establish administrative policies governing the affairs of the association.

    c. Develop a master plan allowing the accomplishment of the association's purposes and for the growth and prosperity of the association.

    d. Transact the general business of the association.

    e. Report business transacted at regular meetings of the association and give an annual report to the membership and at regular meetings of the association.

    f. Act as custodian of the property, securities, and records of the association; select a place for deposit of the funds of the association; provide for the audit of the books of the association; provide for bonding of association officials as it may deem necessary; and provide for payment of authorized expenses.

    g. Establish and dissolve committees, task forces, and appointments for such to accomplish the purposes of this association.

    h. Have the power to fill vacancies except the offices of President and Vice-President.

    i. Decide on the date and place of association meetings.

    j. Perform such other duties as may be assigned elsewhere in these Bylaws or by the association.

Section 6. Retiring Members. All retiring members of the Board shall deliver to the association within one (1) month all association properties in their possession.

Article VI. COMMITTEES

Section 1. Committee Appointments. The association may have standing committees. Each committee shall be chaired by a member of the Board as appointed by the President. The appointed chair shall name additional members with attention to geographic and clinical practice distribution with concurrence by the President. The size of the committee shall be determined by the Board. Committees shall report to the Board and to meetings of the association as requested or as required by these Bylaws.

Section 2. Committees. The association may have, but shall not be limited to, the following committees:

    a. Program Committee. The Program Committee shall plan the general assembly meetings of the association and provide consultation to regional groups and special interest groups desiring to conduct programs of interest to members of the association.

    b. Publications Committee. The Publications Committee shall oversee the publications of the association including but not limited to a regular newsletter, official proceedings of the general assembly, and nursing diagnoses. Recommendations for the editors of these documents shall be submitted to the Board.

    c. Membership Committee. The Membership Committee shall provide for distribution of information for those eligible and interested in association membership. The Committee shall review and accept applications with concurrence of the Board.

    d. Diagnosis Review Committee. The Diagnosis Review Committee shall review proposed diagnoses and recommend acceptance/modification/rejection to the Board. The Committee shall appoint specialized clinical/technical review task forces in specific clinical areas to review diagnoses prior to Committee action; shall designate the format for submission of proposed diagnoses or changes to existing diagnoses; and following meetings of the General Assembly shall prepare proposed diagnoses in final form as recommended for membership voting.

    e. Nominations Committee. The Nominations Committee shall prepare at least six (6) months prior to the elections a slate of at least two nominees for each office and provide for the election according to written policy.

    f. Research Committee. The Research Committee shall promote conducting research studies and review research papers for the publications of the association.

    g. Public Relations Committee. The Public Relations Committee shall promote the relationship with other nursing and health professionals and keep the association abreast of their trends and pertinent activities. The Committee shall serve as the advocate/spokesman for general affairs to the association.

    h. Taxonomy Committee. The Taxonomy Committee shall develop and regularly review a taxonomic system for the diagnoses and submit to the Board for review and action; promote its (taxonomy) use and promote collaboration with groups supporting other established health-related taxonomies.

Section 3. Term of Office. The term of office shall be four (4) years. One half of each of the committees shall be appointed every two (2) years.

Section 4. Automatic Vacancy of Office. If any member of a committee is absent from two regular meetings in succession, unless excused by the Board for valid reasons, the office shall automatically become vacant and the vacancy shall be filled as provided in these Bylaws.

Section 5. Retiring Members. All retiring members of the committees shall deliver to the association within one (1) month all association properties in their possession.

Article VII. ELECTIONS

Section 1. Nominating Committee. In addition to any other committees, the President shall appoint a chair and two members to a Nominating Committee. Two additional members shall be elected by the membership during the regular elections. At the first election, one elected and one appointed member will be given two-year (2) terms, and the remainder four-year (4) terms. All terms shall be four (4) years.

Section 2. Ballot and Election. All elections shall be in accordance with written Board policy and these Bylaws. Election is constituted by a plurality of voting members, and in case of a tie, the choice shall be by lot.

Section 3. Tellers. The President shall appoint tellers one (1) month in advance of elections, who shall serve as inspectors of the election.

Article VIII. GENERAL ASSEMBLY

Section 1. Composition. The composition of the General Assembly shall be the voting members and associate members who are in attendance at the meetings of the association.

Section 2. Authority. The General Assembly shall approve policies and Bylaws to govern the association; and shall review and comment on proposed diagnoses for the Diagnosis Review Committee's actions prior to the submission to the membership for acceptance.

Article IX. MEETINGS

Section 1. Regular meetings. Regular meetings of the General Assembly shall be at least once every thirty (30) months.

Section 2. Special meetings. Special meetings of the General Assembly may be called by the President upon majority vote of the Board or upon the written request of five members each from twenty states.

Article X. QUORUM

Section 1. General Assembly. Twenty percent (20%) of the voting membership of the association shall constitute a quorum at any regular or special meeting of the General Assembly.

Section 2. Board of Directors. A majority of the members of the Board shall constitute a quorum at any meeting of the Board.

Article XI. PARLIAMENTARY AUTHORITY

The rules contained in *Robert's Rules of Order* (newly revised) shall govern meetings of this association in all cases to which they are applicable and in which they are not inconsistent with these Bylaws.

Article XII. AMENDMENTS

Section 1. Amendments. Amendments to these Bylaws must be submitted to the Board prior to submission to the General Assembly.

Section 2. Previous Notice. These Bylaws may be amended at any regular or special meeting of the General Assembly by a two-thirds vote of the members present and voting, provided the proposed amendments have been sent to all members at least two (2) months prior to the meeting.

Section 3. No Notice. These Bylaws may be amended without previous notice at any regular or special meeting of the General Assembly by a 99% vote of those members present and voting.

Article XIII. DISSOLUTION

The association may be dissolved by a two-thirds vote of the members upon recommendation of the General Assembly. Upon dissolution after payment of all liabilities, the remaining assets shall be distributed to any nursing organization provided that no distribution shall be made to any organization not then covered by Section 501 (c) (3) of the Internal Revenue Service Code of 1954 or the corresponding provision of any future federal or applicable tax law.

Article XV. IMPLEMENTATION

On adoption of these Bylaws, the Task Force Officers shall serve for a period of no more than eighteen (18) months as the officers of the association in order to ensure the implementation of these Bylaws.

Choice of language describing licensed nurses remained as proposed by the committee but is referred to the board for further clarification by moving membership to the broader geographic area of North America. It is possible that "license" is not the appropriate limitation, and some other word will have to be identified and submitted for later action.

The original suggestion of the Bylaws Committee would have resulted in a board of directors with an even number of members. An amendment was proposed to ensure an odd number of members to prevent the possibility of deadlock decisions; this was approved.

The participants were interested in more specificity about some activities of the association, including clarification that a variety of special interest groups may arise and be supported and that the clarification and refinement of a taxonomy is of at least as much interest as the creation of the diagnostic entities themselves. Amendments to those effects have been included.

The final change was to change the Nominating Committee from the original proposal that it would be entirely elected by the membership to having appointed as well as elected members on the committee. This combination provides direct feedback from the membership into the nominating process but ensures some continuity and relationship with the ongoing board of directors.

The previous task force was charged with leadership of the association and given a timeframe of no more than 18 months to ensure the first election and organization. Given the level of enthusiasm expressed at the conference and the level of interest in development of nursing diagnoses throughout the profession, there should be no problem in meeting the 18-month deadline.

CHAPTER 9

Future directions and recommendations

MI JA KIM, R.N., PH.D., F.A.A.N.
GERTRUDE K. McFARLAND, R.N., D.N.Sc.
AUDREY M. McLANE, R.N., PH.D.

Future directions for the development of nursing diagnostic taxonomy and the work of the NANDA are offered by the editors of these proceedings. Instead of summarizing the numerous recommendations included in the articles, the editors present their own perspectives.

The publication of these proceedings represents the culmination of the first decade of scholarly work on the development of a system for specifying the domain of nursing. The quality of the process has evolved along with the taxonomy from reliance on retrospective methods to develop and refine diagnostic categories during the early national conferences to provision for research-based presentations before accepting new diagnoses at the Fifth National Conference. The new level of scholarship is reflected not only in the diagnoses accepted at this conference for clinical use and testing but also in the papers presented in the general and research sessions.

We are reminded of the statements by Styles (1982, p. 185):

> What will bring us to the proper realization that practice without verified knowledge must soon be considered unethical? When will we truly understand that we have no freedom to act on our own expert authority until we have developed the science to warrant independent action? How can we be convinced that scientific investigation is not the last thing to be done but the first thing to be done?

Her thinking on the importance of research goes hand in hand with the stance the association has taken on the importance of research. What constitutes adequate research support for provisional summary descriptions of new phenomena must be decided by the association so that rules developed from a research base can be used with confidence to guide the differentiation of one phenomenon from another. Furthermore, the recommendation is made that the association develop research funding to actively support research relevant to the development of nursing diagnoses. Such funding could come from the proceeds of the national conferences, membership fees, and private and public organizational sources.

The diffusion of knowledge about nursing diagnoses has gained momentum but is still uneven, ranging from well-organized local, state, and regional organizations in some parts of the country to the absence of any systematic process for knowledge dissemination in others. NANDA must provide the leadership for creating a network of state and regional groups and resources to facilitate work on generation, validation, and utilization of diagnostic labels. Such local and regional groups and development of resource networks will provide a mechanism for developing future leaders for the national group and for identification of diagnostic experts.

The work that was begun by the group on taxonomy development clearly needs further development. We recommend that this activity continue its articulation with the theorists' proposed framework to give it a fair chance either to be accepted or to be rejected.

The defining characteristics that were added to current nursing diagnoses based on suggestions of the small groups must be further examined and approved by an appropriate mechanism in NANDA. Furthermore, new nursing diagnoses, etiology, and defining characteristics presented in these proceedings must be examined for possible integration into the current diagnoses list.

In keeping with the recommendation of Webster and others, we recommend NANDA to be open minded in the development of a nursing diagnostic taxonomy, leaving the boundaries flexible to accommodate expansion that will occur as nursing science continues to expand its foundation. As the complexity of nursing science and art increases, the threshold of our tolerance for ambiguity must also increase. None of us can afford to operationalize nursing from a personal perspective only. The problems with which nursing deals are complex, and the practice mode of nursing varies depending on the region, specialty area, and function in which nurses are engaged. Hence nursing diagnostic taxonomy should be reflective of the state of the art of nursing practice and be responsive to the clinical needs of nurses.

Although integration of nursing diagnoses into the curriculum both in undergraduate and graduate programs began to appear during the past 2 years, additional efforts in academia are needed.

Faculty teaching in baccalaureate and graduate programs must continue to sharpen their own diagnostic skills so that they can serve as role models for students and can devise curricula to teach the decision-making process at a much more sophisticated level than has been demanded in the past. Models of curricula based on nursing diagnoses must be shared and critiqued. All curricula in schools of nursing should be examined to determine their adequacy for teaching diagnostic skills. Hence we recommend that NANDA take a leadership role in proposing various curriculum models using the concept of nursing diagnoses.

With increased use of nursing diagnoses in the clinical setting, the demand for more programmatic benefits of its use will also increase. With the advent of DRGs and the distinct possibility of incorporating nursing diagnoses into the DRG system, nursing has never been in a better position than now. We recommend that NANDA take an active role in seeking and developing a system by which nursing service can be reimbursed or paid by third-party payers. Success in this endeavor will not only benefit NANDA but, more importantly, will bring lasting and far-reaching contributions to the nursing profession. In addition, further attention must be given to delineating a coding system to facilitate computerization of diagnostic labels. Priority should be given to developing a practical method for gathering and exchanging information about patterns of human responses to health and illness.

The nature of the tasks, questions, and issues with which NANDA is confronted calls for close relationships with ANA and other professional organizations to have a broader base and meaning for the nursing profession. We recommend that the relationships between such organizations be collegial and that they provide for mutual growth and for nursing profession.

REFERENCE

Styles, M.M.:. On nursing: toward a new endowment, St. Louis, 1982, The C.V.Mosby Co.

Appendixes

A. Task Force: National Conference Group for Classification of Nursing Diagnoses

B. Committees

C. Nurse Theorist Group

D. Small Group Leaders and Recorders

E. Participants of the Fifth National Conference on the Classification of Nursing Diagnoses

F. Annotated Bibliographies

National Conference Group for Classification of Nursing Diagnoses

STEERING COMMITTEE

Marjory Gordon, R.N., PhD. *
Chairperson, Task Force
Boston, Massachusetts

Ann Marie Becker, R.N., M.S.N. *
Director, Clearinghouse
St. Louis, Missouri

Mi Ja Kim, R.N., Ph.D. *
Chicago, Illinois

Gertrude K. McFarland, R.N.,
D.N.Sc. *
Oakton, Virginia

Audrey M. McLane, R.N., Ph.D. *
Milwaukee, Wisconsin

MEMBERS

Doris E. Bell, R.N., Ph.D. *
Edwardsville, Illinois

Andrea U. Bircher, R.N., Ph.D. *
Oklahoma City, Oklahoma

Lynda Juall Carpenito, R.N.,
M.S.N. *
Wilmington, Delaware

Maralee Dennis, R.N., M.N.
Rapid City, South Dakota

Marie J. Driever, R.M., M.N.
Portland, Oregon

T. Audean Duesphol, R.N., M.Ed. *
Oil City, Pennsylvania

Lucy Feild, R.N., M.S. *
Brookline, Massachusetts

Garyfallia Forsyth, R.N., Ph.D. *
Chicago, Illinois

Jacqueline Fortin, R.N., M.S.
Cumberland, Rhode Island

Kristine M. Gebbie, R.N., M.S.N. *
Portland, Oregon

Barbara Haas, R.N., M.A.
Yarmouth, Maine

Kathy Hausman, R.N., M.S.N.
Hyattsville, Maryland

Betty Henderson, R.N., M.N.
Houston, Texas

Mary Ann Kelly, R.N., Ed.D. *
Clemson, South Carolina

Mary Lee Kirkland, R.N., M.S.N. *
Charleston, South Carolina

Phyllis B. Kritek, R.N., Ph.D. *
Milwaukee, Wisconsin

Frances M. Lange, R.N., D.S.N. *
Birmingham, Alabama

Nancy Lengel, R.N., M.S.N. *
Bradford, Pennsylvania

Kathleen M. McKeehan
Cleveland, Ohio

Derry Ann Moritz, R.N., M.S.
New Haven, Connecticut

Anne Griffin Perry, R.N., M.S.N.
St. Louis, Missouri

Sue Popkess-Vawter, R.N., Ph.D.
Kansas City, Kansas

Donna L. Ritter, R.N., M.N.
Brookings, South Dakota

Sister Callista Roy, R.N., Ph.D.
Los Angeles, California

Margueritte Rydlewski, R.N.,
D.P.N.P. *
Palatine, Illinois

Elsie Shiramizu, R.N., Ph.D. *
Ogden, Utah

Larry Sieck, R.N., B.S.N. *
Austin, Texas

Lois N. Spencer, R.N., M.S.N.
Kansas City, Missouri

Sandra J. Spotts, R.N., M.S.N. *
Bethlehem, Pennsylvania

Roberta D. Thiry, R.N., Ph.D. *
Pittsburg, Kansas

Mary E. Woods, R.N., M.S.N. *
St. Louis, Missouri

---

*Planning committee members, Fifth National Conference.

Appendix B Committees

Steering Committee
Ann Marie Becker
Marjory Gordon
Mi Ja Kim
Gertrude K. McFarland
Audrey M. McLane

Bylaws committee
Kristine Gebbie
Barbara Haas
Larry Sieck

Nominating committee
Ann Marie Becker
Garyfallia Forsyth
Sylvia Weber
Barbara Haas
Dorothea Jakob

Appendix C Nurse theorist group

Sister Callista Roy, R.N., Ph.D.
Chairperson
Los Angeles, California

Andrea U. Bircher, R.N., Ph.D.
Oklahoma City, Oklahoma

Rosemary Ellis, R.N., Ph.D.
Cleveland, Ohio

Joyce Fitzpatrick, R.N., Ph.D.
Troy, Michigan

Marjory Gordon, R.N., Ph.D.
Boston, Massachusetts

Margaret Hardy, R.N., Ph.D.
Boston, Massachusetts

Imogene King, R.N., Ed.D.
Tampa, Florida

Margaret A. Newman, R.N., Ph.D.
University Park, Pennsylvania

Rosemarie Parse, R.N., Ph.D.
Pittsburgh, Pennsylvania

Martha Rogers, R.N., Sc.D.
New York, New York

Gertrude Torres, R.N., Ed.D.
Buffalo, New York

Small group leaders and recorders

Group 1
Sister Kathleen Krekeler, R.N.,
Ph.D., Leader
Karen Peters, R.N., M.S.N.,
Recorder

Group 2
Susan Ritchie, R.N., M.S.N.,
Leader
Susan Obermeier, R.N., Recorder

Group 3
Richard Fehring, R.N., D.N.S.c.,
Leader
Donna Doro, R.N., M.S.N.,
Recorder

Group 4
Linda Freeman-Grilley, R.N.,
M.S.N., Leader
Joanne Thanovoro, R.N., Recorder

Group 5
Jacqueline Fortin, R.N., M.S.N.,
Leader
Rita Mitchell, R.N., M.S.N.,
Recorder

Group 6
Marion Resler, R.N., M.S.N.,
Leader
Debbie Joshu, R.N., Recorder

Group 7
Anne Perry, R.N., M.S.N., Leader
Susan Keller, R.N., Recorder

Group 8
Laura Rossi, R.N., M.S.N., Leader
Maria S. Poepsel, R.N., Recorder

Group 9
Ruth McShane, R.N., M.N., Leader
Patricia Hobson, R.N. Recorder

Group 10
Peggy McComb, R.N., M.N.,
Leader
Carol Luckey, R.N., Recorder

Group 11
Marty Spies, R.N., M.S.N., Leader
Rosemary Augustyn, R.N.,
Recorder

Group 12
Virginia Luetje, R.N., M.S.N.,
Leader
Kyra Isringhausen, R.N., Recorder

Group 13
Phyllis Kritek, R.N., Ph.D., Leader
Julia Eddins, R.N., Recorder

Participants of the Fifth National Conference on the Classification of Nursing Diagnoses

Wealtha Alex
University of Illinois
Rockford, Illinois

Bonnie Allbaugh
Methodist Hospital
McFarland, Wisconsin

Mary Asazawa
San Jose, California

Mary Aspinall
Huntington Beach, California

Rosemary Augustyn
Wood River, Illinois

Sallyanne Aveni
Columbia Hospital
Milwaukee, Wisconsin

Carol Ann Baer
Boston College
Medfield, Massachusetts

Kathryn Barnard*
University of Washington
Seattle, Washington

Patricia Barry
St. Frances Hospital
West Hartford, Connecticut

Beverly Bartlett
College of Our Lady of the Elms
Graby, Massachusetts

Ann Marie Becker
Saint Louis University
St. Louis, Missouri

Barbara Berkowich
MIEMS
Joppa, Maryland

Michelle Bockrath
University of Pennsylvania
Philadelphia, Pennsylvania

Margaret Briody
University of Rochester
Rochester, New York

Joan Bruce
Bedford V.A.
Bedford, Massachusetts

Barbara Burke
Harden-Grace Hospitals
Detroit, Michigan

Joseph Burley
Sheppard Air Force Base
Sheppard AFB, Texas

Lynda Carpenito
Wilmington Medical Center
Wilmington, Delaware

Janet Carstens
Southwest Missouri State
Cape Girardeau, Missouri

Margaret Carty
Montefiore Hospital and Medical
Center
Bronx, New York

Catherine Castelli
Adventist Health System
Shawnee Mission, Kansas

Anne Marie Cheney
Wauwatosa, Wisconsin

Dianne Christopherson
St. Joseph Mercy Hospital
Ann Arbor, Michigan

Kenneth Cianfrani
University of Illinois
Rock Island, Illinois

Bernadine Cimprich
Memorial Sloan-Kettering
New York, New York

Patricia Clunn
University of Miami
Coral Gables, Florida

Marga Coler
College of Our Lady of the Elms
Chicopee, Massachusetts

Maureen Conrad
Montefiore Hospital and Medical
Center
Bronx, New York

Linda Cooper
Ryerson Polytechnical Institute
Toronto, Ontario

Denise Cost
MIEMS
Baltimore, Maryland

Jennifer Craig
Kellogg Centre
Montreal, Quebec

Laraine Crane
Milwaukee, Wisconsin

Joan Crosley
Long Island Jewish-Hillside
New Hyde Park, L.I. New York

Carolyn Crowell
University of Iowa
Iowa City, Iowa

Marlis Daerr
Columbia Hospital
Milwaukee, Wisconsin

Joanne Dalton
Northwestern University
Boston, Massachusetts

Gail Davis
Harris Hospital
Fort Worth, Texas

Sandra Deli
MIEMS
Baltimore, Maryland

Kathy Dickensheets
St. Joseph Mercy Hospital
Ann Arbor, Michigan

Mary Dokmanovich
Sharp Hospital
San Diego, California

---

*Speakers (not participants).

Donna Doro
Richmond Heights, Missouri

Barbara Dossey
Holistic Nursing Consult.
Dallas, Texas

T. Audean Duespohl
Oil City, Pennsylvania

Kathryn Eckerle
Miami Valley Hospital
Dayton, Ohio

Julie Eddins
St. Louis University
St. Louis, Missouri

Joanne Farley
St. Anselm College
Manchester, New Hampshire

Richard Fehring
Marquette University
Milwaukee, Wisconsin

Lucy Feild
Brigham and Women's Hospital
Boston, Massachusetts

LuAnne Fendrich
Proctor Community Hospital
Peoria, Illinois

Frances Fickess
Loma Linda University
Loma Linda, California

Joan Fitzmaurice*
Boston College
Boston, Massachusetts

Anne Marie Flaherty
Memorial Hospital
New York, New York

Ruby Flesner
Milwaukee County General
Hospital
Milwaukee, Wisconsin

Jacqueline Fortin
University of Rhode Island
Cumberland, Rhode Island

Shirley Frederiksen
St. Joseph Mercy Hospital
Ann Arbor, Michigan

Sheila Fredette
Fitchburg State College
Fitchburg, Massachusetts

Linda Freeman-Grilley
Wausau, Wisconsin

Garyfallia Forsyth
Rush-Presbyterian
Chicago, Illinois

Claudia Gamel-Bentzel
American Association of
Neurosurgical Nurses
Chicago, Illinois

Gramatice Garofallou
Hospital of the Albert Einstein
College of Medicine
Bronx, New York

Kristine Gebbie
Oregon State Health Division
Portland, Oregon

Kathleen Gilbert
Shawnee Mission Medical Center
Shawnee Mission, Kansas

Yvonne Gleiber
National Institutes of Health
Bethesda, Maryland

Lorraine Goodwin
Michael Reese Hospital
Chicago, Illinois

Marjory Gordon
Boston College
Boston, Massachusetts

Faye Gregory
Long Beach City College
Long Beach, California

Elizabeth Gren
Bronson School of Nursing
Kalamazoo, Michigan

Pauline Guay
Labouré Junior College
Boston, Massachusetts

Meg Gulanick
Wooddale, Illinois

Cathie Guzzetta
Catholic University
Washington, D.C.

Barbara Haas
Yarmouth, Maine

Terese Halfmann
University of Wisconsin
Milwaukee, Wisconsin

Margaret Hardy
Boston University
Boston, Massachusetts

Bonnie Hartley
Ryerson Polytechnical Institute
Toronto, Ontario

Donna Hartweg
Illinois Wesleyan
Bloomington, Illinois

Carol Hayes
University of Florida
Gainesville, Florida

Leona Hayes
Olivette Nazarene College
Kankakee, Illinois

Barbara Heater
Southern Illinois University
Edwardsville, Illinois

Patricia Hobson
Washington, D.C.

Lois Hoskins
The Catholic University of
America
Washington, D.C.

Kathy Hubalik
WSUAMC
Chicago, Illinois

Florence Huey
American Journal of Nursing
New York, New York

Mary Hurley
American Association of Critical
Care Nurses
Saddle Brook, New Jersey

Kyra Isringhausen
Saint Louis University
St. Louis, Missouri

Dorothea Jakob
Toronto, Ontario

Dorothy Jones
Boston College
Boston, Massachusetts

Debbie Joshu
St. Louis, Missouri

Joan Kaiser
Memorial Sloan-Kettering, Cancer
Center
New York, New York

Norma Keefer
Miami Valley Hospital
Dayton, Ohio

*Speakers (not participants).

Susan Keller
St. John's Mercy Medical Center
St. Louis, Missouri

Mary Ann Kelly
Clemson University
Clemson, South Carolina

Patricia Kenyon
Arizona Western College
Yuma, Arizona

Barbara Keyes
MIEMS
Baltimore, Maryland

Sybil Kierstead
Kettering Memorial Hospital
Kettering, Ohio

Mi Ja Kim
University of Illinois
Chicago, Illinois

Imogene King
University of South Florida
Tampa, Florida

Mary Lee Kirkland
Medical University of South
Carolina
Charleston, South Carolina

Barbara Krainovich
Garden City, New York

Sister Kathleen Krekeler
St. Louis University
St. Louis, Missouri

Phyllis Kritek
University of Wisconsin
Milwaukee, Wisconsin

Patricia Kucharski
Community Health Nursing
Boston, Massachusetts

Susan Labarthe
McCullough-Hyde Memorial
Hospital
Oxford, Ohio

Jane Lancour
Nurse Consultant
Wauwatosa, Wisconsin

Frances Lange
University of Alabama
Birmingham, Alabama

Margaret Lannon
Neurological Referral Center
Boston, Massachusetts

Marilyn Lanza
ENRVMH
Bedford, Massachusetts

Nancy Lengel
University of Pittsburgh
Bradford, Pennsylvania

Rona Levin
Adelphi University
Garden City, New York

Barbara Levine
Rhode Island Hospital
Providence, Rhode Island

Doris Lister
South Carolina Department of
Health and Environmental Control
Columbia, South Carolina

Jeanette Long
National Institutes of Health
Bethesda, Maryland

Carol Luckey
St. Louis University
St. Louis, Missouri

Virginia Luetje
St. Louis University
St. Louis, Missouri

Margaret Lunney
Hunter College–Bellevue
New York, New York

Louette Lutjens
Bergess Education Medical Center
Kalamazoo, Michigan

Anita Lymburner
Nashua, New Hampshire

Carol Matz
West Chester State College
West Chester, Pennsylvania

Helen Mangan
Clinical Center
Bethesda, Maryland

Agnes Manka
DHHS
Germantown, Maryland

Mary'Vesta Marston-Scott
Boston University
Boston, Massachusetts

Patricia Martin
Miami Valley Hospital
Dayton, Ohio

Joanne McCloskey
University of Iowa
Iowa City, Iowa

Margaret McComb
Dammasch State Hospital
Wilsonville, Oregon

Ann McCourt
NE Sinai Hospital
Stoughton, Massachusetts

Gertrude McFarland
U.S. Department of Health and
Human Services
Rockville, Maryland

Elizabeth McFarlane
Catholic University of America
Washington, D.C.

Audrey McLane
Marquette University
Milwaukee, Wisconsin

Lois McMillin
Adventist Health System
Overland Park, Kansas

Ruth McShane
University of Wisconsin
Milwaukee, Wisconsin

Margaret Mehmert
Davenport, Iowa

Christine Miaskowski
HAECOM
Bronx, New York

Linda Miers
Birmingham, Alabama

Judith Fitzgerald Miller
Marquette University
Milwaukee, Wisconsin

Winnifred Mills
University of British Columbia
Vancouver, British Columbia

Carol Ann Mitchell
Adelphi University
Garden City, New York

Rita Mitchell
St. Louis, Missouri

Martha Montgomery
Henry Ford Community College
Dearborn, Michigan

Therese Mullen
Monson Developmental Center
Palmer, Massachusetts

---

*Speakers (not participants).

Lois Newman
Wesley Medical Center
Wichita, Kansas

Angela Nicoletti
Brigham and Women's Hospital
Boston, Massachusetts

Mary Niemeyer
Ann Arbor, Michigan

Heidi Obermier
St. Louis University
St. Louis, Missouri

Eleanor Pandosh
San Jose, California

Leona Parscenzo
Slippery Rock State College
Slippery Rock, Pennsylvania

Rosemarie Parse
Consultants In Nursing
Pittsburgh, Pennsylvania

Elinor Parsons
VA Westside Hospital
Chicago, Illinois

Karen Peret
Monson Developmental Center
Palmer, Massachusetts

Karen Peters
Cardiovascular Nurse Consultant
Belleville, Illinois

Marcia Petrini
Thiel College
Greenville, Pennsylvania

Susan Pfoutz
Ann Arbor, Michigan

Janice Pigg
Columbia Hospital
Milwaukee, Wisconsin

Maria-Salome Poepsel
St. Louis University
St. Louis, Missouri

Sue Popkess-Vawter
University of Kansas
Kansas City, Kansas

Marie Price
Sault Sainte Marie, Ontario

Precilla Quillen
Oxford, Ohio

Ann Reilly
Bridgewater, Massachusetts

Marion Resler
St. Louis University
St. Louis, Missouri

Linda Rice
Utica, New York

Marilyn Richardson
Nursing Practice Support Service
Oxford, Ohio

Karen Rieder
Naval School of Health Sciences
Bethesda, Maryland

Susan Ritchie
Northwestern Memorial Hospital
Chicago, Illinois

Martha Roark
SMMC
Merriam, Kansas

Laura Rossi
Medway, Massachusetts

Barbara Rottkamp
Westbury, New York

Frances Rowley
Nursing Quality Assurance CHM
Greenfield, Wisconsin

Sister Callista Roy
Mount St. Mary's College
Los Angeles, California

Wanda Ruthven
Case Manager
Fremont, California

Laura Ryan
Clinical Center NIH
Bethesda, Maryland

Margueritte Rydlewski
Palatine, Illinois

Penny Schoenmehl
VA Medical Center
San Diego, California

Pamela Schroeder
St. Luke's Hospital
Milwaukee, Wisconsin

JoAnn Shew
St. Louis University
St. Louis, Missouri

Joyce Shoemaker*
Temple University
Philadelphia, Pennsylvania

Suzanne Sikma
Harborview Medical Center
Seattle, Washington

Sally Silver
Private Practice
Milwaukee, Wisconsin

Susan Simmons
Bethesda, Maryland

Margaret Sipe
New England Deaconess Hospital
Boston, Massachusetts

Diana Smith
University of Alabama
Birmingham, Alabama

Martha Spies
St. Louis University
St. Louis, Missouri

Sandra Spotts
Souderton, Pennsylvania

Margaret Stafford
Northlake, Illinois

Jean Steel
Boston University
Boston, Massachusetts

Jill Streeb
Good Samaritan Hospital and
Medical Center
Portland, Oregon

Rosemarie Suhayda
Woodridge, Illinois

Joanne Thanavaro
Manchester, Missouri

Roberta Thiry
Pittsburgh State University
Pittsburgh, Kansas

Kathleen Thousand
Methodist Hospital
Dane, Wisconsin

Gertrude Torres
D'Youville College
Buffalo, New York

Mary Lynne Toth
MIEMS
Baltimore, Maryland

Rosalinda Toth*
Newark Beth Israel Medical
Center
Newark, New Jersey

*Speakers (not participants).

Sally Tripp
Arnold House—University of
Massachusetts
Amherst, Massachusetts

Barbara Vassallo
Trenton State College
Trenton, New Jersey

Carol Viamontes
Memorial Sloan-Kettering Cancer
Center
New York, New York

Madeline Wake
Marquette University
Milwaukee, Wisconsin

Jane Wall
St. Luke's Hospital
Milwaukee, Wisconsin

Rosemary Wang
University of New Hampshire
Durham, New Hampshire

Judith Warren
University of Hawaii
Honolulu, Hawaii

Carolyn Weber
Wichita State University
Wichita, Kansas

Sylvia Weber
Counseling and Mental Health
Services
Warwick, Rhode Island

Glenn Webster*
University of Colorado
Denver, Colorado

Susan Wessel
Jewish Hospital
Cincinnati, Ohio

Mary Woods
St. Louis University
St. Louis, Missouri

Patricia Woods
Hudson, New Hampshire

Jacqueline Wylie
Bronson Methodist Hospital
Kalamazoo, Michigan

Carolyn Yocom
University of Illinois
Chicago, Illinois

Karen York
Miami Valley Hospital
Dayton, Ohio

Shirley Ziegler
Texas Woman's University
Dallas, Texas

Karin Zuehls
Grand View College
Des Moines, Iowa

EXHIBITORS

American Journal of Nursing
Florence Huey

The Brady Co.
Susan Semmens

McGraw-Hill Book Co.
Sharon Horrell
Tina Pittman

The C.V. Mosby Co.
Barbara Norwitz
Bess Arends
Julie Cardamon

W.B. Saunders Co.
Gordon Landrum
Ilze Rader

*Speakers (not participants).

Annotated bibliographies

These annotations are intended to familiarize beginning practitioners with the literature describing the defining characteristics of specific nursing diagnoses. The list of references has evolved as the nursing diagnoses have been revised and updated. Contributors are nurses from several settings:

Janet Aylward*

Beverly Bartlett**

Michele Bockrath***

Mary Collins***

Joanne Dalton***

Jacqueline Fortin***

Sheila Fredette***

Mary Hanley***

Bette Harbeck***

Hilda Lander***

Dorothy Miller***

Angela Nicoletti***

Kay O'Conner***

Anne Reilly***

Suzanne Reitz***

Laura Rossi, Coordinator***

Judy Thorpe***

Shula Wurmfeldt***

AIRWAY CLEARANCE, INEFFECTIVE

Frame, P.T.: Acute infectious pneumonia in the adult, Basics of RD 10(3):1, Jan 1982.

The defense mechanisms of the respiratory tract are reviewed as well as the etiologies of pneumonias. The most common pathogens and the appropriate antibiotic therapy are discussed. Restorative and preventive therapy are mentioned and supported by an excellent bibliography.

London, R.G.: Cough: a symptom and a sign, Basics of RD 9(3):19, Jan. 1981.

This article describes multiple factors that affect the presence or absence of cough, a major defense mechanism of the respiratory system. The understanding of this vital response will greatly assist the nurse in assessment and clinical decision making. The interested reader is referred to many articles concerning patient care, basic science, and specifically coughing during sleep.

Murphy, R.H., and Holford, S.K.: Lung sounds Basics of RD 8(4):1, March 1980.

This excellent review article on lung sounds clarifies the confusion of auscultatory terminology and the mechanisms producing sounds within the chest. The presentation provides description and interpretation of lung dysfunction and will greatly assist the nurse in the assessment of patients and the evaluation of treatments.

Petty, T.L.: Management of chronic airflow obstruction, Sem. Respir. Med. 1(1):30, July 1979.

This article presents a comprehensive review of the useful modalities of care that comprise pulmonary rehabilitation. They are (but not limited to) the following interventions: patient education, pharmacologic agents, preventive influenza therapy, bronchial hygiene, breathing training, physical reconditioning, and oxygen therapy. The successful results of pulmonary programs are clearly stated and

---

*Cape Cod Conference Group.

**Western Massachusetts Conference Group.

***Massachusetts Conference Group.

illustrated with case studies. The particular approaches for the treatment of chronic bronchitis, emphysema, asthma, cystic fibrosis, and bronchiectasis are also discussed and referenced.

Proceedings of the Conference on the Scientific Basis of In-Hospital Respiratory Therapy, part 2 Am. Rev. Respir. Dis. **122**(5):1, Nov 1980.

This issue presents the summaries and supportive research papers concerning oxygen therapy, aerosol and humidity therapy, mechanical aids to lung expansion, and physical therapy techniques. The summaries discuss the accepted facts, the unknown areas, and recommended studies. This resource will assist the nurse to distinguish the use and abuse of respiratory therapy techniques and to identify outcome criteria by which these treatments can be evaluated.

BREATHING PATTERN, INEFFECTIVE

Belman, M., and Wasserman, K.: Exercise training and testing in patients with chronic obstructive pulmonary disease, Basics of RD **10**(2):1, Nov. 1981.

An excellent review article concerning the physiologic effects of exercise training in normal and COPD patients. The distinctions between cardiovascular and respiratory limitations and benefits are clearly stated. The authors strongly encourage progressive activity training within a comprehensive respiratory care program and provide a variety of exercise techniques, which are referenced for further reading. This article provides specific outcome criteria to evaluate patient care management.

Breslin, E.H.: Prevention and treatment of pulmonary complications in patients after surgery of the upper abdomen, Heart Lung **10**(3):511, May-June 1981.

An excellent review article that will assist the nurse to identify those patients who have postoperative pulmonary complications or who have significant risk factors. Etiologies of ineffective breathing patterns are described in pathophysiologic terms only and specific treatments and outcome criteria are discussed to facilitate evaluation of selected treatments. In addition, the bibliography contains many research articles that will greatly enhance the understanding of this challenging and reversible problem for nursing intervention.

Dudley, D.L., and others: Psychosocial concomitants to rehabilitation in chronic obstructive pulmonary disease, Part 1: psychosocial and psychological considerations Chest **77**(3):413, March 1980.

This article is part one of a three-part series concerning assessment and management of patients with chronic obstructive lung diseases (COPD), with emphasis on anxiety and depression. The classic defenses of isolation, denial, and regression are elucidated within the framework of the psychophysiology of respiratory disease. Patient vignettes and discussions of many research studies illustrate the complexity of the problem of COPD and also the success of individualized treatment plans.

Moser, K.M., and others: Preventive medicine that is effective: rehabilitation for the COPD patients: why, who, when, what, and how? J. Respir. Dis. **1**:42, 1980.

This article describes the personal and social impact of COPD as well as its morbidity and mortality. The authors strongly advocate the early identification and referral of these patients to structured rehabilitation programs to achieve the best physiologic and psychosocial benefits. Health teaching is a major component of the program and is geared toward patient self-care. Examples of individual program goals, a patient disability questionnaire, and suggested readings (annotated) are also provided.

Stein, A.M., and Fuhs, M. eds.: Breathing and breathlessness, Top. Clin. Nurs. **2**(3):1, 1980.

This article presents a variety of topics concerning the adaptation of patients to breathlessness. The authors discuss novel as well as traditional approaches to patient care management. Specific areas of interest are, Eastern and Western theories of breathlessness, home care of children and adult respiratory patients, and weaning the ventilator-dependent patient. Sample nursing assessment forms and care plans are provided with both specific and general outcome criteria to evaluate care.

CARDIAC OUTPUT, ALTERATION IN: DECREASED

Alexy, B.: Monitoring cardiovascular status with noninvasive techniques, Nurs. Clin. North Am. **13**(3):423, Sept. 1978.

The author describes a comprehensive assessment of the cardiovascular system and summarizes diagnostic aids in evaluating the system

Dracup, K.: Unraveling the mysteries of cardiomyopathy, Nursing 79 **9**(5):84, May 1979.

Congestive cardiomyopathy, hypertrophic (obstructive) cardiomyopathy, and restrictive cardiomyopathy are compared and contrasted in terms of etiology, signs and symptoms, treatment, prognosis, and nursing interventions.

Foster, S.B., and Canty, K.A.: Pump failure following myocardial infarction, Heart Lung **9**:293, March-Apr. 1980.

Etiology, signs and symptoms, and assessment of heart failure are discussed. Two cases studies are presented to illustrate clinical interventions.

Kapoor, A., and Dang, N.S.: Reliance on physical signs in acute myocardial infarction and its complications, Heart Lung **7**(6):1020, Nov.-Dec. 1978.

Altered cardiac hemodynamics associated with myocardial infarction include decrease in cardiac output, stroke volume, arterial pressure, and ejection fraction. Signs and symptoms of a decreased cardiac output are addressed.

Rossi, L.P., and Haines, V.M.: Nursing diagnoses related to myocardial infarction, Cardiovasc. Nurs. **15**:11, May-June 1979.

The authors review the diagnostic process and attempt to differentiate between medical and nursing diagnoses. Examples are presented in relation to a patient with a myocardial infarction.

Waxler, R.: The patient with congestive heart failure: teaching implications, Nurs. Clin. North Am. **11**(2):297, June 1976.

The pathophysiology, etiology, signs and symptoms, and medical interventions related to congestive heart failure are addressed in this article in addition to guidelines for educating patients with congestive heart failure.

Pediatric

Agarwala, B., and Baffes, T.: Congestive heart failure in the infant, Heart Lung **5**(1):62, Jan.-Feb. 1976.

The authors state that the etiology of most congestive heart failure in children is congenital cardiac defects and about 90% of all children developing failure are infants. Other causes are discussed as are medical and nursing interventions.

James, F., and Love, E.: Congestive heart failure in infants and children, Heart Lung 3(3):396, May-June 1974.

The authors describe the etiology of congestive heart failure in infants and children, clinical manifestations specific to children, and medical treatment complete with pediatric dosages of digoxin and diuretics.

COMFORT, ALTERATION IN: PAIN

Copp, L.A.: The spectrum of suffering, Am. J. Nurs. **74**:491, March 1974.

A consideration of the characteristics of pain and patients responses taken from the author's clinical study of 148 persons. The subjects in various stages of the pain experience tell what pain is like and how they cope and suggest ways for professionals to help them.

Goodell, H.: Pain: parts I and II: basic concepts and assessment: rationale for intervention, Am. J. Nurs. **66**(5,6):1085; 1345, May-June 1966.

This two-part programmed instruction describes reactions to pain, biologic purposes of pain, and physiologic pathways of the pain response. A pain reaction rating scale is presented. Intervention methods are categorized and examples of each category are given.

Jacox, A.: Pain: a source book for nurses and other health professionals, Boston, 1977, Little, Brown & Co.

The author gives an in depth overview of all aspects of the pain process. The author initially presents pain from a physiologic perspective and then expands to include the psychologic and sociologic components. The author includes methods of assessment of intervention and ends with a discussion of pain and its alleviation in specific patient populations.

McCaffery, M.: Nursing management of the patient with pain, Philadelphia, 1979, J.B. Lippincott Co.

This text is a comprehensive view of pain from a nursing perspective. Contents include definition, nursing assessment of behaviors related to pain, nursing diagnosis of the patient with pain, and nursing intervention and evaluation. Interventions reviewed include behavior therapy, waking-imagined analgesia, decreasing noxious stimuli, providing other sensory input, and being with the patient.

Moss, Q.T., and Meyer, B.: Symposium on pain: a nursing diagnosis, Nurs. Clin. North Am. **12**:609, 1977.

This symposium speaks to each area of the nursing process and its relation to the concept of pain. In addition to executing the nursing process, it focuses on the synthesis of assessment data and the evolution of a nursing diagnosis. Intervention is planned for a cardiac patient, patients in the area of pediatrics, and a terminally ill patient.

COPING, INEFFECTIVE FAMILY: COMPROMISED AND DISABLING

Bell, J.M.: Stressful life events and coping methods in mental illness and wellness behaviors, Nurs. Res. **26**(2):136, March-April 1977.

Descriptive comparative nursing research study uses Selye's stress theory to explore relationship of stressful life events and coping methods with mental illness and wellness. Significant associations are made for all health care professionals.

Giaquinta, B.: Helping families face the crisis of cancer, Am. J. Nurs. **77**(10):1585, Oct. 1977.

This article identifies four stages experienced by families of cancer patients analogous to Kübler-Ross's five stages of dying experienced by the patient: (1) living with cancer, (2) restructuring the living-dying interval, (3) bereavement, and (4) reestablishment. Phases are defined within each stage, and goals of nursing interventions are defined for each phase.

Hall, J.E., and Weaver, B.R.: Nursing of families in crisis, Philadelphia, 1974, J.B. Lippincott Co.

Encompassing anthology that views the family unit in both situational and maturational crises. A few articles review crisis theory, but most are specific examples of a nurse's role interacting within a particular crisis. Good resource for focusing on nursing intervention in situations that require coping.

Moos, R.H., ed.: Coping with physical illness, New York, 1977, Plenum Publishing Corp.

Identifies major adaptive tasks and coping skills used by families and patients sharing the crises and stresses of serious physical illness. Discusses maladaptive behaviors and suggests supportive interventions for professionals.

Porth, C.: Physiological coping: a model for teaching pathophysiology, Nurs. Outlook **25**:781, Dec. 1977.

This article propounds a physiologic coping model that supports the forming of nursing diagnoses rather than medical diagnoses. Observed physiologic coping behaviors are correlated with underlying pathophysiology (rather than with a specific disease state), thus stimulating creative thinking about nursing actions that would relieve or immunize the disorder.

Sullivan, B.P.: Patient responses to BOG therapy for malignant melanoma, Am. J. Nurs. **79**(2):230, Feb. 1979.

Case history following a young woman's course through treatment for terminal cancer. The nurse-author focuses on individual and family perceptions and coping behaviors, including detailed background, strengths, weaknesses, and professional supportive approaches.

COPING, INEFFECTIVE INDIVIDUAL

Coehlo, G.V., Hamburg, D.A., and Adams, J.E.: Coping and adaptation, New York, 1974, Basic Books, Inc.

The authors describe strategies of coping that depend on such factors as genetic constitution, experience, phase of life, and environment and provide explicit and implicit methods of assessing coping abilities. They give background for both diagnosis of and intervention for maladaptive individual and group coping processes.

Cohen, F., and Lazarus R.S.: Active coping processes, coping dispositions, and recovery from surgery, Psychosom. Med. **35**:375, Sept.-Oct. 1973.

A study of 61 patients undergoing elective surgery investigated coping behavior as it affected four measures: the number of hospital days, pain medications used, minor complications, and negative psychologic reactions. Three coping behaviors were identified: avoidance/denial, vigilance (seeking information), and a mixture of both. The most vigilant showed the most complicated recovery: it was higher in all measures but number of pain medications. The authors postulated that elective surgery might be better handled by denial for example, although many threats exist, few materialize.

Fontana, A.F., and others: Coping with interpersonal conflict through life events and hospitalization, J. Nerv. Ment. Dis. **162:**88, 1976.

The authors discuss a model used for predicting a patient's ability to cope with post hospital adjustment using events in the prehospital experience. Great detail is given to describing the model, and two case histories are used to illustrate its applicability.

Hamburg, D.A.: Coping behavior in life-threatening circumstances, Psychother. Psychosom. **23:**13, 1974.

Inspired by the lack of systematic research on the subject, the author has gathered data exploring the coping tasks and strategies of patients with severe physical impairment and their psychologic response. He explores the primary adaptive tasks and the underlying human needs associated with injury and illness and deals with the way medical practice can be enhanced by a more in-depth understanding of the psychosomatic process. The author summarizes information on coping behavior used under stress and suggests similarities that can be used in different situations.

Murphy, L.B., and Moriarity, A.E.: Vulnerability, coping and growth, New Haven, Conn., 1976, Yale University Press.

Longitudinal study of a group of children from Topeka, Kansas, from infancy through adolescence is reported. The development of these children is followed, with emphasis on the contribution of coping efforts to growth processes.

DEPENDENCE-INDEPENDENCE CONFLICT

Cook, R.L.: Psychosocial responses to myocardial infarction, Heart Lung **1:**130, 1979.

In Cook's discussion of the psychosocial reactions to a myocardial infarction, she describes the regression to childlike patterns of coping as dependency and explains the reward system as a method of dealing with dependent behavior.

Mayou, R., and others: The psychological and social effects of myocardial infarction on wives, Br. Med. J. **1:**699, 1978.

Throughout this article, the results of the conflict of independence versus dependence as they relate to the patients, their wives, and their relationships as couples are discussed. Signs and symptoms are described as well as specific outcomes of the conflict. Criteria for successful long-term adjustments are also described.

Minckley, B., and others: Myocardial infarct stress of transfer inventory: development of a research tool, Nurs. Res. **28:**4, 1979.

In discussing the rationale for the Myocardial Infarct Stress of Transfer Inventory (MISTI), Minckley describes the influences of transfer anxiety, a special type of separation anxiety, on the patient's ability to become independent. The deleterious effects of transfer anxiety coupled with fear and stress reaction promote dependence on staff and others to meet gratification of needs. Use of the MISTI has shown a significant reduction in these anxiety levels and better rehabilitative success of the patients.

Raines, F., and others: Helping a young cardiac patient accept limitations without scaring him—balancing act, Nursing 77 **11**:56, 1977.

In describing the unusual protectiveness of the staff toward the young MI patient, references are made to the increasing dependency imposed on the patient by the action of the nurses. Some signs and symptoms are identified. The effects of this behavior on the progress of the patient are also expressed.

Wash, M.G.: Home dialysis: a family copes with a patient on a kidney machine at home, Nurs. Times **75**:449, 1979.

In this article's discussion of the preparation of the patient and her family for home dialysis, several references to the conflict of independence and dependence related to dialysis are described. Some signs and symptoms specific to the dialysis patient and the home dialysis process are given.

GAS EXCHANGE, IMPAIRED

Ferrer, M. I.: Management of patients with cor pulmonale, Med. Clin. North Am. **63**(1):251, Jan. 1979.

This article describes the multiple diseases that cause right-sided heart failure, cor pulmonale, in both adults and children. The reversible and irreversible factors contributing to pulmonary hypertension are clearly defined. Physiologic assessment criteria and management are discussed. The medical advances in the prevention and treatment of this debilitating complication are emphasized. This report provides a strong and optimistic base from which nursing interventions concerning pulmonary toilet, activity prescription, and teaching self-care can evolve.

Flenley, D.C.: Blood gas and acid base interpretation, Basics of RD **10**(1):1, Sept. 1981.

This article succinctly describes the clinical manifestations of hypoxemia and hypercapnia and the need and use of arterial blood gas measurements in the assessment and treatment of impaired gas exchange. The five mechanisms contributing to hypoxemia are reviewed as well as the distinguishing features between acute and chronic respiratory failure. Although the multiple etiologies of respiratory failure are merely highlighted, the reader is provided with a variety of comprehensive references on specific treatments and outcome criteria.

Hopewell, P.C.: Adult respiratory distress syndrome, Basics of RD **7**(4):16, March 1979.

The multiple disorders associated with adult respiratory distress syndrome are merely listed; however, the common abnormalities of pulmonary function are discussed in depth. The assessment and management of alveolar capillary membrane injury are fully described and supported by references. The controversies concerning fluid treatment, PEEP, steroids, and heparin are discussed. The article provides the physiologic assessment and outcome criteria by which the nurse can develop realistic interventions for this patient population, which is associated with a 50% to 60% mortality.

Nocturnal Oxygen Therapy Trial Group: Continuous or nocturnal oxygen therapy in hypoxemic chronic obstructive lung disease, Ann. Int. Med. **93**(3):391, Sept. 1980.

This article is a landmark study concerning the use of continuous low-flow oxygen therapy in patients with chronic obstructive lung disease and hypoxemia. Earlier studies indicated that chronic intermittent oxygen therapy resulted in improved exercise tolerance, decreased pulmonary hypertension and erythrocytosis, and improved neuropsychologic function, but this study showed a striking difference in mortality. The intermittent group was 1.94 times greater than the continuous oxygen group. This article provides a strong physiologic basis for nursing interventions concerning health teaching compliance in patients with severe chronic impaired gas exchange.

GRIEVING: ANTICIPATORY AND DYSFUNCTIONAL

Brue, C., and Dracup, K.: Helping the spouses of critically ill patients, Am. J. Nurs., **78**(1):50, Jan. 1978.

The author provides an example of a nursing care plan for the grieving spouse. The plan focuses on the spouse's need for relief of initial anxiety, need for information, need to be with the patient, need to be helpful to the patient, and need for support and ventilation. Specific nursing interventions are identified.

Carlson, C.E., and Blackwell, B., eds.: Behavioral concepts and nursing intervention, pp. 72-111, Philadelphia, 1978, J.B. Lippincott Co.

This book contains consecutive chapters on loss and grief, followed by a framework for assessment and understanding of the behaviors. Knowledge about the stages of grief provides a general guide for assessment that can be effective only when viewed as a set of generalizations that will apply to some, but not all, who grieve. Extensive references.

Crate, M.A.: Nursing functions in adaptation to chronic illness, Am. J. Nurs. **65**(10):72, Oct. 1965.

A model of adaptation to chronic illness following the events of the grieving process is presented. The author describes behaviors that manifest progressive adaptation: disbelief, awareness, reorganization, resolution, and identity change. Nurse behaviors should support and guide the client as he moves toward a way of life that accommodates the illness.

Humpe, S.O.: Needs of the grieving spouse in a hospital setting, Nurs. Res. **24**(2):113, March-Apr. 1975.

This paper reports a study to determine whether the spouse whose mate is terminally ill or had died can recognize own needs and whether she/he perceives being helped by nurses. Twenty-seven spouses were interviewed during the terminal illness of their mates. Fourteen of the spouses were interviewed again after the death of their mate. Eight needs of grieving spouses were noted. Twenty references are included.

Lawrence, S.A., and Lawrence, R.M.: A model of adaptation to the stress of chronic illness, Nurs. Forum **18**(1):33, 1979.

A model of adaptation is described consisting of three stages: shock and disbelief, developing awareness, and resolution of the loss. Behavioral outcomes of adaptation are described as self-dependency, understanding one's illness, and knowing when and where to go for needed help. Suggested nursing actions assist the client toward developing self-dependency.

Roberts, S.L.: Behavioral concepts and nursing throughout the life span, pp. 145-171, Englewood Cliffs, N.J., 1978, Prentice-Hall, Inc.

> In this chapter, the components of loss that are defined involve death, dying, grief, and mourning. The author reviews the stages of grieving as identified by Engel, Kübler-Ross, and Lipowski and emphasizes the unique behavioral response of each person who experiences a loss. Nursing implications involve assessment of the internal and external influencing factors or variables in adaptation to loss and interventions directed toward altering, maintaining, and strengthening these variables.

INJURY, POTENTIAL FOR

Brown, M.H., and Kiss, M.E.: A problem-focused approach to nursing audit: cancer falls, Cancer Nurs. **5**(2):389, Oct. 1979.

> These authors use the nursing audit to identify circumstances surrounding patient fall. Although described in terms of the cancer patient, the focus is useful for evaluating a patient's potential for physical injury in a variety of settings.

Kilikiwski, E.: A study of accidents in a hospital, Superv. Nurse **10**:44, July 1979.

> The author reviews a study exploring types of accidents occurring in the hospital setting. It provides interesting discussion for nursing staff at all levels.

Walshe, A., and Rosen, H.: A study of patient falls from bed, J. Nurs. Administration **9**(5):31, May 1979.

> The study provides examples of an investigation of patient falls from bed. Implications for nursing in preventing as well as treating this common problem are discussed.

Witte, N.: Why the elderly fall, Am. J. Nurs. **79**(11):1950, Nov. 1979.

> This article delineates criteria that may be used as defining characteristics for this diagnosis. Although the cues require clinical testing, they provide a useful basis for patient assessment.

KNOWLEDGE DEFICIT

Cohen, N.: Three steps to better patient teaching, Nursing 80 **10**(2):72, Feb. 1980.

> A brief overview is given of three steps to be taken before teaching is begun. Emphasis is on step two, "assess the patient learner," and includes data to be obtained about the patient to identify content to be taught. Included is level of knowledge, patient goals for learning, readiness, and ability to learn.

Miller, V.: Rudiments of care; helping the patient learn, Nurs. Times **75**(24):1016, June 14, 1979.

> Items to consider in determining what the patient needs to learn are reviewed, including knowledge, skill, and attitudes. Consideration is given to the processes of teaching and evaluating the learning.

Redman, B.: Curriculum in patient education, Am. J. Nurs. **78**(8):1363, Aug. 1978.

> The need for differentiation and categorization of patient's learning needs is described. Proposed categories based on priorities are acute, preventive, and mainte-

nance educational needs. Five classes of difficulty proposed range from profound difficulty to delayed readiness causing variable difficulty. These classifications predict learning ability and nursing time needed for effective teaching.

Redman, B.K.: The process of patient education, St. Louis, 1984, The C.V. Mosby Co.

This comprehensive text explores the phases of patient education. The teaching-learning process is reviewed as well as assessment of readiness for health education and objectives of health teaching in nursing. Teaching tool information and an overview of delivery and development of patient education are presented.

MOBILITY, IMPAIRED PHYSICAL

Aspinall, M.J. and Tanner, C.A.: Decision making for patient care, pp. 231-263, New York, 1981, Appleton-Century-Crofts.

Assessment parameters indicative of deviations from normal movement are outlined. The major physiologic and psychologic alterations experienced by the person with altered mobility are presented. Included is a table depicting the abnormal initiating mechanism or clinical state, a brief statement describing the pathophysiology, and the identifying characteristics of disturbed mobility. Interventions are presented in the following categories: exercise, positioning, diet, elimination, intake, and patient involvement. A case study concludes the chapter.

Beland, I.L., and Passos, J.Y.: Clinical nursing, ed. 4, New York, 1981, Macmillan Publishing Co.

Chapter 49 "Problems Associated with Disuse Syndromes—Including the Integument," discusses the effect of prolonged bedrest and inactivity on motor function, elimination, peripheral circulation, and cardiovascular and respiratory function. Considerable attention is given to pressure sores—etiology, predisposing factors, and prevention. Nursing interventions are described. A comprehensive bibliography is included at the end of the chapter.

Hirschberg, G.G., Lewis, L., and Vaughan, P.: Promoting patient mobility, Nursing **7**:42, May 1977.

This article is adapted from a text by these authors entitled *Rehabilitation—A Manual for the Care of the Disabled and Elderly*, ed. 2, (Philadelphia, 1976, J.B. Lippincott Co.). Paralysis as the cause of immobility is the focus. Disabilities secondary to disuse or inactivity are described. Characteristics of muscle and joint degeneration and metabolic and circulatory disturbances are delineated. Interventions include active exercises, passive mobilization, frequent position changes, and bowel and bladder routines.

Lentz, M.: Selected aspects of deconditioning secondary to immobilization, Nurs. Clin. North Am. **16**:729, Dec. 1981.

The focus of this article is on the major deconditioning changes that occur in the cardiovascular and musculoskeletal systems as a result of immobility. Changes affecting the cardiovascular system are decreased venous flow, decreased orthostatic tolerance, and decreased work capacity. Changes related to the musculoskeletal system are bone demineralization, altered joint function, and loss of muscle mass, strength, and tone. The goal of the suggested nursing interventions and rationale is to minimize the deconditioning that occurs with immobilization.

Murray, R.B., Wilson Huelskoetter, M. M., and Lueckerath-O'Driscoll, D. The nursing process in later maturity, pp. 380-414, Englewood Cliffs, N.J., 1980, Prentice-Hall Inc.

Chapter 15 applies the nursing process to the person with the nursing diagnosis of limited mobility regardless of underlying pathogenesis. Included are assessment guides for range of motion, muscle strength, reflexes, gait, and posture and activities of daily living. Nursing interventions are presented that are applicable to all persons with limited mobility. Specific nursing interventions are directed toward impaired mobility of muscular origin, arising from joint pathology, and resulting from fractures and orthopedic surgery.

NONCOMPLIANCE

Connolly, C.E.: Patient compliance: a review of the research with implications for psychiatric-mental health nursing, J. Psychiatr. Nurs. **16**:15, 1978.

The article reviews current research according to Marston's three variables, which have been identified by researchers studying patient/client compliance. These variables are demographic, illness-related, and psychosocial factors. The two factors that were found to influence compliance pertinent to psychiatric and mental health nursing were the practitioner/client relationship and the continuity of care.

Komaroff, A.L.: The practitioner and the compliant patient, Am. J. Public Health **66**:833, 1976.

The author reviews many factors that may influence patient drug-taking behavior: social characteristics, patient personality, patient understanding of illness and treatment, patient/practitioner relationship, and practitioner's attitudes. Komaroff then presents suggestions for the practitioner to encourage compliance. He stresses the importance of the patient's knowledge and understanding of the need for medication and the practitioner's role in this process.

Marston, M.V.: Compliance with medical regimes: a review of the literature, Nurs. Res. **19**:312, 1970.

The author presents a summary of studies of compliance behavior. She reviews the various methods that have been used to study compliance and the relationship of rates of compliance to the methods of collection of the basic data. Three variables related to compliance are identified: demographic, illness, and social-psychologic behavior. Treatment must consider the interaction of all three variables.

Sackett, D.L., and Haynes, R.B.: Compliance with therapeutic regimes, Baltimore, 1976, John Hopkins University Press.

This book provides a comprehensive review of the significant issues related to patient compliance including effects of education, socio-behavioral determinants and treatment strategies. An analysis of research methods and an annotated bibliography are also provided.

Scherwitz, L., and Leventhal, H.: Strategies for increasing patient compliance, Health Values **2**:301, 1978.

The authors review several approaches to understanding noncompliance. They present a theoretic model that may be used in selecting and coordinating interventions and evaluating their impact on compliance with medication regimens. Suggestions regarding message content and techniques that may be used to increase compliance are provided.

NUTRITION ALTERATION IN: LESS THAN BODY REQUIREMENTS

Grant, A.: Nutritional assessment guidelines, ed. 2, Berkeley, 1979, Cutter Medical Laboratories.

This book provides guidelines for the assessment of nutritional status. Not intended to be a complete review of literature, this manual is a compilation of information that may be useful in making a nutritional assessment of the hospitalized patient. Other sources of information are required to formulate a plan of therapy.

Green, M.L., and Harry, J., eds.: Nutrition in contemporary nursing practice, New York, 1981, John Wiley & Sons, Inc.

This textbook, co-authored by a nurse and a dietitian, is intended for use in all types of basic nursing curricula. It is also intended to serve as a reference for both registered nurses and licensed practical nurses. It is divided into two sections, one focuses on the basic theory of nutrition, the other applies nutrition to nursing practice. The steps of the nursing process serve as a framework for discussing nutritional care. Included is a set of nutritional nursing diagnoses developed by Claire Campbell in her book, *Nursing Diagnosis and Intervention in Nursing Practice,* New York, 1978, John Wiley & Sons, Inc.

Krause, M., and Mahan, L.K.: Food nutrition and diet therapy, ed. 6, Philadelphia, 1979, W.B. Saunders Co.

A reference for both nurses and dietitians, this text is divided into three sections. The first section discusses the basics of nutrition, focusing on nutrients and the metabolic processes of cells. The major portion of the book follows and discusses diet therapy and nutritional care associated with the various disease processes. It takes a clinical approach to nutritional therapy. The final section focuses on the proper nourishment provided by combination of food as well as the way food meets the psychosocial needs of the client.

Weisner, R.L., Butterworth, C.E., and Sahm, D.N.: Handbook of clinical nutrition, Birmingham, 1977, Department of Nutrition, University of Alabama in Birmingham, Schools of Public and Allied Health, Medicine and Dentistry.

Just as the title states, this is a handbook. It is a tool for evaluating the nutritional status of patients, especially hospitalized patients. It gives special attention to nutritional assessment and to identifying high-risk patients. Nutritional support is discussed from a general approach to the more specific approaches of therapeutic diets, tube feedings, and total parenteral nutrition. Included also are discussions of drug nutrient interactions and reference tables, which are easily readable.

NUTRITION, ALTERATION IN: MORE THAN BODY REQUIREMENTS

Braden, B.: Disturbances in ingestion. In Jones, D.A., Dunbar, C.F., and Jirovec, M.M., eds.: Medical surgical nursing: a conceptual approach, New York, 1978, McGraw Hill Book Co.

The author discusses the criteria of 10% and 20% over ideal height and weight as defining characteristics of obesity. Also mentioned is the triceps skinfold measurement. Pathophysiology, causes, and medical treatment of obsese individuals are discussed, as well as nursing interventions.

Ellis, C.: Morbid obesity: a comparative study, Nurs. Times 5(8):17, 1980.

This article focuses on the characteristics of the American life-style that predispose the population to a higher incidence of obesity than in the United Kingdom. The defining characteristic of sedentary life-style is discussed in relationship to domestic boredom of Americans.

Halpern, S.L.: Quick reference to clinical nutrition, pp. 244-246, Philadelphia, 1979, J.B. Lippincott Co.

In discussing the etiology of obesity, the author states that regardless of the etiology, the cause of obesity is always an imbalance of calorie intake and calorie expenditure by the body. Three etiologies are identified: genetics, lack of nutritional knowledge, and modern life-style, which results in decreased walking and increased automation.

Norris, C.M.: Body image: its relevance to professional nursing. In Carlson, C.E., and Blackwell B., eds.: Behavioral concepts and nursing intervention, ed. 2, Philadelphia, 1978, J.B. Lippincott Co.

The discussion is on body image and obesity, identifying how obese individuals feel about themselves. Identified are the defining characteristics of dysfunctional eating patterns, sedentary activity level, and weight over 20% of ideal for height and frame.

Sundberg, M.C.: Framework for nursing intervention in the treatment of obesity, Issues Ment. Health Nurs. 1:25, 1978.

This article incorporates nursing process in a therapeutic nursing intervention model for obese individuals. Dysfunctional eating patterns are discussed under the dynamics of obesity. An etiology of energy intake vs. energy expenditure imbalance is identified.

Wineman, N.M.: Obesity: locus of control, body image, weight loss, and age of onset, Nurs. Res. 29(4):231, 1980.

This article discusses a retrospective study into the psychologic characteristics of the obese to assist in determining more effective individualized nursing interventions. Dysfunctional eating patterns are identified under stimulus-binding hypotheses regarding obesity.

PARENTING, ALTERATION IN: ACTUAL AND POTENTIAL

Bishop, B.: A guide to assessing parenting capabilities, Matern. Child Nurs. J. 76(11):1784, Nov. 1976.

Written from a clinical perspective, this article enumerates the factors that influence parenting skills in the mother. A nursing assessment outlining key parental behaviors indicative of impaired parenting is proposed.

Clark, A.: Recognizing discord between mother and child, and changing it to harmony, Matern. Child Nurs. J. 1(2):100, March-Apr. 1976.

The article offers several tools for detecting an impaired mother-infant relationship and for monitoring the effect of interventions. A case example of use of these tools and the interventions employed is described.

Clark, A., and Affonso, D.: Infant behavior and maternal attachment: two sides to the coin, Matern. Child Nurs. J. **1**(2):95, March-Apr. 1976.

This article focuses on the attachment process during the early postpartum period. The process is interactional, similar to the acquaintance process, with both mother and infant influencing the ease and strength of attachment. They also discuss specific factors in both parties that influence the attachment.

Josten, L.: Prenatal assessment guide for illuminating possible problems with parenting, Matern. Child Nurs. J. **6**(1):113, March-Apr. 1981.

This is an excellent article focusing on prenatal factors that may predict an impaired parenting. Half of the assessment tool being proposed is shown in the body of the article, the second half is discussed in detail. Success in predicting parenting problems is cited.

Reiser, S. LeF.: A tool to facilitate mother-infant attachment, JOGN, Nurs. **10**(4):294, July-Aug. 1981.

A brief explanation of the formation and use of this tool is given, along with the tool. The tool is intended to be used during the early postpartum period.

Sullivan, B.J., and Selvaggio, E.: Negative evaluations, how they affect the child, Matern. Child Nurs. J. **8**(3):173, Fall 1979.

Emotional disturbances of children are often the result of impaired parent-child interactions. Parenting patterns involving negative reinforcements that lower the child's self-esteem are discussed. Several examples of the results of such patterns are given.

SELF-CONCEPT: DISTURBANCE IN

Fisher, S., and Cleveland, S.E.: Body image and personality, New York, 1968, Dover Publications Inc.

After an initial survey of body image theory, the book turns to the dimension of body image boundary. Discussions include the development of boundaries as well as associated behavioral variation and physiologic reactions to body image boundary. The book contains frequent references to research, numerous case studies, and an extensive bibliography.

Gentry, W.D., and Williams, R.N.: Psychological aspects of myocardial infarction and coronary care, St. Louis, 1979, The C.V. Mosby Co.

Gruendemann, B.J.: The impact of surgery on body image, Nurs. Clin. North Am. **10**:635, Dec. 1975.

Although this article is written from the perspective of the operating room nurse, it offers concrete suggestions for assessment and intervention of altered body image in the surgical patient that should be useful to all nurses. Also included are a definition of body image and a discussion of the potential threats to the body image that are posed by surgery.

McCloskey, J.C.: How to make the most of body image theory in nursing practice, Nursing 76, **6**(5):68, May 1976.

This article provides a basic introduction to body image theory for practicing nurses. After listing the determinants of body image, the author discusses the two major etiologies of altered body image seen in hospitalized patients, relying on numerous common examples to illustrate points. She includes a short tool for subjective and objective assessment of body image and six vignettes that provide an opportunity to apply the theory presented to clinical situations.

Murray, R.: Symposium on the concept of body image, Nurs. Clin. North Am. **7**:593, Dec. 1972.

This symposium focuses on expanding the nurse's understanding of body image theory and increasing skills in nursing process with patients who experience an alteration in body image. The first three articles discuss the development of body image throughout the life cycle, using Erikson's developmental stages as an organizing framework. Subsequent articles deal with specific health situations in which body image alterations may occur.

Shontz, F.C.: Body image and its disorders, Int. J. Psy. Med. **5**(4):461, 1974.

The author discusses body image in terms of the functions it serves and the levels at which it is experienced and describes four treatment approaches effective in patients with alterations in body image. Although written for the physician, the article contains much information useful to nursing.

SENSORY-PERCEPTUAL ALTERATION

Ashworth, P.: Sensory deprivation: the acutely ill, Nurs. Times **75**(7):290, Feb. 15, 1979.

This article reviews different interpretations of sensory deprivation. An excellent description of effects of sensory deprivation in intensive care units with specific interventions is offered.

Kratz, C.: Sensory deprivation in the elderly, Nurs. Times **75**(8):330, Feb. 22, 1979.

The gradual onset of sensory deprivation is correlated with the aging process in an innovative way. The author provides a theoretic framework for viewing sensory deprivation using the unitary man/human framework.

Oster, C.: Sensory deprivation in geriatric patients, J. Am. Geriatr. Soc. **24**:461, Oct. 1976.

The physiologic processes associated with sensory deprivation are outlined. It provides a basis for differential diagnosis and their varying physiologic responses.

Shelby, J.: Sensory deprivation, Image **10**:49, June 1978.

This paper provides a historic background about sensory deprivation. It includes an in-depth description of the pathophysiologic causes and effects of sensory deprivation with a case study portraying these concepts.

Solomon, P.: Sensory deprivation, Boston, 1961, Harvard University Press.

This book provides articles from diverse disciplines on the clinical research involving sensory deprivation. Experimental designs and methodologies are specifically and technically described.

SEXUAL DYSFUNCTION

Carey, P.: Temporary sexual dysfunction in reversible health limitations, Nurs. Clin. North Am. **10**(3):575, Sept. 1975.

Types of male and female sexual dysfunction are identified and defined. The author has suggested the following classifications of etiologies for the purpose of discussion: (1) a disease process, surgical procedure, or change in health status that alters physical status and/or body image; (2) a drug or other treatment that causes physiologic change; (3) fatigue that causes one or both partners performance difficulties; (4) anxiety that interferes with sexual response; (5) depression or grief that alters libido or sex drive; (6) physical separation that prevents normal sexual activity and requires adjustment. Nursing interventions specific to these etiologies are identified.

Macrae, I., and Henderson, M.: Sexuality and irreversible health limitations, Nurs. Clin. North Am. **10**(3):587, Sept. 1975.

The authors begin by justifying the importance of including sexuality in patient care. Guidelines for effective therapy when dealing with a patient's sexual needs and desires are provided. The nursing process is applied to two specific etiologies of sexual dysfunction: spinal cord injuries in a male and arthritis in a female. Suggestions for change of focus with other irreversible conditions are also discussed.

Masters, W.H., and Johnson, V.E.: Human sexual inadequacy, Boston, 1970, Little, Brown, & Co.

Masters, W.H., and Johnson, V.E.: The pleasure bond, Boston, 1970, Little, Brown, & Co.

Puksta, N.S.: All about sex after a coronary, Am. J. Nurs. **77**(4):602, Apr. 1977.

The author discusses the physical demands of sex for the postcoronary patient. Points to assess before counseling the patient are suggested. Areas for concern for teaching/counseling sessions are identified. The author lists recommendations for postcoronary sexual counseling programs.

Woods, N.F.: Human sexuality in health and illness, ed. 4, St. Louis, 1984, The C.V. Mosby Co.

The author deals with all aspects of sexuality throughout the life span. Normal life events that threaten sexual integrity, for example, pregnancy, and aging, are discussed as well as those illnesses that interfere with sexuality and sexual function. The nursing process is addressed in terms of assessment and appropriate nursing interventions for problems identified. Although the scope of the book is broad, it provides a good baseline from which to begin a more in-depth specific study.

SKIN INTEGRITY, IMPAIRMENT OF: ACTUAL AND POTENTIAL

Beeson, P., and others: Textbook of medicine, Philadelphia, 1979, W.B. Saunders Co.

Anatomy and physiology of skin and associated appendages are discussed along with common pathologic alterations. The procedure of examination of the skin is discussed in terms of general concepts of the skin as a total organ (pp. 2266-2273). (More detailed abnormalities of the skin and appendages are discussed on pp. 2278-2373.)

Berecek, K.: The etiology of decubitus ulcer, Nrs. Clin. North Am. **10**:157, March 1975.

The author describes characteristics and mechanisms of ulcer formation. A classification of decubitus ulcers is provided.

Peacock, V.W.: Wound repair, Philadelphia, 1976, W.B. Saunders Co.

> The text discusses the body's normal attempt to seal and heal injuries resulting from minimal trauma, extensive trauma, and surgical intervention (pp. 1-145). The remaining text gives excellent reviews of wound healing involving structures other than skin.

Van Ort, S.R., and Gerber, R.M.: Topical application of insulin on decubitus ulcers, Nurs. Res. **25:**9, Jan.-Feb. 1976.

> This study examined the effects of insulin on the rate of healing for decubitus ulcers in 29 patients. The report identifies characteristics of ulcers and factors that interfere with healing.

Williams, A.: A study of factors contributing to skin breakdown, Nurs. Res. **21:**238, May-June 1972.

> Patients were classified to determine which factors affected the development of skin breakdown. A scale was proposed to assist in the identification of patients at high risk.

EEP PATTERN DISTURBANCE

Association of Sleep Disorders Centers: Diagnostic classification of sleep and arousal disorders, Sleep **2:**5, 1979.

> This comprehensive reference provides a detailed diagnostic classification system of sleep disorders. Use of this standardized terminology will be helpful in developing a taxonomy for clinical use by professional nurses.

Davies, D.R.: Individual differences in sleep patterns, Postgrad. Med. J. **52:**10, Jan. 1976.

> This paper reviews individual differences in sleep patterns. The author discusses the methods of defining and measuring sleep patterns, the relationship between objective and subjective reports of sleep quality, and the individual and personality characteristics.

Johns, W.: Methods for assessing human sleep, Arch. Int. Med. **127:**484, March 1971.

> Most of the subjective and objective methods for assessing the duration and the quality of sleep are briefly discussed. The author suggests that the choice of method depends on the objectives of the user.

Kales, A., and Kales, J.D.: Sleep disorders, N. Engl. J. Med. **290:**487, Feb. 28, 1974.

> This article provides a comprehensive review of the sleep laboratory studies and current methods for evaluating and treating six sleep disorders. The authors also review the sleep pattern disturbances that may be associated with specific underlying illnesses.

Monroe, L.J.: Psychological and physiological differences between good and poor sleepers, J. Abnorm. Psychol. **72:**255, 1967.

> The investigator has defined characteristics of good and poor sleepers. Physiologic, personality, and EEG patterns of the two groups are compared. Significant differences are noted.

Taub, J.M., and Berger, R.J.: The effects of changing the phase and duration of sleep, J. Exp. Psychol. **2:**30, Feb. 1976.

The study is concerned with the effects of shifting habitual sleep time. The authors conclude that disrupting the sleep-wakefulness cycle produces degradation in performance independent of total sleep time.

THOUGHT PROCESSES, ALTERATION IN

Davidhizar, R., and Grunden, E.W.D.: Recognizing and caring for the delirious patient, J. Psychiatr. Nurs. Ment. Health Serv. **16**:38, May 1978.

Definitions of clinical features and etiology of delirium (acute brain syndrome) concisely delineated as a foundation for nursing actions. These suggested nursing actions deal with normalizing the environmental stimuli and protecting the patient from self-harm. A useful table summarizes variables that are possible sources for delirium such as sensory input, milieu, activity, culture, personality, and general circumstances. These variables can be used to evaluate the causes and effects of delirium.

Dodd, M.J.: Assessing mental status, Am. J. Nurs. **78**(9):1501, Sept. 1978.

Using behavioral descriptions by means of an assessment tool that defines the behavioral characteristics of mental status categories of orientation, confusion, disorientation, and delirium, this article presents a concise, clinically useful guide for assessing mental status. The patient behaviors to be observed and categorized within the above framework are orientation to place, perception of pain, recognition of visual stimuli, recognition of tactile stimuli, and memory and performance of tasks on requests. This assessment tool is adaptable to pocket-size file cards a bedside recording sheet.

Drummond, L.K., and Scarbrough, D.: A practical guide to reality orientation: a treatment approach for confusion and disorientation, Gerontologist, **18**:568, Dec. 1978.

A reality orientation program developed from working with the staff on two long-term care units in a neuropsychiatric hospital is described. Questions answered are: Who needs orientation? What is a 24-hour reality orientation? What are examples of time, place, person, and environmental orientation? The authors briefly explain classroom reality orientation including topics such as choosing the leader and class members and how to conduct both basic and advanced orientation classes. Reality orientation at the beginning phase or rehabilitation is differentiated from maintenance intervention.

Trockman, G.: Caring for the confused or delirious patient, Am. J. Nurs. **78**:1495, Sept. 1978.

This article focuses mainly on acute confusional states that can be identified and treated by the nurse and is especially useful for the direct care giver. Specific nursing interventions include orienting measures, communication guides, finding familiar ground, stressing what the person can do, calming effects of a nonanxious staff, and explaining what has happened only when the patient indicates a readiness to know. The use of medication and safety measures is briefly mentioned.

Voelkel, D.: A study of reality orientation and resocialization groups with confused elderly, J. Gerontol. Nurs. **4**:13, May-June 1978.

Voelkel presents reality orientation as a method for treating the confused person by attacking the processes of confusion, disorientation, and memory loss through continual, stimulating repetitive orientation to person, place, and time. A study describing two methods used to orient elderly nursing home patients concluded that a group social experience improved mental status more effectively than merely giving constant reminders of current information. The explanation of group functioning is useful as a nursing intervention for practitioners.

Wilkinson, O.: Out of touch with reality, Am. J. Nurs. **78**(9):1492, Sept. 1978.

This personal account written by a nurse who endured 6 months of mental confusion vividly describes fuzzy perceptions of occurrences, descriptions that are useful to heighten any nurse's sensitivity to and empathy for the confused patient. Her summarizing statement that "people in the health care professions had the least understanding . . . little consideration was given to what the person must deal with in relearning how to become a person, a human being," prompts one to do some soul-searching concerning the nursing care given to the delirious patient.

URINARY ELIMINATION, ALTERATION IN PATTERNS

Bates, P.: A trouble-shooter's guide to indwelling catheters, RN, **44**(3):62, March 1981.

This reference provides an illustrated guide to managing catheters, teaching patients, problem solving, and preventing complications.

Bielski, M.: Preventing infection in the catheterized patient, Nurs. Clin. North Am. **15**(4):703, 1980.

Sources of urinary tract infections are discussed. Suggestions for control such as catheter care, alternatives to indwelling catheterization and patient education are discussed.

Blaivas, G.: Management of bladder dysfunction in multiple sclerosis, Neurology **30**:12, July 1980.

A prospective study of 67 multiple sclerosis (MS) patients admitted to the urodynamic laboratory at Tufts–New England Medical Center for diagnosis and treatment of bladder symptoms in MS. Based on results of urodynamic testing, patients' symptoms were described as failure to store urine (30%), failure to empty the bladder (18%) or both (50%). Treatment was based on the underlying pathophysiology and included intermittent catheterization (21%), none (20%), surgical (12%), drugs (9%), voiding maneuvers (6%), and condom drainage (6%). In 18%, permanent indwelling catheters were required after failure of other methods. Clinical signs and symptoms were often found to be poor predictors of actual urodynamic function. The article defined the potential urinary signs and symptoms in the patient with MS and the varieties of medical treatment.

Felder, L.: Neurogenic bladder dysfunction, J. Neurosurg. Nurs. **2**:94, June 1979.

Felder first defines *neurogenic bladder* as "a dysfunction of micturition resulting from lesions of the peripheral and central nervous system." The article emphasizes the scientific basis for nursing assessment and care approach for the patient with bladder dysfunction, including a review of the normal anatomy and physiology of the bladder, pathophysiology, description of urodynamic studies, and medical and nursing management based on the etiology of the dysfunction. The author stresses that accurate nursing assessment is based on multiple factors, not only disease process and type of bladder dysfunction but also on the patients' total life situation and capabilities. Goals of management and alternative solutions for specific bladder dysfunctions are explored.

Gault, P.L.: How to break the kidney stone cycle, Nursing 78 8(12):24, 1978.

Types of kidney stones, signs and symptoms, management, preoperative and postoperative care, and patient education and counseling.

Hartman, M.: Intermittent self catheterization, Nursing 78 8(11):72, 1978.

Review of a successful ISC program on a rehabilitation unit includes patient diet and fluid regimen and illustrated teaching guides for male and female patients.

Johnson, J.: Rehabilitative aspects of neurological bladder dysfunction, Nurs. Clin. North Am. **15**:293, June 1980.

The author emphasizes that reconditioning programs for patients with bladder dysfunction must be based on knowledge of normal micturition and accurate assessment of the patient's specific dysfunction. Physiology of micturition and categories of bladder dysfunction are outlined, followed by general goals of bladder reconditioning and goals specific to each category. Complications (infection, calculi, overdistention) and their prevention are discussed. Specific questions pertinent to a nursing assessment of bladder function are described along with appropriate nursing and medical management.

Mahoney, J.: What you should know about ostomies, Nursing 78 8(5):74, 1978.

The author provides guidelines for general stoma care and also specific types of ostomies, including urinary diversions. Selected from Mahoney's book *Guide to Ostomy Nursing Care*, Boston, 1976, Little, Brown, & Co.

VALUE CONFLICT

Anger, D., and Anger, D.W.: Dialysis ambivalence: a matter of life and death, Am. J. Nurs. **76**(2):276, 1976.

Quality of life on dialysis is discussed as a source of conflict for patients and staff. The staff's role in explaining options open to the patient is described.

Bayles, M.D.: The value of life—by what standard? Am. J. Nurs. **80**(12):2226, 1980.

This thought-provoking article discusses ethical theories and applies theories to individual cases. Stress is placed on the nurse's role in assessing the patient's value of life and assisting to maximize the value of that life.

Beard, B.H.: Fear of death and fear of life, Arch. Gen. Psychiatry **21**:373, 1969.

This study of 14 patients with chronic renal failure describes the signs and symptoms caused by the dilemma over fear of an unacceptable life vs. fear of death.

Coombs, A.W., Avila, D.L., and Purkey, W.W.: Helping relationships: basic concepts for the helping professions, ed. 2, Newton, Mass., 1978, Allyn & Bacon, Inc.

Davis, A.J., and Aroskar, M.A.: Ethical dilemmas and nursing practice, New York, 1978, Appleton-Century-Crofts.

Ryden, M.B.: An approach to ethical decision making, Nurs. Outlook **26**(11):705, Nov. 1978.

Patient's and nurse's roles in the decision-making process are explored. Discussion includes examples of assisting student nurses in learning strategies to use in helping relationships.

Shirley, M.S., and Harmon, V.M.: Values clarification in nursing, New York, 1979, Appleton-Century-Crofts.

Uustal, D.: Values clarification in nursing: application to practice, Am. J. Nurs. **78**(12):2058, 1978.

The need for nurses to understand their personal value system to give sensitive care to others is stressed. Values clarification theory and examples of strategies are highlighted.

INDEX